Parasitic Helminths and Zoonoses - From Basic to Applied Research

Edited by Jorge Morales-Montor, Victor Hugo Del Río-Araiza and Romel Hernandéz-Bello

Published in London, United Kingdom

Parasitic Helminths and Zoonoses - From Basic to Applied Research
http://dx.doi.org/10.5772/intechopen.98178
Edited by Jorge Morales-Montor, Victor Hugo Del Río-Araiza and Romel Hernandéz-Bello

Contributors
Adetayo Olorunlana, Katia Cristina Oliveira, Ednilson Hilário Lopes-Junior, Claudio Romero Bertevello, Rafaella Pontes Marques, Sarir Ahmad, Mehrab Khan, Ikram Ullah, Jay R. Stauffer, Jr., Henry Madsen, Koushik Das, Neeraj Mahindroo, Shashi Upadhyay, Muhammad Tahir Aleem, Ruofeng Yan, Asad Khan, Rida Asrar, Amna Shakoor, Areej Asif, Zhaohai Wen, Zhengqing Yu, Muhammad Abdullah Malik, Tauseef Ur-Rehman, Rao Zahid Abbas, Muhammad Mohsin, Xiaokai Song, Lixin Xu, Xiangrui Li, James-Paul Kretchy, Abdallah Zacharia, Anne H. Outwater, Twilumba Makene, Eliza Lupenza, Alex J. Joseph Mujuni, Agustin Plancarte, Gabriela Nava, Meghan May, Evangeline Green, Priyanka Ravichandran, Meagan Short, Vrushabh Ashok Daga, Osama M. Darwesh, Hoda Samir El-Sayed, Jorge-Luis de-la-Rosa-Arana, Christian-Irene Irene Nevarez-Lechuga, Antonio Meza-Lucas, Alejandro Escobar-Gutiérrez, Carlos Wong-Baeza, Isabel Baeza, Muhammad Sohail Sajid, Faisal Rasheed Anjum, Muhammad Farhab, Mahvish Maqbool, Muhammad Zeeshan, Kashif Hussain, Namrah Rehman, Rana Hamid Ali Nisar, Hafiz Muhammad Rizwan, Urfa Bin Tahir, Gabriela Alvite, Adriana Esteves, Stefan L. L. Debbert, Ezra J. Marker, Jesuthas Ajendra, Marc P. Hübner, Achim Hoerauf, Michael A. Steele, Carolyn Mahan, Marco Antonio Muñoz-Guzmán, Fernando Alba-Hurtado, Jorge Morales-Montor, Víctor Hugo Del Río-Araiza, Romel Hernandéz-Bello

First published in London, United Kingdom, 2022 by IntechOpen
IntechOpen is the global imprint of INTECHOPEN LIMITED, registered in England and Wales, registration number: 11086078, 5 Princes Gate Court, London, SW7 2QJ, United Kingdom

British Library Cataloguing-in-Publication Data
A catalogue record for this book is available from the British Library

Additional hard and PDF copies can be obtained from orders@intechopen.com

Parasitic Helminths and Zoonoses - From Basic to Applied Research
Edited by Jorge Morales-Montor, Victor Hugo Del Río-Araiza and Romel Hernandéz-Bello
p. cm.
Print ISBN 978-1-80355-567-6
Online ISBN 978-1-80355-568-3
eBook (PDF) ISBN 978-1-80355-569-0

For EU product safety concerns:
IN TECH d.o.o., Prolaz Marije Krucifikse Kozulić 3, 51000 Rijeka, Croatia,
info@intechopen.com or visit our website at intechopen.com.

Meet the editors

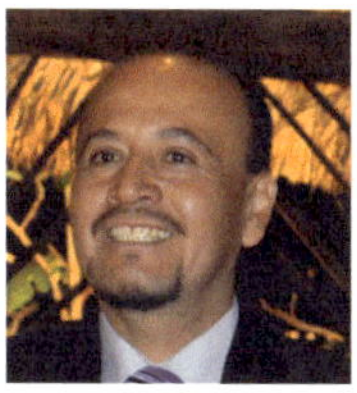

Dr. Jorge Morales-Montor's doctoral thesis was recognized with the Lola and Igo Flisser PUIS Award for the best graduate thesis at the national level in the field of parasitology. He received a fellowship from the Fogarty Foundation to perform a post-doctoral research stay at the University of Georgia, USA. He has 153 journal articles to his credit. He has also edited several books and written more than fifty-five book chapters. He is a member of the Mexican Academy of Sciences, Latin American Academy of Sciences, and the National Academy of Medicine. Dr. Morales-Montor has won more than thirty-five awards and has graduated thirty-five bachelor's, eight master's, and twelve doctorate students. He was previously the president of the Mexican Society of Parasitology.

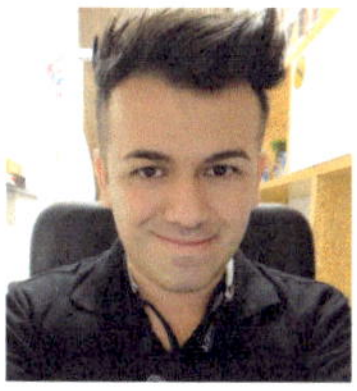

Dr. Victor Hugo Del Río-Araiza graduated in Veterinary Medicine at Universidad Nacional Autónoma de México (UNAM). He obtained his master's degree and Ph.D. in Biomedical Sciences from the same university. He is a professor-researcher at the Faculty of Veterinary Medicine and Zootechnics, UNAM, where he is responsible for the Laboratory of Endocrine-Immune Interactions in Parasitic Diseases. He has seventeen scientific publications and seven book chapters to his credit. He is MVZ certified by CONCERVET in Parasitology and a member of the Mexican Association of Veterinary Parasitologists and the Mexican Society of Neuroimmunoendocrinology.

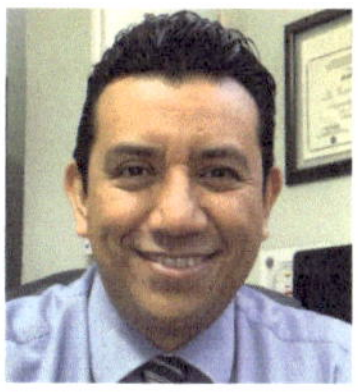

Dr. Romel Hernandez-Bello obtained his BSc and MSc in Biology at the Universidad Nacional Autónoma de México (UNAM). He obtained a Ph.D. in Molecular Biology and Genetics from the Centro de Investigación y de Estudios Avanzados. He was a research fellow in the Department of Immunology, National Autonomous University of México. He is the recipient of the Lola and Igo Flisser Award for research in parasitology and the 1st Prize in Basic Biomedical Research from the Universidad Autónma de Nuevo León. He has graduated four master's and two doctorate students. Dr. Hernandez-Bello has more than thirty peer-reviewed publications to his credit.

Contents

Preface **XI**

Section 1
Therapeutic Approaches in Helminth Infections **1**

Chapter 1 **3**
Therapeutic Properties of *Trichinella spiralis* (Nematoda) in Chronic Degenerative Diseases
by Christian-Irene Nevárez-Lechuga, Antonio Meza-Lucas, Alejandro Escobar-Gutiérrez, Carlos Wong-Baeza, Isabel Baeza and Jorge-Luis de-la-Rosa-Arana

Chapter 2 **25**
Anthelmintic Drug Resistance in Livestock: Current Understanding and Future Trends
by Muhammad Abdullah Malik, Muhammad Sohail Sajid, Rao Zahid Abbas, Muhammad Tahir Aleem, Faisal Rasheed Anjum, Asad Khan, Muhammad Farhab, Mahvish Maqbool, Muhammad Zeeshan, Kashif Hussain, Namrah Rehman, Rana Hamid Ali Nisar, Hafiz Muhammad Rizwan and Urfa Bin Tahir

Chapter 3 **49**
Recent Advances in Anti-Schistosomiasis Drug Discovery
by Ezra J. Marker and Stefan L. Debbert

Chapter 4 **75**
Perspective Chapter: Application of Probiotics to Inactivate Helminth Parasitic Zoonosis
by Osama M. Darwesh and Hoda Samir El-Sayed

Chapter 5 **91**
New Uses for Old Drugs and Their Application in Helminthology
by Victor Hugo Del Río-Araiza, Romel Hernandéz-Bello and Jorge Morales-Montor

Section 2
Advances in the Molecular and Immune Response in Helminth Infection **111**

Chapter 6 **113**
Perspective Chapter: Parasitic Platyhelminthes Nuclear Receptors as Molecular Crossroads
by Adriana Esteves and Gabriela Alvite

Chapter 7 **131**
Perspective Chapter: Molecular Crosstalk and Signal Transduction between Platyhelminths and Their Hosts
by Ednilson Hilário Lopes-Junior, Rafaella Pontes Marques, Claudio Romero Bertevello and Katia Cristina Oliveira

Chapter 8 **149**
Helminths Derived Immune-Modulatory Molecules: Implications in Host-Parasite Interaction
by Koushik Das, Shashi Upadhyay and Neeraj Mahindroo

Chapter 9 **165**
Oxygen and Redox Reactions Contribute to the Protection of Free-Living and Parasite Helminths against Pathogens and/or Host Response
by Agustin Plancarte and Gabriela Nava

Section 3
One Health Approach to Study Helminth Infections **185**

Chapter 10 **187**
Toxocariosis: From a One Health Perspective
by Fernando Alba-Hurtado and Marco Antonio Muñoz-Guzmán

Chapter 11 **207**
Schistosoma Hybridizations and Risk of Emerging Zoonosis in Africa: Time to Think of a One Health Approach for Sustainable Schistosomiasis Control and Elimination
by Abdallah Zacharia, Anne H. Outwater, Eliza Lupenza, Alex J. Mujuni and Twilumba Makene

Chapter 12 **231**
Dancing in a Cycle: Global Health Agenda and *Schistosomiasis* Control in Africa
by Adetayo Olorunlana

Section 4
Management, Biology and Control Strategies in Helminth Infections **253**

Chapter 13 **255**
Perspective Chapter: Integrated Root-Knot Nematodes (*Meloidogyne*) Management Approaches
by Sarir Ahmad, Mehrab Khan and Ikram Ullah

Chapter 14 269
Perspective Chapter: The Potential Role of Nematode Parasites in Wildlife Decline – Evidence from Allegheny Woodrats (*Neotoma magister*), Northern Flying Squirrels (*Glaucomys sabrinus*) and Now the Eurasian Red Squirrel (*Sciurus vulgaris*)
by Carolyn Mahan and Michael Steele

Chapter 15 279
Soil-Transmissible Helminths Infections; Diagnosis, Transmission Dynamics, and Disease Management Strategies in Low-and Middle-Income Countries
by James-Paul Kretchy

Chapter 16 291
Zoonotic Trematode Infections; Their Biology, Intermediate Hosts and Control
by Henry Madsen and Jay R. Stauffer, Jr.

Chapter 17 327
Biology of the Human Filariases
by Jesuthas Ajendra, Achim Hoerauf and Marc P. Hübner

Section 5
Advances in Vaccines against Helminth Parasites **349**

Chapter 18 351
Perspective Chapter: Advances in the Development of Anti-*Trichinella spiralis* Vaccine, Challenges, and Future Prospective
by Muhammad Tahir Aleem, Ruofeng Yan, Asad Khan, Rida Asrar, Amna Shakoor, Areej Asif, Zhaohai Wen, Zhengqing Yu, Muhammad Abdullah Malik, Tauseef-ur-Rehman, Rao Zahid Abbas, Muhammad Mohsin, Xiaokai Song, Lixin Xu and Xiangrui Li

Chapter 19 369
Perspective Chapter: Multi-Omic Approaches to Vaccine Development against Helminth Diseases
by Vrushabh Daga, Evangeline Green, Priyanka Ravichandran, Meagan Short and Meghan May

Preface

Helminthiases, caused by the larval or adult stage of various genera of worms, are a serious health and veterinary problem in many developing countries and are considered the most important neglected tropical diseases (NTDs) in developed countries. A great deal of scientific advances have occurred in this field, including in vaccination, epidemiology, drug design, management and diagnostics, and host–parasite interaction at all levels. Recently, the One Health approach has been proposed as a global way to treat and control helminthiasis. This book provides a comprehensive overview of the current state of the art in helminthiases. It highlights the most recent advances in the study of helminth infections, addressing topics such as clinical disease, vaccines, immune response, new possible drug targets, and basic molecular research.

The book is divided into five sections:

- Section 1: "Therapeutic Approaches in Helminth Infections"
- Section 2: "Advances in the Molecular and Immune Response in Helminth Infection"
- Section 3: "One Health Approach to Study Helminth Infections"
- Section 4. "Management, Biology and Control Strategies in Helminth Infections"
- Section 5: "Advances in Vaccines against Helminth Parasites"

Section 1 includes five chapters. Chapter 1, "Therapeutic Properties of *Trichinella spiralis* (Nematoda) in Chronic Degenerative Diseases" by Nevárez-Lechuga et al., discusses diseases produced by helminth parasites. These diseases occur frequently in underdeveloped countries where they present a serious public health problem. However, these regions exhibit a low rate of autoimmune and allergic diseases. As such, some researchers have proposed that some helminths, such as *Trichinella spiralis* or its proteins, have strong anti-inflammatory potential, or have assessed them as modulating agents of the immune response. *T. spiralis* shifts the host immune response from a Th1 profile, characterized by pro-inflammatory cytokines, to a Th2 profile, characterized by the release of different cytokines with anti-inflammatory properties. Thus, the chapter authors point out that this parasite has shown high therapeutic potential in a wide variety of disease models. In one of the most promising, the experimental lupus model in mice, the release of anti-inflammatory cytokines IL-4 and IL-10 and delayed onset of the key clinical features of the experimental lupus model for at least 5 months were observed, when previously parasitized. This is the first study to date that focuses on the use of *T. spiralis* as an immunomodulator in lupus disease. The authors conclude that further study of the immune response generated by the parasite is necessary to advance the development of new therapies for inflammatory diseases.

Chapter 2, "Anthelmintic Drug Resistance in Livestock: Current Understanding and Future Trends" by Muhammad Abdullah Malik et al., discusses how anthelmintic, ectoparasiticides (insecticides, acaricides) and antiprotozoal chemotherapeutic drugs target parasites. *Chenopodium* oil-like alkaloids, arsenic compounds, cupric sulfate, nicotine, and cupric silicate have been used to destroy nematodes. Unfortunately, these chemicals are less effective and less safe for livestock. The four major groups of broad-spectrum antinematodal compounds are macrocyclic lactones such as milbemycins/ivermectin, benzimidazole/pro-benzimidazole, tetrahydro pyrimidines such as morantel, pyrantel tartrate, and imidazothiazoles such as tetramisole and levamisole. The various factors responsible for gastrointestinal parasitism make it difficult to develop effective control measures. Hence, an effective strategy for the control of parasitic diseases that does not solely rely on anthelmintic therapies needs to be developed at the regional level, based on the epidemiology of the disease.

Chapter 3, "Recent Advances in Anti-Schistosomiasis Drug Discovery" by Ezra J. Marker and Stefan L. Debbert, discusses schistosomiasis, a parasitic disease caused by infection by helminths of the *Schistosoma* genus that affects more than 200 million people, primarily in the developing world. Treatment of this disease largely relies on one drug, praziquantel. Although this drug is cheap, safe, and effective, the looming prospect of drug resistance makes the development of a pipeline of anti-schistosomiasis drugs a priority. Many new drug leads have arisen from screening existing sets of compounds such as the Open Access Boxes developed by the Medicines for Malaria Venture (MMV) in collaboration with the Drugs for Neglected Diseases Initiative (DNDI). Other leads have been found through work focused on druggable targets such as kinases, histone deacetylases, proteases, and others. Thus, the chapter discusses recent work concerning the discovery and development of novel anti-schistosomiasis drug leads from many sources.

Chapter 4, "Perspective Chapter: Application of Probiotics to Inactivate Helminth Parasitic Zoonosis" by Osama M. Darwesh and Hoda Samir El-Sayed, discusses zoonotic infections, which are animal infections that might be transmissible to people. The infection may be transmitted through ingestion of contaminated food, infected soil, skin penetration, or direct animal contact. Parasitic helminths are a group of parasites that remain poorly studied in comparison to viruses and bacteria but may pose considerable future risk to humans. Zoonotic parasites may be separated into four classes: direct-zoonotic, meta-zoonotic, cyclo-zoonotic, and sapro-zoonotic. It is possible to prevent helminth parasitic zoonosis via proper hygiene and sanitation or regular deworming with anthelmintic pills. However, because of the lack of effective vaccines and anthelmintic resistance to medication, suppression of parasitic infestation requires new techniques. One potential treatment involves probiotics, which are exogenous residing microorganisms that are beneficial to the host's fitness when administered inside the digestive tract. The most extensively used microorganisms for this purpose are of the genus *Lactobacillus* and *Enterococcus*, along with a few fungi and yeasts.

Chapter 5, "New Uses for Old Drugs and their Application in Helminthology" by Del Río-Araiza et al., examines parasitic infection research performed on both humans and domestic animals. This research has focused mostly on vaccines, diagnostic methods, epidemiology, and the evolutionary origins of parasites, thanks to the emergence of genomics and proteomics. However, the basic biology of the host–parasite interactions of several important medical and veterinary parasites has not been fully studied. Limited information has been obtained on the intricate neuroimmunoendocrine effects of host–parasite interplay. Therefore, the consequences of these interactions, and their possible therapeutic applications, need to be thoroughly investigated. The chapter reviews the available literature on the host–parasite neuroimmunoendocrine network and discusses how this basic research can be used to design new treatments using hormones, anti-hormones, and hormone analogues as a novel therapy against parasitic diseases. In addition, these studies may also contribute to identifying alternative treatments for parasitic diseases in the future. The complex immune-endocrine network may also help in explaining the frequently conflicting results observed in infections with regards to host sex and age and offer helpful insight into other research avenues besides parasite treatment and control strategies. Finally, several natural products isolated from plants, used in traditional medicine, offer an alternative approach for natural products in the preparation of inexpensive and effective antiparasitic drugs.

Section 2 includes four chapters. Chapter 6, "Perspective Chapter: Parasitic Platyhelminthes Nuclear Receptors as Molecular Crossroads" by Adriana Esteves and Gabriela Alvite, discusses research directed at identifying the nuclear receptors (NRs) set expressed by parasitic platyhelminths. Important gaps concerning NRs mechanism of action, ligands, co-regulator proteins, and DNA binding sequences on target genes need to be addressed. Several in vitro effects of host steroid hormones on *Taenia* and *Echinococcus* species have been observed, but the classical mammalian estrogen, androgen, or progesterone receptors couldn't be identified in databases. Nonetheless, novel nuclear receptors and related proteins and genes are being identified and characterized. The elucidation of NRs gene targets as well as ligands in parasitic platyhelminths could allow for the discovery of new and specific pathways differing from those of their hosts. In this sense, these parasitic proteins seem to be good putative targets of new drugs.

Chapter 7, "Perspective Chapter: Molecular Crosstalk and Signal Transduction between Platyhelminths and their Hosts" by Ednilson Hilário Lopes-Junior et al., highlights that parasitic infection is an intimate relationship between host and parasites with an exchange of signal and complex signaling systems involved in these organisms' molecular crosstalk. With the advances of knowledge due to the genomic and transcriptomics projects in the last decades, several genes and the molecular mechanism involved in the biological function of platyhelminths have been described. Cytokines, hormones, and other molecules from the host have influenced the growth, development, and reproduction of platyhelminths. Thus, the authors review the effects of host cytokines (IL-1, IL-4, IL-12, IL-7, TGF-β, TNF-α) and hormones (T4, estrogen, progesterone, and androgens) that directly or indirectly affect parasite development and reproduction and the possible associated signaling pathways.

Chapter 8, “Helminths Derived Immune-Modulatory Molecules: Implications in Host-Parasite Interaction” by Das et al., points out that the parasitic life cycle of helminths greatly relies on sophisticated manipulation of the host environment and successful evasion of the host defense. Helminths produce a repertoire of secretory molecules (extracellular vesicles and/or exosomes) to invade and generate habitable host environments and modulate the host immune responses in such a way that ensures their prolonged survival within the host. The authors present an outline on helminths derived immune-modulatory molecules and their implications in host–parasite crosstalk.

Chapter 9, “Oxygen and Redox Reactions Contribute to the Protection of Free-Living and Parasite Helminths against Pathogens and/or Host Response” by Agustin Plancarte and Gabriela Nava discuss how millions of years ago, the reductive atmosphere environment of Earth was replaced by an oxidative one as a result of oxidation-reduction reactions (redox reactions), which increase the concentration of oxygen. These oxidative conditions allowed aerobic organisms to populate the planet, which acquired mechanisms to both control the toxicity of oxygen and obtain from it via redox reactions energy, both situations, through their aerobic metabolism. In addition, aerobic organisms began to produce reactive oxygen species (ROS) via redox reactions of oxygen molecules. In aerobic organisms, some ROS such as H_2O_2 function as second messengers in cell signal transduction, allowing for the development of metabolic processes, including gene control. Free-living helminths appeared in the early Paleozoic era and parasite helminths appeared later in the same era. Because of their ancient origins, these organisms represent an excellent research area for biological models. Free-living helminths, such as *Caenorhabditis elegans* and earthworms, have been used as host models to understand their micro pathogen defenses, particularly those associated with ROS. The chapter discusses the evolution of oxygen molecules and redox reactions, as well as of Earth’s atmosphere, and changes over time in the protection mechanisms of helminths.

Section 3 includes three chapters. Chapter 10, “Toxocariasis: From a One Health Perspective” by Fernando Alba-Hurtado and Marco Antonio Muñoz-Guzmán, discusses toxocariasis, which is a neglected zoonotic infection caused by the nematodes *Toxocara canis* and *Toxocara cati*. The distribution of the disease is worldwide and mainly affects dogs and cats. Its larval stage can cause human infection with serious repercussions on the health of its hosts. The infection causes developmental delays, digestive disorders, nonspecific nervous manifestations, and occasionally death associated with hyperparasitosis in some puppies and kittens. In humans, the infection produces clinical syndromes known as visceral larva migrans (VLM), ocular larva migrans (OLM), neurotoxocarosis, and covert toxocariasis. The close contact of people with their pets and the environmental conditions that favor the transmission of this disease place it within the context of one health. The One Health concept is defined as the collaborative efforts of multiple disciplines (medical personnel, veterinarians, researchers, etc.) that work locally, nationally, and globally to achieve optimal health for people, animals, and the environment. From this perspective, toxocariasis is a study model in which classic and recent knowledge of the medical and veterinary area must be combined for its full understanding, with a goal of establishing integrative criteria for its treatment, control, and prevention.

Chapter 11, "*Schistosoma* Hybridizations and Risk of Emerging Zoonosis in Africa: Time to Think of a One Health Approach for Sustainable Schistosomiasis Control and Elimination" by Zacharia et al., discusses the current control of human schistosomiasis in Africa, which is based on preventive chemotherapy and whereby populations are mass-treated with the anthelminthic medication praziquantel. The World Health Organization (WHO) has set a goal of eliminating schistosomiasis as a public health problem and, ultimately, eliminating transmission in all countries where schistosomiasis is endemic by 2030. However, recurrent hybridization between *Schistosoma* species is an emerging public health concern that has a major impact on distribution of the disease and ultimately may derail elimination efforts. The One Health approach recognizes interconnections between the health of humans, animals, and the environment, and encourages collaborative efforts toward the best outcomes. Thus, this chapter explains how the One Health approach can accelerate the control and elimination of schistosomiasis in Africa.

Chapter 12, "Dancing in a Cycle: Global Health Agenda and *Schistosomiasis* Control in Africa" by Adetayo Olorunlana, discusses that schistosomiasis and other NTDs affect about 2 billion people globally. Africa shares approximately 90% of the global burden of schistosomiasis disease. Despite, WHO efforts to control the disease, it remains neglected in most African countries. Control programs exclude adults in Mass Drug Administration (MDAs), and water, sanitation, and hygiene (WASH) because the drug praziquantel is used for treatment. However, migratory patterns of the neglected population and the interplay of social, economic, political, and cultural factors have introduced the disease into previously eliminated and/or new areas. The question is whether Africa can achieve the new goals of the WHO NTDs 2021–2030 Roadmap for schistosomiasis elimination. The chapter compares and contrasts Africa's current top-down approach to schistosomiasis control to a dynamic approach. Or if the previous pattern of late implementation, dependent on only one drug and shifting focus to other diseases of relevance continues. If a new approach is not adopted the dance in the cycle has just begun.

Section 4 includes five chapters. Chapter 13, "Perspective Chapter: Integrated Root-Knot Nematodes (*Meloidogyne*) Management Approaches" by Ahmad et al., describes the *Meloidogyne* genus, which contains the most prevalent and harmful worms formally known as root-knot nematode species. They attack a wide range of plants belonging to different plant families. In the infective second stage, juveniles (J-II) feed on the plant's roots and, as a result, the host plant roots become swollen/produce galls. The attack plant shows stunted growth and in extreme cases the plant dies. An integrated pest management (IPM) approach is required to tackle these harmful nematodes spp. The integrated tactics include cultural/agronomic practices as well as biological and chemical control. A sole management method is not enough to deal with the root-knot nematode. Therefore, a proper IPM package is required for the farmer to gain good health for the crops.

Chapter 14, "Perspective Chapter: The Potential Role of Nematode Parasites in Wildlife Decline – Evidence from Allegheny Woodrats (*Neotoma magister*), Northern Flying Squirrels (*Glaucomys sabrinus*) and now the Eurasian Red Squirrel (*Sciurus vulgaris*)" by Carolyn Mahan and Michael Steele points out that global climate change and human-induced habitat loss alter the landscape for native wildlife, resulting in shifts in geographic ranges, occupation of smaller, remnant habitat patches, or use of novel environments. These processes often lead to sympatry between species that historically occupied non-overlapping ranges and habitats. Such interactions may result in increased competition for resources and expose species to novel parasites that adversely affect a species' fitness, leading to wildlife declines. The chapter explores these interactions in two species of endangered North American rodents: Northern flying squirrels (*Glaucomys sabrinus*) and Allegheny woodrats (*Neotoma magister*). Northern flying squirrels are declining in the eastern United States due to competition with its congener, southern flying squirrels (*Glaucomys volans*). Increasing evidence indicates that this competition is mediated by a shared intestinal nematode, *Strongyloides robustus*. Transmission of this nematode to the endangered northern flying squirrel may be increasing due to habitat loss, forest fragmentation, and climate change. Climate change causes the northward range expansion of southern flying squirrels and adversely affects the health of coniferous forests, which is the preferred habitat of northern flying squirrels. The chapter authors also note the most recent discovery of *S. robustus* as a factor in the decline of the European red squirrel (*Sciurus vulgaris*). *S. robustus* is a novel parasite to this host in Europe and was introduced along with the invasive eastern gray squirrel (*Sciurus carolinensis*) that is native to North America. Likewise, in Allegheny woodrats, shrinking habitat and landscape changes have resulted in increased range overlap with raccoons (*Procyon lotor*), which harbor a nematode fatal to woodrats. The chapter also discusses the subsequent transmission of this nematode, *Baylisascaris procyonis*, to woodrats as a contributing factor to their decline throughout the Appalachian Mountains.

Chapter 15, "Soil-Transmissible Helminths Infections; Diagnosis, Transmission Dynamics, and Disease Management Strategies in Low-and Middle-Income Countries" by James-Paul Kretchy, examines soil-transmissible helminthes (STHs) infections, which are among the most common sanitation-related public health problems among people living in poor settlements of tropical and sub-tropical regions in low- and middle-income countries (LMICs). Though available data suggest occurrence of disease in adults, children of school-going age bear the greatest burden, as these infections affect their cognitive development and physical growth. The characteristic high levels of poverty, poor environmental hygiene, open defecation practices, and inadequate sanitation and waste management systems expose residents to the risks of STH infections. Walking bare-footed, inappropriate hand hygiene behavior, and the unavailability/improper use of personal protective equipment (PPE) can impact transmission risks in endemic communities and among occupational risk groups. These must be properly investigated and managed, and appropriate interventions must be communicated to decision-makers.

Chapter 16, "Zoonotic Trematode Infections; Their Biology, Intermediate Hosts and Control" by Henry Madsen and Jay R. Stauffer, Jr., point out that many diseases linked with trematodes are zoonotic, including liver flukes (*Fasciola spp.*, *Clonorchis*, and *Opistorchis* are the most common), intestinal flukes (some species of *Heterophyidae*), lung flukes (*Paragonimus* spp.), and the blood flukes (*Schistosome* species). A characteristic of all these species is that they have a vertebrate as the final host and freshwater snail species as the first intermediate host. The foodborne trematodes also have a second intermediate host where their infective stage (metacercariae) lodge or in case of the Fasciolidae, cercariae encyst on aquatic or semi-aquatic plants. The chapter describes the biology of transmission with emphasis on the intermediate snail hosts and their control.

Chapter 17, "Biology of the Human Filariases" by Jesuthas Ajendra, Achim Hoerauf, and Marc P. Hübner discusses filarial nematodes, which are parasitic worms transmitted by blood-feeding insects. They cause some of the most debilitating infectious diseases known to humankind. Mainly found in tropical and subtropical areas of the developing world, diseases such as lymphatic filariasis and onchocerciasis represent major public health issues. With millions of people infected and billions at risk of infection, these diseases can stun economic growth and impair quality of life of the affected regions. As such, the WHO has classified both lymphatic filariasis and onchocerciasis as NTDs. The lesser-known filarial disease loiasis not only affects millions of people, but also represents a huge obstacle during mass drug administration programs targeting other filarial diseases. Even less is known about mansonellosis, potentially the most widespread of the human filariases but underestimated due to the lack of clinical symptoms. Large-scale intervention as well as mass drug administration programs are undertaken with the long-term goal of eliminating filarial diseases, as declared in the WHO roadmap 2021–2030. However, there is still neither a vaccination nor short-term macrofilaricidal treatments available. Many drugs have side effects or are not suitable for all patients and thus there are still billions of people living in areas with a high risk of infection.

Section 5 includes two chapters. Chapter 18, "Perspective Chapter: Advances in the Development of Anti-*Trichinella spiralis* Vaccine, Challenges, and Future Prospective" by Aleem et al., discusses trichinellosis, which is a very important foodborne zoonosis caused by *Trichinella spiralis*. This is an important disease and its causative agent is prevalent throughout the world (cosmopolitan). More clinical awareness of trichinellosis is required due to its many outbreaks and the increase in the consumption of pork meat and its byproducts. Trichinellosis is epizootic in nature and its economic burden is associated with the prevention of this disease from the human food chain. This disease is transmitted from animals to humans through the consumption of raw or undercooked meat containing encapsulated muscle larvae of *T. spiralis*. This chapter demonstrates the direct effect of progesterone (P4) and mifepristone (RU486) on the progesterone receptors of *T. spiralis*. It also examines the challenges in the preparation of DNA and recombinant protein vaccination to control trichinellosis.

Finally, Chapter 19, "Perspective Chapter: Multi-Omic Approaches to Vaccine Development against Helminth Diseases" by Daga et al., discusses the need for protective vaccines for humans and livestock against helminth diseases. The "-omics" era has led to renewed interest in vaccine development against helminth diseases, as candidate vaccines can now be designed, evaluated, and refined in a fraction of the time previously required. In this chapter, the authors describe and review genomic, transcriptomic, and proteomic approaches to the design of vaccines against helminth diseases.

We hope that readers find this book helpful and informative. It is our attempt to compile novel and important information about diseases and parasites that are a health burden in underdeveloped countries and an emerging health problem in developed ones.

Jorge Morales-Montor
Departamento de Inmunología,
Instituto de Investigaciones Biomédicas,
Universidad Nacional Autónoma de México,
Mexico City, Mexico

Victor Hugo Del Río-Araiza
Facultad de Medicina,
Departamento de Microbiología y Parasitología,
Veterinaria y Zootecnia,
Universidad Nacional Autónoma de México,
Mexico City, Mexico

Romel Hernandéz-Bello
Facultad de Medicina,
Departmento de Microbiología,
Universidad Autónoma de Nuevo León,
San Nicolás de los Garza, Mexico

Section 1

Therapeutic Approaches in Helminth Infections

Chapter 1

Therapeutic Properties of *Trichinella spiralis* (Nematoda) in Chronic Degenerative Diseases

Christian-Irene Nevárez-Lechuga, Antonio Meza-Lucas, Alejandro Escobar-Gutiérrez, Carlos Wong-Baeza, Isabel Baeza and Jorge-Luis de-la-Rosa-Arana

Abstract

Diseases produced by helminth parasites occur frequently in underdeveloped countries where they present a serious public health problem. At the same time, in these regions, a lower rate of autoimmune and allergic diseases has been observed. Due to these observations, some researchers have proposed that some helminths, such as *Trichinella spiralis* or its proteins, have strong anti-inflammatory potential, or have assessed them as modulating agents of the immune response. *T. spiralis* shifts the host immune response from a Th1 profile, characterized by pro-inflammatory cytokines, to a Th2 profile, characterized by the release of different cytokines with anti-inflammatory properties. This parasite has shown high therapeutic potential in a wide variety of disease models. In one of the most promising, the experimental lupus model in mice, the release of anti-inflammatory cytokines IL-4 and IL-10 and delayed onset of the key clinical features of the experimental lupus model for at least 5 months were observed, when previously parasitized. This is the first study to date that focuses on the use of *T. spiralis* as an immunomodulator in lupus disease. In conclusion, further study of the immune response generated by the parasite is necessary to advance the development of new therapies for inflammatory diseases.

Keywords: *Trichinella*, immunomodulation, chronic degenerative diseases, lupus, helminths

1. Introduction

1.1 Helminths and parasitosis

Helminthiases are parasitic diseases caused by helminths, which are colloquially called "parasitic worms". Although a great biodiversity of helminths exists, the most relevant in public and veterinary health are the cestodes (tapeworms), trematodes (flukeworms) and nematodes (roundworms). Helminthiases affect more than 2 billion people worldwide, which can become chronic infections when untreated and persist for the rest of their host's life [1–3]. The population affected by helminthiases is mostly found in tropical and subtropical areas, where precarious health systems and poor sanitation prevail. This situation contributes to an increase in their prevalence due to global climate change that has caused parasites to undergo evolutionary changes to adapt over time, which in turn generate resistance to antiparasitic treatments [3]. Although the immune system could eliminate the helminth from the host's body, parasites can often evade the immune response and, in the worst-case scenario, the host suffers collateral damage, consequence of the immunopathology caused by the immune attack against helminths, as an attenuated immune response can trigger a tolerance towards the helminth [2].

1.2 T-helper immune response

In vertebrate animals, the immune response is divided in innate- and adaptive immunity. The first one acts in a non-specific but immediate manner, while in the second is antigen-specific and can be classified as cellular (T cells) or humoral (B cells). The adaptive immune response develops antigen-specific immunological memory and drives both inflammation and tissue repair. The cellular immune response play a key role in the development and progression of chronic inflammatory diseases [4]. T cells are divided into several groups, the two most important are the T helper cell and the cytotoxic T cells, both respectively distinguished by CD4+ and CD8+ cell surface markers. The helper (Th) immune response initiates with the interaction of a CD4+ T cell and an antigen-presenting cell. The T-cell receptor, which is in the surface of the CD4 + T cells, bounds with the major histocompatibility complex type II, which is on the cell membrane of an antigen-presenting cell (B cells, dendritic cells, among others). This interaction leads to the differentiation of B cells into plasma cells that produce antibodies. Various cytokines and other co-stimulatory molecules can stimulate the CD4+ T cell population to divide itself into cell subsets, which elicit a different antigen-specific response, as Th1, Th2, Th9, Th17, and Treg [5]. Each subset has specific characteristics and specialized properties. The Th1 response express pro-inflammatory cytokines, as interferon-gamma (IFN-γ), interleukin 2 (IL-2) and tumor necrosis factor beta (TNF-β). Th1 cells respond against intracellular parasites including protozoa, bacteria, viruses, and fungi. Overexpression of Th1 cells can lead to the development of autoimmune diseases such as hypersensitivity, arthritis, and type 1 diabetes. The Th2 express anti-inflammatory cytokines, as IL-4, IL-5 and IL-13; the Th2 is induced as response to helminth parasites, but its over-activation leads to systemic autoimmune inflammatory diseases, such as allergies and atopic dermatitis. Overexpression of Th9 and Th17 cells is also involved in the development of autoimmune and inflammatory disorders. In the case of Treg cells, they regulate the differentiation and proliferation of effector T cells and promote tolerance, thereby limiting the development of autoimmune diseases [5].

1.3 Hygiene hypothesis

In humans, the immune system has adapted to recurrent infections caused by numerous non-pathogenic organisms. Through exposure to environments rich in microorganisms, this adaptation leads to a more effective immune response to invasion by pathogens. However, the elimination of these "microbial allies" from environments in industrialized cities because of advances in medical care, and improvements in hygiene and urbanization, has been associated with a dramatic increase in autoimmune, allergic, and chronic degenerative conditions of inflammatory origin [6, 7]. In 1989, at the London School of Hygiene and Tropical Medicine, the research group led by Dr. Strachan found an inverse relationship between the number of children in British families, their quality of life, and the rate of hay fever in their children. In other words, the incidence of this disease is higher in families with fewer children and better hygienic conditions; thus, family members have a more limited exposure to the various antigens found in the environment, and this probably leads to a lack of stimulation of the immune system at an early age [6]. However, it was not the first study with these observations; previously, in 1968, a study showed that the Swedish urban population was more susceptible to developing bronchial asthma and chronic bronchitis compared to Swedes living in rural areas [7]. In 1976, another study performed in Canada reported that the prevalence of some atopic diseases, as asthma, eczema, and urticarial was higher in the white community respect to a native community called Metis, which showed an elevated serum IgE level and a higher prevalence of helminthiases, in addition to untreated viral and bacterial diseases [8]. These studies comprise the origin of the so-called "hygiene hypothesis" as we know it today.

Several studies have documented the existence of an inverse relationship between the increased incidence of inflammatory and metabolic diseases and a decreased prevalence of parasitic helminthiases, such as filariasis, where helminths mildly immunosuppress the host in a chronic and non-specific manner [9]. This modulation is associated with the development of a particular immune mechanism referred to as Th2 (T helper 2) response. Derived from the hypothesis that helminths have evolved in parallel with their hosts, it is possible to think that helminths can survive and perpetuate their life cycle because they "control" the host's immune response. Helminths can live for prolonged periods by maintaining their hosts as asymptomatic carriers. It is likely that their surface proteins, as well as those secreted, excreted, and shed from the parasite, play a significant role in immunomodulation, which, collaterally, can benefit the host by reducing the consequences of exacerbated inflammatory responses from a Th1 response. This mechanism is a normally occurring part of many autoimmune disorders. Parasitic infections have also been observed to have beneficial effects on clinical outcomes of allergy patients [1, 10, 11]. The relationship between Th1 and Th2 immune response mechanisms can be understood, considering the immune system as a dynamic but regulated entity within a balance between these Th1 and Th2 antagonistic responses. Naturally, there are certain cells, such as T regulatory lymphocytes (Tregs), which upon receiving certain stimuli can suppress competing responses and maintain the system balance [5].

2. Use of helminths in experimental therapies

Data from tropical and subtropical countries have shown that inflammatory and autoimmune diseases are rare, but helminthiases are very abundant there. However, in those regions, the anthelmintic treatment is associated with an increased rate of chronic degenerative diseases [1]. These findings have suggested that helminths or their products may be useful to control inflammatory diseases amending the host immune response from Th1 to Th2. The Th2 response is characterized by the production of anti-inflammatory cytokines (IL-4, IL-5, IL-10, and IL-13), non-specific and parasite-specific IgEs, as well as the mobilization of mast cells, basophils, and eosinophils. During infection, Treg cells release cytokines (Il-10 and TGF-β) that negatively regulate the Th1 cell subset [3, 12].

Helminths secrete enzymes and hormones, along with their debris, these molecules are the excretory and secretory products (ESP). ESP are the main mechanism of immune response evasion due to their high antigenicity and ability to migrate away from the helminth, "distracting" the immune response and ensuring parasite survival [3, 13]. Studies on helminth immunomodulation derived from this observation have raised interest in the use of total extracts, ESP or even, recombinant proteins as immunomodulatory treatment in animal models and human clinical trials. Most of these studies have reported clinical improvement, but do not address the molecular mechanisms involved in the process [1, 12].

A vast variety of parasites and their ESP have been used in studies that seek to find emerging therapies for many diseases, for example the findings on *Trichuris suis* ova (TSO). This approach has shown therapeutic effects in diseases such as rheumatoid arthritis, inflammatory bowel disease, or multiple sclerosis, with phase 1 and 2 clinical studies being carried out. Patients received a controlled treatment of 2500 TSO units every 2 weeks for 12 months and a low clinical efficacy was obtained, with just small variations in the immune response of the patients receiving the parasite [14]. Another trial used the nematodes *Trichuris vulpis* and *Uncinaria stenocephala* as a treatment in a model of atopic dermatitis in dogs, which were infected with larval eggs of *T. vulpis* (two groups with 500, and 2500 eggs respectively) or *U. stenocephala* (three groups with 100, 500, and 2500 eggs respectively). The results showed that all dogs improved their lesions; however, there was no change in the inflammation caused by subcutaneous infiltrates. In a subsequent randomized study with *T. vulpis*, no difference was found between parasitized dogs and those receiving a placebo, and it was concluded that *T. vulpis* did not generate significant changes [15]. There are few examples of parasites used as disease modulators and how parasites or molecules derived from them can induce an anti-inflammatory response through Th2/regulatory responses directly associated with the established helminth response.

3. *Trichinella spiralis*

Trichinella is a nematode genus comprised of 12 species and 3 genotypes. *Trichinella spiralis*, *T. nativa*, *T. murrelli*, *T. britovi*, *T. patagoniensis*, *T. nelsoni* species and T6, T8 and T9 genotypes are distinguished by encapsulation in the host muscle tissues, while *T. pseudospiralis*, *T. papuae* and *T. zimbabwensis* species do not induce capsule formation. The genus *Trichinella* is cosmopolitan and parasitizes more than 150 species of domestic and wild vertebrates, mostly carnivorous mammals. All *Trichinella* species can be transmitted zoonotically, although the one most frequently related to human disease is *T. spiralis*. The parasite load is correlated with the severity of the disease and is the cause host death [13, 16–19].

3.1 Life cycle, physiopathology and diagnosis

The adult worm settles in the small intestine, while the larvae inhabits the skeletal muscle, this is the muscle larva (ML) which lives inside of a myocyte surrounded by a collagen capsule. In general, there is one ML per myocyte but, sometimes two or more larvae are found [20]. The enteric phase occurs during the first week after infection and is associated with gastroenteritis, diarrhea, and abdominal pain. The life cycle begins when the host ingests raw or undercooked meat with viable ML. In the stomach, the ML is released from the collagen capsule. In the duodenum, the ML invade the epithelial columnar cells and molt four times to become adult. At 90 hours after copulation, females deposit the first larval stage, called newborn larva (NBL), which enters the bloodstream. The migration and invasion phase continues during 3 to 7 days and at the end of 30 days post infection, the NBL matured into ML, and the invaded myocyte was repaired, but does not recovered its contractile functions; on the contrary, the glycocalyx hypertrophies, generating a collagen capsule and surrounding itself with a network of new blood capillaries. This new structure is the nurse cell (NC), which allows to the ML remains in hypobiosis for months or years to be transmitted by ingestion to a new host to complete the life cycle. During this last phase, fever, myalgia, and arthralgia are observed; however, individuals with a low parasite load may remain asymptomatic [4]. The diagnostic methods are (1) trichinoscopy, where the ML and the NC are sought by microscopic examination of striated muscle; this technique is used in *post-mortem* studies and food safety protocols. (2) The artificial enzymatic digestion allows isolate ML from meat samples; this method is used in food safety. (3) Antigen detection seeks parasite proteins as biomarkers, mainly in experimental issues (4). Nowadays ELISA and Western blotting are used to determine parasite-specific antibodies in the host serum; this is the gold standard to corroborate clinical suspicion. (5) The molecular diagnosis uses diagnostic probes specific to unique DNA sequences of the parasite for taxonomic purposes [21, 22].

3.2 Immunobiology

ESP from ML and intestinal larval stages as well as from adult helminths play an important role in a successful infection and trigger an early immune response in the host. Many of these proteins are glycosylated and have an N-terminal signal peptide indicating that they are secreted proteins. The high immunogenicity is due to these glycosylations being formed by repetitive chains of oligosaccharides, such as tyvelose and fucose, that confer them modulating properties of the host immune response. Tyvelose is the main antigenic component of ESP and is part of the ML immunodominant antigens [13, 23, 24]. Proteomics and immunoproteomics analyses have shown that some of these proteins are serine proteases, a family of proteolytic enzymes with varied biological functions during a parasite infection. These functions involve host tissue invasion, migration, and proteolysis by helminths. Serine proteases purified from ESP participate in the degradation of host intestinal tissues. They also allow the penetration of a wide range of tissues for acquiring nutrients, and mediate apoptosis-like cell death and phagocytosis, which contributes to a higher parasite-mediated immunosuppression. ESP may play an important regulatory activity by controlling host immune reaction and recognition. In addition to serine proteases, different studies have found other functional proteins involved in the interactions between *T. spiralis* and its host, such as multiple DNase II isoforms that could function as immunomodulators [25].

4. Therapeutic potential of *Trichinella spiralis*

4.1 Therapeutic potential on cancer

In 1970, Weatherly and collaborators [26] conducted one of the first studies where the therapeutic potential of *T. spiralis* was assessed. The authors observed that parasitized mice survived for longer according to the dose of parasites administered, as well as having a decrease in breast tumor size compared to non-parasitized mice. Since then, many aspects of the inhibitory effect of *T. spiralis* on cancer have been studied and described, both in animal and *in vitro* models with promising results, ranging from the induction of apoptosis in cancer cells to the total or partial inhibition of the growth of some of the tumors studied. The increase in the survival rate of subjects has also been observed *in vivo* in different experimental models, such as in mice that have been parasitized with ML and inoculated with sarcoma 180 tumor cells, where the suppressive effects on cancer development were observed [27–29]. Inhibition of tumor cell growth has also been observed in experimentally infected mice and rats; the inhibition of the development of B16 melanoma, mammary gland cancer, and the number of histiocytomas appears to be directly proportional to the dose of infection [30–34]. The antitumor effects of *T. spiralis* ML have been tested in BALB/c mice with A549 lung cancer, HCT-8 human colorectal carcinoma and C6 glioma [35–37]. In ICR mice, the mouse esophageal carcinoma and mouse ascitic hepatoma (H22) were studied, while in C57BL/6 mice, the hepatoma by Hepa1–6 carcinoma cells were studied [29, 38, 39]. In all experiments, an inhibitory effect of cancer was reported. In addition, studies have been conducted in mouse models of SP2/0 myeloma and colon cancer also immunized with extracts of the parasite and with their ESPs, which immune- modulate the development of both types of cancer [40–42].

ESPs contain some bioactive substances with known antitumor properties, such as the translationally controlled tumor-protein (TCTP) associated with growth, cell cycle regulation and antiapoptotic and immunomodulatory properties. The presence of caveolin-1 (cav-1), an essential protein component of caveolae that acts as a tumor suppressor, has also been described. Other proteins with antitumor properties are some heat shock proteins (HSPS), such as sHSP, HSP60, HSP70, and H3 and H2B histones, involved in fold stability, intracellular arrangement, and proteolytic turnover of many key regulators of growth, differentiation, and survival; they are vital to prevent cell death and maintain homeostasis in *T. spiralis* [20]. The antitumor properties of ESP and ML extracts were also studied in *in vitro* models of esophageal carcinoma, sarcoma 180, chronic myeloid leukemia, hepatomas, lung cancer, B16 melanoma, human cervical carcinoma, and Graffi myeloid tumor. The incubation of cell cultures with ESP or parasite extract showed results that ranged from tumor apoptosis to inhibitory effect on the proliferation of carcinogenic cells [29, 33, 43–47]. These reports are detailed in **Table 1**.

4.2 Therapeutic potential in autoimmune and allergic diseases

Currently, more than 80 autoimmune diseases have been described, such as rheumatoid arthritis, systemic lupus erythematosus (SLE), and type I diabetes. Autoimmune diseases affect between 5 and 9% of the world's population and arise from the loss of immune tolerance to self-antigens. Loss of immune tolerance leads to the development of autoreactive T and B cells and the attack of the body's own tissues; for example, an organ-specific attack is presented in rheumatoid arthritis where the target organ is the joints, or it can occur systemically as is the case in SLE [48]. Because *T. spiralis* can induce a Th2-type response in its host to limit the inflammation within the tissue where it is, many studies are focused on the search for new therapies for autoimmune diseases based on these properties. The same happens for allergic diseases, where *T. spiralis* and its ESPs have also shown encouraging results. That is the case of some studies conducted in animal models of allergic asthma, a chronic inflammatory disorder of the respiratory tract with a strong relationship with an exacerbated Th2 response [49].

	Model	Parasite dose	Duration	Effect	Author
In vivo	Sarcoma 180 in (1) HaM/ICR mice, (2) ICR/CD-1 mice & (3) ICR mice	(1) 3000 ML (2) 50–400 ML (3) 400 ML, oral	(1) 28 & 56 days (2) 2–8 & 34 weeks (3) 7 days	(1) Increased survival, no effect on tumor growth (2) Protection in the first weeks (3) Suppression of cancer development	(1) Lubiniecki et al. [27] (2) Molinari and Carric [28] (3) Wang et al. [29]
	B16 melanoma in (1) B6D2F1/J mice (2) & (3) C57Bl/6 mice (4) variant B16-F10 in C57Bl/6 mice	(1) 200 ML, (2) 5 & 20 larvae/g, (3) & (4) different ML doses, oral	(1) 176 days (2) 2 months (3) variable (4) 40 days	(1) & (2) No signs of tumor growth (3) & (4) Suppression of melanoma development	(1) Molinari and Ebersole [30] (2) Pocock and Meerovitch [31] (3) Kang et al. [32] (4) Vasilev et al. [33]
	Malignant fibrous histiocytoma and mammary gland cancer in rats	Prophylactic infection with ML	—	Decreased number of histiocytomas. Suppression of mammary gland cancer	Apanasevich and Britov [34]
	Lung cancer with A549 cells in BALB/c mice	Different doses, attenuated and non-attenuated ML, oral	7 & 11 days	Inhibition of cancer development with attenuated and non-attenuated ML	Gong et al. [35]
	HCT-8 carcinoma in BALB/c mice	Different ML doses, oral	20 days	Decrease in size and weight of tumors	Li et al. [36]
	C6 Glioma in BALB/c mice	Different ML doses, oral	11 days	Parasite load-dependent antitumor effect	Liu et al. [37]
	Esophageal carcinoma in ICR mice	400 ML, oral	7 days	Suppression of cancer development	Wang et al. [29]
	Hepatoma (1) & (2) H22 in ICR mice (3) Hepa1-6 in C57BL/6 mice	(1) 400 ML (2) & (3) different ML doses, oral	(1) 7 days, (2) & (3) variable	Suppression of cancer development	(1) Wang et al. [29] (2) Ding et al. [38] (3) Zhang et al. [39]
	(1) & (2) Myeloma SP2/0 in BALB/c mice	(1) Immunized with crude extract & ESP (2) parasitosis with oral ML	(1) 30 days, (2) 11 days	(1) Induction of protective immunity with antitumor effect (2) Suppression of myeloma development	(1) Gong et al. [40] (2) Deng et al. [41]
	Mouse model of colon cancer induced by 1,2-dimethylhydrazine	Immunized with ESP	—	Enhanced immunomodulation in cancer development	Eissa et al. [42]

	Model	Parasite dose	Duration	Effect	Author
In vitro	Esophageal carcinoma, hepatoma H22, sarcoma 180, human chronic myeloid leukemia (K562)	Incubation with crude extract	—	Inhibition of carcinogenic cell proliferation	Wang et al. [29]
	Human hepatoma (1) & (2) H7402 (3) HepG2	Incubation with (1) & (2) crude extract (3) ESP	24 h	(1) Tumor apoptosis (2) & (3) Inhibition of carcinogenic cell proliferation	(1) Wang et al. [43] (2) Wang et al. [29] (3) Liu et al. [44]
	Lung cancer in (1) NCI-H446 cells (2) SCLC-H446 cells	Incubation with ESP	(1) 24 h, (2) 12, 24 & 48 h	Dose- and time-dependent inhibitory effect on cancer cells.	(1) Chang et al. [45] (2) Luo et al. [46]
	B16 melanoma	Incubation with crude extract	—	Tumor apoptosis	Vasilev et al. [33]
	Graffi myeloid tumor cells, human cervical carcinoma (HeLa)	Biological active substances from Wistar rats parasitized with 1000 ML orally administered	24 h	Inhibitory effect on Graffi myeloid tumor cells, milder growth of HeLa cells.	Tsocheva-Gaytandzhieva et al. [47]

Muscle l(ML), excretory and secretory products (ESP).

Table 1.
Therapeutic effects of T. spiralis *on cancer.*

Among the existent animal models for autoimmune diseases, a model of type 1 diabetes in non-obese mice, when parasitized with ML, showed a decrease in the number of cytotoxic pancreatic cells, which in turn, delayed the disease progression up to 37 weeks [50]. Likewise, a suppressive effect on the disease was observed in parasitized animals with experimental autoimmune encephalomyelitis (EAE) in a study of new treatments for multiple sclerosis; here, there was an increase in the expression of the Th2 profile and a suppression of the disease signs and symptoms [51–53]. In the case of chronic intestinal disease, immunization with recombinant proteins derived from the TsP53, Cystatin-B and paramyosin proteins of *T. spiralis* (rTsP53, Tsp_03420, and rTsPmy, respectively) led to a decrease in the expression of Th1-type cytokines and disease progression [54–56]; in addition, ML parasitosis and ESP immunization also showed anti-inflammatory effects [57–60]. Another animal model used to observe the therapeutic potential of *T. spiralis* is the collagen-induced rheumatoid arthritis model, where parasitosis with ML and immunizations with its extracts and the rTsPmy protein decreased disease progression, inflammation, and histopathological damage in the synovial tissue of the joint cavities [10, 61, 62].

In the case of allergic diseases, the use of ESPs from *T. spiralis* has also shown promising results in animal models of allergic asthma, a chronic inflammatory respiratory disorder triggered by an exacerbated Th2 response. In some cases, ML and its soluble extracts were used in mice with airway inflammation; as a result, improvements were observed in the disease progression, observed by the reduction of the levels of infiltrated eosinophils and ovalbumin-specific IgE, the decrease in IL-4, and the increase in IL-10 and TGF-β [49, 63]. This modulation was also observed in a mouse model of sepsis-induced acute lung injury where immunization with ESP from the parasite increased survival by 50% and reduced inflammation by a decreased production of pro-inflammatory cytokines [64]. These studies on autoimmune and allergic diseases are mentioned in **Table 2**.

4.3 Therapeutic potential of T. spiralis and other nematodes on experimental lupus mice models

SLE is a chronic autoimmune disease that can affect all organs and tissues of the body due to a set of alterations in the innate and adaptive immune system, such as inefficient removal of apoptotic bodies, generation of autoantibodies that activate the complement cascade, and deposition of immune complexes in tissues that triggers an uncontrolled inflammatory process [65]. Renal, dermatological, and cardiovascular symptoms may occur as clinical features. It has an estimated worldwide prevalence between 6.5 and 178.0 per 100,000 people while its incidence varies from 0.3 to 23.7 cases per 100,000 people per year. The disease occurs in the young population, mainly females (9:1 ratio) [66]. SLE is a social and public health problem because 10–25% of patients who develop SLE die within 10 years of diagnosis. Currently, many of these patients die due to the uncontrolled inflammatory activity associated to the disease or because of the immunosuppressive treatment to which they are subjected [67]. Although the etiology of the disease is not completely known, its clinical heterogeneity suggests that different subsets of immune cells play a vital role in its pathogenesis, especially autoreactive B cells and autoantibody-producing plasma cells. Likewise, T cells play a fundamental role in the progression of the disease due to the loss of the delicate balance between Th1 and Th2 responses [68]. Another pivotal part in this disease is the increased levels of a variety of pro-inflammatory cytokines, such as type I (IFN-α, IFN-β, IFN-κ), type II (IFN-γ) and

	Disease	Mouse model	Parasite dose	Effect	Author
Autoimmune diseases	Type 1 diabetes mellitus	Non-obese diabetic mice	Parasitosis with ML orally administered	Infection protected animals from disease for <37 weeks. Mediated by increased CD4+ T cell numbers and decreased CD8+ and NK T cell numbers in the pancreas.	Saunders et al. [50]
	Multiple sclerosis	Experimental autoimmune encephalomyelitis (EAE)	(1) & (2) Parasitosis with ML orally administered (2) Transfer of T cells from parasitized rats to rats with EAE (3) Immunized with ESP	(1) Parasitosis decreased disease in a dose-dependent manner. (2) Infection maintained a Th2 profile immunity after EAE treatment. T cell transfer protected from disease. (3) ESP caused significant suppression of clinical signs in EAE.	(1) Gruden-Movsesijan et al. [51] (2) Gruden-Movsesijan et al. [52] (3) Kuijk et al. [53]
	Inflammatory bowel disease	Colon damage by dinitrobenzene sulfonate or trinitrobenzene sulfonate	Immunized with recombinant proteins (1) 53 kDa protein rTsP53, (2) Cystatin-B (Tsp_03420) & (3) paramyosin (rTsPmy) of *T. spiralis* (4), (5) & (6) parasitosis with ML orally administered (7) Immunized with ESP of adult worms	(1) RTsP53 significantly improved the disease progression and decreased Th1-type cytokines. (2) A better Th1 / Th2 response balance was observed, and it improved the disease outcome. (3) & (4) *T. spiralis* infection and use of rTsPmy inhibited colitis and increased regulatory cytokines and Treg cells. (5) & (6) Colon damage was reduced through an increased Th2 response. (7) ESP immunization showed anti-inflammatory therapeutic effects.	(1) Du et al. [54] (2) Xu et al. [55] (3) Hao et al. [56] (4) Cho et al. [57] (5) Zhao et al. [58] (6) Xu et al. [59] (7) Yang et al. [60]
	Rheumatoid arthritis	Collagen-induced arthritis	(1) Immunized with soluble ML extract (2) Parasitosis with ML orally administered (3) Immunized with recombinant paramyosin protein (rTsPmy)	(1) Decreased clinical disease progression. (2) Inhibition of Th1/Th17 pro-inflammatory responses and polarization to Th2/Treg. (3) Decreased inflammation, histopathological damage and complement deposition in joints.	(1) Eissa et al. [61] (2) Cheng et al. [10] (3) Chen et al. [62]
Allergic diseases	Asthma	Allergy-induced airway inflammation model in BALB/c mice	(1) Parasitosis with ML orally administered (2) Immunized with adult parasite extract.	(1) Improved lung function and decreased inflammation through the increase of regulatory cytokines IL-10 and TGF-β in parasitized mice. (2) Reduced allergic airway inflammation by an IL-4-mediated upregulation of IL-10 and TGF-β, which in turn stimulated a Th2/Treg response.	(1) Park et al. [63] (2) Sun et al. [49]
	Acute lung injury	Experimental lung injury induced by sepsis	Immunized with ESP	Improved survival of mice by 50% and decreased pro-inflammatory cytokine production, which reduced inflammation and lung tissue injury.	Li et al. [64]

Muscle larvae (ML), excretory and secretory products (ESP).

Table 2.
Therapeutic effects of T. spiralis *on autoimmune and allergic diseases.*

type III (IFN-λ1, IFN -λ2, IFN -λ3 and IFN -λ4) interferons, tumor necrosis factor α (TNF-α), interleukins (IL)-1, IL-2, IL-6, IL-10, IL-12, IL-16, IL-17, IL-23, and others. Due to their correlation with the disease, they have been proposed as therapeutic candidates since there is a lack of effective treatments [69]. Thus, the study of new therapies based on immunomodulation that can ameliorate the symptoms and severity of the disease and improve the quality of life of patients has become highly relevant. To date, the few published reports focus on the therapeutic potential of the nematode *Acanthocheilonema viteae* in SLE, based on the use of a dominant ESP protein called ES-62, a widely tested glycoprotein with therapeutic effects in inflammatory diseases such as arthritis and asthma. This glycoprotein, administered in the MRL/Lpr lupus model, induced a decrease in the production of antinuclear autoantibodies, reduced aortic atherosclerotic lesions, and diminished fibrosis by up to 60%. These results have encouraged the use of drug-like small molecule analogs (SMAs) based on the active phosphorylcholine found on the N-glycans of ES-62, with similar outcomes to those obtained by the original protein, setting up a novel approach to control atherosclerosis in SLE [70, 71].

Phosphorylcholine effect on the intestinal microbiome was also studied in mice from the MRL/Lpr lupus model that received a synthetic conjugate called TPC (Tuftsin-Phosphorylcholine); this is made up of a tetrapeptide with immunostimulatory effects called Tuftsin, part of an IgG molecule, and phosphorylcholine. The mice treated with TPC had significant changes in the intestinal microbiome, such as the increase of the populations of beneficial bacteria of the genera *Turicibacter, Bifidobacterium, Mogibacteriaceae, Clostridiaceae, Adlercreutzia, Allobaculum* and *Anaeroplasma* and the reduction of pro-inflammatory bacteria, like the genus *Akkermansia*. Furthermore, TPC treatment was related to a significant decrease in proteinuria levels and an improvement in the disease progression [72].

Due to the immunomodulatory properties shown above, it is important that further studies be carried out, focused on other parasites or their derivatives with a potential therapeutic effect in lupus disease, like *T. spiralis*.

In 2004, Baeza et al. developed a murine model of experimental lupus that shares strikingly similar characteristics to the human disease, such as the presence of anti-histone, anti-nuclear and anti-coagulant antibodies, as well as anti-cardiolipin and anti non-bilayer phospholipid arrangements (NPA). NPA are three-dimensional structures in the cell membrane, different from the canonical bilayer, formed by the polar fractions of the phospholipids; this rearrangement causes the generation of auto antibodies. The lupus mice present glomerulonephritis, splenomegaly, arthritis-like joint lesions, alopecia and facial lesions resembling human malar erythema. IgG anti-NPA antibodies are found in lupus model mice and in some human patients with anti-phospholipid antibody syndrome [73–75].

The influence of *T. spiralis* infection have been studied in the experimental lupus murine model to find out whether the parasite had a therapeutic effect on the progression and outcome of this inflammatory disease. One of our experiments consisted in study mice were orally infected with 100 ML and at day 30 *post* infection induce lupus by intrasplenic administration of 100 μL of liposomes incubated with the promazine to trigger the formation of non bilayer phospholipid arrangement or NPA [76, 77]. The NPA administration was weekly by intraperitoneal until the end of the experiment. Blood samples were taken every 30 days for 6 months to determine the presence of pro- (IL-1α, IL-17a, IFN-γ and TNF-α) and anti-inflammatory cytokines (IL-4 and IL-10) by flow cytometry. In addition, body weight, clinical lesions and, antibodies to the ML were evaluated by ELISA [22].

The levels of IFN-γ and IL-1α did not show significant differences between experimental groups. **Figure 1** shows that first month *post-infection*, low levels of IL-4 and IL-10 were observed in mice with lupus and lupus infected mice respect to infected. However, unexpected at fifth moth *post-infection*, the lupus infected mice group increased the IL-4 levels (**Figure 1a**); in accordance with data published in different experimental models of inflammatory diseases for arthritis, colitis and airway inflammations [2], is possible that a modulation towards an anti-inflammatory-type response by IL-4 along with the induction of Tregs initiated by IL-10 (**Figure 1b**) were observed. In our observations, levels of IL-17a were higher in the lupus infected mice respected to lupus mice (**Figure 1c**), which contrasts with data shown by Cheng and collaborators, who found that the decrease in this cytokine did not produce any effect in an arthritis model [10]. IL-17a is commonly related to an inflammatory response, but also participate in tissue regeneration [78]. The overexpression of TNF-α in the infected mice and lupus infected mice (**Figure 1d**) is in accordance with results reported by Kim and Moudgil in 2008, using an arthritis model developed by the administration of heat-killed *M. tuberculosis* in rats and subsequently administered with TNF-α and IFN-γ. Authors observed that high levels of TNF-α had a protective effect against arthritis progression [79]. Our data shows absence of arthritis-like lesions in lupus infected mice in concordance with data reported by Cheng and collaborators in 2018, where a therapeutic effect of *T. spiralis*

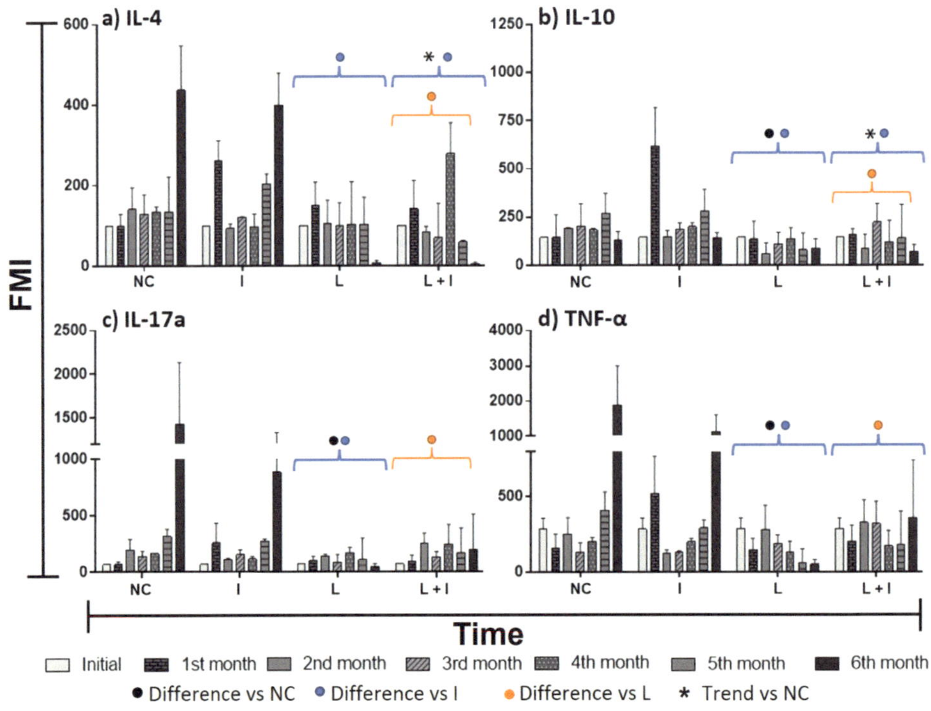

Figure 1.
FMI levels of intracellular cytokines in peripheral blood of the experimental mice. Bar graphs show the levels of cytokines IL-4, IL-10, IL-17a, and TNF-α. Untreated (NC, negative control), infected (I), lupus (L), and lupus infected (L + I) mice. Circles indicate significant differences, asterisks trends between study groups, and square brackets the time during which the statistical difference is valid. Orange color stands for 5 months and blue color for 6 months of study. To determine the differences (p < 0.05), a two-way ANOVA for independent samples was performed. FMI stands for fluorescence mean intensity.

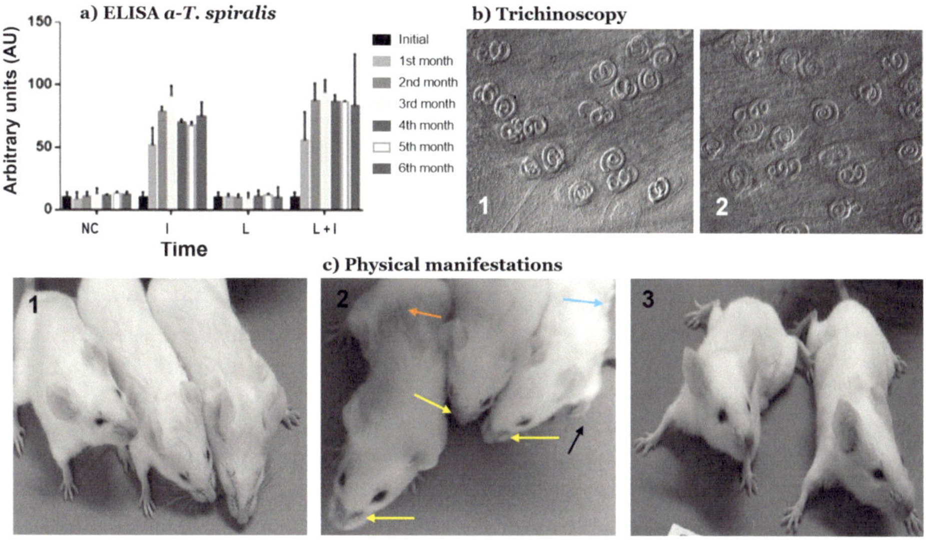

Figure 2.
Physical and clinical characteristics of the mice studied. (a) Bar graphs show serum levels of antibodies specific for T. spiralis. Untreated (NC, negative control), infected (I), lupus (L) and lupus infected (L+I) mice. Circles indicate significant differences between groups. To determine differences (p < 0.05), a two-way ANOVA for independent samples was performed. (b) Trichinoscopies of mouse diaphragms from the P (b1) and P+L (b2) groups analyzed by optic microscopy. (c) Photos show some of the lesions presented by mice at the end of the study, indicated by colored arrows; black arrows show joint lesions, yellow arrows facial lesions, orange arrows alopecia spots, and blue arrows piloerection. (c1) infected (I), (c2) lupus (L), and (c3) lupus infected (L+I) mice.

in a collagen-induced arthritis mouse model was observed by promoting tolerance, suppressing inflammatory T-cell activity and reducing tissue damage [10]. IgG serum antibodies to *T. spiralis* was similar between infected and lupus infected mice (**Figure 2a**). Trichinoscopy of all infected mice showed similar parasite loads in diaphragms (**Figure 2b**). Clinical lesions were only observed in lupus mice (**Figure 2c**). At the beginning of the third month, half of the L group had developed alopecia and facial lesions, and more than half of these mice showed arthritis-like articular lesions.

In conclusion, data suggest a *T. spiralis* a protective effect during 5 months through the production of anti-inflammatory cytokines; this effect can delay or reduce the appearance of some of the lupus-related signs. It is imperative to continue the research to gather more data on the mechanisms of immunomodulation triggered by *T. spiralis* to look out for future lupus therapies.

5. Risks of treatment with helminths or helminth products

Nowadays, there are number for alternative therapies to autoimmune disorders, including the use helminth infection; however, these "treatment" is neither attractive nor etic because the use of live worms. Indeed, in the experimental approach, there are many unanswered questions such as appropriate dosing regimens and optimal timing of treatment, in addition to how host genetics, diet, and environment influence disease progression [80, 81]. Because helminth-enabled immunomodulation can extend to other unknown effects on the immune response to other pathogens or vaccines, these interactions can induce immune downregulation and may lead to predispositions to other types of infections, such as those caused by *Mycobacterium tuberculosis* or malaria [1]. Even though some helminths reduce the risk of developing adenocarcinoma associated with *Helicobacter pylori*, others increase the development of several types of cancer, such as trematodes of genus *Opisthorchis*. In this case, it is important to consider that although all vermiform organisms are considered helminths, there are notable metabolic differences between them; in flatworms (e.g., *Opisthorchis*), the parasite–host contact is carried out through their tegument and involves a whole range of surface proteins. On the other hand, nemathelminths (e.g., *Trichinella*) contact its host through the cuticle that surrounds the parasite, mainly made up of chitin, and turning the ESP into the main antigens recognized by the immune response [1].

In the case of *T. spiralis*, there are some concerns about its use as a therapeutic reagent, the most important being the possible induction of an antibody response, which may reduce the efficacy of its ESP. Even though many of the reports do not use adjuvants or the administrations are intraperitoneally given for short time periods, limiting the response against the parasite proteins, the efficacy could be negatively affected if they are used repeatedly or for prolonged time periods due to the probable production of neutralizing antibodies. Another problem that has arisen from this kind of treatment is the complex composition of the ESP itself, which may lead to the occurrence of side effects or immunological interference, if ESP are used in their entirety. This complexity in composition also represents a problem for scaling their production, limiting ESP clinical use; thus, the characterization of each component that has immunoregulatory properties is of upmost importance [64].

6. Conclusion

Although helminths are different, both biologically and morphologically, most have developed similar strategies to evade innate and adaptive host immune responses, allowing them to establish prolonged parasitism. Among these strategies, the capacity of immunosuppression or immunomodulation stands out, turning helminths into a focus of attention for the study of new therapeutic strategies that allow improving the quality of life during chronic degenerative diseases. The study of *Trichinella spiralis* has shown to have immunomodulatory potential in experimental models of cancer, allergy and autoimmune diseases. In the case of experimental murine lupus, infection with *Trichinella* delayed the presence of signs of disease for 5 months and increased the levels of the cytokines IL-10 and IL-4. To our knowledge, this is the only work reporting the therapeutic effects of *T. spiralis* in an experimental mouse model of lupus.

Acknowledgements

The authors thank Carla Landa-Saldivar and Sandra Sánchez-Barbosa for their technical assistance and Institute for Diagnostic and Epidemiological Reference animal house veterinary technicians for the excellent animal care. This study was grant supported by National Polytechnic Institute (Instituto Politécnico Nacional), Mexico

(SIP20210418 to IB and SIP 20210382 to CWB) and National Council for Science and Technology (CONACYT), Mexico (Internal number 818877). Authors are National System of Researchers fellows (CONACYT). The native speaker Sandra Sánchez-Barbosa conducted the critical review of the English language.

Conflict of interest

The authors declare no conflict of interest.

Author details

Christian-Irene Nevárez-Lechuga[1,2], Antonio Meza-Lucas[2], Alejandro Escobar-Gutiérrez[2], Carlos Wong-Baeza[1], Isabel Baeza[1] and Jorge-Luis de-la-Rosa-Arana[2,3]*

1 Escuela Nacional de Ciencias Biológicas, Instituto Politécnico Nacional (National School of Biological Sciences, National Polytechnic Institute), Mexico City, Mexico

2 Ministry of Health, Institute for Diagnostic and Epidemiological Reference, Mexico City, Mexico

3 Faculty of Advanced Studies Cuautitlán, National Autonomous University of Mexico, Mexico City, Mexico

*Address all correspondence to: delarosa.jorgeluis@yahoo.com

References

[1] Homan EJ, Bremel RD. A role for epitope networking in immunomodulation by helminths. Frontiers in Immunology. 2018;**9**:1763. DOI: 10.3389/fimmu.2018.01763

[2] Maizels RM, Smits HH, McSorley HJ. Modulation of host immunity by helminths: The expanding repertoire of parasite effector molecules. Immunity. 2018;**49**(5):801-818. DOI: 10.1016/j.immuni.2018.10.016

[3] Idris OA, Wintola OA, Afolayan AJ. Helminthiases; prevalence, transmission, host-parasite interactions, resistance to common synthetic drugs and treatment. Heliyon. 2019;**5**(1):e01161. DOI: 10.1016/j.heliyon.2019.e01161

[4] Sun L, Wang X, Saredy J, Yuan Z, Yang X, Wang H. Innate-adaptive immunity interplay and redox regulation in immune response. Redox Biology. 2020;**37**:101759. DOI: 10.1016/j.redox.2020.101759

[5] Kumar S, Jeong Y, Ashraf MU, Bae Y-S. Dendritic cell-mediated Th2 immunity and immune disorders. International Journal of Molecular Sciences. 2019;**20**(9):2159. DOI: 10.3390/ijms20092159

[6] De-La-Rosa-Arana J-L, Tapia-Romero R. Triquinelosis, Parasitosis Más Comunes En La Población Mexicana. La Población Mexicana. In: Morales-Montor J. PMCE, Terrazas-Valdes L-I, (Eds). Tendencias H-BR, editors. Triquinelosis. 2015;**6**:159-192

[7] Moulson AJ, Av-Gay Y. BCG immunomodulation: From the "hygiene hypothesis" to COVID-19. Immunobiology. 2021;**226**(1):152052. DOI: 10.1016/j.imbio.2020.152052

[8] Strachan DP. Hay fever, hygiene, and household size. BMJ. 1989;**299**(6710):1259-1260. DOI: 10.1136/bmj.299.6710.1259

[9] Irnell L, Kiviloog J. Bronchial asthma and chronic bronchitis in a Swedish urban and rural population. With special reference to prevalence, respiratory function and socio-medical condition. Scandinavian Journal of Respiratory Diseases. Supplementum. 1968;**66**:1-86

[10] Gerrard JW, Geddes CA, Reggin PL, Gerrard CD, Horne S. Serum IgE levels in white and metis communities in Saskatchewan. Annals of Allergy. 1976;**37**(2):91-100

[11] Aravindhan V, Anand G. Cell Type-specific immunomodulation induced by helminthes: Effect on meta-inflammation, insulin resistance and Type-2 diabetes. The American Journal of Tropical Medicine and Hygiene. 2017;**97**(6):1650-1661. DOI: 10.4269/ajtmh.17-0236

[12] Cheng Y, Zhu X, Wang X, Zhuang Q, Huyan X, Sun X, et al. *Trichinella spiralis* infection mitigates collagen-induced arthritis via programmed death 1-mediated immunomodulation. Frontiers in Immunology. 2018;**9**:1566. DOI: 10.3389/fimmu.2018.01566

[13] Yue X, Sun XY, Liu F, Hu CX, Bai Y, Da Yang Q, et al. Molecular characterization of a *Trichinella spiralis* serine proteinase. Veterinary Research. 2020;**51**(1):125. DOI: 10.1186/s13567-020-00847-0

[14] Yordanova IA, Ebner F, Schulz AR, Steinfelder S, Rosche B, Bolze A, et al. The worm-specific immune response in multiple sclerosis patients

receiving controlled *Trichuris suis ova* immunotherapy. Life (Basel). 2021;**11**(2):101. DOI: 10.3390/life11020101

[15] Mueller RS, Specht L, Helmer M, Epe C, Wolken S, Denk D, et al. The effect of nematode administration on canine atopic dermatitis. Veterinary Parasitology. 2011;**181**(2-4):203-209. DOI: 10.1016/j.vetpar.2011.05.001

[16] Pozio E. New patterns of *Trichinella* infection. Veterinary Parasitology. 2001;**98**(1-3):133-148. DOI: 10.1016/s0304-4017(01)00427-7

[17] Pozio E, Darwin MK. Systematics and epidemiology of *Trichinella*. Advances in Parasitology. 2006;**63**: 367-439. DOI: 10.1016/S0065-308X(06)63005-4

[18] de-la-Rosa JL, Aranda JG, Padilla E, Correa D. Prevalence and risk factors associated with serum antibodies against *Trichinella spiralis*. International Journal for Parasitology. 1998;**28**(2):317-321. DOI: 10.1016/s0020-7519(97)00163-x

[19] Solís-Hernández D, Saucedo-Gutiérrez K-L, Meza-Lucas A, Gómez-de-Anda F-R, Medina-Lerena M-S, García-Rodea R, et al. Statistical approach to *Trichinella* infection in horses handled by rural slaughterhouses across five distinctive socioeconomic regions in Mexico. Revista Argentina de Microbiología. 2020;**52**(4):288-292. DOI: 10.1016/j.ram.2020.04.001

[20] Ramírez-Melgar C, Gómez-Priego A, De-la-Rosa J-L. Application of Giemsa stain for easy detection of *Trichinella spiralis* muscle larvae. The Korean Journal of Parasitology. 2007;**45**(1):65-68. DOI: 10.3347/kjp.2007.45.1.65

[21] de-la-Rosa JL, Gómez-Priego A. Triquinelosis. In: Becerril-Flores MA, García MA, editors. Parasitología médica. 5th ed. Cd. de México: McGraw-Hill Interamericana; 2019

[22] Zumaquero-Ríos J-L, García-Juarez J, De-La-Rosa-Arana J-L, Marcet R, Sarracent-Pérez J. *Trichinella spiralis*: Monoclonal antibody against the muscular larvae for the detection of circulating and fecal antigens in experimentally infected rats. Experimental Parasitology. 2012;**132**(4):444-449

[23] Sofronic-Milosavljevic L, Ilic N, Pinelli E, Gruden-Movsesijan A. Secretory products of *Trichinella spiralis* muscle larvae and immunomodulation: Implication for autoimmune diseases, allergies, and malignancies. Journal of Immunology Research. 2015;**2015**:523875. DOI: 10.1155/2015/523875

[24] Braasch J, Ostermann S, Mackiewicz M, Bardot C, Pagneux C, Borchardt-Lohölter V, et al. *Trichinella spiralis*-New method for sample preparation and objective detection of specific antigens using a chemiluminescence immunoassay. Veterinary Parasitology. 2020;**X**:4

[25] Wang Y, Bai X, Zhu H, Wang X, Shi H, Tang B, et al. Immunoproteomic analysis of the excretory-secretory products of *Trichinella pseudospiralis* adult worms and newborn larvae. Parasit Vectors. 2017;**10**(1):579. DOI: 10.1186/s13071-017-2522-9

[26] Weatherly NF. Increased survival of Swiss mice given sublethal infections of *Trichinella spiralis*. The Journal of Parasitology. 1970;**56**(4):748-752. http://dx.doi.org/10.2307/3277722

[27] Lubiniecki AS, Cypess RH. Quantitative study of the effect of previous *Trichinella spiralis* infection on sarcoma 180 ascitic tumor formation in

mice. Tropenmedizin und Parasitologie. 1975;**26**(3):329-334

[28] Molinari JA, Carrick L Jr, Lubiniecki AS. Influence of *Trichinella spiralis* infection on development of sarcoma-180 ascites tumors. Tropenmedizin und Parasitologie. 1979;**30**(4):429-433

[29] Wang XL, Fu BQ, Yang SJ, Wu XP, Cui GZ, Liu MF, et al. *Trichinella spiralis*—A potential anti-tumor agent. Veterinary Parasitology. 2009;**159**(3-4):249-252. DOI: 10.1016/j.vetpar.2008.10.052

[30] Molinari JA, Ebersole JL. Antineoplastic effects of long-term *Trichinella spiralis* infection on B-16 melanoma. International Archives of Allergy and Applied Immunology. 1977;**55**(1-6):444-448. DOI: 10.1159/000231956

[31] Pocock D, Meerovitch E. The anti-neoplastic effect of trichinellosis in a syngeneic murine model. Parasitology. 1982;**84**(3):463-473. DOI: 10.1017/s0031182000052768

[32] Kang Y-J, Jo J-O, Cho M-K, Yu H-S, Leem S-H, Song KS, et al. *Trichinella spiralis* infection reduces tumor growth and metastasis of B16-F10 melanoma cells. Veterinary Parasitology. 2013;**196**(1-2):106-113. DOI: 10.1016/j.vetpar.2013.02.021

[33] Vasilev S, Ilic N, Gruden-Movsesijan A, Vasilijic S, Bosic M, Sofronic-Milosavljevic L. Necrosis and apoptosis in *Trichinella spiralis*-mediated tumour reduction. Central European Journal of Immunology. 2015;**40**(1):42-53

[34] Apanasevich VI, Britov VA, Zban' IV. Antitumor cross-resistance of trichinosis. Voprosy Onkologii. 2002;**48**(2):223-226

[35] Gong PT, Zhang XC, Li JH, Zhang GC, Yang J, Cao LL36, et al. Observation of anti-tumer effect of *Trichinella spirialis* in mice on A549 lung cancer cell. Journal of Pathogen Biology. 2008;**3**:200-202

[36] Li X, Zhang G, Zhang XC, Li J, Yang J, Gong P, et al. Effect of *Trichinella* on growth of human colorectal carcinoma HCT-8 cells in BALB/c mice. Chinese Journal of Biology. 2008;**4**:285-287

[37] Liu YJ, Xu J, Huang HY, Xu GQ. Inhibitory effect of the excretory/secretory proteins of *Trichinella spiralis* on proliferation of human hepatocellular carcinoma HepG2 cell line. Chinese Journal of Parasitology & Parasitic Diseases. 2015;**33**:315-317

[38] Ding J, Tang B, Liu X, Bai X, Wang Y, Li S, et al. Excretory-secretory product of *Trichinella spiralis* inhibits tumor cell growth by regulating the immune response and inducing apoptosis. Acta Tropica. 2022;**225**:106172. DOI: 10.1016/j.actatropica.2021.106172

[39] Zhang YY, Gong PT, Zhang XC, Li JH, Yang J, Zhang GC. Anti-tumor effect of *Trichinella spirialis* on Hepal-6 hepatoma carcinoma cell in the C57BL/6 mice. Journal of Pathogen Biology. 2009;**4**:24-26

[40] Gong P, Zhang J, Cao L, Nan Z, Li J, Yang J, et al. Identification and characterization of myeloma-associated antigens in *Trichinella spiralis*. Experimental Parasitology. 2011;**127**(4):784-788. DOI: 10.1016/j.exppara.2010.12.001

[41] Deng B, Gong P, Li J, Cheng B, Ren W, Yang J, et al. Identification of the differentially expressed genes in SP2/0 myeloma cells from Balb/c mice infected with *Trichinella spiralis*. Veterinary

Parasitology. 2013;**194**(2-4):179-182. DOI: 10.1016/j.vetpar.2013.01.050

[42] Eissa MM, Ismail CA, El-Azzouni MZ, Ghazy AA, Hadi MA. Immuno-therapeutic potential of *Schistosoma mansoni* and *Trichinella spiralis* antigens in a murine model of colon cancer. Investigational New Drugs. 2019;**37**(1):47-56. DOI: 10.1007/s10637-018-0609-6

[43] Wang XL, Liu MY, Sun SM, Liu XL, Yu L, Wang XR, et al. An anti-tumor protein produced by *Trichinella spiralis* induces apoptosis in human hepatoma H7402 cells. Veterinary Parasitology. 2013;**194**(2-4):186-188. DOI: 10.1016/j.vetpar.2013.01.052

[44] Liu J, Sun JH, Liu LD. Observation of *Trichinella* on C6 glioma in BALB/c mice. Journal of Apoplexy and Nervous Diseases. 2008;**6**:722-724

[45] Chang HM, Zhao L, Wang XJ, Fang YH, Li D, Luo JM, et al. Effect of the excretory/secretory proteins from *Trichinella spiralis* on apoptosis of NCI-H446 small-cell lung cancer cells. Chinese Journal of Parasitology & Parasitic Diseases. 2014;**32**:299-303

[46] Luo J, Yu LI, Xie G, Li D, Su M, Zhao X, et al. Study on the mitochondrial apoptosis pathways of small cell lung cancer H446 cells induced by *Trichinella spiralis* muscle larvae ESPs. Parasitology. 2017;**144**(6):793-800. DOI: 10.1017/S0031182016002535

[47] Tsocheva-Gaytandzhieva N, Toshkova R, Gardeva E, Yossifova L, Petkova S, Nanev V. Antiproliferative activity against tumour cells of biologically active substances isolated from livers of healthy and *Trichinella spiralis* infected rats. Comptes Rendus de L'Academie Bulgare des Sciences. 2016;**69**(11):1443-1448

[48] Paulendran B, Davis MM. The science and medicine of human immunology. Science. 2020;**6511**:eaay4014

[49] Sun S, Li H, Yuan Y, Wang L, He W, Xie H, et al. Preventive and therapeutic effects of *Trichinella spiralis* adult extracts on allergic inflammation in an experimental asthma mouse model. Parasites & Vectors. 2019;**12**(1):326. DOI: 10.1186/s13071-019-3561-1

[50] Saunders KA, Raine T, Cooke A, Lawrence CE. Inhibition of autoimmune type 1 diabetes by gastrointestinal helminth infection. Infection and Immunity. 2007;**75**(1):397-407. DOI: 10.1128/IAI.00664-06

[51] Gruden-Movsesijan A, Ilic N, Mostarica-Stojkovic M, Stosic-Grujicic S, Milic M, Sofronic-Milosavljevic L. *Trichinella spiralis*: modulation of experimental autoimmune encephalomyelitis in DA rats. Experimental Parasitology. 2008;**118**(4):641-647. DOI: 10.1016/j.exppara.2007.12.003

[52] Gruden-Movsesijan A, Ilic N, Mostarica-Stojkovic M, Stosic-Grujicic S, Milic M, Sofronic-Milosavljevic L. Mechanisms of modulation of experimental autoimmune encephalomyelitis by chronic *Trichinella spiralis* infection in Dark Agouti rats: Modulation of EAE by *T. spiralis* infection. Parasite Immunology. 2010;**32**(6):450-459. DOI: 10.1111/j.1365-3024.2010.01207

[53] Kuijk LM, Klaver EJ, Kooij G, van der Pol SMA, Heijnen P, Bruijns SCM, et al. Soluble helminth products suppress clinical signs in murine experimental autoimmune encephalomyelitis and differentially modulate human dendritic cell activation. Molecular Immunology. 2012;**51**(2):210-218. DOI: 10.1016/j.molimm.2012.03.020

[54] Du L, Tang H, Ma Z, Xu J, Gao W, Chen J, et al. The protective effect of the recombinant 53-kDa protein of *Trichinella spiralis* on experimental colitis in mice. Digestive Diseases and Sciences. 2011;**56**(10):2810-2817. DOI: 10.1007/s10620-011-1689-8

[55] Xu J, Liu M, Yu P, Wu L, Lu Y. Effect of recombinant *Trichinella spiralis* cysteine proteinase inhibitor on NCBS-induced experimental inflammatory bowel disease in mice. International Immunopharmacology. 2019;**66**:28-40

[56] Hao C, Wang W, Zhan B, Wang Z, Huang J, Sun X, et al. *Trichinella spiralis* paramyosin induces colonic regulatory T cells to mitigate inflammatory bowel disease. Frontiers in Cell and Development Biology. 2021;**9**:695015. DOI: 10.3389/fcell.2021.695015

[57] Cho MK, Park MK, Kang SA, Choi SH, Ahn SC, Yu HS. *Trichinella spiralis* infection suppressed gut inflammation with CD4(+) CD25(+) Foxp3(+) T cell recruitment. Korean Journal. 2012;**50**:385-390

[58] Zhao Y, Liu MY, Wang XL, Liu XL, Yang Y, Zou HB, et al. Modulation of inflammatory bowel disease in a mouse model following infection with *Trichinella spiralis*. Veterinary Parasitology. 2013;**194**(2-4):211-216. DOI: 10.1016/j.vetpar.2013.01.058

[59] Xu J, Yu P, Wu L, Liu M, Lu Y. Effect of *Trichinella spiralis* intervention on NCBS-induced experimental colitis in mice. Immunobiology. 2019;**224**:147-153

[60] Yang X, Yang Y, Wang Y, Zhan B, Gu Y, Cheng Y, et al. Excretory/secretory products from *Trichinella spiralis* adult worms ameliorate DSS-induced colitis in mice. PLoS One. 2014;**9**(5):e96454. DOI: 10.1371/journal.pone.0096454

[61] Eissa MM, Mostafa DK, Ghazy AA, El Azzouni MZ, Boulos LM, Younis LK. Anti-arthritic activity of *Schistosoma mansoni* and *Trichinella spiralis* derived-antigens in adjuvant arthritis in rats: Role of FOXP3+ Treg Cells. PLoS One. 2016;**11**(11):e0165916. DOI: 10.1371/journal.pone.0165916

[62] Chen Y, Shao S, Huang J, Gu Y, Cheng Y, Zhu X. Therapeutic efficacy of a *Trichinella spiralis* paramyosin-derived peptide modified with a membrane-targeting signal in mice with antigen-induced arthritis. Frontiers in Microbiology. 2020;**11**:608380. DOI: 10.3389/fmicb.2020.608380

[63] Park H-K, Cho MK, Choi SH, Kim YS, Yu HS. *Trichinella spiralis*: infection reduces airway allergic inflammation in mice. Experimental Parasitology. 2011;**127**(2):539-544. DOI: 10.1016/j.exppara.2010.10.004

[64] Li H, Qiu D, Yang H, Yuan Y, Wu L, Chu L, et al. Therapeutic efficacy of excretory-secretory products of *Trichinella spiralis* adult worms on sepsis-induced acute lung injury in a mouse model. Frontiers in Cellular and Infection Microbiology. 2021;**11**:653843. DOI: 10.3389/fcimb.2021.653843

[65] Fava A, Petri M. Systemic lupus erythematosus: Diagnosis and clinical management. Journal of Autoimmunity. 2019;**96**:1-13. DOI: 10.1016/j.jaut.2018.11.001

[66] Islam MA, Khandker SS, Kotyla PJ, Hassan R. Immunomodulatory effects of diet and nutrients in systemic lupus erythematosus (SLE): A systematic review. Frontiers in Immunology. 2020;**11**:1477. DOI: 10.3389/fimmu.2020.01477

[67] Montiel D, Cacace P. Mortalidad y causas de muerte en pacientes con lupus

eritematoso sistémico. Revista paraguaya de reumatologia. 2019;**5**(2):51-57

[68] Katsuyama T, Tsokos GC, Moulton VR. Aberrant T cell signaling and subsets in systemic lupus erythematosus. Frontiers in Immunology. 2018;**9**:1088. DOI: 10.3389/fimmu.2018.01088

[69] Idborg H, Oke V. Cytokines as biomarkers in systemic Lupus Erythematosus: Value for diagnosis and drug therapy. International Journal of Molecular Sciences. 2021;**22**(21):11327. DOI: 10.3390/ijms222111327

[70] Aprahamian TR, Zhong X, Amir S, Binder CJ, Chiang LK, Al-Riyami L, et al. The immunomodulatory parasitic worm product ES-62 reduces lupus-associated accelerated atherosclerosis in a mouse model. International Journal for Parasitology. 2015;**45**(4):203-207. DOI: 10.1016/j.ijpara.2014.12.006

[71] Rodgers DT, Pineda MA, Suckling CJ, Harnett W, Harnett MM. Drug-like analogues of the parasitic worm-derived immunomodulator ES-62 are therapeutic in the MRL/Lpr model of systemic lupus erythematosus. Lupus. 2015;**24**(13):1437-1442. DOI: 10.1177/0961203315591031

[72] Neuman H, Mor H, Bashi T, Givol O, Watad A, Shemer A, et al. Helminth-based product and the microbiome of mice with lupus. mSystems. 2019;**4**(1):e00160-18. DOI: 10.1128/mSystems.00160-18

[73] Baeza I, Leyva E, Campos B, Lara M, Ibanez M, Farfan N, et al. Antibodies to non-bilayer phospholipid arrangements induce a murine autoimmune disease resembling human lupus. European Journal of Immunology. 2004;**34**:576-586

[74] Wong-Baeza C, Hernández-Pando R, Reséndiz A, Tescucano A, Bustos I, Ibáñez M, et al. Molecular organization of the non-bilayer phospholipid arrangements that induce an autoimmune disease resembling human lupus in mice. Molecular Membrane Biology. 2012;**29**(2):52-67. DOI: 10.3109/09687688.2012.667577

[75] Wong-Baeza C, Reséndiz-Mora A, Donis-Maturano L, Wong-Baeza I, Zárate-Neira L, Yam-Puc JC, et al. Anti-lipid IgG antibodies are produced via germinal centers in a Murine model resembling human lupus. Frontiers in Immunology. 2016;7:396. DOI: 10.3389/fimmu.2016.00396

[76] Aguilar L, Ortega-Pierres G, Campos B, Fonseca R, Ibáñez M, Wong C, et al. Phospholipid membranes form specific nonbilayer molecular arrangements that are antigenic. The Journal of Biological Chemistry. 1999;**274**(36):25193-25196. DOI: 10.1074/jbc.274.36.25193

[77] Reséndiz-Mora A, Wong-Baeza C, Nevárez-Lechuga I, Landa-Saldívar C, Molina-Gómez E, Hernández-Pando R, et al. Interleukin 4 deficiency limits the development of a lupus-like disease in mice triggered by phospholipids in a non-bilayer arrangement. Scandinavian Journal of Immunology. 2021;**93**(3):e13002. DOI: 10.1111/sji.13002

[78] Flores-García Y, Talamás-Rohana P. Interleucina 17, funciones Biológicas y su Receptor. Revista de Educacion Bioquimica. 2012;**31**(1):3-9

[79] Kim EY, Moudgil KD. Regulation of autoimmune inflammation by pro-inflammatory cytokines. Immunology Letters. 2008;**120**(1-2):1-5. DOI: 10.1016/j.imlet.2008.07.008

[80] Liao C, Cheng X, Liu M, Wang X, Boireau P. *Trichinella spiralis* and tumors:

Cause, coincidence or treatment? Anti-Cancer Agents in Medicinal Chemistry. 2018;**18**(8):1091-1099. DOI: 10.2174/1871520617666171121115847

[81] Long SR, Liu RD, Kumar DV, Wang ZQ, Su C-W. Immune protection of a helminth protein in the DSS-induced colitis model in mice. Frontiers in Immunology. 2021;**12**:1438. DOI: 10.3389/fimmu.2021.664998

Chapter 2

Anthelmintic Drug Resistance in Livestock: Current Understanding and Future Trends

Muhammad Abdullah Malik, Muhammad Sohail Sajid, Rao Zahid Abbas, Muhammad Tahir Aleem, Faisal Rasheed Anjum, Asad Khan, Muhammad Farhab, Mahvish Maqbool, Muhammad Zeeshan, Kashif Hussain, Namrah Rehman, Rana Hamid Ali Nisar, Hafiz Muhammad Rizwan and Urfa Bin Tahir

Abstract

Anthelmintic, ectoparasiticides (insecticides, acaricides), and antiprotozoal chemotherapeutic drugs target parasites. Chenopodium oil like alkaloids, arsenic compounds, cupric sulfate, nicotine, and cupric silicate were used to destroy nematodes. Unfortunately, these chemicals were less effective and less safe for livestock. The four major groups of broad-spectrum antinematodal compounds are macrocyclic lactones such as milbemycins/ivermectin, benzimidazole/pro-benzimidazole, tetrahydro pyrimidines such as morantel, pyrantel tartrate, and imidazothiazoles such as tetramisole and levamisole. The various factors responsible for gastrointestinal (GI) parasitism make it difficult to develop effective control measures, to the best of our knowledge. Hence, an effective strategy for the control of parasitic diseases that do not solely rely on anthelmintic therapies needs to be developed at the regional level, based on the epidemiology of the disease. This book chapter aims to elaborate on the various other ways to control parasitic diseases due to Anthelmintic drug resistance.

Keywords: gastrointestinal parasitism, anthelmintic resistance, chemical Control, alternative control, future trends in livestock

1. Introduction

Antiparasitic chemotherapeutics can be categorized as anthelmintics, ectoparasiticides (insecticides and acaricides), and antiprotozoals. Anthelmintics are those agents used to destroy worms and are used as anticestodal, antinematodal, and antinematodal agents [1].

The use of chemical agents against nematodes traced back to the 1990s and those agents were having less effectiveness. Chemicals used for nematode destruction were arsenic compounds, cupric sulfate, nicotine, Chenopodium oil like alkaloids. These chemical compounds were found less effective and more toxic for livestock. Synthetic drug phenothiazine antinematodal characteristics were first reported in the United States and were used as broad-spectrum medicine for nematode treatment in horses, ruminants, and chickens. Phenothiazine is removed from the therapeutic inventory in many countries [1].

From that time scientists were trying to produce an ideal anthelmintic drug that could be used as broad-spectrum dewormers and result in the use of organophosphorus compounds, imidazoles, and tetrahydro pyrimidines. Thiabendazole (TBZ) was developed in 1961 after two decades, and this drug is having high efficiency and safety and broad-spectrum. It was the first-generation benzimidazole group and used against a wide range of hosts, i.e., goats, poultry, sheep, cattle, pigs, horses, and humans against gastrointestinal nematodes, and it shows ovicidal, larvicidal, and adulticidal activities. After TBZ's success, it was planned to structurally modify it toward evolving drugs with excellent properties. Levamisole was discovered in 1966 and was marketed with the name of hydrochloride (HCL) salt having broad-spectrum antinematodal activities and immunomodulator effects [2].

Macrocyclic lactone derivatives including ivermectin (IVM) were discovered in 1981 broad-spectrum insecticidal activities. After this in 2009 after 28 years, monepantel was commercially released [3]. Broad-spectrum antinematodal synthetic compounds are divided into four major groups, i.e., macrocyclic lactone derivatives including milbemycins/ivermectin, benzimidazole/pro-benzimidazole group, tetrahydro pyrimidines group including morantel, pyrantel tartrate, and imidazothiazoles group including tetramisole and levamisole [1].

Commonly used chemotherapeutic groups are briefly reviewed in this review.

2. Benzimidazoles/pro-benzimidazoles and their mode of action

Compounds of this group are metabolized in the body and activate BZ metabolites. Members of this group are oxfendazole, ricobendazole, albendazole, thiabendazole, mebendazole, triclabendazole, oxibendazole, cambendazole, and other chemicals belonging to pro-benzimidazole, i.e., thiophanate, febantel, and netobimin [1].

Benzimidazole is effective against adult nematodes in ruminants and also has ovicidal and larvicidal activities. Some benzimidazole also exhibits anti-trematode and anticestodal activities. They are used in various hosts such as bovine, canine, equine, ovine, feline, reptiles, caprine, birds, and human species. In the case of humans, thiabendazole, mebendazole, and albendazole are used. They are having low toxicity and in some cases can be drenched 10 times than the calculated standard dose rate [2, 4].

All members of this group are having the same mode of action and disturb the energy metabolism of parasitic nematodes through binding with tubulin protein (alpha and beta molecules). This protein is present in plasma and microtubules and forms heterodimers and constructs blocks in polymeric microtubules [1]. Microtubules formation is a dynamic process affected by tubulin ring polymerization and depolymerization. Microtubules play an important role in cell division, energy metabolism, shape, and transport of substrate and protein assemblage. Benzimidazole group members bundle with β-tubulin, and this complex integrates

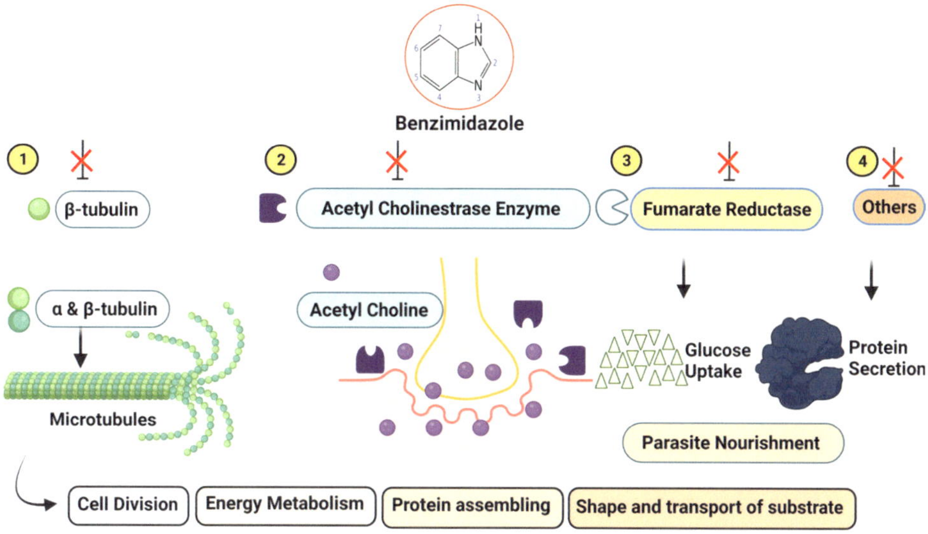

Figure 1.
Illustration of four different mechanisms of action by benzimidazoles against GI parasites.

at the propagating ends of the microtubules and inhibits the assemblage of extra microtubules. This whole process is known as capping [5–7].

They cause parasite undernourishment (due to failure in glucose uptake, the proliferation of microtubules, and protein secretion), reduction in acetylcholinesterase enzyme secretion, reduction in carbohydrate catabolism through fumarate reductase enzyme. Histological investigation of benzimidazole pharmacodynamics also reports their role in disturbance of microtubule aggregation in nematodes at those concentrations that do not influence mammalian cells (**Figure 1**) [1, 6, 8].

3. Imidazothiazoles and their mode of action

Imidazothiazoles consist of two drugs, i.e., tetramisole and levamisole HCL (LEV). Levamisole is a Levo isomer and has true antinematodal activity while tetramisole is a mixture of Levo and destroys forms. That is why the calculated dose of levamisole is half that of tetramisole.

Levamisole is mostly used in goats, sheep, swine, and cattle while in the case of horses, it is contraindicated. This drug is having potency against both mature and immature stages. That's why the calculated dosage of LEV is half that of tetramisole with a safety index of twice.

In sheep, goat, cattle, and swine, LEV is administrated, and in horses, mostly it is contraindicated. In several mature and immature stages of alimentary tract nematodes and lungworms, LEV has shown great potential. Whereas LEV is not anticestodal nor it is anti-trematode. LEV has not shown any ovicidal activity such as BZs. Whereas the remedial index of LEV is relatively lower than that of other antinematodal. LEV has also been found effective against hypobiotic larvae of the sheep parasitic nematode, *H. contortus* [1, 4].

The working mode of action of levamisoles has depicted that it works as a cholinergic agonist; it acts as nicotinic acetylcholine receptors on the surface of the nematode muscle cells along with neuromuscular junction. The antinematodal potential of

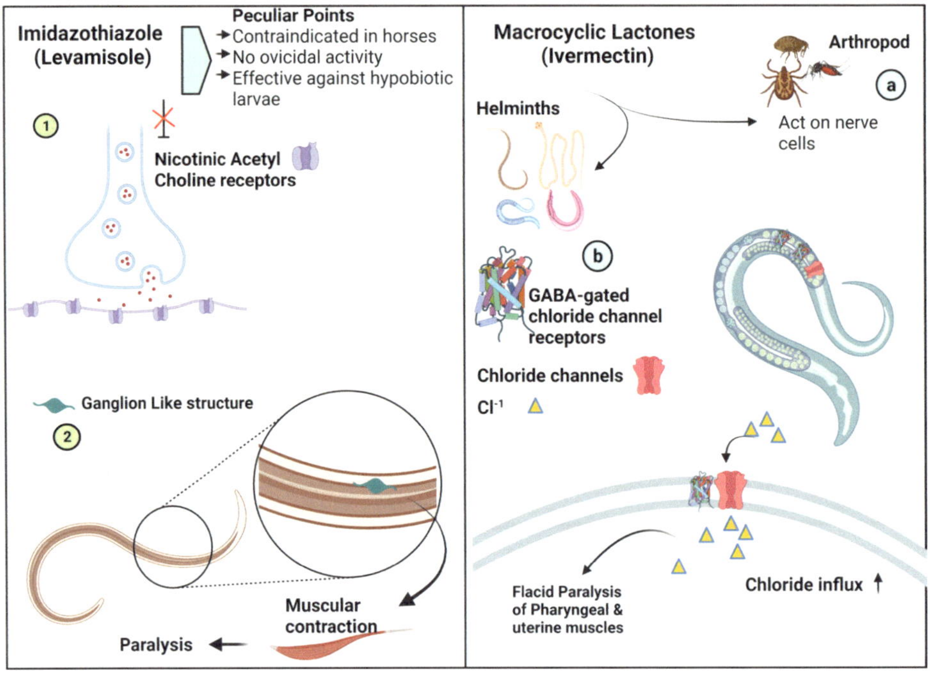

Figure 2.
Illustration of the mechanism of actions of levamisole and ivermectin against GI parasites.

LEV is mostly associated with its ganglion stimulant activity. It induces ganglion-like structure in somatic muscle cells of nematodes. The induction ultimately results in determining muscle contractions that are in line with the depolarizing barricades causing paralysis.

The pharmacodynamics of the compound plays an important role in the paralysis that leads to the elimination of helminths promptly through normal intestinal peristalsis (**Figure 2**) [1, 2].

4. Macrocyclic lactones (avermectins/milbemycins) and their mode of action

Macrocyclic lactones have different commercialized products that show insecticidal activity against a broad range of parasitic nematodes and ectoparasites (ticks, mites, lice) that infest domestic animals [9, 10]. Avermectins that include doramectin, ivermectin, abamectin, and eprinomectin are the fermented products of actinomycete *Streptomyces avermitilis*. On the other hand, milbemectins including moxidectin and selamectin are the fermented products of *Streptomyces cyanogriseus*. On a chemical basis, avermectins differ based on the side chain of the lactone ring while milbemycins differ from each other because of the lactone skeleton [1].

The unequal larvicidal and adulticidal activity of IVM against Gastro-Intestinal Tract (GIT) roundworms and lungworms of ruminantia, porcine, and equine is its main factor of characterization [10, 11]. The control of microfilariae of canine heartworm *Dirofilaria immitis* is also achieved by the same chemical [1]. These chemicals do not have any anticestodal or antitrematodal activity nor are they ovicidal.

Because of the nematicidal, acaricidal, and insecticidal activity of IVM, it is frequently used in sheep in different countries [4].

IVM along with other ML derivatives such as moxidectin is frequently used against haemonchosis in sheep due to its mode of action [1]. This increases their influence by binding to glutamate and GABA-gated chloride channel receptors in nematode and arthropod nerve cells. The whole process results in the opening of the channel and allows the entry of chloride ions (Cl^-). This will lead to the paralysis of the body wall, pharyngeal muscles, and uterine muscles in nematodes [12]. It is stated that the sensitivity of dissimilar chloride channel subunits to MLs and expression location are variable characters, and it can be accounted for the paralytic effect of different concentrations of MLs on the neuromuscular systems. It is also stated that nematode paralysis and body wall muscle paralysis can be proved serious for prompt exclusion, also pharyngeal muscle paralysis is more sensitive [13]. It has also been revealed that MLs cause the flaccid paralysis of the pharynx of nematodes along with moxidectin and IVM as it is more sensitive than somatic musculature, which shows that the target is the nervous system of parasites. If the concentration of MLs drops, then the motility of the parasites can be recuperated. As compared with somatic muscles, the paralysis of the pharyngeal muscles, as well as consequential inhibition of nourishing, can be longer. The reason for the ineffectiveness of ML derivatives against trematode and cestode parasites is that these worms do not have receptors at their glutamate-gated chloride channel.

5. Anthelmintic resistance of GIT nematodes

Resistance development against anthelmintics consists of a certain phase, i.e., during first phase, number of parasites developing resistance against specific anthelmintics is less; there is a gradual increase, and heterozygous parasites develop resistance and lead to the final phase where individuals become resistant against those anthelmintics, and the population becomes homozygous parasites population. It is also observed that parasite resistance against a specific anthelmintic also brings resistance against some other anthelmintics groups [14].

Resistance is a drug tolerance ability of a worm and survives in the recommended doses of anthelmintics that are normally an effective dose [15]. Parasitic resistance was first described in 1957, and firstly studied anthelmintic agents were organophosphates, phenothiazine, rafoxanide, thiabendazole, and macrocyclic lactones [16]. Recently different GIT parasites especially *H. contortus* resistance are studied against different anthelmintics groups, i.e., rafoxanide, macrocyclic lactones, phenothiazine, organophosphates, levamisole, ivermectin, and thiabendazole in small ruminants [17]. It is also noted that resistance development started after a few years of drug development especially in *H. contortus* [18]. But, the resistance of the parasites against a broad spectrum of anthelmintics is increasing gradually within days; multiple factors are involved in developing resistance such as excessive and repeated use of the same anthelmintic, underdosing, poor management, etc. [19, 20]. Resistance of some GI parasites, specifically of *H. Contortus* against diverse groups of drugs, namely rafoxanide, organophosphates, phenothiazine, macrocyclic lactones (ivermectin), thiabendazole, and levamisole in small ruminants, has been reported worldwide [18]. Currently, numerous tests are available for the detection of anthelmintic resistance of GI parasites including *in vitro* egg hatch assay, fecal egg count reduction test, *in vivo* anthelmintic efficiency assay (AEA), and tubulin binding assay (TBA) [21].

Imidazothiazoles (Levamisole HCL)	**Benzimidazoles** (most members)	**Tetrahydropyrimidines** (Morantel and Pyrantel)
Common	Very common	Less common
Salicylanilides (Closantel)	**Avermectines** (Ivermectin and Moxidectin)	**Amino acetonitrile derivatives** (Monepantel)
Common	Common	Less common

Table 1.
The renowned anthelmintic classes (with drug examples) reported resistance [3, 22].

The prominent anthelmintic classes reported for resistance of *H. contortus* in sheep [3, 22] have been presented in the **Table 1**.

6. Geographic regions where resistance has developed

Initially, the development of resistance against nematicidal drugs was reported in the Southern hemisphere, and the most resistant was studied on *H. contortus*

Country	**Anthelmintic drugs**	**Reference(s)**
Argentina	BZs, LEV, IVM	[24]
Australia	Ops, BZs, LEV, TBZ, OXF, Closantel, Morantel	[19, 20]
Belgium	BZs	[25]
Brazil	BZs, LEV, IVM, Closantel	[24]
France	BZs, LEV	[26]
Germany	IVM,BZs, Pyrantel tarterate, FEN, Febantel, OXF, LEV, TBZ, ALB, MBZ	[27]
India	BZs, IVM, FEN, Morantel, Closantel, LEV, Thiophanate,	[28]
Kenya	BZs, LEV, RAF, FEN, IVM	[29]
Malaysia	BM_Z, LEV_S, IVM, Moxidectin, Closantel	[25]
Netherlands	OXF_S, LEV_S, BM_Z, IVM	[30]
New Zealand	BM_Z, LEV_S, IVM	[18, 31]
Pakistan	OXF_S, LEV_S, ALB, IVM	[32, 33]
Paraguay	BM_Z, LEV_S, IVM	[34]
South Africa	BM_Z, IVM, RAF, Closantel	[35]
Uruguay	BM_Z, LEV_S, IVM	[36]
United State of America	FEN, IVM, Pyrantel pamoate, LEV_S, TB_Z,	[37, 38]
Zimbabwe	RAF, BM_Z, LEV_S,	[39]

ALB = Albendazole, BM_Z = Benzimidazoles, FEN=Fenbendazole, IVM = Ivermectin, LEV_s = Levamisole, OXF_S=Oxfendazoles, RAF = Rafoxanide, and TB_Z = Thiabendazole.

Table 2.
Geographical distribution of anthelmintic resistance developed by helminths in different parts of the world (selected references).

nematode. The development of resistance has differed geographically based on various factors such as weather conditions, species of parasite, mode of therapy, use of variable drugs, etc. The resistance rate is slightly lower in temperate zones in the Northern hemisphere [1, 23]. Prominently in the previous three decades, anthelmintic resistance is reaching its peak and becoming a great issue in livestock development, and the resistance is being reported around the globe including South Pacific, Australia, Latin America, North America, Africa, Eastern Union, and Southeast Asia [23]. Several studies reporting the occurrence of antinematodal resistance against various chemotherapeutic agents residing in sheep abomasa from different parts of the world are shown in **Table 2**:

Hence, the growing anthelmintic resistance is threatening livestock production, increasing the toxic level in the environment, and ultimately reducing the food availability for human beings [23, 40]. Therefore, the scientists and parasitologists are performing the duty to raise one's hope by launching alternatives to overcome the developing resistance such as biological control (phytotherapy) [33].

7. Globally applicable gastrointestinal nematodes control measures/strategies

Control of gastrointestinal nematode parasite (GINP).

Numerous techniques and plans have been utilized to lower the gastrointestinal (GI) nematode parasites of small ruminants across the world. Some of the techniques and methods are appropriate, and a few of them have limitations. Moreover, new methods and new approaches are being evaluated and established. The prime methodologies that have been used routinely to reduce the burden of GI nematodes are reviewed here.

7.1 Chemical control methods

7.1.1 Chemotherapy (anthelmintic)

Anthelmintics are those drugs that kill the helminths and are playing a toxic role to the worms and can be achieved by exposing the nematodes to a higher concentration of anthelmintics. This higher concentration is for worms not for the host body cells. This higher concentration inhibits the vital metabolic processes of the worms and kills the worm either by starving it or paralyzing it [23]. Resistance is a reduction in the efficacy of certain anthelmintics against parasites that are susceptible to anthelmintics in normal conditions [41]. Chemotherapeutic application is a very common and primitive method (conventional) to control the GINP around the globe. The agents have been used for both therapy and prophylaxis. Benzimidazole, Ivermectin, and Imidathiazole are three major chemical groups that have been used frequently for decades.

Several reports are published that demonstrate the resistance generation of GI nematodes to these chemicals worldwide [23]. Few studies reported the higher level of resistance produced against the broad-spectrum anthelmintics and also reported the side effects at higher dose levels [41]. A higher level of resistance in *H. contortus* is developed in the endemic areas of haemonchosis. Nevertheless, the side effects and resistance produced by the excessive use urged scientists to adapt alternative GI nematode control methods to reduce the risk of environmental pollution.

The consumer requested "clean and green" by-products that are free from residuals and growth promoters and cost-effective, and scientists were appealed to work for the launching of new and effective drugs and strategies [23]. Various factors such as frequent dosing of the same brand to infected and noninfected without discrimination, wrong choice, inappropriate administration massively involved in the development of resistance and reoccurrence of disease with re-exposure of the parasites [41]. *H. contortus* (roundworm) has been reported as resistant to all broad-spectrum families of anthelmintics [33, 35, 42].

Resistance is a global issue, and some regions are more exposed to it as compared with others, e.g., tropical and subtropical regions are more affected by the resistance of GI nematodes [33]. Soli *et al.*, [40] reported multiple anthelmintic resistance in goats from Punjab Pakistan, and various other researchers also reported anthelmintic resistance in goats [33, 35, 42]. The most extensively used model for the control of nematode parasites is the use of chemical agents, and among these the most commonly used chemicals are benzimidazoles and avermectin. However, resistance development against these anthelmintics results in difficulty in the use of these chemicals as a control measure at the farm level [23]. High-degree resistance is reported in parasites against multiple chemical agents [43]. Along with *H. contortus*, some other nematode parasites develop resistance and are studied well, e.g., *Trichostrongylus* spp. and *Ostertagia* spp. [23]. Due to resistance development, the introduction of new administered drugs shows reduced efficacy [41].

Regions where haemonchosis is endemic and anthelmintic treatment is frequently used at the farm level are exhibiting more resistance in *H. contortus*. So, the use of alternative strategies is the necessity of time to control parasite burden at farm level, and also consumer demand is changed; they need cost-effective and residual-free strategies for control [23]. Some other methods are also used for the control of parasites in the animal industry, which are still underutilized and can be a more successful alternative against resistance development issues.

7.1.2 Copper oxide wire particles

In grazing ruminants, copper is administered along with diet as a feed additive to overcome the deficiency symptoms. The use of copper started in the 1900s, in various forms to minimize the worm load (SCSRPC). The use of copper oxide wire particles (COWPs) was found more successful in reducing nematodes, more precisely *H. contortus* [40, 43]. Following administration of COWP, it enters the abomasum along with the ingesta and sticks to the mucosal folds [44]. In the acidic conditions of the abomasum, stuck elements take several weeks to dissolve, and free copper is released slowly, which augments the soluble copper concentrations. Ultimately, copper reserve of the liver increases. The copper mode of action is yet to be understood, but researchers assumed that it alters the abomasum conditions that hinder nematode attachment and cause their death or expulsion. Following the COWP ingestion, an increase in packed cell volume (PCV) and a decline in EFC have been observed. The efficacy of COWP is higher against adult worms of abomasum but ineffective in the case of intestinal helminths [43]. Therefore, fecal culture is recommended to explore the higher population of *H. contortus,* before COWP administration [45]. The COWP is found to be equally effective against nematodes in both sheep and goats [40].

For administration in cattle, COWP boluses (Copasure©) of 12.5 and 25 g are available and for small ruminants, smaller dosages of 0.5–2 g are used [40, 43]. The recommended COWP dosage for cattle of weight above 227 kilograms was 12.5 g [45]. The sensitivity of sheep is higher against copper, and a little higher dosage may lead to toxicity although COWP is released slowly. Risk factors of copper toxicity that should be considered during administration are animal breed, age, health status, and other minerals deficiency such as molybdenum, poultry litter exposure [46]. Investigation on the use of COWP among exotic artiodactyls has been performed at Disney's Animal Kingdom® Lodge. During the trials, four artiodactyl species included roan antelope, blesbuck, scimitar-horned oryx, and blackbuck. The corollary of their study indicated a marked reduction in EFC (above 90%) on day 7 post-COWP therapy. The animal species variations, liver health status, copper level, interaction level with other minerals, and history of copper supplementation should be considered before the implementation of the COWP GIN control program in exotic animals. Before the use of COWP in an integrated pest management program, the impact of COWP on reproduction, accumulation level, and sensitivity level among species should be investigated [45].

7.2 Nonchemical methods to control GI parasitism

7.2.1 Biological control

In this perspective, the naturally found pest antagonist organisms are used to control the pest population. Grønvold *et al.* [47] ascertain the role of fungi as nematophagous, earthworm, and dung beetle as anthelmintic [48], and these are potentially effective biological agents. Biological control is an effective way of overcoming the GI helminths. Mainly nematophagous fungus, *Duddingtonia flagrans*, is used to control the nematodes infesting GI tract. During the field trial, it shows encouraging results toward sheep and goats' GI nematode parasite control [42]. The fungal spores are fed to animals along with a diet that passes through the GI tract without harming the gut mucosa. Fungus sporulates in animal feces and their hyphae kill the nematode larvae in fecal material; hence, diminished the pasture burden of nematodes larval stage [49–52]. The use of nematophagous fungi is an effective alternative approach, but there is a limitation regarding delivery to animals and antagonist role of other drugs, namely benzimidazole as an antifungal agent. *Duddingtonia flagrans* also show their effectiveness toward the larvae that escape out after the COWP treatment, which proposes another application of biological control for helminths [43].

The biological control strategies were proposed to reduce the parasite population below the economic threshold and clinical level above that considerable production losses are there. High efficacy of *D. flagrans* was noticed against larval stages of various nematodes of cattle [47], sheep [53], and horses [52]. It has been proven by field trials that among grazing animals, daily fungal spores feeding for 3–4 months hinder the build-up of various larvae up to dangerous levels on pasture.

Sheep feeding supplemented with *D. flagrans* chlamydospores lowers the egg counts and improves animal weight gain in comparison with untreated animals [54]. For the application of nematode-trapping fungi against GINs of ruminants, a strategy was formulated [55]. *D. flagrans* can produce a large quantity of thick-walled chlamydospores, which makes them more effective against nematodes in comparison with other nematode-trapping fungi [56]. *D. flagrans* is used as a biological agent against nematode such as *H. contortus* in grazing animals [42].

7.3 Control through monitoring

7.3.1 Parasite monitoring strategies

Strategies for worm load investigation: FEC, larval developmental assays (LDA), FEC reduction test, and fecal larval culture (FLC) have proved valuable linkage with monitoring and control of worm infection. Mainly FEC is used for monitoring and management of GIN parasites. LDA is used for nematode species identification and to explore the resistance level [57]. FLC helps in identifying worm species, seasonal variation, and enclosure of GIN population. FECRT is the most authentic approach to determine anthelmintic resistance, but it is expensive and labor-intensive [57]. The demands for the exploration of alternative strategies toward helminth control have been augmented due to the lack of new anthelmintics. The applications of plants having condensed tannins, COWP, nematophagous fungi, and other biological approaches in combination with anthelmintics, animal management, control of ecological factors, and GIN level monitoring strategies could be effective to overcome GIN resistance in small ruminants.

7.3.2 FAMACHA chart and mac master technique

Among TST methods FAMACHA chart and McMaster are mainly used way to identify the worm-infected animals and require treatment. The former method is used to diagnose anemic animals by comparing their eye (conjunctiva) color with the chart. The latter method provides a real-time picture of parasite burden via egg counting in fecal material. In the McMaster method, fecal material is suspended in floatation solution and supernatants are taken on a specific glass slide (Mc Master chamber) and observed under a microscope for egg counting. For reducing anthelmintic resistance among GI parasites, selective therapy is highly effective. By using the aforementioned methods, medicinal cost of animals declines because they selectively purchase few anthelmintics and animals are responsive against these drugs. On the other hand, selective therapy is laborious and time-taking, farmers have to perform the FAMACHA check once a month. Routine-wise performance of McMaster is mandatory because sometimes with FAMACHA check animals found healthy while through McMaster they were found with high worm burden, and such animals should be treated because these animals may act as a source for others. The FAMACHA score system is found to be highly effective in the selection of worm-resilient animal breeds [58].

7.4 Control through management

7.4.1 Pasture management, grazing management, rotational grazing

For the control of GI nematodes infections, two most commonly used methods include the use of anthelmintics and pasture management; they are associated with reduction of production losses because of nematodes infections. Two ways of producing safe pastures and reducing the infectivity of pasture include rotational grazing and pasture spelling, this strategy is very [59]. In rotational grazing, it is assumed that significant larval mortality occurs because of break-in grazing. But, unfortunately, the period in between animal rotations makes the best use of available and nutritious forage coincides with the period during that high concentration of L3 becoming available for reinfection. In the United States, a study was conducted at a farm and reported that lambs raised under a rotational grazing system were highly infested with helminths in comparison with others. Most of them were infected with nematodes, *H. contortus*, and gained less weight in comparison with control (non-grazing). It is therefore concluded that rotational grazing is not a good option in sheep. In some situations, it is recommended to extend the periods between the rotations of (60–90 days) as it may significantly lessen the parasitic infection. Rotation of younger susceptible animals with highly resistant older animals may prove to be beneficial. But such a strategy may not be possible due to practical restraints [35].

7.4.2 Manipulating supplementation of nutrients

With the provision of a good and high level of nutrition, the productivity of animals can be improved with an increase in the immune response against parasites. With an increase in the level of proteins in the diet, an increase in the resistance and resilience of lamb against *H. contortus* has been observed [60]. The supplementation of a meal with sorghum and soybean for the grazing kids has shown increased resilience against helminth parasites [61]. Indeed, improvement in nutrition is an efficient strategy to lessen and compensate for the negative impacts of parasitic infection. Whereas approach to urea molasses increases both resistance and resilience in grazing East African goat kids in an environment overshadowed by *H. contortus* [62]. In a review by Hoste et al., [63], it has been discussed that the supplementary feeding to the goats has shown an increased response concerning resilience, whereas the effects on host resistance were less prominent.

7.5 Control through medicinal plants

In ethnoveterinary medicine, medicinal plants are used for the prevention and treatment of gastrointestinal parasitism. There is a wide range of medicinal plants or plant extracts that are used to treat almost every kind of livestock disease related to parasites. There are so many studies and available literature on the anthelmintic properties of plants and their extracts, which confirms the antinematodal effects of these plants [33, 42, 64–67]. In comparison to synthetic drugs the herbal preparations are way cheaper and easily available and thus have been used for a long time in the therapy of livestock diseases of helminth parasites [68].

Many plants and herbs are used as control agents for human and veterinary endoparasites, and the efficacy of each plant depends upon the chemical composition and secondary metabolites composition. The composition of a plant is a variable character depending upon soil properties, climatic conditions, geographical variability, and environmental conditions. Anthelmintic activity of a plant is variable in different areas of the world and depends upon the harvest of the plant, plant parts, which are used as anthelmintics, storage of the plant, and combination of different plant extracts [68]. Choice of extraction solvent is also an important factor that affects the solubility of secondary metabolites of the target plants usually water and methanol are used as extraction solvents. Ethanolic extracts are considered a better choice as they can easily enter the body of the parasite through absorption [69].

To determine the plant properties, two different study types are used. i.e., in vitro and in vivo, and each study type has some merits and demerits. In vitro studies are cost-effective and can study a variety of plants at the same time, allowing the study of specific parasites and their lifecycle stages [70]. While in vivo studies are lengthy processes and can study a single plant at a time. Sometimes the result of the in vivo and in vitro can be different as the outcome of the study depends on the internal factor of the host and plant species, e.g., the digestive system of the host [71].

Till today 25% of modern pharmacopeia use plant-derived drugs and some semi-synthetic using plant as prototype compound [72]. Anthelmintic efficacy of plants is derived from different parts, e.g., saponins (can cause teguments degradation and vacuolization), tannins, and polyphenols can form a protein complex in the rumen and increase the protein supply, interfere with energy generation, reduction in gastrointestinal metabolism, and ultimately death of the helminth and alkaloids (effect the transport of sucrose transfer from the stomach to the intestine and helminth glucose support is disturbed causing paralysis) [73].

7.5.1 Condensed tannins

Tannins are compounds that attach with proteins and other molecules and are used as a biological alternative against chemical anthelmintic; many plants naturally contain condensed tannins. There are two main groups in which tannins are divided: one is hydrolyzable tannins (HTs) and the other one is condensed tannins (CTs). Among the two of these groups, condensed tannins are more abundant and are naturally present in browse, legumes, plants, and forage. The concentration of CT, type of animal consuming CT, the plant itself, and the concentration of CT in the plant are the factors that stimulate the effects of CTs. The high concentration of CT can have negative effects, and the noticeable negative effect is reduced palatability that ultimately causes a reduction in intake and digestion, which exerts a negative impact on productivity [46]. There are several benefits of CT intake that include increased wool growth and growth rate, increased amount of bypass protein, reduced bloating, high milk production, as well as a high rate of ovulation.

The prominent and most important benefit of CTs is their positive impact on the GIN infection. It has been observed that CTs specifically *H. contortus* reduce the GIN infection, it also reduces the overall egg output through the reduction in female fecundity. In addition to this, there is also a decrease in the GIN egg hatchability and the development of larva in the feces. Concerning reduction in GIN infection, the most important and researched CTs include big trefoil, sericea lespedeza, sulla, and sanfoin [46]. When the animals are allowed to graze SL management benefits have been observed that are less exposure to GIN as the plant grows off the ground, and since there is also an increase in the level of proteins that causes a potential increase in the resilience and resistance.

7.5.2 Plants as nutraceuticals

The nutritional combination of animal feed affects the biodiversity of GIT fauna, which may affect the parasite fitness by altering the intestinal environment in which the parasites propagate [63]. Tannins, flavonol glycosides, sesquiterpene, and secondary metabolites are potential candidates for integrated nematode control at the farms level [63, 74, 75]. The plants having these properties are known as nutraceuticals, which are considered for both the nutritional value and as an anthelmintic. It has been reported that supplementation of bioactive plants to goats played role in the regulation of bionomics of resistant parasitic populations along with enhancing the ability of the goat to withstand negative effects of the pathophysiology of parasitic infections [63]. An increase in post-ruminal protein availability playing role in reducing the parasitic infections in large ruminants has also been reported, which may be attributed to the availability of condensed tannins (CTs) or proanthocyanidins and polymers of flavonoid units [48].

7.6 Control through immunological interventions

7.6.1 Vaccines (immunization and vaccination)

The most effective way of controlling infection is vaccination; therefore, demand for vaccine development against GI parasites rises. In disparity with vaccines of viral and bacterial pathogens, vaccine development against parasites did not gain similar success although parasitologists are working in this regard for the last 30 years. The vaccine has been developed against tapeworm and lungworm sheep and cattle respectively. Studies have been conducted in the identification of various antigens of nematodes as vaccine agents [76]. Gut-associated antigens have been reported as vaccine candidates, namely H-gal-GP and H11 of *H. contortus* [77]. Fecal egg count has been markedly declined in goat kids with the use of vaccine candidates. Secretory and excretory products of parasites have been found as effective vaccine candidates. It has been reported that the use of secretory and excretory antigens as vaccine candidates in infection of *H. contortus* results in enhancing the immunity of the host, thereby reducing the FEC and worm burden by 70% [78]. It has been reported that the use of H-11 and H-gal reduces 60–75% of worm burden and 80–90% FEC, and they can be good candidates for vaccine development [79]. Both of these candidates have been reported to induce protective immunity in terms of IgG production, PCV maintenance, FEC, and worm burden reduction in lambs and kids [77].

Traditional use of chemotherapeutic agents against infection of ectoparasites as well as endoparasites leads to the development of resistance against these therapeutic agents. It converges the scientists for exploring the nontraditional ways of controlling GI parasites; development of a resistant breed of the host through selective breeding, vaccine development, implementation of other control measures (alternate pasture grazing and rotational grazing), and synergistic use of anthelmintics [80].

In vaccines, acquired immunity plays a pivotal role in the protection of the host against pathogens, and it needs to be explored for the development of a vaccine. In the case of parasites, the role of acquired immune response is not fully explored. Therefore, vaccine development against GI parasites for protection remains ineffective [81].

Some fungi of *Arthrobottrys* spp. have been reported to attack and kill the larvae of nematodes in fecal pats, but these fungi are being killed by passage through the gut and therefore are of no great importance, but nowadays, a new fungus *D. flagrans* has been reported, which will grow and pass through the gut harmlessly and is active against larvae of nematodes in fecal pats [13].

8. Alternatives

Gastrointestinal nematode resistance to anthelmintics has been growing day by day, gaining currency to consider it for adopting control measures shortly of the domestic livestock industry. The use of chemical anthelmintics in combination with bioactive plants as nutraceuticals seems to be a potential strategy for parasitic control. Alternate strategies, i.e., use of plants containing condensed tannins, plant-based vaccines, COWP, and biological control through nematode-trapping fungi along with husbandry management may prove helpful in minimizing the mortality and morbidity of parasitic diseases in small ruminants. However, animal breeds selected based on their response to nematodes present in the gastrointestinal tract are an alternate control strategy toward minimizing gastrointestinal problems in goats [43].

8.1 Breeding for resistance

Identification of resistant individuals is necessary for the production of parasitic-resistant breeds. Two parameters are mostly reported for the selection of resistant breeds, i.e., FEC, which is an indirect parameter for measurement of the relative level of infection [82]. Hematocrit and PCV are being used for the identification of worm burden, especially in the case of *H. contortus*. In Australia, FEC both in natural and artificial infections has been used for many years to select the animals for parasitic resistance [83].

The researchers cannot divide the magnitude of resistance into discrete genetic units; therefore, the resistance is described in the form of heritability estimates [84]. The phenotype of quantitative traits is regulated by the additive effect of specialized genes [85], which are yet to be identified. The resulting resistance may be attributed to the effect of a combination of many small genes or a group of major genes that are being regulated not only by additive effects but also by the environmental effects [84].

8.2 Genetic and phenotypic parameters for worm resistance

Packed cell volume and fecal egg count are the most useful markers/parameters to estimate the response of host challenge and natural infection with nematodes present in GI in general and specifically *H. contortus*. Both PCV and FEC are heritable traits. Heritability of FEC ranges from 0.04 to 0.37. Morris *et al.* [86] described a heritability estimate of 0.05 in Saanen goats at the age of 12 months in New Zealand, and Woolaston *et al.* [87] described a heritability estimate of 0.04 and 0.08 in Fijian goats at 12 months of age in Fiji. [88]. Similar studies have been conducted in Kenya where they found FEC heritability estimates of 0.15, 0.16, and 0.12 in small East African goats at the age of 4, 5, 8, and 10 months, respectively. Some more studies have been conducted by Vagenas *et al.*, [89] in Scotland, and they found 0.37 and 0.32 estimates of heritability for FEC in Scottish Cashmere goat's breed.

8.3 Genetic and phenotypic correlation between resistant traits

Estimations of phenotypic and genetic correlation explained the amount to which genes affect two different traits and the phenotypic correlation guides the number of relations between two traits. Correlation evaluations are important in the measurement of the appropriateness of indicator traits as indirect criteria in programs related to breeding. Mandonnet *et al.*, [88] under tropical conditions, stated positive

(0.37–0.58) and negative (0.56–0.79) genetic correlations between FEC and PCV and eosinophil and FEC amount in goats. Costa *et al.*, [66] in Brazil also describe a highly negative and significant relationship between changed PCV and FEC or hemoglobin −0.53 and − 0.45 in *H. contortus* infected goats. Very strong negative correlations between IgA activity and FEC have been found in *Teladorsagia circumcincta* infected Scottish Blackface lambs (−0.97, s.e. 0.11 and − 0.78, s.e. 0.18, respectively) and also in resistance-related traits and burdens of worms [90].

8.4 Genetic and phenotypic parameters for production traits

Host live weight is a production trait that has been considered as an important parameter while assessing the genetic resistances of the host toward GI nematode parasites. The heritability estimates of live weight (LWT) varied widely ranging from 0.13 in Australian Angora goats to 0.50 in Texan Angora goats [91]. Likewise, heritability estimates have been reported in South Africa goats breed as 0.29 and 0.35 [92]. It has been shown that resistance to infection by nematode parasites may not necessarily equate to resistance to the effects of the parasite challenge in grazing animals [86]. The association between FEC and productivity varies in magnitude and direction depending on the breed and the environment in which the evaluation was done. The genetic correlations between packed cell volume (PCV) and packed cell volume decline (PCVD) and production (live weight and wool growth) are either negligible or favorable [93].

Several studies around the globe have been conducted to assess the genetic potential of sheep and goats breeds that are resistant to gastrointestinal nematodes in the last three to four decades [82, 83, 87, 93]. The selection of breeds that are resistant to gastrointestinal nematode parasites is assuming the most promising alternate control method of gastrointestinal nematodes. Improved resistance toward nematodes control leads to reduced cost of anthelmintic treatment and diminished production losses associated with worm burden. Australia and New Zealand initiate programs on breeding for resistance and adopt them successfully by utilizing phenotypic markers [94]. Approximately 96% of the world's goat population is kept by smallholders in developing countries, and genetic improvement programs are rare [95].

8.5 Phenotypic traits as indicators of GI resistance

Host selection for resistance has based mostly on quantitative measurement of phenotypic traits. These traits have been measured to check the response of the host being evaluated for resistance, which are biochemical, immunological, parasitological, and pathological features [84]. For the development of high-resistant breeds, it is necessary to identify the high-resistant individuals. Criteria for the selection of parasitic resistance are commonly based on two traits, i.e., packed cell volume, which indicates anemia, and fecal egg count, which measures the amount of infection. There is variation in the development of resistance between the animals of different breeds and within the same breeds, which is because of their genetic makeup. The scientists are working to investigate the cause of the development of resistance, and up to some extent they succeeded in finding some reasons while the others are under investigation [84].

9. Conclusion

According to the best of our knowledge about different factors that are responsible for GI parasitism, it is hard to develop control measures. So, the epidemiology of each parasitic disease is needed to be studied at the regional level to recommend an effective strategy for the control of parasitic diseases, which is not completely dependent on anthelmintic therapy [11]. Keeping in mind the subtropical and tropical areas in which dry seasons are more might be grazing management, rational use of anthelmintics, and use of resistant breeds.

Acknowledgements

The author wishes to thank all other coauthors for providing guidance and support.

Conflict of interest

The authors declare that they have no conflict of interest.

Author details

Muhammad Abdullah Malik[1*], Muhammad Sohail Sajid[1], Rao Zahid Abbas[1], Muhammad Tahir Aleem[2], Faisal Rasheed Anjum[3,4], Asad Khan[2], Muhammad Farhab[5], Mahvish Maqbool[1], Muhammad Zeeshan[1], Kashif Hussain[1], Namrah Rehman[3], Rana Hamid Ali Nisar[1], Hafiz Muhammad Rizwan[6] and Urfa Bin Tahir[1]

1 Faculty of Veterinary Science, Department of Parasitology, University of Agriculture, Faisalabad, Pakistan

2 MOE Joint International Research Laboratory of Animal Health and Food Safety, College of Veterinary Medicine, Nanjing Agricultural University, Nanjing, P.R. China

3 Faculty of Veterinary Science, Department of Epidemiology and Public Health, University of Agriculture, Faisalabad, Pakistan

4 Faculty of Veterinary Science, Institute of Microbiology, University of Agriculture, Faisalabad, Pakistan

5 College of Veterinary Medicine, Yangzhou University, China

6 Department of Pathobiology, Section of Parasitology, KBCMA College of Veterinary and Animal Sciences, Narowal, Sub-campus UVAS, Lahore

*Address all correspondence to: abdullahmalik42@gmail.com

References

[1] Taylor MA, Coop RL, Wall RL, editors. Veterinary Parasitology. 4th ed. London: Blackwell Publishing; 2007. pp. 356-447

[2] Einstein R, Jones RS, Knifton A, Starmer GA. Hypnotics and sedatives. In: Principles of veterinary therapeutics. England: Longman Scientific & Technical; 1994:121124

[3] Beech RN, Silvestre A. Mutations associated with anthelmintic drug resistance. Anti-Infective Agents Med Chem (Formerly Curr Med Chem Agents). 2010;**9**(3):105-112

[4] Soulsby EJL. Helminths. Arthropods and Protozoa of Domesticated Animals. 7th Ed., London, UK: Bailliere Tindall; 1982:1-430

[5] Friedman PA. The Molecular Mechanism of Action of Benzimidazole Drugs in Embryos of Ascaris Suum. Riverside: University of California; 1979

[6] Lacey E. The role of the cytoskeletal protein, tubulin, in the mode of action and mechanism of drug resistance to benzimidazoles. International Journal for Parasitology. 1988;**18**(7):885-936

[7] von Samson-Himmelstjerna G. Molecular diagnosis of anthelmintic resistance. Veterinary Parasitology. 2006;**136**(2):99-107

[8] Davidse LC. Benzimidazole fungicides: Mechanism of action and biological impact. Annual Review of Phytopathology. 1986;**24**(1):43-65

[9] Campbell WC, Fisher MH, Stapley EO, Albers-Schonberg G, Jacob TA. Ivermectin: A potent new antiparasitic agent. Science. 1983;**221**(4613):823-828

[10] Qa M, Benchaoui HA. Avermectins and milbemycins. Journal of Veterinary Pharmacology and Therapeutics. 1996;**19**:331-351

[11] Arundel JH, Gay CC, Radostits OM. Veterinary Medicine: A Textbook of the Diseases of Cattle, Sheep, Pigs, Goats, and Horses. London; Toronto: Baillière Tindall; 1989

[12] Feng X, Hayashi J, Beech RN, Prichard RK. Study of the nematode putative GABA type-a receptor subunits: Evidence for modulation by ivermectin. Journal of Neurochemistry. 2002;**83**(4):870-878

[13] TmG G, SIMs SM, Thomas EM, Vanover L, Davis JP, Winterrowd CA, et al. Haemonchus contortus: Ivermectin-induced paralysis of the pharynx. Experimental Parasitology. 1993;**77**(1):88-96

[14] Calvete C, Calavia R, Ferrer LM, Ramos JJ, Lacasta D, Uriarte J. Management and environmental factors related to benzimidazole resistance in sheep nematodes in Northeast Spain. Veterinary Parasitology. 2012;**184**(2-4):193-203

[15] Good B, Hanrahan JP, de Waal DT, Patten T, Kinsella A, Lynch CO. Anthelmintic-resistant nematodes in Irish commercial sheep flocks-the state of play. Irish Veterinary Journal. 2012;**65**(1):1-5

[16] George N, Persad K, Sagam R, Offiah VN, Adesiyun AA, Harewood W, et al. Efficacy of commonly used anthelmintics: First report of multiple drug resistance in gastrointestinal nematodes of sheep in Trinidad. Veterinary Parasitology. 2011;**183**(1-2):194-197

[17] Chagas ACS, Katiki LM, Silva IC, Gigliotti R, Esteves SN, Oliveira MCS, et al. Haemonchus contortus: A multiple-resistant Brazilian isolate and the costs for its characterization and maintenance for research use. Parasitology International. 2013;**62**(1):1-6

[18] McKenna PB, Badger SB, McKinley RL, Taylor DE. Simultaneous resistance to two or more broad-spectrum anthelmintics by gastrointestinal nematode parasites of sheep and goats. New Zealand Veterinary Journal. 1990;**38**(3):114-117

[19] Webb RF, Ottaway SJ. The prevalence of anthelmintic resistance in sheep nematodes on the central tablelands of New South Wales. Australian Veterinary Journal. 1986;**63**(1):13-16

[20] Love SC, Johns WH, Coverdale OR. Anthelmintic resistance in sheep nematodes in the New England region of New South Wales. Australian Veterinary Journal. 1992;**69**(8):196-197

[21] Coles GC, Bauer C, Borgsteede FHM, Geerts S, Klei TR, Taylor MA, et al. World Association for the Advancement of veterinary parasitology (WAAVP) methods for the detection of anthelmintic resistance in nematodes of veterinary importance. Veterinary Parasitology. 1992;**44**(1-2):35-44

[22] Sangster NC, Riley FL, Wiley LJ. Binding of [3H] m-aminolevamisole to receptors in levamisole-susceptible and-resistant Haemonchus contortus. International Journal for Parasitology. 1998;**28**(5):707-717

[23] Waller DA. The role of surgery in diagnosis and treatment of malignant pleural mesothelioma. Current Opinion in Oncology. 2003;**15**(2):139-143

[24] Waller PJ, Echevarria F, Eddi C, Maciel S, Nari A, Hansen JW. The prevalence of anthelmintic resistance in nematode parasites of sheep in Southern Latin America: General overview. Veterinary Parasitology. 1996;**62**(3-4):181-187

[25] Sivaraj S, Dorny P, Vercruysse J, Pandey VS. Multiple and multigeneric anthelmintic resistance on a sheep farm in Malaysia. Veterinary Parasitology. 1994;**55**(1-2):159-165

[26] Kerboeuf D, Beaumont-Schwartz C, Hubert J, Maillon M. Resistance des strongles gastrointestinaux aux anthelminthiques chez les petits ruminants. Resultats d'une enquete dans le Val de Loire. Recueil de Medecine Veterinaire. 1988;**164**(12):1001-1006

[27] Düwel D, Schmid K, Bechmann G. Benzimidazole-resistant Haemonchus contortus in sheep in West Germany. Berliner und Münchener Tierärztliche Wochenschrift. 1987;**100**(4):120-123

[28] Uppal RP, Yadav CL, Godara P, Rana ZS. Multiple anthelmintic resistance in a field strain of Haemonchus contortus in goats. Veterinary Research Communications. 1992;**16**(3):195-198

[29] Waruiru RM, Kogi JK, Weda EH, Ngotho JW. Multiple anthelmintic resistance on a goat farm in Kenya. Veterinary Parasitology. 1998;**75**(2-3):191-197

[30] Borgsteede FHM, Pekelder JJ, Dercksen DP, Sol J, Vellema P, Gaasenbeek CPH, et al. A survey of anthelmintic resistance in nematodes of sheep in the Netherlands. The Veterinary Quarterly. 1997;**19**(4):167-171

[31] Kettle PR, Vlassoff A, Ayling JM, McMurtry LW, Smith SJ, Watson AJ. A survey of nematode control measures used by sheep farmers and of anthelmintic resistance on their farms

Part 2: South Island excluding the Nelson region. New Zealand Veterinary Journal. 1982;**30**(6):79-81

[32] Afaq M. Parasite control practices and anthelmintic resistance against gastrointestinal nematodes of sheep. Ph.D. thesis, Department of Veterinary Parasitology, University of Agriculture; 2003

[33] Jabbar A, Zaman MA, Iqbal Z, Yaseen M, Shamim A. Anthelmintic activity of Chenopodium album (L.) and Caesalpinia crista (L.) against trichostrongylid nematodes of sheep. Journal of Ethnopharmacology. 2007;**114**(1):86-91

[34] Maciel S, Giménez AM, Gaona C, Waller PJ, Hansen JW. The prevalence of anthelmintic resistance in nematode parasites of sheep in Southern Latin America: Paraguay. Veterinary Parasitology. 1996;**62**(3-4):207-212

[35] Van Wyk JA, Malan FS, Randles JL. How long before resistance makes it impossible to control some field strains of Haemonchus contortus in South Africa with any of the modern anthelmintics? Veterinary Parasitology. 1997;**70**(1-3):111-122

[36] Nari A, Salles J, Gil A, Waller PJ, Hansen JW. The prevalence of anthelmintic resistance in nematode parasites of sheep in Southern Latin America: Uruguay. Veterinary Parasitology. 1996;**62**(3-4):213-222

[37] Miller JE, Baker NF. Thiabendazole-resistant strains of Haemonchus and Ostertagia in California lambs. American Journal of Veterinary Research. 1980;**41**(10):1674-1676

[38] Uhlinger C, Fleming S, Moncol D. Survey for drug-resistant gastrointestinal nematodes in 13 commercial sheep flocks. Journal of the American Veterinary Medical Association. 1992;**201**(1):77-80

[39] Boersema JH, Pandey VS. Anthelmintic resistance of trichostrongylids in sheep in the highveld of Zimbabwe. Veterinary Parasitology. 1997;**68**(4):383-388

[40] Soli F, Terrill TH, Shaik SA, Getz WR, Miller JE, Vanguru M, et al. Efficacy of copper oxide wire particles against gastrointestinal nematodes in sheep and goats. Veterinary Parasitology. 2010;**168**(1-2):93-96

[41] Wooster MJ, Woodgate RG, Chick BF. Reduced efficacy of ivermectin, abamectin, and moxidectin against field isolates of Haemonchus contortus. Australian Veterinary Journal. 2001;**79**(12):840-842

[42] Chandrawathani P, Brelin D, Nor Fasihah S, Adnan M, Jamnah O, Sani RA, et al. Evaluation of the neem tree (Azadirachta indica) as a herbal anthelmintic for nematode parasite control in small ruminants in Malaysia. Tropical Biomedicine. 2002;**19**(1&2):41-48

[43] Burke JM, Miller JE, Larsen M, Terrill TH. Interaction between copper oxide wire particles and Duddingtonia flagrans in lambs. Veterinary Parasitology. 2005;**134**(1-2):141-146

[44] Vatta AF, Waller PJ, Githiori JB, Medley GF. The potential to control Haemonchus contortus in indigenous South African goats with copper oxide wire particles. Veterinary Parasitology. 2009;**162**(3-4):306-313

[45] Fontenot ME, Miller JE, Peña MT, Larsen M, Gillespie A. Efficiency of feeding Duddingtonia flagrans chlamydospores to grazing ewes on

reducing availability of parasitic nematode larvae on pasture. Veterinary Parasitology. 2003;**118**(3-4):203-213

[46] Coffey L, Hale M, Terrill T, Mosjidis J, Miller J, Burke J. Tools for managing internal parasites in small ruminants: Sericea Lespedeza. ATTRA. 2007

[47] Grønvold J, Henriksen SA, Larsen M, Nansen P, Wolstrup J. Biological control aspects of biological control—With special reference to arthropods, protozoans, and helminths of domesticated animals. Veterinary Parasitology. 1996;**64**(1-2):47-64

[48] Waghorn TS, Leathwick DM, Chen L-Y, Skipp RA. Efficacy of the nematode-trapping fungus Duddingtonia flagrans against three species of gastro-intestinal nematodes in laboratory faecal cultures from sheep and goats. Veterinary Parasitology. 2003;**118**(3-4):227-234

[49] Wolstrup J, Grønvold J, Henriksen SA, Nansen P, Larsen M, Bøgh HO, et al. An attempt to implement the nematode-trapping fungus Duddingtonia flagrans in biological control of trichostrongyle infections of first-year grazing calves. Journal of Helminthology. 1994;**68**(2):175-180

[50] Nansen P, Larsen M, Grønvold J, Wolstrup J, Zorn A, Henriksen SA. Prevention of clinical trichostrongylidosis in calves by strategic feeding with the predacious fungus Duddingtonia flagrans. Parasitology Research. 1995;**81**(5):371-374

[51] Larsen M. Prospects for controlling animal parasitic nematodes by predacious micro fungi. Parasitology. 2000;**120**(7):121-131

[52] Fernandez AS, Henningsen E, Larsen M, Nansen R, Grønvold J, Søndergaard J. A new isolate of the nematophagous fungus Duddingtonia flagrans as a biological control agent against free-living larvae of horse strongyles. Equine Veterinary Journal. 1999;**31**(6):488-491

[53] Peloille M. Selection of nematode-trapping fungi for use in biological control. Bulletin OILB SROP. 1991;**14**(2):13-17

[54] Knox MR, Faedo M. Biological control of field infections of nematode parasites of young sheep with Duddingtonia flagrans and effects of spore intake on efficacy. Veterinary Parasitology. 2001;**101**(2):155-160

[55] Sanyal PK. Mycological control of nematode parasites of livestock: From academic interest to reality. Proceedings of the National Academy of Sciences, India Section B. 2005;**75**:263-271

[56] de Oliveira VV, Furlong J, de Freitas GM, Dolinski C, Aguillera MM, Rodrigues RCD, et al. Steinernema glaseri Santa Rosa strain (Rhabditida: Steinernematidae) and Heterorhabditis bacteriophora CCA strain (Rhabditida: Heterorhabditidae) as biological control agents of Boophilus microplus (Acari: Ixodidae). Parasitology Research. 2004;**94**(3):201-206

[57] Kaplan RM. Drug resistance in nematodes of veterinary importance: A status report. Trends in Parasitology. 2004;**20**(10):477-481

[58] Burke JM, Miller JE. Use of FAMACHA system to evaluate gastrointestinal nematode resistance/resilience in offspring of stud rams. Veterinary Parasitology. 2008;**153**(1-2):85-92

[59] Morley FHW, Donald AD. Farm management, and systems of helminth

control. Veterinary Parasitology. 1980;**6**(1-3):105-134

[60] Bricarello PA, Amarante AFT, Rocha RA, Cabral Filho SL, Huntley JF, Houdijk JGM, et al. Influence of dietary protein supply on resistance to experimental infections with Haemonchus contortus in Ile de France and Santa Ines lambs. Veterinary Parasitology. 2005;**134**(1-2):99-109

[61] Torres-Acosta JFJ, Aguilar-Caballero AJ. Epidemiología, prevención y control de nematodos gastrointestinales en rumiantes. Enfermedades importancia económica en Prod Anim McGraw-Hill-UADY. México: DF México; 2005. pp. 145-173

[62] Waruiru RM, Kyvsgaard NC, Thamsborg SM, Nansen P, Bøgh HO, Munyua WK, et al. The prevalence and intensity of helminth and coccidial infections in dairy cattle in Central Kenya. Veterinary Research Communications. 2000;**24**(1):39-53

[63] Hoste H, Gaillard L, Le Frileux Y. Consequences of the regular distribution of sainfoin hay on gastrointestinal parasitism with nematodes and milk production in dairy goats. Small Ruminant Research. 2005;**59**(2-3): 265-271

[64] Iqbal Z, Lateef M, Jabbar A, Ghayur MN, Gilani AH. In vitro and in vivo anthelmintic activity of Nicotiana tabacum L. leaves against gastrointestinal nematodes of sheep. Phytotherapy Research: An International Journal Devoted to Pharmacological and Toxicological Evaluation of Natural Product Derivatives. 2006;**20**(1):46-48

[65] Alawa CBI, Adamu AM, Gefu JO, Ajanusi OJ, Abdu PA, Chiezey NP, et al. In vitro screening of two Nigerian medicinal plants (Vernonia amygdalina and Annona senegalensis) for anthelmintic activity. Veterinary Parasitology. 2003;**113**(1):73-81

[66] Costa ES, Hiruma-Lima CA, Lima EO, Sucupira GC, Bertolin AO, Lolis SF, et al. Antimicrobial activity of some medicinal plants of the Cerrado, Brazil. Phytotherapy Research: An International Journal Devoted to Pharmacological and Toxicological Evaluation of Natural Product Derivatives. 2008;**22**(5):705-707

[67] Githiori JB, Höglund J, Waller PJ, Baker RL. Evaluation of anthelmintic properties of some plants used as livestock dewormers against Haemonchus contortus infections in sheep. Parasitology. 2004;**129**(2):245-253

[68] Athanasiadou S, Githiori J, Kyriazakis I. Medicinal plants for helminth parasite control: Facts and fiction. Animal. 2007;**1**(9):1392-1400

[69] Tariq KA, Chishti MZ, Ahmad F, Shawl AS. Anthelmintic activity of extracts of Artemisia absinthium against ovine nematodes. Veterinary Parasitology. 2009;**160**(1-2):83-88

[70] Githiori JB, Athanasiadou S, Thamsborg SM. Use of plants in novel approaches for control of gastrointestinal helminths in livestock with emphasis on small ruminants. Veterinary Parasitology. 2006;**139**(4):308-320

[71] Fomum WS, Nsahlai VI. In vitro evaluation of anthelmintic efficacy of some plant species possessing proteinases and/or other Nitroge-nous compounds in small ruminants. Journal of Alternative and Complementary Medicine. 2017;**3**:38

[72] Surya S, Salam AD, Tomy DV, Carla B, Kumar RA, Sunil C. Diabetes mellitus and medicinal plants-a review.

Asian Pacific Journal of Tropical Disease. 2014;**4**(5):337-347

[73] Tiwari P, Kumar B, Kaur M, Kaur G, Kaur H. Phytochemical screening and extraction: A review. Internationale pharmaceutica sciencia. 2011;**1**(1):98-106

[74] Terrill TH, Dykes GS, Shaik SA, Miller JE, Kouakou B, Kannan G, et al. Efficacy of sericea lespedeza hay as a natural dewormer in goats: Dose titration study. Veterinary Parasitology. 2009;**163**(1-2):52-56

[75] Terrill TH, Mosjidis JA, Moore DA, Shaik SA, Miller JE, Burke JM, et al. Effect of pelleting on efficacy of sericea lespedeza hay as a natural dewormer in goats. Veterinary Parasitology. 2007;**146**(1-2):117-122

[76] Secoy DM, Smith AE. Use of plants in the control of agricultural and domestic pests. Economic Botany. 1983;**37**(1): 28-57

[77] Kabagambe EK, Wells SJ, Garber LP, Salman MD, Wagner B, Fedorka-Cray PJ. Risk factors for fecal shedding of Salmonella in 91 US dairy herds in 1996. Preventive Veterinary Medicine. 2000;**43**(3):177-194

[78] Schallig H, Van Leeuwen MAW. Protective immunity to the blood-feeding nematode Haemonchus contortus induced by vaccination with parasite low molecular weight antigens. Parasitology. 1997;**114**(3):293-299

[79] Newton SE, Meeusen ENT. Progress and new technologies for developing vaccines against gastrointestinal nematode parasites of sheep. Parasite Immunology. 2003;**25**(5):283-296

[80] Fraser D, Bernon DE, Ball RO. Enhanced attraction to blood by pigs with inadequate dietary protein supplementation. Canadian Journal of Animal Science. 1991;**71**(3):611-619

[81] O'Brien DJ. Anthelmintics and other measures to control helminth parasites of livestock. Veterinary Surgery. 1993;**15**:25

[82] Gray GD. The use of genetically resistant sheep to control nematode parasitism. Veterinary Parasitology. 1997;**72**(3-4):345-366

[83] Kemper KE, Elwin RL, Bishop SC, Goddard ME, Woolaston RR. Haemonchus contortus and Trichostrongylus colubriformis did not adapt to long-term exposure to sheep that were genetically resistant or susceptible to nematode infections. International Journal for Parasitology. 2009;**39**(5):607-614

[84] Beh KJ, Maddox JF. Prospects for the development of genetic markers for resistance to gastrointestinal parasite infection in sheep. International Journal for Parasitology. 1996;**26**(8-9):879-897

[85] Canales M, Enriquez A, Ramos E, Cabrera D, Dandie H, Soto A, et al. Large-scale production in Pichia pastoris of the recombinant vaccine Gavac™ against cattle tick. Vaccine. 1997;**15**(4):414-422

[86] Morris CA, Vlassoff A, Bisset SA, Baker RL, Watson TG. Direct responses to selection for divergence in fecal nematode egg count in young Romney and Perendale sheep. In: Proc Assoc Adv Anim Breed Genet. Hamilton, New Zealand: Ruakura Agricultural Research Centre; 1997. pp. 413-416

[87] Woolaston RR, Elwin RL, Barger IA. No adaptation of Haemonchus contortus to genetically resistant sheep. International Journal for Parasitology. 1992;**22**(3):377-380

[88] Mandonnet N, Aumont G, Fleury J, Arquet R, Varo H, Gruner L, et al. Assessment of genetic variability of resistance to gastrointestinal nematode parasites in creole goats in the humid tropics. Journal of Animal Science. 2001;**79**(7):1706-1712

[89] Vagenas D, Jackson F, Russel AJF, Merchant M, Wright IA, Bishop SC. Genetic control of resistance to gastro-intestinal parasites in crossbred cashmere-producing goats: Responses to selection, genetic parameters, and relationships with production traits. Animal Science. 2002;**74**(2):199-208

[90] de Monteiro CMO, da Matos RS, Araújo LX, de Perinotto WMS, Bittencourt VREP, Dolinski C, et al. First report of pathogenicity of entomopathogenic nematodes of the genus Heterorhabditis on partially engorged females of Dermacentor nitens (Acari: Ixodidae). Biological Control. 2014;**69**:78-81

[91] Shelton M, Bassett JW. Estimate of certain genetic parameters relating to angora goats. Texas Agricultural Station Research Reports. 1970:38-41

[92] Georges K, Ezeokoli CD, Newaj-Fyzul A, Campbell M, Mootoo N, Mutani A, et al. The application of PCR and reverse line blot hybridization to detect arthropod-borne hemopathogens of dogs and cats in Trinidad. Annals of the New York Academy of Sciences. 2008;**1149**(1):196-199

[93] Albers GAA, Gray GD, Piper LR, Barker JSF, Le Jambre LF, Barger IA. The genetics of resistance and resilience to Haemonchus contortus infection in young merino sheep. International Journal for Parasitology. 1987;**17**(7):1355-1363

[94] Gray GD. Genetic resistance to haemonchosis in sheep. Parasitology Today. 1987;**3**(8):253-255

[95] Opara MN, Nwaobasi JK, Okoli IC. Occurrence of parasitic helminths among small ruminants reared under traditional husbandry system in Owerri, South East NigeriaPresence des helminthes chez les petits ruminants en elevage traditionnel a Owerri dans le Sud-Est du Nigeria. Bulletin of Animal Health Production Africa. 2005;**53**(4):226-233

Chapter 3

Recent Advances in Anti-Schistosomiasis Drug Discovery

Ezra J. Marker and Stefan L. Debbert

Abstract

Schistosomiasis, a parasitic disease caused by infection by helminths of the *Schistosoma* genus, affects over 200 million people, primarily in the developing world. Treatment of this disease largely relies on one drug, praziquantel. Although this drug is cheap, safe, and effective, the looming prospect of drug resistance makes the development of a pipeline of anti-schistosomiasis drugs a priority. Many new drug leads have arisen from screening existing sets of compounds such as the Open Access Boxes developed by the Medicines for Malaria Venture (MMV) in collaboration with the Drugs for Neglected Diseases Initiative (DNDI). Other leads have been found through work focused on druggable targets such as kinases, histone deacetylases, proteases, and others. This chapter will discuss recent work concerning the discovery and development of novel anti-schistosomiasis drug leads from many sources.

Keywords: schistosomiasis, drug discovery, praziquantel, antiparasitic medicinal chemistry, drug screening, enzyme inhibitors

1. Introduction

Schistosomiasis is a neglected tropical disease that affects hundreds of millions of people, primarily in the developing world [1, 2]. The disease is caused by blood flukes of the genus *Schistosoma*; the three main infectious species are *S. mansoni* (in Africa and tropical South America), *S. japonicum* (in China and the Philippines), and *S. haematobium* (in Africa) [1]. Infections occur when parasites in their cercariae stage swim from their freshwater snail hosts and penetrate human skin. The cercariae then lose their tails and migrate to the intestinal or urogenital area. There they mature to adult worms, form male-female pairs, and lay eggs prolifically; the host's disease symptoms are due to an immune response to these eggs [3]. Eggs shed into a water source by human defecation hatch and release miracidia, which infect the intermediate snail host and continue the cycle.

Chronic schistosomiasis is associated with diseases of the kidneys, spleen, liver, bladder and intestine [3]. In endemic areas, up to 75% of the incidence of bladder cancer has been attributed to infection with *S. haematobium*; [4, 5] the link between *S. mansoni* infection and cancer is still being investigated [6]. In all, the global burden

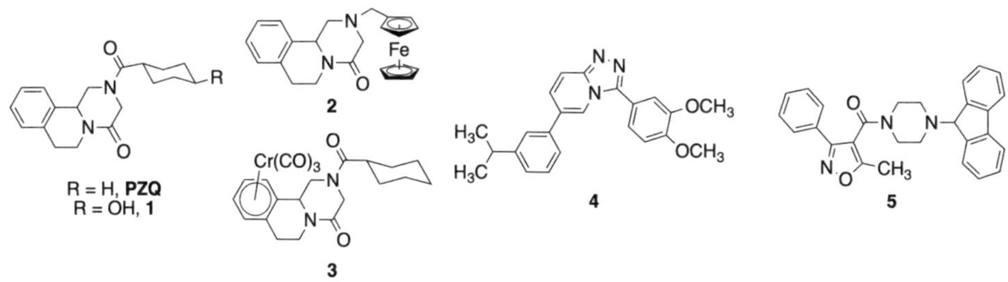

Figure 1.
*Praziquantel (***PZQ***), its primary metabolite (***1***), and related compounds* **2–5***.*

due to schistosomiasis, in terms of disability-adjusted life years (DALYs, which combine premature mortality data with years lived with a disability) has been estimated at 1.7–4.5 million [7].

Current treatment of this disease relies almost exclusively on one drug: praziquantel (**PZQ**, **Figure 1**). While PZQ has so far proven effective against adult *Schistosoma* worms of all species, the specter of drug resistance, as well as PZQ's ineffectiveness against immature parasites, have motivated the search for new antischistosomals. Several excellent reviews have recently been published on these efforts [8–13]. In this chapter, I will briefly discuss current antischistosomals in use, antimalarials with antischistosomiasis potential, and finally, the discovery of novel scaffolds for drug development, by screening for phenotypic changes or against a specific biological target.

2. Praziquantel

In 1972, Merck and Bayer tested **PZQ** among 400 other drugs, in efforts to develop a commercialized treatment against schistosomiasis [14]. It was first approved and used as a veterinary treatment against the disease, but in the 1980s, it was transitioned into treatment against infections in humans [15]. It is regarded as a safe and highly effective drug against all adult *Schistosoma* worms [16]. **PZQ**'s main metabolite is its 4-*trans*-cyclohexanol derivative **1**, which is 4 to 10 times less effective against *S. mansoni* than **PZQ** itself [17, 18].

PZQ analogs derivatized with ferrocenyl groups at various positions, including **2**, were determined to have only moderate *in vitro* activity against *S. mansoni* [19]. Tricarbonylchromium **PZQ** derivatives such as **3**, however, have demonstrated *in vitro* anti-schistosomiasis activity on par with that of **PZQ** itself [20]. Further work established that chromium derivatives of *R*-**PZQ** were more effective than derivatives of *S*-**PZQ**, but still only effected low worm burden reductions (WBRs) *in vivo* [21].

PZQ appears to owe its activity to its activation of a Ca^{2+}-permeable ion channel in *S. mansoni* that belongs to a family of transient receptor potential (TRP) channels, which are non-selective cation channels [22, 23]. This target has been widely exploited by other antihelmintics [24, 25] as well as therapies for respiratory diseases, cancer and other conditions [26–28]. By activating this ion channel, **PZQ** effects a rapid calcium uptake across the ion channel, with deleterious effect to the parasite's morphology [29].

Since **PZQ** has been found to target a TRP channel, TRP channels have been further studied as druggable targets for schistosomiasis. A high-throughput screen of about 16,000 compounds against a TRP channel in the melastatin family yielded **4** as a strong receptor agonist (EC_{50} = 1.6 ± 0.3 μM) and 32 potential receptor antagonists, including **5** [22].

DOI: http://dx.doi.org/10.5772/intechopen.103056

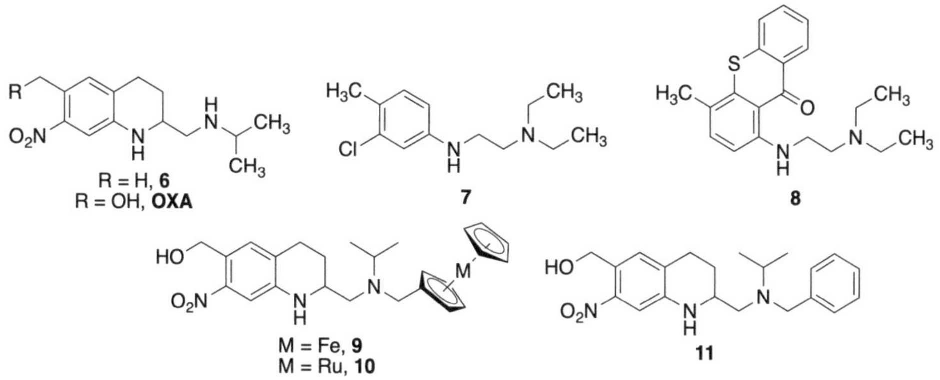

Figure 2.
*Oxamniquine (***OXA***) and related compounds (***6–11***).*

3. Oxamniquine

The development of oxamniquine (**OXA**, **Figure 2**) as an anti-schistosomiasis drug began with the study of Pfizer compound UK 3883 (**6**) [30, 31], a conformationally restricted analog of Mirasan (**7**), which was itself a simplified version of the early anti-schistosomiasis drug lucanthone (**8**). Mirasan proved effective against *S. mansoni* in mice but not in primates, suggesting that it and its analogs were acting as prodrugs activated by metabolic oxidation at their benzylic positions. The hydroxymethyl metabolite of **6**, **OXA**, has showed excellent anti-schistosomiasis activity in both mice and humans [32].

Although **OXA** can be easily absorbed orally, is active against both intestinal and liver infections, and has a lower cost than **PZQ** [18], it remains the second choice when compared to **PZQ** for a variety of reasons. **OXA** is only effective against *S. mansoni*, whereas **PZQ** is effective against all major forms that manifest in humans [33]. **OXA** also can cause a wide variety of side effects, such as nausea, dizziness, drowsiness, and headache [18]. **OXA** is a prodrug, converted into its reactive sulfate ester form by an *S. mansoni* sulfotransferase enzyme (Smp089320, or *Sm*SULT-OR) [34, 35]. Recent work guided by the crystal structure of this enzyme has led to the development of **OXA** derivatives with greater efficacy not only against *S. mansoni*, but *S. japonium* and *S. hematobium* as well [36].

Ferrocenyl and ruthenocenyl derivatives of **OXA** (**9–10**) were also synthesized and found to be roughly as active as the parent **OXA** against *S. mansoni*, but significantly more active in *in vitro* testing than **OXA** against *S. haematobium* and *S. japonicum* [37–39]. Notably, this work also found a benzylated **OXA**, **11**, to be effective against all three parasites *in vitro* [37]. However, the *in vivo* efficacy against the parasites was limited, in part due to their instability in acidic media [39].

4. Antischistosomal antimalarials

4.1 Artemisinins

Artemisinin (**12**, **Figure 3**) and its congeners are the active ingredients in the extracts of *Artemisia annua*, which have been used as traditional Chinese medicine for a variety

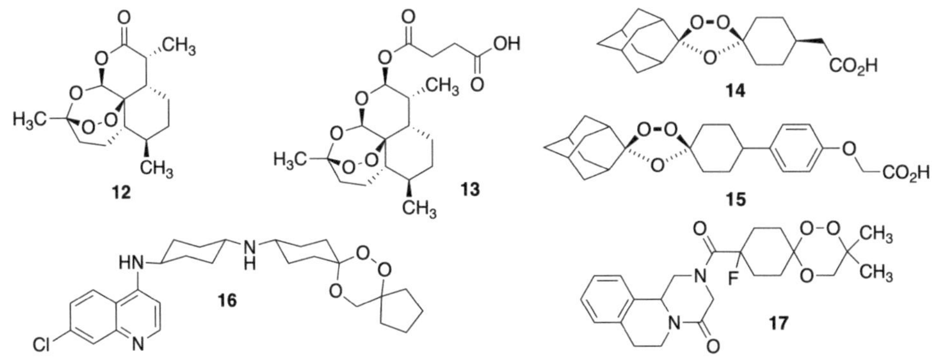

Figure 3.
Artemisinin derivatives (12–13) and synthetic endoperoxides with antischistosomal potential (14–17).

of ailments for thousands of years [40]. The disclosure of the artemisinins' antimalarial potential in 1979 [41] was followed closely by a 1980 report on their antischistosomal activity [42]. The schistosomicidal activity of **12** and similar antimalarials may stem from their ability to interfere with the blood-feeding parasite's ability to detoxify heme [43].

Artemisinins such as **12** and artesunate (**13**) have demonstrated high *in vivo* efficacy against juvenile schistosomes and moderate *in vivo* efficacy against adult schistosomes [43], suggesting that simultaneous treatment with artemisinins and **PZQ** may prove complementary [40]. Although one study did find synergistic effects when artemisinins were combined with **PZQ**, this treatment method would have to be administered repeatedly to prevent reinfection [44].

4.2 Trioxolanes

The success of artemisinins as antiparasitic agents has motivated the development of fully synthetic derivatives [45]. OZ78 (**14, Figure 3**) is a carboxylic acid trioxolane that achieves high WBRs (greater than 80%) against juvenile *S. mansoni* in mice [46]. Its endoperoxide moiety appears to be necessary for its antischistosomal activity, as non-peroxidic analogs showed no activity. Another trioxolane, OZ418 (**15**), is orally active and targets multiple developmental stages of *S. mansoni*. With a single oral dose of 200 mg/kg, infections of juvenile *S. mansoni* were completely cured, and an 80% WBR was achieved [43]. Antimalarial hybrids of trioxolanes with quinine derivatives (e.g. the "trioxaquine" **16**) have also demonstrated promising antischistosomal activity [8, 43], as have similar trioxolane-PZQ hybrids (e.g., the "trioxaquantel" **17**) [47].

4.3 Other antimalarials

Other antimalarials, including mefloquine (**18, Figure 4**), have also shown broad antischistosomal activity [48]. Recent work has added pyronaridine (**19**) and methylene blue (**20**) to the list of antimalarial compounds that show promise against schistosomiasis; both demonstrated sub-micromolar IC_{50} values against schistosomula, as well as complete killing of adult worms at 30 μM [49]. Pyronaridine was found to be active against juvenile *S. mansoni* but not the adult parasite [48], while methylene blue showed good activity against adult worms *in vivo*. In a small observational trial in Gabon, three out of four children with an *S. haematobium* infection were cured with Pyramax, a combination of pyronaridine and artesunate (**13**) [49].

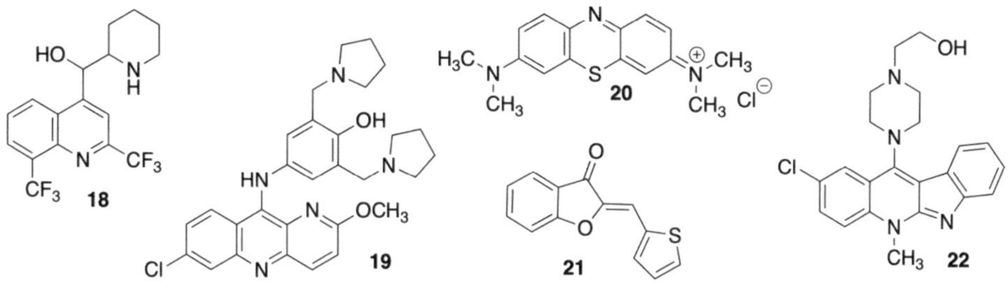

Figure 4.
Antimalarials/antiparasitics with anti-schistosomiasis activity (18–22).

Many natural products have demonstrated anti-schistosomiasis activity [10, 50–52]. The aurone scaffold is another source of antimalarial compounds [53, 54] that has been investigated for anti-schistosomiasis potential [55, 56]. Aurone **21** proved efficacious against *S. mansoni* in an *in vivo* mouse model (against both juvenile (21-day-old) and adult (49-day-old) parasites) and caused a marked decrease in both immature and mature eggs eliminated in feces by infected mice [55].

Cryptolepines, isolated from the roots of *Cryptolepis sanguinolenta,* have been used as traditional medicine in Central and West Africa, and more recently have studies as an antimalarial treatment [57]. Piperazinyl-substituted norneocryptolepines such as **22** have been shown to have high antischistosomal activity (IC_{50} < 5 μM against adult *S. mansoni*); six out of sixteen neocryptolepines showed 100% worm mortality at a concentration of 5 μg/mL after five days [58].

5. New antischistosomals found by phenotypic screening

5.1 Medium-throughput phenotypic screening results

In vitro phenotypic screening of selected compound sets has provided several new drug leads for further optimization [8, 59]. Compound sets prepared by the Medicines for Malaria Venture (MMV) have proven particularly fruitful in this regard. The first of these sets to be assessed was the Malaria Box, which contained 400 diverse, commercially available compounds, 200 of which were "drug-like" according to Lipinski's Rule of Five, all with confirmed *in vitro* activity against the blood stage of *P. falciparum* [60]. *In vitro* screening of these compounds against newly transformed schistosomula (NTS) was followed by similar testing against adult parasites; the five most active of these compounds (**23–27, Figure 5**) were then tested *in vivo* for efficacy and pharmacokinetic properties [61]. While three of the five were ineffective *in vivo* (WBR <20%), compounds **26** and **27** were able to reduce worm burdens in infected mice by 52.5% and 40.8%, respectively, with a single 400 mg/kg dose [61].

The diarylurea MMV665852 (**26**) above stood out for its good *in vivo* activity and its ease of synthesis, so it was chosen for further development. A set of MMV665852 analogs, including bissulfonamide, oxalamide, thiourea, carbamate, imidazolidinone, and pyrazine central moieties, was assessed against *S. japonicum* [62]. The parent MMV665852, along with six urea analogs, demonstrated IC_{50}'s under 10 μM for both juvenile and adult parasites in *in vitro* testing, but none of them produced WBR values above 35% in mice harboring either a juvenile or an adult *S. japonicum* infection.

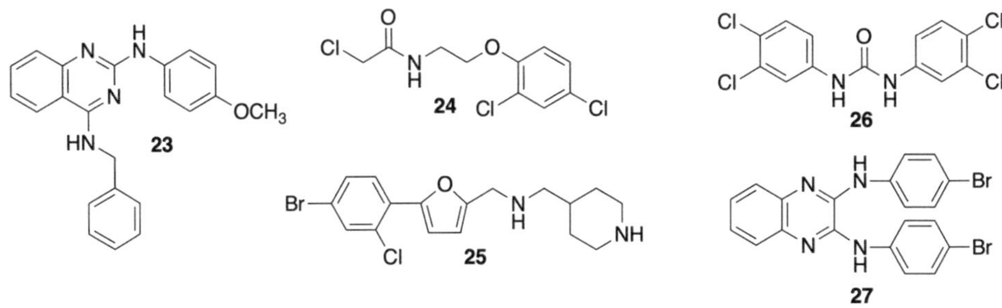

Figure 5.
Antischistosomal hits from the MMV malaria box (23–27).

Commercially available analogs of **26**, including ureas (25), benzamides (17), and carbamates (4), were screened for activity against *S. mansoni* as above [63]. While nine of these compounds had IC_{90}'s of <10 μM against adult worms, only the salicylanilide **28** (**Figure 6**) demonstrated significant *in vivo* activity. While its worm burden reduction was greater than that of the lead compound **26**, its cytotoxicity (as measured against L6 cells), and the resulting poor selectivity index (4.9), may preclude its further development as antischistosomal lead.

Further exploration of the diarylurea chemotype resulted in the synthesis and testing of 20 new analogs designed with aqueous solubility and chemical diversity in mind. Seven of these analogs demonstrated sub-micromolar IC_{50}'s against adult *S. mansoni* with high antischistosomal selectivities [64]. Three of these (**29**–**31**), all bearing 4-fluoro-3-trifluoromethylaniline moieties, showed modest *in vivo* activity, with WBRs between 37% and 50%. Pharmacokinetic data suggest that **31** has significantly higher overall systemic exposure than the other two, perhaps due to the pyridine substituent. N,N′-diarylureas bearing pentafluorosulfanyl ($-SF_5$) groups, such as **32**, have also been synthesized and assessed; like the other ureas tested, they demonstrated excellent activity *in vitro* (IC_{50}'s as low as 0.6 μM against *S. mansoni* NTS) but marginal efficacy *in vivo* [65].

Another of the leads from the Malaria Box screening, the dianilinoquinoxaline MMV007204 (**27**), was also selected for further development. Quinoxaline compounds have previously demonstrated utility against other parasitic diseases such

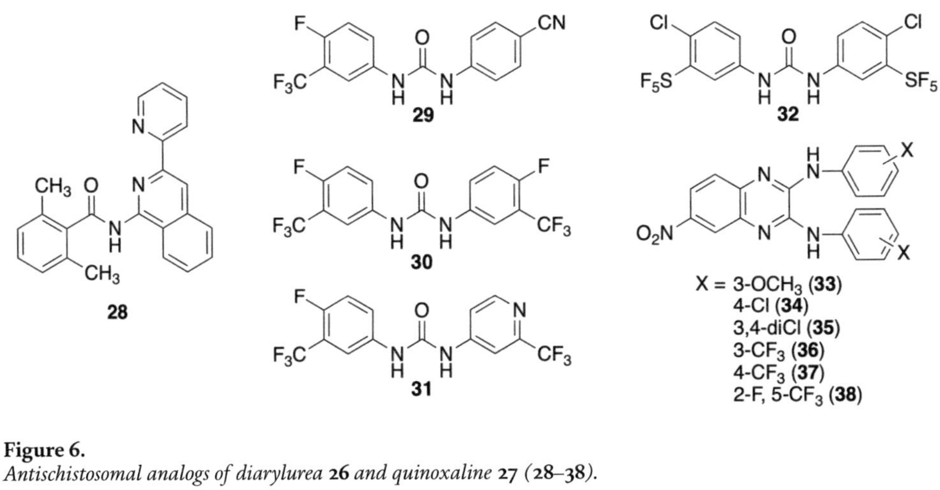

Figure 6.
Antischistosomal analogs of diarylurea **26** *and quinoxaline* **27** *(28–38).*

as malaria, Chagas disease, leishmaniasis, amebiasis, giardiasis, and filariasis [66]. Analogs of quinoxaline **27** (47, including 12 triazoloquinoxalines) were screened as above; three nitroquinoxalines (**33**–**35**) showed IC_{50}'s of under 0.31 μM against adult *S. mansoni* worms. Again, the *in vivo* potency of these compounds was underwhelming, with highest WBR among them 46.3% for compound **35** [67]. In a separate contemporaneous study, other quinoxaline analogs of **36** bearing nitro, amine and amide functionalities were screened for both phenotypic and motility effects on schistosomula [68]. Compared to compound **27**, compounds **36**, **37** and **38** showed significantly greater efficacy against the adult worms; the latter two compounds also showed excellent activity against *S. japonicum* and *S. haematobium* adults [68].

The MMV Stasis Box, containing 400 compounds that whose development as drugs was stopped at an advanced stage for various reasons, was also explored as a source of new chemotypes for anti-schistosomiasis drug development [69]. Eleven of these compounds showed an *in vitro* effect against adults of least 75%, with four demonstrating complete lethality, but the only compound to have an *in vivo* effect on worm burden over 50% was MMV690534, (**39**, **Figure** 7) with a 51.4% WBR. Compound **39** is a TGF-β receptor I kinase inhibitor developed for cancer chemotherapy; [70] other kinase inhibitors with anti-schistosomiasis activity will be discussed later in this review.

The MMV also prepared a Pathogen Box containing 400 compounds with activity against various neglected diseases, including malaria, tuberculosis, toxoplasmosis, and schistosomiasis. Three institutions explored this compound set for anti-schistosomiasis activity; teams at the Swiss Tropical and Public Health (TPH) [71] and the University of California-San Diego (UCSD) conducted *in vitro* phenotypic assays of these compounds against *S. mansoni* NTS, while a team at the Fundação Oswaldo Cruz (FIOCRUZ) used a metabolic activity indicator to assess schistosomula viability [72]. The two phenotypic assays showed a strong 87% concordance, but the inclusion of the FIOCRUZ assay only lowered the overall concordance slightly, to 74%. At 72 h drug treatment, 35 compounds in the Pathogen Box, including the antimalarial mefloquine (**18**), registered as "active" on all three screens against schistosomula. Five of those common hits demonstrated moderate *in vivo* activity in mice infected with *S. mansoni*: MMV022478 (**40**, 70.7% WBR), MMV022029 (**41**, 67.8%), MMV688761 (**42**, 55.2%), MMV687273 (**43**, 22.4%), and MMV690102 (**44**, 32.8%) (**Figure** 7) [71].

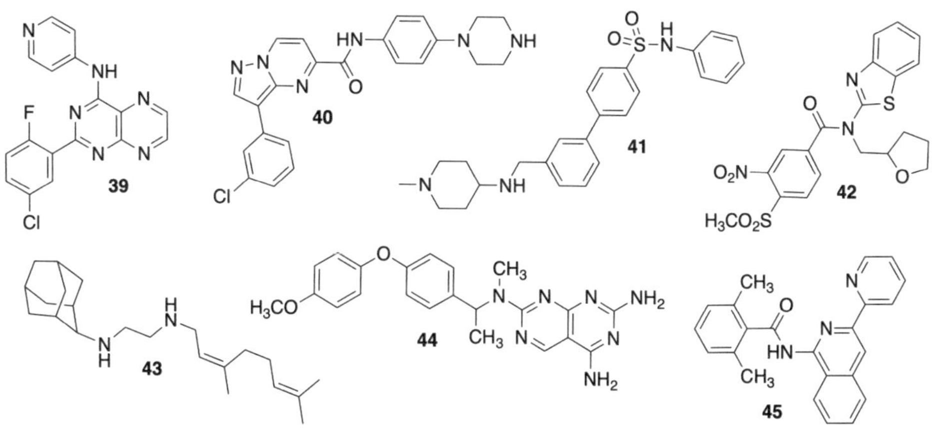

Figure 7.
Antischistosomal hits from the MMV Statis, pathogen and pandemic response boxes (39–45).

Notably, **PZQ** was *not* one of those 35 common hits, showing only borderline activity in the Swiss TPH screen and no activity in the FIOCRUZ screen. This reminds us that overreliance on obvious phenotypic signs in screening might be keeping us from discovering anti-schistosomiasis compounds with more subtle modes of action, especially modes that rely on the host immune response. A recent essay by Zamanian and Chan recommends the further development of *in vitro* screens to more closely model *in vivo* environments [73].

The most recent MMV Box to be assessed for anti-schistosomiasis activity was the Pandemic Response Box, a set of compounds with antibacterial, antiviral and/or antifungal activity [74]. Phenotypic screening found 17 of these 400 compounds to have at least moderate activity (>66%) against adult *S. mansoni in* vitro. The most promising of these compounds was found to be the isoquinoline MMV1581558 (**45**), with an EC_{50} of 0.18 ± 0.01 μM against adult *S. mansoni*, and a WBR of 42 ± 25% in *in vivo* testing.

Phenotypic screening of a set of 2160 compounds purchased from Microsource Discovery Systems, containing 821 FDA-approved drugs, against *S. mansoni* NTS yielded about 100 hits, which were narrowed by subsequent screening against adult worms as well as consideration of known compound toxicity and side effects [75]. The ionophoric antibiotic lasalocid sodium **46** (**Figure 8**) effected moderate reductions in worm burden (~40%) and egg burden as well as improvements in spleen and liver pathology in the same model [75]. The anthelminthic niclosamide (**47**) demonstrated excellent *in vitro* activity but no WBR in infected mice; among related salicylanilides that were tested, rafoxanide (**48**) reduced WBRs by half at a 50 mg/kg dose [75].

Recently, a set of 73 non-steroidal anti-inflammatory drugs (NSAIDs) was screened for activity against *S. mansoni* [76]; this was in part motivated by the reported antischistosomal activity of the NSAID diclofenac (**49**), which is structurally similar to PZQ [77]. The most active NSAID in the set proved to be mefenamic acid (**50**), with good activity *in vitro* (EC_{50} = 11.1 μM) and *in vivo* (at 400 mg/kg, >70% reduction in both worm and egg burden) [76].

5.2 High-throughput screening results

Development of reliable high-throughput screening (HTS) tools promises to accelerate the identification of novel anti-schistosomiasis chemotypes [78]. Using a previously developed high-throughput protocol for screening NTS [79], Mansour et al. tested over 294,000 compounds taken from MMV, Pfizer, European Screening

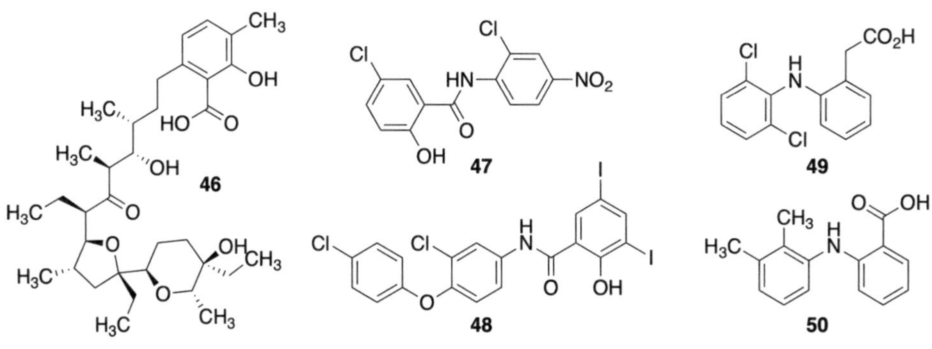

Figure 8.
Other hits from phenotypic screening (46–50).

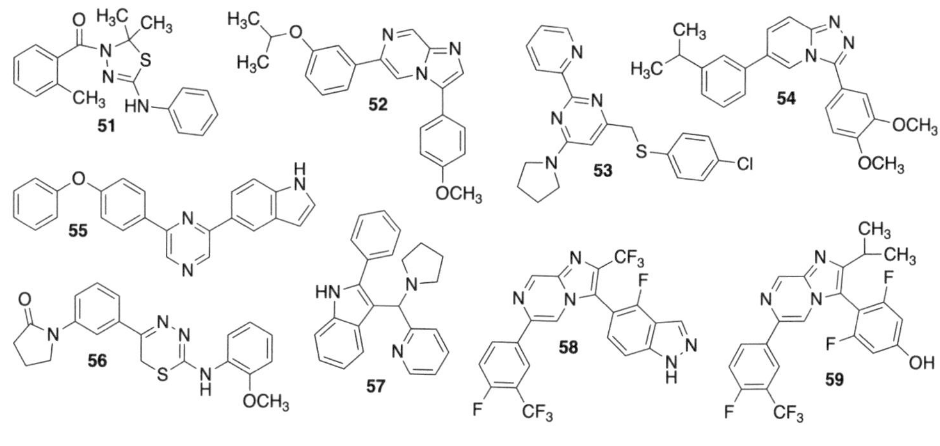

Figure 9.
Leads resulting from a large high-throughput screening experiment (**51–59**).

Port, GSK (the Tres Cantos Antimalarial Set), and Enamine [80]. The compounds from this set selected for further development, compounds **51–57** (**Figure 9**) and the previously mentioned TRP channel ligand **4**, demonstrated EC_{50} values under 7 μM for NTS, and under 15 μM for juvenile and adult worms.

Several of these leads bear indole or azaindole (e.g., triazolopyridine) units; indoles similar to **57** have also demonstrated activity against *S. mansoni* peroxiredoxin Prx2 and TGR in other high-throughput screening assays [81, 82]. Further development of the lead compound **52** led to the development of a series of pyrazolopyrimidines and imidazopyrazines, the latter typified by compounds **58** and **59** [83]. Compound **58** combined exceptional potency in *in vitro* testing (EC_{50} 27 nM against juvenile worms, and 46 nM against adult worms) with decent metabolic stability and good *in vivo* efficacy.

Another HTS strategy uses ATP quantitation to assess test compounds' effect on the number and viability of schistosomula in a sample [84]. Applying this screen to a 40,000-sample set, followed by clustering and retesting, led to compounds **60–62** (**Figure 10**) being identified as the most promising leads [85]. The latter of those, perhexiline maleate (**62**), is an anti-angina drug whose efficacy against schistosomiasis had been studied previously [86, 87]. Starting from those three hits, pharmacophore

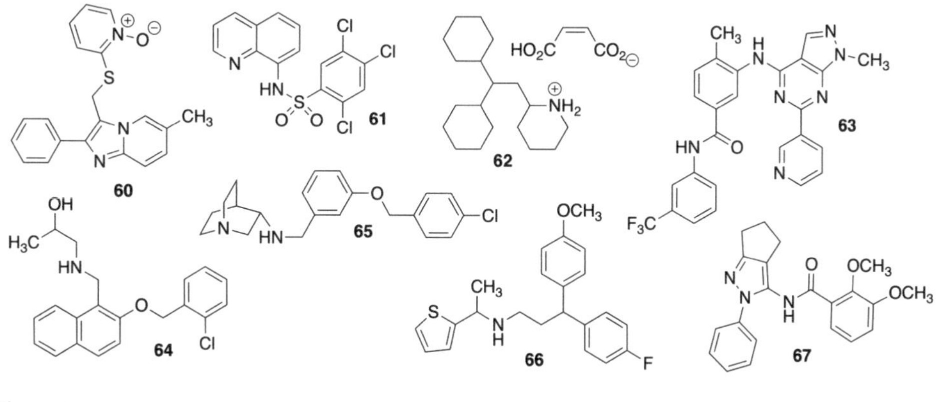

Figure 10.
Leads resulting from a high throughput screen using ATP quantitation (**60–67**).

modeling resulted in the selection of compounds **63–67** as novel scaffolds for potential development. All eight of these compounds not only proved efficacious, *in vitro* and *in vivo*, against both juvenile and adult worms at 10 μM, but strongly impaired egg production in *S. mansoni* at sub-lethal doses (2.5–5 μM) [85].

6. Target based approaches

6.1 Targeting thioredoxin glutathione reductase

The redox system of *Schistosoma* parasites depends on the enzyme thioredoxin glutathione reductase (TGR), This enzyme is critical to the redox homeostasis of schistosomes as it acts in the detoxification of reactive oxygen species present in the host. Inhibitors of this enzyme have been sought and assessed for antischistosomal potential [88–91]. The silencing of *S. mansoni* TGR (*Sm*TGR) expression with RNAi led to parasite death within 4 d in an *in vitro* study [89]. Though **PZQ** does not inhibit this enzyme, two previously studied antischistomals, potassium antimonyl tartrate (**69**, **Figure 11**) and oltipraz (**70**), were found to be effective *Sm*TGR inhibitors.

Auranofin (**71**), a gold complex widely used to treat rheumatoid arthritis, strongly inhibited the enzyme (IC_{50} < 10 nM) and effected good WBRs (~60%) in infected mice [89]. Further work has established that treatment with **71** causes cysteine-gold-cysteine bridges to form in *Sm*TGR, and that this process may be catalyzed by the selenocysteine present in the enzyme [92].

Early HTS efforts in this vein revealed the oxadiazole 2-oxide scaffold as a promising lead for novel *Sm*TGR inhibitors [81]. Treatment with furoxan derivative **72** at 10 μM caused 100% parasite death in adult *S. mansoni, S. japonicum* and *S. haematobium* within 24 h in *in vitro* studies, and was highly effective *in vivo* (>88% WBR at 10 mg/kg dosage) [93]. The parasite's phenotypic response to treatment with **72** resembled the effects of RNAi silencing of *SmTGR* expression [89]. The addition of a nitric oxide (NO) scavenger to the system slowed the schistosomal activity of **72** considerably, indicating that **72**'s release of NO in the presence of *SmTGR*

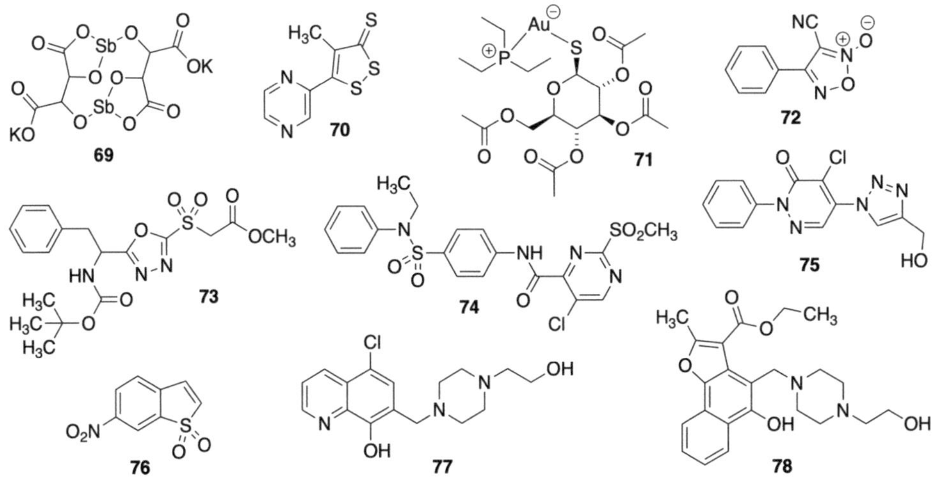

Figure 11.
Inhibitors of S. mansoni thioredoxin glutathione reductase (SmTGR) (**69–78**).

contributes to its potency [93]. Further structure-activity relationship (SAR) work established the 3-cyano-1,2,5-oxadiazole-2-oxide moiety as the pharmacophore of interest [94]. Testing several aryl-substituted furoxans against *S. japonicum* yielded several active compounds, but no correlations between antischistosomal activity and either TGR inhibition or NO release rate [95].

HTS efforts to find other *Sm*TGR inhibitors yielded a set of eight hits with IC_{50} values under 10 μM [96]. Four of these, **73–76**, showed consistent antischistosomal activity against *S. mansoni*, *S. japonicum*, and *S. haematobium*, rapidly killing at least half the adult worms present at a 10 μM dose [96].

A secondary "doorstop pocket" binding site in *Sm*TGR has recently been identified; binding to this site appears to preclude NADPH binding elsewhere in the enzyme [97]. Piperazine derivatives **77** and **78** were predicted to bind tightly to this pocket in binding studies, and in fact proved to be good *Sm*TGR inhibitors with antischistosomal activity against adult worms *in vitro* [97].

6.2 Targeting kinases

Kinases play critical roles in regulating vital functions like cell proliferation, differentiation, apoptosis, and migration in various organisms. The use of protein-kinase-targeting drugs against *S. mansoni* and *S. japonicum* has been reviewed recently [98–100]. *S. mansoni* has 357 kinases; 351 of those are transcribed in adults with 268 being protein kinases (PKs) [99]. Phenotypic screening of a set of 114 approved oncology drugs against *S. mansoni* NTS revealed several kinase inhibitors with good activity against both NTS and adult *S. mansoni* (IC_{50} < 10 μM) *in vitro* [101]. Six of those compounds (**Figure 12**)— trametinib (**79**), bosutinib (**80**), ponatinib (**81**), afatinib (**82**), sunitinib (**83**), and vandetanib (**84**)—were then assessed for *in vivo* activity. In a murine model, only **79** and **84** showed *in vivo* efficacy, with WBR values of 63.6% and 48.1%, respectively [101].

Protein tyrosine kinases (PTKs) are involved in angiogenesis, reproduction, cell proliferation, and many other processes [102]. Many PTK inhibitors (or "tyrphostins", for tyrosine phosphorylation inhibitors [103]) are able to inhibit multiple PTKs, including receptor tyrosine kinases (RTKs) like growth factor receptors, insulin receptors, (IR) and Venus kinase receptors (VKR). Among the RTK inhibitors that have demonstrated

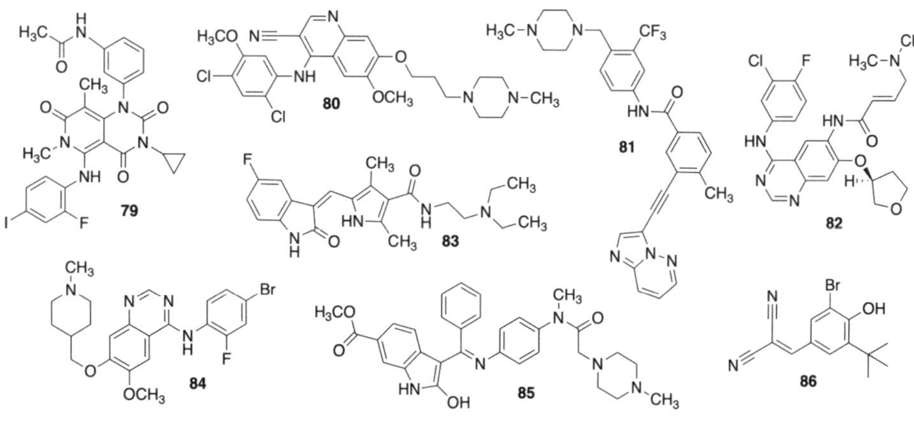

Figure 12.
Anti-schistosomiasis kinase inhibitors (79–86).

antischistosomal activity is BIBF1120 (**85**), which inhibits fibroblast growth factor receptors in *S. mansoni* (*Sm*FGFR-A and -B) and which, in *in vitro* testing, caused unpairing of coupled worms at 5 μM and complete worm death within 48 h at 10 μM [104]. Another is tyrphostin AG1024 (**86**), which inhibits both insulin receptors and VKRs in *S. mansoni*, induces death in both schistosomula and adult worms at 10 μM [105].

Other kinases that have been studied as antischistosomal targets include mitogen-activated protein kinases (MAPKs) [106, 107], Polo-like kinases (PLKs) [108], Abl-kinase [109], and *Sm*TAO and *Sm*STK25, two protein kinases discovered in a recent large-scale RNAi screen to be critical to worm survival [110].

6.3 Targeting hemozoin formation

Like other blood-feeding parasites, *S. mansoni* must free themselves of toxic free heme, and do so by polymerizing heme to crystalline hemozoin [111, 112]. Inhibiting the parasites' heme polymerization, then, presents another anti-schistosomiasis strategy; this is considered to be the antischistosomal mode of action for several antimalarials [113, 114]. However, recent work showing that some hemozoin in the *Schistosoma* gut is actually consumed to yield free iron for egg development indicates that there is more to learn about hemozoin formation in this parasite [115].

A series of pyrido[1,2-*a*]benzimidazoles, some of which with demonstrated inhibition of heme polymerization in *P. falciparum*, were screened against *S. mansoni* [116]. A majority of the compounds tested (48 of 57) showed good activity against NTS, with 19 of those demonstrating IC_{50} values below 3 μM against adult worms. However, the correlation between hemozoin inhibition and antischistosomal activity was weak ($R^2 < 0.05$ for both NTS and adults).

Further investigation of this scaffold led to analogs **87** and **88**, with IC_{50}'s under 0.4 μM against adult *S. mansoni* and moderately good WBR effects in infected mice (62.2% and 69.1%, respectively) [117], and to the chiral 1-phenylethylamine derivative **89**, which combined excellent WBR activity (89.6%) at 50 mg/kg with some toxicity concerns (**Figure 13**) [118].

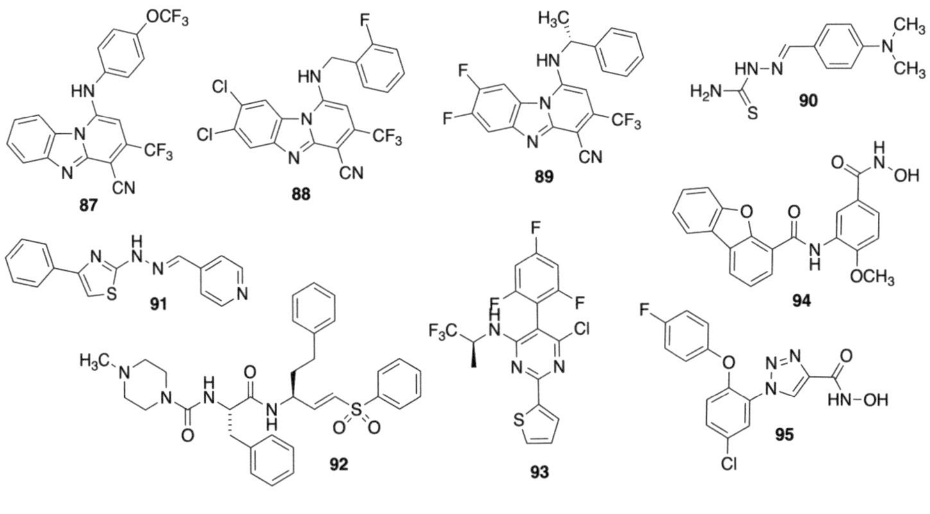

Figure 13.
Antischistosomals targeting hemozoin formation (87–89), cysteine proteases (90–92), tubulin (93), and histone deacetylase (94–95).

6.4 Targeting cysteine proteases

Cysteine proteases are integral to metabolism, nutrition and immune invasion in several parasites, including *Trypanosoma cruzi, Trypanosoma brucei, and S. mansoni* [119, 120]. In particular, *S. mansoni* cathepsin B1 (*Sm*CB1) inhibitors have been assessed for anti-schistosomiasis activity. A series of thiosemicarbazone and thiazoles were assessed for *Sm*CB1 inhibitory activity and screened for phenotypic effect on *S. mansoni* schistosomula and adult worms [121]. The best *Sm*CB1 inhibitor found, thiosemicarbazole **90** (IC_{50} = 1.5 ± 0.4 μM), displayed no activity against the parasite *in vitro*, while thiazole **91**, which showed no *Sm*CB1 inhibition, was the most active compound against schistosomula, and the only one active against adult worms, in the set [121]. However, a series of peptidomimetic vinyl sulfones including K11777 (**92**) has demonstrated both excellent *Sm*CB1 inhibitory efficacy (IC_{50} = 2.09 ± 0.08 nM for **92**) and good activity against schistosomula *in vitro* [122, 123].

6.5 Targeting tubulin

Tubulin, and tubulin-containing cellular components like microtubules, which are essential for cell division and many other functions of the eukaryotic cell, have long been considered druggable targets in *S. mansoni* [124, 125]. In 1977, colchicine and vinblastine were shown to inhibit red blood cell ingestion and microtubule formation in the parasite [126]. However, the cytotoxicity of these natural products preclude their wider application as anti-schistosomiasis agents.

Phenotypic screening of a library of tubulin-binding compounds led to the further exploration of the phenylpyrimidine scaffold as a source of new leads [127]. Further development resulted in thiophene-substituted phenylpyrimidines such as **93**, which reduced worm movement by over 90% at 5 μM but lacked the mammalian cell cytotoxicity of other tubulin-targeting compounds [127].

6.6 Targeting histone deacetylase

Histone deacetylase (HDAC) inhibitors, developed for epigenetic cancer chemotherapy [128], have shown effectiveness against *S. mansoni* at all stages [129–131]. In target validation studies, reducing expression of *S. mansoni* HDAC8 (*Sm*HDAC8) leads to decreased worm and egg counts in infected mice [132]. A series of hydroxamic acid *Sm*HDAC8 inhibitors has been developed [133, 134]; the most potent of these, dibenzofuran **94**, strongly inhibited *Sm*HDAC8 (IC_{50} = 270 nM) and killed >98% of *S. mansoni* schistosomula at 10 μM, but its poor solubility foiled efforts to test its *in vivo* activity [134]. Triazole hydroxamic acids such as **95** were found to have similar *in vitro* activity [135]. Related enzyme studied as *S. mansoni* drug targets have included *Sm*HDAC6 [136], histone methyltransferase EZH2 [137], and some sirtuins (particularly *Sm*Sirt1 and *Sm*Sirt2) [138, 139].

6.7 Other targets

Other *S. mansoni* targets being investigated for new antischistosomal drugs include phosphodiesterase-4 [140–142], dihydroorotate dehydrogenase [143], 3-hydroxy-3-methylglutaryl coenzyme A (HMG-CoA) reductase [144, 145], farnesyl transferase [146], carbonic anhydrase [147], NAD+ catabolizing enzyme [148], cytochrome P450 (CYP3050A1) [149] and aldose reductase [9, 150, 151].

7. Conclusion

The drawbacks of global schistosomiasis monotherapy with **PZQ** have motivated considerable work to generate a pipeline of new drug leads for further development. In recent years, screening studies agnostic on candidates' modes of action have complemented more target-focused work. The limits of both approaches are evident, as hit compounds with excellent *in vitro* activity often fail to ameliorate a *Schistosoma* infection in *in vivo* models. This calls for better understanding of the pharmacokinetics required of effective schistosomicides, better screening techniques to approximate *in vivo* conditions, and more research into host-parasite interaction. The embrace of these challenges by the drug development community is encouraging.

Acknowledgements

We thank Judith Humphries and Clayton Agler for helpful discussions.

Author details

Ezra J. Marker and Stefan L. Debbert*
Department of Chemistry, Lawrence University, Appleton, Wisconsin, USA

*Address all correspondence to: stefan.debbert@lawrence.edu

References

[1] McManus DP, Dunne DW, Sacko M, Utzinger J, Vennervald BJ, Zhou X. Schistosomiasis. Nature Reviews Disease Primers. 2018;**4**(1):13

[2] Steinmann P, Keiser J, Bos R, Tanner M, Utzinger J. Schistosomiasis and water resources development: Systematic review, meta-analysis, and estimates of people at risk. The Lancet Infectious Diseases. 2006;**6**(7):411-425

[3] Gray DJ, Ross AG, Li YS, McManus DP. Diagnosis and management of schistosomiasis. BMJ. 2011;**342**:d2651

[4] Van Tong H, Brindley PJ, Meyer CG, Velavan TP. Parasite infection, carcinogenesis and human malignancy. eBioMedicine. 2017;**15**:12-23

[5] Bhagwandeen S. Schistosomiasis and carcinoma of the bladder in Zambia. South African Medical Journal. 1976;**50**(41):1616-1620

[6] von Bulow V, Lichtenberger J, Grevelding CG, Falcone FH, Roeb E, Roderfeld M. Does *Schistosoma Mansoni* facilitate carcinogenesis? Cells. 2021;**10**(8):1982. DOI: 10.3390/cells10081982

[7] Lopez AD, Mathers CD, Ezzati M, Jamison DT, Murray CJ, editors. Global Burden of Disease and Risk Factors. Washington, DC: World Bank and Oxford University Press; 2006

[8] Dziwornu GA, Attram HD, Gachuhi S, Chibale K. Chemotherapy for human schistosomiasis: How far have we come? What's new? Where do we go from here? RSC Medicinal Chemistry. 2020;**11**(4):455-490

[9] Caffrey CR, El-Sakkary N, Mäder P, Krieg R, Becker K, Schlitzer M, et al. Drug discovery and development for schistosomiasis. Neglected Tropical Diseases: Drug Discovery and Development. 2019:187-225

[10] Gemma S, Federico S, Brogi S, Brindisi M, Butini S, Campiani G. Dealing with schistosomiasis: Current drug discovery strategies. Annual Reports in Medicinal Chemistry. 2019;**2019**(53):107-138

[11] Thétiot-Laurent SA, Boissier J, Robert A, Meunier B. Schistosomiasis chemotherapy. Angewandte Chemie International Edition. 2013;**52**(31):7936-7956

[12] Mader P, Rennar GA, Ventura AMP, Grevelding CG, Schlitzer M. Chemotherapy for fighting schistosomiasis: Past, present and future. ChemMedChem. 2018;**13**(22):2374-2389

[13] Lago EM, Xavier RP, Teixeira TR, Silva LM, da Silva Filho AA, de Moraes J. Antischistosomal agents: State of art and perspectives. Future Medicinal Chemistry. 2018;**10**(1):89-120

[14] Novaes M, Souza JPD, Araújo HCD. Síntese do anti-helmíntico praziquantel, a partir da glicina. Química Nova. 1999;**22**(1):5-10

[15] Sinha S, Sharma B. Neurocysticercosis: A review of current status and management. Journal of Clinical Neuroscience. 2009;**16**(7):867-876

[16] Guglielmo S, Cortese D, Vottero F, Rolando B, Kommer VP, Williams DL, et al. New praziquantel derivatives containing NO-donor furoxans and related furazans as active agents against *Schistosoma mansoni*. Eur J Med Chem. 2014;**84**:135-145

[17] Wang H, Fang Z, Zheng Y, Zhou K, Hu C, Krausz KW, et al. Metabolic profiling of praziquantel enantiomers. Biochemical Pharmacology. 2014;**90**(2):166-178

[18] da Silva VBR, Campos BRKL, de Oliveira JF, Decout JL, do Carmo Alves de Lima M. Medicinal chemistry of antischistosomal drugs: Praziquantel and oxamniquine. Bioorganic & Medicinal Chemistry. 2017;**25**(13):3259-3277

[19] Patra M, Ingram K, Pierroz V, Ferrari S, Spingler B, Keiser J, et al. Ferrocenyl derivatives of the anthelmintic praziquantel: Design, synthesis, and biological evaluation. Journal of Medicinal Chemistry. 2012;**55**(20):8790-8798

[20] Patra M, Ingram K, Pierroz V, Ferrari S, Spingler B, Gasser RB, et al. [(η^6-Praziquantel)$Cr(CO)_3$] derivatives with remarkable *in vitro* antischistosomal activity. Chemistry: A European Journal. 2013;**19**(7):2232-2235

[21] Patra M, Ingram K, Leonidova A, Pierroz V, Ferrari S, Robertson MN, et al. *In vitro* metabolic profile and *in vivo* antischistosomal activity studies of (η^6-praziquantel)$Cr(CO)_3$ derivatives. Journal of Medicinal Chemistry. 2013;**56**(22):9192-9198

[22] Chulkov EG, Smith E, Rohr CM, Yahya NA, Park S, Scampavia L, et al. Identification of novel modulators of a schistosome transient receptor potential channel targeted by praziquantel. PLoS Neglected Tropical Diseases. 2021;**15**(11):e0009898

[23] Park SK, Gunaratne GS, Chulkov EG, Moehring F, McCusker P, Dosa PI, et al. The anthelmintic drug praziquantel activates a schistosome transient receptor potential channel. The Journal of Biological Chemistry. 2019;**294**(49):18873-18880

[24] Bais S, Greenberg RM. Schistosome TRP channels: An appraisal. International Journal for Parasitology: Drugs and Drug Resistance. 2020;**13**:1-7

[25] Bais S, Greenberg RM. TRP channels as potential targets for antischistosomals. International Journal for Parasitology: Drugs and Drug Resistance. 2018;**8**(3):511-517

[26] Nilius B, Szallasi A. Transient receptor potential channels as drug targets: From the science of basic research to the art of medicine. Pharmacological Reviews. 2014;**66**(3):676-814

[27] Moran MM. TRP channels as potential drug targets. Annual Review of Pharmacology and Toxicology. 2018;**58**:309-330

[28] Li S, Westwick J, Poll C. Transient receptor potential (TRP) channels as potential drug targets in respiratory disease. Cell Calcium. 2003;**33**(5-6):551-558

[29] Pax R, Bennett J, Fetterer R. A benzodiazepine derivative and praziquantel: Effects on musculature of *Schistosoma mansoni* and *Schistosoma japonicum*. Naunyn-Schmiedeberg's Archives of Pharmacology. 1978;**304**(3): 309-315

[30] Richards HC, Foster R. A new series of 2-aminomethyltetrahydroquinoline derivatives displaying schistosomicidal activity in rodents and primates. Nature. 1969;**222**(5193):581-582

[31] Foster R, Cheetham B, King D, Mesmer E. The action of UK 3883, a novel 2-aminomethyltetrahydroquinoline derivative, against mature schistosomes

in rodents and primates. Annals of Tropical Medicine and Parasitology. 1971;**65**(1):59-70

[32] Kaye B, Woolhouse N. The metabolism of a new schistosomicide 2-isopropylaminomethyl-6-methyl-7-nitro-1,2,3,4-tetrahydroquinoline (UK 3883). Xenobiotica. 1972;**2**(2):169-178

[33] Rugel AR, Guzman MA, Taylor AB, Chevalier FD, Tarpley RS, McHardy SF, et al. Why does oxamniquine kill *Schistosoma mansoni* and not *S. haematobium* and *S. japonicum*? International Journal for Parasitology: Drugs and Drug Resistance. 2020;**13**:8-15

[34] Valentim CL, Cioli D, Chevalier FD, Cao X, Taylor AB, Holloway SP, et al. Genetic and molecular basis of drug resistance and species-specific drug action in schistosome parasites. Science. 2013;**342**(6164):1385-1389

[35] Taylor AB, Roberts KM, Cao X, Clark NE, Holloway SP, Donati E, et al. Structural and enzymatic insights into species-specific resistance to schistosome parasite drug therapy. The Journal of Biological Chemistry. 2017;**292**(27):11154-11164

[36] Guzman MA, Rugel AR, Tarpley RS, Alwan SN, Chevalier FD, Kovalskyy DP, et al. An iterative process produces oxamniquine derivatives that kill the major species of schistosomes infecting humans. PLoS Neglected Tropical Diseases. 2020;**14**(8):e0008517

[37] Hess J, Panic G, Patra M, Mastrobuoni L, Spingler B, Roy S, et al. Ferrocenyl, ruthenocenyl, and benzyl oxamniquine derivatives with cross-species activity against *Schistosoma mansoni* and *Schistosoma haematobium*. ACS Infectious Diseases. 2017;**3**(9): 645-652

[38] Buchter V, Hess J, Gasser G, Keiser J. Assessment of tegumental damage to *Schistosoma mansoni* and S. *haematobium* after *in vitro* exposure to ferrocenyl, ruthenocenyl and benzyl derivatives of oxamniquine using scanning electron microscopy. Parasites & Vectors. 2018;**11**:580

[39] Buchter V, Ong YC, Mouvet F, Ladaycia A, Lepeltier E, Rothlisberger U, et al. Multidisciplinary preclinical investigations on three oxamniquine analogues as new drug candidates for schistosomiasis. Chemistry: A European Journal. 2020;**26**(66):15232-15241

[40] Tu Y. The discovery of artemisinin (qinghaosu) and gifts from Chinese medicine. Nature Medicine. 2011;**17**(10):1217-1220

[41] Qinghaosu Antimalarial Coordinating Research Group. Antimalarial studies on qinghaosu. Chinese Medical Journal. 1979;**92**:811-816

[42] Chen D, Fu L, Shao P, Wu F, Fan C, Shu H, et al. Experimental studies on antischistosomal activity of qinghaosu. Chinese Medical Journal. 1980;**60**:422-425

[43] Keiser J, Utzinger J. Antimalarials in the treatment of schistosomiasis. Current Pharmaceutical Design. 2012;**18**(24):3531-3538

[44] Bergquist R, Utzinger J, Keiser J. Controlling schistosomiasis with praziquantel: How much longer without a viable alternative? Infectious Diseases of Poverty. 2017;**6**(1):74

[45] Panic G, Duthaler U, Speich B, Keiser J. Repurposing drugs for the treatment and control of helminth infections. International Journal for Parasitology: Drugs and Drug Resistance. 2014;**4**(3):185-200

[46] Xiao SH, Keiser J, Chollet J, Utzinger J, Dong Y, Endriss Y, et al. *In vitro* and *in vivo* activities of synthetic trioxolanes against major human schistosome species. Antimicrobial Agents and Chemotherapy. 2007;**51**(4):1440-1445

[47] Laurent SA, Boissier J, Coslédan F, Gornitzka H, Robert A, Meunier B. Synthesis of "trioxaquantel"® derivatives as potential new antischistosomal drugs. European Journal of Organic Chemistry. 2008;**2008**(5):895-913

[48] Keiser J, Chollet J, Xiao S, Mei J, Jiao P, Utzinger J, et al. Mefloquine—An aminoalcohol with promising antischistosomal properties in mice. PLoS Neglected Tropical Diseases. 2009;**3**(1):e350

[49] Koehne E, Zander N, Rodi M, Held J, Hoffmann W, Zoleko-Manego R, et al. Evidence for *in vitro* and *in vivo* activity of the antimalarial pyronaridine against *Schistosoma*. PLoS Neglected Tropical Diseases. 2021;**15**(6):e0009511

[50] de Moraes J. Natural products with antischistosomal activity. Future Medicinal Chemistry. 2015;**7**(6):801-820

[51] de Carvalho LSA, Silva LM, de Souza VC, da Silva MPN, Capriles PVSZ, de Faria PP, et al. Cardamonin presents *in vivo* activity against *Schistosoma mansoni* and inhibits potato apyrase. Chemistry & Biodiversity. 2021;**18**(11):e2100604

[52] Simoben CV, Ntie-Kang F, Akone SH, Sippl W. Compounds from African medicinal plants with activities against selected parasitic diseases: Schistosomiasis, trypanosomiasis and leishmaniasis. Natural Products and Bioprospecting. 2018;**8**(3):151-169

[53] Carrasco MP, Newton AS, Goncalves L, Gois A, Machado M, Gut J, et al. Probing the aurone scaffold against *Plasmodium falciparum*: Design, synthesis and antimalarial activity. European Journal of Medicinal Chemistry. 2014;**80**:523-534

[54] Kayser O, Kiderlen AF, Croft SL. Natural products as antiparasitic drugs. Parasitology Research. 2003;**90** (Suppl. 2):S55-S62

[55] Pereira VRD, da Silveira LS, Mengarda AC, Alves Junior IJ, da Silva OOZ, Miguel FB, et al. Antischistosomal properties of aurone derivatives against juvenile and adult worms of *Schistosoma mansoni*. Acta Tropica. 2021;**213**:105741

[56] Silva Torres D, Alves de Oliveira B, Souza D, Silveira L, Paulo da Silva M, Rodrigues Duraes Pereira V, et al. Synthetic aurones: New features for *Schistosoma mansoni* therapy. Chemistry Biodiversity. 2021;**18**(11):e2100439

[57] Wright CW. Recent developments in naturally derived antimalarials: Cryptolepine analogues. The Journal of Pharmacy and Pharmacology. 2007;**59**(6):899-904

[58] El Bardicy S, El Sayed I, Yousif F, Van der Veken P, Haemers A, Augustyns K, et al. Schistosomicidal and molluscicidal activities of aminoalkylamino substituted neo- and norneocryptolepine derivatives. Pharmaceutical Biology. 2012;**50**(2):134-140

[59] Marxer M, Ingram K, Keiser J. Development of an *in vitro* drug screening assay using *Schistosoma haematobium* schistosomula. Parasites & Vectors. 2012;**5**:165

[60] Spangenberg T, Burrows JN, Kowalczyk P, McDonald S, Wells TN, Willis P. The open access malaria box: A drug discovery catalyst for neglected diseases. PLoS One. 2013;**8**(6):e62906

[61] Ingram-Sieber K, Cowan N, Panic G, Vargas M, Mansour NR, Bickle QD, et al. Orally active antischistosomal early leads identified from the open access malaria box. PLoS Neglected Tropical Diseases. 2014;**8**(1):e2610

[62] Yao H, Liu F, Chen J, Li Y, Cui J, Qiao C. Antischistosomal activity of N, N′-arylurea analogs against *Schistosoma japonicum*. Bioorganic & Medicinal Chemistry Letters. 2016;**26**(5):1386-1390

[63] Cowan N, Dätwyler P, Ernst B, Wang C, Vennerstrom JL, Spangenberg T, et al. Activities of N,N′-diarylurea MMV665852 analogs against *Schistosoma mansoni*. Antimicrobial Agents and Chemotherapy. 2015;**59**(4):1935-1941

[64] Wu J, Wang C, Leas D, Vargas M, White KL, Shackleford DM, et al. Progress in antischistosomal N,N'-diaryl urea SAR. Bioorganic & Medicinal Chemistry Letters. 2018;**28**(3):244-248

[65] Probst A, Pujol E, Häberli C, Keiser J, Vazquez S. *In vitro*, *in vivo*, and absorption, distribution, metabolism, and excretion evaluation of SF_5-Containing N,N'-diarylureas as antischistosomal agents. Antimicrobial Agents and Chemotherapy. 2021;**65**(10):e0061521

[66] Soto-Sánchez J, Ospina-Villa JD. Current status of quinoxaline and quinoxaline 1,4-di-N-oxides derivatives as potential antiparasitic agents. Chemical Biology & Drug Design. 2021;**98**(4):683-699

[67] Debbert SL, Hintz MJ, Bell CJ, Earl KR, Forsythe GE, Häberli C, et al. Activities of quinoxaline, nitroquinoxaline, and [1,2,4]triazolo[4,3-a]quinoxaline analogs of MMV007204 against *Schistosoma mansoni*. Antimicrobial Agents and Chemotherapy. 2021;**65**(3):e01370-20. DOI: 10.1128/AAC.01370-20

[68] Padalino G, El-Sakkary N, Liu LJ, Liu C, Harte DSG, Barnes RE, et al. Anti-schistosomal activities of quinoxaline-containing compounds: From hit identification to lead optimisation. European Journal of Medicinal Chemistry. 2021;**226**:113823

[69] Pasche V, Laleu B, Keiser J. Screening a repurposing library, the Medicines for Malaria Venture Stasis Box, against *Schistosoma mansoni*. Parasites & Vectors 2018;11(1):1-8.

[70] Uhl M, Aulwurm S, Wischhusen J, Weiler M, Ma JY, Almirez R, et al. SD-208, a novel transforming growth factor beta receptor I kinase inhibitor, inhibits growth and invasiveness and enhances immunogenicity of murine and human glioma cells *in vitro* and *in vivo*. Cancer Research. 2004;**64**(21):7954-7961

[71] Pasche V, Laleu B, Keiser J. Early antischistosomal leads identified from *in vitro* and *in vivo* screening of the Medicines for Malaria Venture Pathogen Box. ACS Infect Dis. 2019;**5**(1):102-110

[72] Maccesi M, Aguiar PHN, Pasche V, Padilla M, Suzuki BM, Montefusco S, et al. Multi-center screening of the Pathogen Box collection for schistosomiasis drug discovery. Parasites & Vectors. 2019;**12**(1):493

[73] Zamanian M, Chan JD. High-content approaches to anthelmintic drug screening. Trends in Parasitology. 2021;**37**(9):780-789

[74] Biendl S, Häberli C, Keiser J. Discovery of novel antischistosomal scaffolds from the open access Pandemic Response Box. Expert Review of Anti-Infective Therapy. 2021:1-9

[75] Abdulla M, Ruelas DS, Wolff B, Snedecor J, Lim K, Xu F, et al. Drug discovery for schistosomiasis: Hit and

lead compounds identified in a library of known drugs by medium-throughput phenotypic screening. PLoS Neglected Tropical Diseases. 2009;**3**(7):e478

[76] Lago EM, Silva MP, Queiroz TG, Mazloum SF, Rodrigues VC, Carnauba PU, et al. Phenotypic screening of nonsteroidal anti-inflammatory drugs identified mefenamic acid as a drug for the treatment of schistosomiasis. eBioMedicine. 2019;**43**:370-379

[77] Carvalho AA, Mafud AC, Pinto PL, Mascarenhas YP, de Moraes J. Schistosomicidal effect of the anti-inflammatory drug diclofenac and its structural correlation with praziquantel. International Journal of Antimicrobial Agents. 2014;**44**(4):372-374

[78] Neves BJ, Muratov E, Machado RB, Andrade CH, Cravo PVL. Modern approaches to accelerate discovery of new antischistosomal drugs. Expert Opinion on Drug Discovery. 2016;**11**(6):557-567

[79] Paveley RA, Mansour NR, Hallyburton I, Bleicher LS, Benn AE, Mikic I, et al. Whole organism high-content screening by label-free, image-based Bayesian classification for parasitic diseases. PLoS Neglected Tropical Diseases. 2012;**6**(7):e1762

[80] Mansour NR, Paveley R, Gardner JMF, Bell AS, Parkinson T, Bickle Q. High throughput screening identifies novel lead compounds with activity against larval, juvenile and adult *Schistosoma mansoni*. PLoS Neglected Tropical Diseases. 2016;**10**(4):e0004659

[81] Simeonov A, Jadhav A, Sayed AA, Wang Y, Nelson ME, Thomas CJ, et al. Quantitative high-throughput screen identifies inhibitors of the *Schistosoma mansoni* redox cascade. PLoS Neglected Tropical Diseases. 2008;**2**(1):e127

[82] Lea WA, Jadhav A, Rai G, Sayed AA, Cass CL, Inglese J, et al. A 1,536-well-based kinetic HTS assay for inhibitors of *Schistosoma mansoni* thioredoxin glutathione reductase. Assay and Drug Development Technologies. 202;**6**(4):551-555

[83] Gardner JMF, Mansour NR, Bell AS, Helmby H, Bickle Q. The discovery of a novel series of compounds with single-dose efficacy against juvenile and adult *Schistosoma* species. PLoS Neglected Tropical Diseases. 2021;**15**(7):e0009490

[84] Lalli C, Guidi A, Gennari N, Altamura S, Bresciani A, Ruberti G. Development and validation of a luminescence-based, medium-throughput assay for drug screening in *Schistosoma mansoni*. PLoS Neglected Tropical Diseases. 2015;**9**(1):e0003484

[85] Guidi A, Lalli C, Gimmelli R, Nizi E, Andreini M, Gennari N, et al. Discovery by organism based high-throughput screening of new multi-stage compounds affecting *Schistosoma mansoni* viability, egg formation and production. PLoS Neglected Tropical Diseases. 2017;**11**(10):e0005994

[86] Guidi A, Lalli C, Perlas E, Bolasco G, Nibbio M, Monteagudo E, et al. Discovery and characterization of novel anti-schistosomal properties of the anti-anginal drug, perhexiline and its impact on *Schistosoma mansoni* male and female reproductive systems. PLoS Neglected Tropical Diseases. 2016;**10**(8):e0004928

[87] Guidi A, Saraswati AP, Relitti N, Gimmelli R, Saccoccia F, Sirignano C, et al. ( )-(R)-and (−)-(S)-Perhexiline maleate: Enantioselective synthesis and functional studies on *Schistosoma mansoni* larval and adult stages. Bioorganic Chemistry. 2020;**102**:104067

[88] Alger HM, Williams DL. The disulfide redox system of *Schistosoma*

mansoni and the importance of a multifunctional enzyme, thioredoxin glutathione reductase. Molecular and Biochemical Parasitology. 2002;**121**(1):129-139

[89] Kuntz AN, Davioud-Charvet E, Sayed AA, Califf LL, Dessolin J, Arnér ESJ, et al. Thioredoxin glutathione reductase from *Schistosoma mansoni*: An essential parasite enzyme and a key drug target. PLoS Medicine. 2007;**4**(6):e206

[90] Song L, Li J, Xie S, Qian C, Wang J, Zhang W, et al. Thioredoxin glutathione reductase as a novel drug target: Evidence from *Schistosoma japonicum*. PLoS One. 2012;**7**(2):e31456

[91] Perbandt M, Ndjonka D, Liebau E. Protective mechanisms of helminths against reactive oxygen species are highly promising drug targets. Current Medicinal Chemistry. 2014;**21**(15):1794-1808

[92] Angelucci F, Sayed AA, Williams DL, Boumis G, Brunori M, Dimastrogiovanni D, et al. Inhibition of *Schistosoma mansoni* thioredoxin-glutathione reductase by auranofin: Structural and kinetic aspects. The Journal of Biological Chemistry. 2009;**284**(42):28977-28985

[93] Sayed AA, Simeonov A, Thomas CJ, Inglese J, Austin CP, Williams DL. Identification of oxadiazoles as new drug leads for the control of schistosomiasis. Nature Medicine. 2008;**14**(4):407-412

[94] Rai G, Sayed AA, Lea WA, Luecke HF, Chakrapani H, Prast-Nielsen S, et al. Structure mechanism insights and the role of nitric oxide donation guide the development of oxadiazole-2-oxides as therapeutic agents against schistosomiasis. Journal of Medicinal Chemistry. 2009;**52**(20):6474-6483

[95] Song L, Luo H, Fan W, Wang G, Yin X, Shen S, et al. Oxadiazole-2-oxides may have other functional targets, in addition to SjTGR, through which they cause mortality in *Schistosoma japonicum*. Parasites & Vectors. 2016;**9**(1):1-12

[96] Lyu H, Petukhov PA, Banta PR, Jadhav A, Lea WA, Cheng Q, et al. Characterization of lead compounds targeting the selenoprotein thioredoxin glutathione reductase for treatment of schistosomiasis. ACS infectious diseases. 2020;**6**(3):393-405

[97] Silvestri I, Lyu H, Fata F, Boumis G, Miele AE, Ardini M, et al. Fragment-based discovery of a regulatory site in thioredoxin glutathione reductase acting as "doorstop" for NADPH entry. ACS Chemical Biology. 2018;**13**(8):2190-2202

[98] Morel M, Vanderstraete M, Hahnel S, Grevelding CG, Dissous C. Receptor tyrosine kinases and schistosome reproduction: New targets for chemotherapy. Frontiers in Genetics. 2014;**5**:238

[99] Grevelding CG, Langner S, Dissous C. Kinases: Molecular stage directors for schistosome development and differentiation. Trends in Parasitology. 2018;**34**(3):246-260

[100] Wu K, Zhai X, Huang S, Jiang L, Yu Z, Huang J. Protein kinases: Potential drug targets against *Schistosoma japonicum*. Frontiers in Cellular and Infection Microbiology. 2021;**11**:691757

[101] Cowan N, Keiser J. Repurposing of anticancer drugs: *in vitro* and *in vivo* activities against *Schistosoma mansoni*. Parasites & Vectors. 2015;**8**(1):1-9

[102] Kapp K, Knobloch J, Schüßler P, Sroka S, Lammers R, Kunz W, et al. The *Schistosoma mansoni* Src kinase TK3 is expressed in the gonads and likely

involved in cytoskeletal organization. Molecular and Biochemical Parasitology. 2004;**138**(2):171-182

[103] Levitzki A, Mishani E. Tyrphostins and other tyrosine kinase inhibitors. Annual Review of Biochemistry. 2006;**75**:93-109

[104] Hahnel S, Quack T, Parker-Manuel SJ, Lu Z, Vanderstraete M, Morel M, et al. Gonad RNA-specific qRT-PCR analyses identify genes with potential functions in schistosome reproduction such as SmFz1 and SmFGFRs. Frontiers in Genetics. 2014;**5**:170

[105] Vanderstraete M, Gouignard N, Cailliau K, Morel M, Lancelot J, Bodart J, et al. Dual targeting of insulin and venus kinase receptors of *Schistosoma mansoni* for novel anti-schistosome therapy. PLoS Neglected Tropical Diseases. 2013;**7**(5):e2226

[106] Avelar LDGA, Gava SG, Neves RH, MCS S, Araújo N, Tavares NC, et al. Smp38 MAP kinase regulation in *Schistosoma mansoni*: Roles in survival, oviposition, and protection against oxidative stress. Frontiers in Immunology. 2019;**10**:21

[107] Andrade LF, Mourao MM, Geraldo JA, Coelho FS, Silva LL, Neves RH, et al. Regulation of *Schistosoma mansoni* development and reproduction by the mitogen-activated protein kinase signaling pathway. PLoS Neglected Tropical Diseases. 2014;**8**(6):e2949

[108] Long T, Neitz RJ, Beasley R, Kalyanaraman C, Suzuki BM, Jacobson MP, et al. Structure-bioactivity relationship for benzimidazole thiophene inhibitors of polo-like kinase 1 (PLK1), a potential drug target in *Schistosoma mansoni*. PLoS Neglected Tropical Diseases. 2016;**10**(1):e0004356

[109] Buro C, Beckmann S, Oliveira KC, Dissous C, Cailliau K, Marhöfer RJ, et al. Imatinib treatment causes substantial transcriptional changes in adult *Schistosoma mansoni in vitro* exhibiting pleiotropic effects. PLoS Neglected Tropical Diseases. 2014;**8**(6):e2923

[110] Wang J, Paz C, Padalino G, Coghlan A, Lu Z, Gradinaru I, et al. Large-scale RNAi screening uncovers therapeutic targets in the parasite *Schistosoma mansoni*. Science. 2020;**369**(6511):1649-1653

[111] Oliveira MF, d'Avila JC, Torres CR, Oliveira PL, Tempone AJ, Rumjanek FD, et al. Haemozoin in *Schistosoma mansoni*. Molecular and Biochemical Parasitology. 2000;**111**(1):217-221

[112] Xiao S, Sun J. *Schistosoma* hemozoin and its possible roles. International Journal for Parasitology. 2017;**47**(4):171-183

[113] Correa Soares JB, Menezes D, Vannier-Santos MA, Ferreira-Pereira A, Almeida GT, Venancio TM, et al. Interference with hemozoin formation represents an important mechanism of schistosomicidal action of antimalarial quinoline methanols. PLoS Neglected Tropical Diseases. 2009;**3**(7):e477

[114] De Villiers KA, Egan TJ. Recent advances in the discovery of haem-targeting drugs for malaria and schistosomiasis. Molecules. 2009;**14**(8):2868-2887

[115] Sun J, Li C, Wang S. Organism-like formation of *Schistosoma* hemozoin and its function suggest a mechanism for anti-malarial action of artemisinin. Scientific Reports. 2016;**6**(1):1-10

[116] Okombo J, Singh K, Mayoka G, Ndubi F, Barnard L, Njogu PM, et al. Antischistosomal activity of pyrido[1,2-a] benzimidazole derivatives and correlation with inhibition of beta-hematin formation. ACS Infect Dis. 2017;**3**(6):411-420

[117] Mayoka G, Keiser J, Häberli C, Chibale K. Structure-activity relationship and *in vitro* absorption, distribution, metabolism, excretion, and toxicity (ADMET) studies of N-aryl-3-trifluoromethyl pyrido[1,2-a] benzimidazoles that are efficacious in a mouse model of schistosomiasis. ACS Infectious Diseases. 2019;**5**(3):418-429

[118] Probst A, Chisanga K, Dziwornu GA, Haeberli C, Keiser J, Chibale K. Expanding the activity profile of pyrido[1,2-a]benzimidazoles: Synthesis and evaluation of novel N^1-1-phenylethanamine derivatives against *Schistosoma mansoni*. ACS Infectious Diseases. 2021;**7**(5):1032-1043

[119] McKerrow JH. Development of cysteine protease inhibitors as chemotherapy for parasitic diseases: Insights on safety, target validation, and mechanism of action. International Journal for Parasitology. 1999;**29**(6):833-837

[120] Sajid M, McKerrow JH. Cysteine proteases of parasitic organisms. Molecular and Biochemical Parasitology. 2002;**120**(1):1-21

[121] Fonseca NC, da Cruz LF, da Silva VF, do Nascimento Pereira GA, de Siqueira-Neto JL, Kellar D, et al. Synthesis of a sugar-based thiosemicarbazone series and structure-activity relationship versus the parasite cysteine proteases rhodesain, cruzain, and *Schistosoma mansoni* cathepsin B1. Antimicrobial Agents and Chemotherapy. 2015;**59**(5):2666-2677

[122] Abdulla M, Lim K, Sajid M, McKerrow JH, Caffrey CR. Schistosomiasis *mansoni*: Novel chemotherapy using a cysteine protease inhibitor. PLoS Medicine. 2007;**4**(1):e14

[123] Jilkova A, Rezacova P, Lepsik M, Horn M, Vachova J, Fanfrlik J, et al. Structural basis for inhibition of cathepsin B drug target from the human blood fluke, *Schistosoma mansoni*. Journal of Biological Chemistry. 2011;**286**(41):35770-35781

[124] Fennell B, Naughton J, Barlow J, Brennan G, Fairweather I, Hoey E, et al. Microtubules as antiparasitic drug targets. Expert Opinion on Drug Discovery. 2008;**3**(5):501-518

[125] Chatterji BP, Jindal B, Srivastava S, Panda D. Microtubules as antifungal and antiparasitic drug targets. Expert Opinion on Therapeutic Patents. 2011;**21**(2):167-186

[126] Bogitsh BJ. *Schistosoma mansoni*: Colchicine and vinblastine effects on schistosomule digestive tract development *in vitro*. Experimental Parasitology. 1977;**43**(1):180-188

[127] Monti L, Cornec AS, Oukoloff K, Kovalevich J, Prijs K, Alle T, et al. Congeners derived from microtubule-active phenylpyrimidines produce a potent and long-lasting paralysis of *Schistosoma mansoni in vitro*. ACS Infectious Diseases. 2021;7(5):1089-1103

[128] Monneret C. Histone deacetylase inhibitors for epigenetic therapy of cancer. Anti-Cancer Drugs. 2007;**18**(4):363-370

[129] Dubois F, Caby S, Oger F, Cosseau C, Capron M, Grunau C, et al. Histone deacetylase inhibitors induce apoptosis, histone hyperacetylation

and up-regulation of gene transcription in *Schistosoma mansoni*. Molecular and Biochemical Parasitology. 2009;**168**(1):7-15

[130] Oger F, Dubois F, Caby S, Noel C, Cornette J, Bertin B, et al. The class I histone deacetylases of the platyhelminth parasite *Schistosoma mansoni*. Biochemical and Biophysical Research Communications. 2008;**377**(4):1079-1084

[131] Pierce J, Dubois-Abdesselem F, Lancelot J, Andrade L, Oliveira G. Targeting schistosome histone modifying enzymes for drug development. Current Pharmaceutical Design. 2012;**18**(24):3567-3578

[132] Marek M, Kannan S, Hauser AT, Moraes Mourao M, Caby S, Cura V, et al. Structural basis for the inhibition of histone deacetylase 8 (HDAC8), a key epigenetic player in the blood fluke *Schistosoma mansoni*. PLoS Pathogens. 2013;**9**(9):e1003645

[133] Heimburg T, Chakrabarti A, Lancelot J, Marek M, Melesina J, Hauser AT, et al. Structure-based design and synthesis of novel inhibitors targeting HDAC8 from *Schistosoma mansoni* for the treatment of schistosomiasis. Journal of Medicinal Chemistry. 2016;**59**(6):2423-2435

[134] Ghazy E, Heimburg T, Lancelot J, Zeyen P, Schmidtkunz K, Truhn A, et al. Synthesis, structure-activity relationships, cocrystallization and cellular characterization of novel smHDAC8 inhibitors for the treatment of schistosomiasis. European Journal of Medicinal Chemistry. 2021;**225**:113745

[135] Kalinin DV, Jana SK, Pfafenrot M, Chakrabarti A, Melesina J, Shaik TB, et al. Structure-based design, synthesis, and biological evaluation of triazole-based smHDAC8 inhibitors. ChemMedChem. 2020;**15**(7):571-584

[136] Vogerl K, Ong N, Senger J, Herp D, Schmidtkunz K, Marek M, et al. Synthesis and biological investigation of phenothiazine-based benzhydroxamic acids as selective histone deacetylase 6 inhibitors. Journal of Medicinal Chemistry. 2019;**62**(3):1138-1166

[137] Pereira AS, Amaral MS, Vasconcelos EJ, Pires DS, Asif H, da Silva LF, et al. Inhibition of histone methyltransferase EZH2 in *Schistosoma mansoni in vitro* by GSK343 reduces egg laying and decreases the expression of genes implicated in DNA replication and noncoding RNA metabolism. PLoS Neglected Tropical Diseases. 2018;**12**(10):e0006873

[138] Lancelot J, Caby S, Dubois-Abdesselem F, Vanderstraete M, Trolet J, Oliveira G, et al. *Schistosoma mansoni* sirtuins: Characterization and potential as chemotherapeutic targets. PLoS Neglected Tropical Diseases. 2013;**7**(9):e2428

[139] Monaldi D, Rotili D, Lancelot J, Marek M, Wossner N, Lucidi A, et al. Structure-reactivity relationships on substrates and inhibitors of the lysine deacylase sirtuin 2 from *Schistosoma mansoni* (SmSirt2). Journal of Medicinal Chemistry. 2019;**62**(19):8733-8759

[140] Long T, Rojo-Arreola L, Shi D, El-Sakkary N, Jarnagin K, Rock F, et al. Phenotypic, chemical and functional characterization of cyclic nucleotide phosphodiesterase 4 (PDE4) as a potential anthelmintic drug target. PLoS Neglected Tropical Diseases. 2017;**11**(7):e0005680

[141] Botros SS, William S, Sabra AA, El-Lakkany NM, Seif El-Din SH, Garcia-Rubia A, et al. Screening of

a PDE-focused library identifies imidazoles with *in vitro* and *in vivo* antischistosomal activity. International Journal for Parasitology: Drugs and Drug Resistance. 2019;**9**:35-43

[142] Sebastián-Pérez V, Schroeder S, Munday JC, Van Der Meer T, Zaldívar-Díez J, Siderius M, et al. Discovery of novel *Schistosoma mansoni* PDE4A inhibitors as potential agents against schistosomiasis. Future Medicinal Chemistry. 2019;**11**(14):1703-1720

[143] Calil FA, David JS, Chiappetta ER, Fumagalli F, Mello RB, Leite FH, et al. Ligand-based design, synthesis and biochemical evaluation of potent and selective inhibitors of *Schistosoma mansoni* dihydroorotate dehydrogenase. European Journal of Medicinal Chemistry. 2019;**167**:357-366

[144] Chen G, Foster L, Bennett JL. Antischistosomal action of mevinolin: Evidence that 3-hydroxy-methylglutaryl coenzyme A reductase activity in *Schistosoma mansoni* is vital for parasite survival. Naunyn-Schmiedeberg's Archives of Pharmacology. 1990;**342**(4): 477-482

[145] Rojo-Arreola L, Long T, Asarnow D, Suzuki BM, Singh R, Caffrey CR. Chemical and genetic validation of the statin drug target to treat the helminth disease, schistosomiasis. PLoS One. 2014;**9**(1):e87594

[146] Probst A, Nguyen TN, El-Sakkary N, Skinner D, Suzuki BM, Buckner FS, et al. Bioactivity of farnesyltransferase inhibitors against *Entamoeba histolytica* and *Schistosoma mansoni*. Frontiers in Cellular and Infection Microbiology. 2019;**9**:180

[147] Da'dara AA, Angeli A, Ferraroni M, Supuran CT, Skelly PJ. Crystal structure and chemical inhibition of essential schistosome host-interactive virulence factor carbonic anhydrase SmCA. Common Biology. 2019;**2**(1):1-11

[148] Jacques SA, Kuhn I, Koniev O, Schuber F, Lund FE, Wagner A, et al. Discovery of potent inhibitors of *Schistosoma mansoni* NAD catabolizing enzyme. Journal of Medicinal Chemistry. 2015;**58**(8):3582-3592

[149] Ziniel PD, Karumudi B, Barnard AH, Fisher EM, Thatcher GR, Podust LM, et al. The *Schistosoma mansoni* Cytochrome P450 (CYP3050A1) is essential for worm survival and egg development. PLoS Neglected Tropical Diseases. 2015;**9**(12):e0004279

[150] Mader P, Blohm AS, Quack T, Lange-Grunweller K, Grunweller A, Hartmann RK, et al. Biarylalkyl carboxylic acid derivatives as novel antischistosomal agents. ChemMedChem. 2016;**11**(13):1459-1468

[151] Blohm AS, Mäder P, Quack T, Lu Z, Hahnel S, Schlitzer M, et al. Derivatives of biarylalkyl carboxylic acid induce pleiotropic phenotypes in adult *Schistosoma mansoni in vitro*. Parasitology Research. 2016;**115**(10):3831-3842

Chapter 4

Perspective Chapter: Application of Probiotics to Inactivate Helminth Parasitic Zoonosis

Osama M. Darwesh and Hoda Samir El-Sayed

Abstract

Zoonotic infections may be defined as infections of animals that might be obviously transmissible to people. The contamination may transfer from ingestion of infective level of worms with food, infected soil, skin penetration, or direct animal contact. Parasitic helminths are a group of parasites that remains poorly studied in comparison to viruses and bacteria but may pose a considerable future risk to humans. Zoonotic parasites may be separated into four classes—direct-zoonotic, meta-zoonotic, cyclo-zoonotic, and sapro-zoonotic. Helminth parasitic zoonosis is possible to prevent and manage by simple service of hygiene and sanitation or regular deworming with anthelmintic pills. However, because of the lack of effective vaccines and appeared of anthelmintic resistance to medication, suppression of parasitic infestation still lingers a venture, which needs to improve the new possibility techniques. As a result, the hobby of exploiting probiotics as an alternative to pills has accelerated significantly during the last couple of years. Probiotics are exogenous residing microorganisms, which are beneficial to the host's fitness when administered inside the digestive tract. The most extensively used microorganisms, for this reason, are microorganisms of the genus *Lactobacillus* and *Enterococcus*, and a few fungi and yeasts. The current chapter is proposed to summarize some topics related to the use of probiotics toward helminth parasitic zoonosis.

Keywords: probiotics, anti-parasite, helminth parasitic zoonosis, environmental protection, hygiene

1. Introduction

Zoonotic infections may be defined as infections of animals that might be obviously transmissible to people. As such, they are worldwide and frequently unfold with humans via their partner and home animals [1, 2]. Zoonotic infections are among the most not unusual on earth and are accountable for over 60% of human infectious sicknesses, some of which can be as a result of helminth parasites. Contamination may also result from ingestion of infective levels of worms with food, infected soil; skin penetration, or direct animal contact. Parasites, such as helminths and protists, are considered pathogenic organisms that occur in developed and developing areas, which are responsible for both foods—water-borne diseases. Their international prevalence is tough to estimate, however the world health organization (WHO) has indicated the worldwide disorder burden of 11 waterborne and foodborne parasitic illnesses, is liable for inflicting over 407 million ailments ensuing in an estimated 94 passable deaths and 11 million disability-adjusted life years [3, 4]. Parasitic helminths are followed by the parasites group that still need more studied as viruses and bacteria, which may pose a future risk to humans. Helminths are macro-parasites, commonly tapeworms (cestodes), roundworms (nematodes), or flatworms (trematodes), and are usually recognized for persistent infections of the gastrointestinal tract, although helminths can infect nearly all human tissues [5, 6].

Helminths include one of the most diverse and geographically widespread groups of parasites that infect humans and animals. Approximately 100 species had been mentioned from humans, generally generating asymptomatic infection or mild signs and symptoms. However, approximately 20 species are of public health significance inflicting severe or maybe fatal infections. Some of the most important and well-known human zoonoses are caused by worm or helminth parasites, including species of nematodes (trichinellosis), cestodes (cysticercosis, echinococcosis), and trematodes (schistosomiasis) [7, 8]. Others include intestinal capillariasis, anisakidosis, eosinophilic enteritis, oesophagostomiasis, and gnathostomiasis [9]. The change of surroundings via wars, famine and the ever expanding and increasingly population brings people into close contact with new environments and flora and fauna species which makes the observe and manage of zoonoses is special interest and complexity [10].

Those zoonotic helminths can cause human diseases and be transferred from consuming food. This food may be meat contaminated with the parasite (taeniasis; trichinosis); fish (diphyllobothriasis; Diplogonorus granidis; clonorchiasis; anisakiasis); invertebrates (paragonimiasis; angiostrongyliasis) or ingestion of the infective degree of the germ with contaminated soil (toxocariasis; hydatid) water or salad (fascioliasis; fasciolopsiasis; hydatid; toxocariasis); pores and skin contact with infected soil/water containing energetic infective larvae and subsequent pores and skin penetration (cutaneous larva migrans; cercarial dermatitis); from direct animal touch (hydatid; toxocariasis) or thru insect vectors/intermediate hosts thru ingestion (dipylidiasis; Hymenolepis diminuta or Inermicapsifer contamination) or injection by way of a mosquito (dirofilariasis; Brugia contamination) [1, 11]. Numerous parasites have been observed on ready-to-consume produce, indicating that modern-day sanitation tactics utilized in the manufacturing of, for example, salads, do not always bring about a product this is free of parasites of fecal origin [12, 13]. This displays that parasite transmission stages within the surroundings are typically incredibly proof against the sanitation approaches normally used inside the food chain. Moreover, as those organisms often have low infectious doses, they may constitute the main danger for customers. A worldwide ranking of foodborne parasites of public fitness significance prepare through the food and Agriculture enterprise (FAO)/WHO become launched in 2014 [14].

Zoonotic parasites may be divided into four classes: direct-zoonotic, meta-zoonotic, cyclo-zoonotic, and sapro-zoonotic. Direct zoonotic parasites infect people directly from animals and involve Entamoeba histolytica, *Cryptosporidium parvum*, *Toxoplasma gondii*, and *Sarcoptes scabiei*. Meta-zoonotic parasites, which contain *Fasciola* spp. and *Schistosoma* spp. can infect human beings from invertebrate intermediate hosts. Cyclo-zoonotic parasites have vertebrate intermediate hosts and consist of *Echinococcus granulosus*, *Taenia saginata*, and *Taenia solium*. Saprozoonotic parasites can infect people from soil or water and consist of *Ancylostoma caninum* and *Strongyloides stercoralis* [15, 16].

Because of the zoonotic nature of so sufficiently of those food or water-borne parasites, one health recognition technique is needed for controlling and preventing most of those infections. The one health method for tackling zoonotic illnesses desires to take into account the mitigation and prevention of ailment risks that originate at the interface among humans, animals (domestic and wild), and their environments. Accordingly, veterinarians, collectively with other meals and environmental experts worried about the production of food and agricultural and consuming water, play an extensive function in safeguarding food safety [17, 18].

2. Use of probiotics toward helminth parasitic zoonosis

Helminth parasitic zoonosis is simply controlled and prevented by using hygiene and sanitation or regular deworming with anthelmintic pills. However, the vaccines not found to control the helminth parasitic infection, also, the occurrence of anthelmintic medication resistance so, the suppression of parasitic infestation are still needed improvement with new strategies. As a result, the used probiotics was considered the new alternative way instead of on pills or beside the medication which had a significant effect occur in the last couple of years.

Probiotics are anaerobic or aerobic microorganisms found naturally in the raw food and able to isolate simply, which are helpful to the host when consumed with a sufficient amount inside the gastrointestinal tract. These "Good Microorganisms" can be obtained from various dairy products and non-dairy products. The most broadly used microorganisms are used for this purpose, the genus of *Lactobacillus* and *Enterococcus*, also, a few fungi and yeasts could be used (**Figure 1**, [19]). The protective effect of probiotics is by the competition between probiotics and pathogens against colonization or antagonistic elimination within the intestine. An extra mechanism for probiotics is the ability to produce antimicrobial substances, such as bacteriocins or oxygen peroxide, some acids as lactic acid, or through immunomodulation [20, 21].

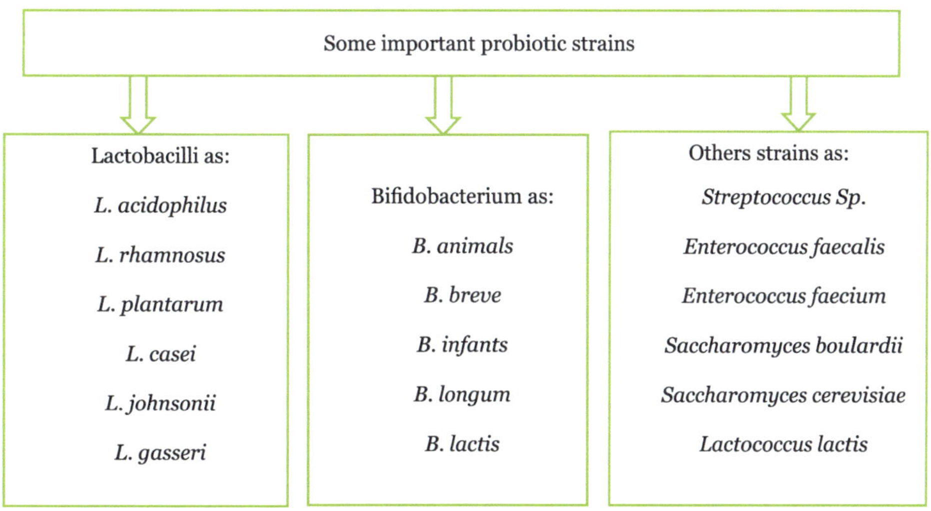

Figure 1.
Important probiotic strains.

Similarly, probiotics may also inhibit and opposite the working of parasites inside the intestine. Additionally, their productions could have anthelmintic values and may reduce many parasites' virulence. Also, probiotic strains play a wide range in the host body as decreasing illnesses and stress, enhancing immunity, modulation of gut microbiota, and nutritional assistance. From this point, probiotics may be used as a new and imperative strategy to control helminth parasites [22].

A suitable probiotic strain requirement to confer beneficial belongings (stimulate the immune, antimicrobial activity against pathogens, production of metabolism as bacteriocins and other compounds, and many others.), also, confirmed the probiotic strains to be not pathogenic, able to survive at low pH and acid conditions, thereby continuing within the intestine, and able to colonized and adhered inside the intestine epithelium [23, 24]. Approximately 50 traces similar to 26 species satisfy these standards. Probiotic strains are gram-positive bacteria, isolated from the human intestine microflora or numerous dairy products. However, the beneficial effects of probiotics were more usually tested in model animals than thru direct therapeutic indications and depended largely on the dose consumed. The dose of probiotics is suggested at least 5 billion colonies forming per day for a minimum of 5 days to give their effect [23]. This minimal dose takes under consideration the survival capability of the ingested probiotics inside the gastrointestinal tract, where they may be in opposition with the resident bacteria [25]. Three principal advantages are pronounced: Modulation of the intestinal surroundings, through probiotics having the capacity to manipulate the proliferation of surrounding microorganisms, and/or by using opposition for the occupancy of a common biotope (e.g., get entry to nutriments) [23]. As an example, iron is a proscribing nutriment—it is miles important for maximum bacteria and probiotics can compete for its availability. *Lactobacillus* can bind ferric hydroxide and reduces iron unavailability for pathogenic microorganisms [26] or by secreting siderophores that chelate and shipping iron [25]. Some probiotics are also capable to influence the composition and balance of the gut microflora [27]. For instance, in probiotic therapy, the use of a mixture of probiotics became shown to grow the whole number of intestinal microorganisms and to repair the variety of the bacterial microbiota in patients [28].

In the end, probiotics also can manage their biotic environment via regulation of intestinal motility and mucus secretion [23, 29]. Secretion of the energetic compounds (such as bacteriocins, antibiotics, loose fatty acids, and hydrogen peroxide) that could manage the boom and/or survival of surrounding microorganisms. Bacteriocins are secreted peptides or proteins that commonly kill closely associated bacteria by using penetrating their membranes or by means of interfering with vital enzymes [28]. Lots of them are produced with the aid of *Lactobacillus* probiotic lines (lactacin B, lactacin F, nisin, and so forth.). *Lactobacillus reuteri* produces reuterin (three-hydroxypropionaldehyde), an extensive-spectrum antibiotic, lively against bacteria, yeast, fungi, protozoa, and viruses [30]. By means of lowering the nearby intestinal pH with lactic acid, probiotics can also regulate the increase of acid-sensitive organisms [28]. Also, different probiotics were able to stimulate the reaction of the host immune to an expansion of pathogens to create immunity modulation. Within the intestine, probiotics join with the epithelial cells; Peyer's patches cells, and immune cells. Those interactions result in a boom within the quantity of IgA producing cells followed by a way of development of IgM and secretory IgA which might be particularly crucial in mucosal immunity, contributing to the barrier against pathogenic organisms [31, 32]. In addition, probiotics can also affect dendritic cells, which might be accountable for the collection of antigens from the intestine and their presentation to native T cells, leading to their differentiation to T-helper (Th1, Th2) or T-regulatory lymphocytes. Probiotic molecules implicated in dendritic cellular induction are poorly characterized, one exception being the S layer protein A of *Lactobacillus acidophilus* NCFM that regulates maturation of dendritic cells and T cell features [33]. Probiotics have additionally been shown to modulate cytokine release (TNF-α IFN-γ, IL-10, IL-12) [34]. Those cytokines play a valuable function in retaining the delicate balance between important and excessive protection mechanisms. For example, polysaccharide A, synthesized by *Bacillus fragilis* NCTC 9343, protects in opposition to experimental colitis via an adequate induction of IL-10 manufacturing [35].

3. Some examples for the effect of probiotics in helminth parasitic zoonosis

3.1 Effect of probiotic on Cryptosporidium

Cryptosporidium is an abdominal pathogen followed by the Alveolata group. It could cause overwhelming contamination of gastrointestinal in immunosuppressed humans. In the surroundings, the infective form Cryptosporidium is determined as oocyst found in water. After consumption, the oocysts passage through the gut lumen to the small intestine, in which they release the motile sporozoites that adhere and attack the epithelial intestine cells. The sporozoites are disrupting the microvilli and penetrate to the cells of the host to arrange their intracellular position, wherein they continue to be in a further cytoplasmic vacuole. After replication of parasite and elusion, oocysts are produced and excreted within the faces [36, 37]. Intestinal epithelial cells, inflamed by way of *Cryptosporidium parvum*, show lessened sodium ions and water absorption as well as greater chloride ion secretion, leading to diarrhea. Also, the use of paromomycin and azithromycin or nitazoxanide is the handiest powerful in mixture with immune restoring agents [38]. Beneficial outcomes of probiotics upon cryptosporidiosis have been tested—female mice were fed day-by-day for 4 weeks vintage with *L. reuteri* traces 4000 and 4020 or *L. acidophilus* NCFM provided reduced oocyst dropping [39, 40]. Waters et al. [41] recommended that protection becomes due to secretion of as yet unidentified antimicrobial products. Curiously, *in vitro* research tested the inhibitory results of cellular-unfastened supernatants of *L. acidophilus* NCFM and *L. reuteri* stress 23,272 on *C. parvum* and *C. hominis* viability and infectivity [42, 43]. In addition, mobile-unfastened supernatants of *Bacillus brevis*, *Enterococcus faecium,* and *Pseudomonas alcaligenes* reduce *C. parvum* oocyst persistence by inducing oocyst premature excystation [44, 45]. The compounds at the basis of such inhibition are under investigation. Pickerd and Tuthill, [46] resolved diarrhea due to *Cryptosporidium oocysts* via probiotic lines *Lactobacillus rhamnosus* GG 10^9 CFU/day and *Lactobacillus casei* Shirota 6.56 X 10^9 CFU/day during 4-week. Within 10 days of beginning, the pain was decreased and the pattern of stool unfastened from Cryptosporidium after 4 weeks after beginning with probiotics.

Also, Sanad et al. [47] studied the therapeutic effects of daily administration of a mixture of *L. acidophilus, L. helveticus,* and *Bifidobacterium bifidum against C. parvum* infection in an immunosuppressed mouse model. The parasite was not achieved by eradication. But, the infection of the probiotics used caused a significant reduction in parasite burden, ultrastructural changes with respect to parasite attachment, internalization into epithelial cells, partial compensation of the mucosal damage caused by the parasite, and an increase in serum level IFN. These results reveal the beneficial effects of probiotics on cryptosporidiosis and suggest that they can help to reduce the risk of serious disease in immunosuppressed patients.

Moreover, Del Coco et al. [48] studied the treated *C. parvum* infection by oral administration of *Enterococcus faecalis* CECT 7121 as probiotic strain in immunosuppressed mice. Also, studied the effect of *C. parvum* infection in the intestinal mucosa and counted at each part of the intestine. The results were established that when both *E. faecalis* and *C. parvum* were present in the same intestinal location happened interfered with them. Also, proposing that supplementation of *E. faecalis* can improve the harmful effects on infection of *C. parvum*. Also, Glass et al. [42] recognized that *L. acidophilus* (LA) and *L. reuteri* (LR) cell-free supernatants able to diminish about 21–42% and 30–35%, respectively of the infection of bovine *C. parvum* and *C. hominis* in a cell-culture immunofluorescence (CCIF) test. Moreover, reduction of oocyst viability reached 40–80% at 24 h incubation of bovine *C. parvum* oocysts in the bacterial cell-free supernatants and this reduction was evaluated by flow cytometric analysis and the infectivity of oocyst reached up to 95% by the CCIF analysis. So, the production of antimicrobial compounds secreted from LA and LR had a harmful effect on bovine *C. parvum* and *C. hominis*. Likewise, Khalifa [49] evaluated a study consisting of 70 mice as; 60 mice were infected with *Cryptosporidium oocysts and* immune-suppressed, other 10 mice were not infected and left immune-competent. Formerly, the mice were divided into three groups; group (1) infected mice were treated with *L. casei*, group (2) infected mice were treated with yogurt, and group (3) infected mice but not treated as control. The counts of oocyst in the mice stools were determined to evaluate the cryptosporidiosis progress and measured by the developmental stages in histopathological sections of ilea. The results found that the parasitic burden in mice was reduced by regular administration of yogurt and *L. casei* in comparison with the control group. Moreover, the use of yogurt daily was more effective than *L. casei* where the yogurt was stopped oocyst shedding previous than *L. casei* and the counts of oocyst were lesser during the experiment duration in comparison with infected mice that treated with *L. casei*. Previous studies indicated that the used probiotics are promising and hopeful to control and treated the parasite's development.

In contracts, Guitard et al. [50] studied the feeding rates with *L. casei* daily with 2×10^7 CFU before 2 days of the infection until the spontaneous clearance of the parasite. Effects on weight gain, parasite burden, mucosal histology, and production of mucosal cytokines (IFNγ, IL10, and TNFα). The authors also indicated that administration of probiotic strains through the infection course was not significantly affected the weight gain, parasite burden, mucosal damage, or mucosal cytokines kinetics. Overall, the studied model data revealed that the use of *L. casei* as regular administration was unable to eradicate the parasite. Other studies established that treatment the cryptosporidiosis by probiotic strains did not eradicate the parasite, but resulted in a moderate benefit with a decrease in parasite burden and mucosal damage, and these results were obtained after long-term feeding (7–28 days) or prolonged pre-feeding (≥7 days) before infection [51–55].

3.2 Effect of probiotics on Giardia

Giardia lamblia (also known as *Giardia intestinalis* or *Giardia duodenalis*) is an intestinal pathogenic protozoan parasite belonging to the Diplomonad institution that reasons ~280 million symptomatic human infections in line with 12 months [56]. This monoxenous waterborne parasite has the capability to contaminate an extensive variety of hosts. To initiate the infection for humans need, 10 environmentally resistant cysts to infect. When the cysts passage through the gastrointestinal, they unlock and replicates to form trophozoites. These trophozoites had the ability to reproduce inside the gut lumen and adhere to the epithelium. These proliferate of trophozoites in the gut was associated with the disorder symptoms, such as watery diarrhea, epigastric pain, nausea, vomiting, and weight drop, which appeared during 6–15 days after cyst consumption, but half of the infections stay asymptomatic. The infection was mainly treated by metronidazole and nitroimidazole, but infections can also solve spontaneously. The immune response T cells, neutrophils, macrophages also with IgM, IgG, and IgA antibodies are major players for the decision of giardiasis. *L. casei* MTCC 1423 stress as well as *E. faecium* SF68 were additionally effective in eliminating Giardia contamination from mice [53, 57]. Protection becomes related to a diminution of atrophied villi and infiltrating cells inside the small gut of probiotic-handled mice [57] or with an enhancement of the immune response for the reason that production of specific anti-Giardia intestinal IgA and IgG was noticed in dealing with mice. *In vivo* experimentation on malnourished mice showed that day-by-day pretreatment with *L. casei* MTCC1423 effectively decreased severity and period of giardiasis, as compared to non-probiotic-fed malnourished mice [58, 59].

Shukla et al. [60] determined the acid-tolerated strains of probiotics *L. casei* or *Lactobacillus* yogurt when found in the gastrointestinal tract. The authors have studied the possibility of these isolates to therapeutic treated the infected mice with the Giardia. After 1 day of Giardia infection, it was found that supplementation of probiotics either *L. casei* or L. yogurt were eliminated the infection severity comparison with Giardia infected mice. All changes in the Pathophysiologically, the morphological and cellular changes of the small intestine were slightest in treated mice with probiotics in compared to harshly inflamed, edematous, vacuolated epithelial cells in infected mice with Giardia. The results concluded that L. yogurt possessed better probiotic properties and has the possibility to diminish the severity of infection in mice with Giardia. Also, Goyal et al. [61] investigated the efficiency of four probiotic strains (*L. rhamnosus* GG (LGG), *L. acidophilus*, *L. plantarum*, and *L. casei*) against the murine giardiasis modulation. The daily strain was received around 10^9 CFU for single animal via orogastric gavage. The more effective strain was LGG, which proved more effect in decreasing the duration of *G. lamblia* cycle, by eliminating the active trophozoite number in the intestine, increasing cyst excretion, and leading to suppression of the disease around 13 days after trial inoculation. Amer et al. [62] evaluated *in vitro* and *in vivo* the beneficial effectiveness of bacteriocins that resulted from new Egyptian probiotic Lactobacilli strains [*L. acidophilus* (P106) and *L. plantarum* (P164)] against *G. lamblia*. The results showed that 50 μg of bacteriocin from *L. acidophilus* eliminated the trophozoites adherence and the counts around 58.3 ± 4.04%. Oral feeding of 50 μg/mouse of bacteriocin from *L. acidophilus* every 5 days was able to reduce the density of parasites inside the intestines and enhance the strength of the gut disease system of infected mice. The authors established that bacteriocin from strain *L. acidophilus* (P106) had a promising potential therapeutic outcome and alternative safety way instead of present commercial drugs to treat *G. lamblia*.

In the same line, the Bifidobacterium efficiency can be evaluated in an experiment against infected mice with *G. lamblia* infection. The single-dose about 0.1 ml of Bifidobacterium cells for every day significantly eliminated the *G. lamblia* cysts shedding in feces, and this infection was disappeared totally at the 5 days of probiotic Bifidobacterium inoculation. Also, in the mice group that used metronidazole, the authors found that Giardia cysts were reduced and infection cured on the day 17th of treatment, in comparison with the control group that showed parasite shedding cysts. Moreover, for histopathological results, *in vivo* by gut cells, the Bifidobacterium has prevented inflection of the Giardia colonization and able to reduce the infection with this parasite [63]. Generally, the usage of probiotic strains, such as *Lactobacillus* and *Saccharomyces*, had a positive influence to reduce gastrointestinal symptoms time and repair the damages, especially for giardiasis. Probiotics had the ability to control the composition of commensal microbiota and balance which lead to therapeutic impact. According to pre-clinical and clinical searches, different probiotic strains can increase the antioxidant capacity, destroy oxidative products, regulate the systemic, and activate the responses of mucosal immune as well as reduce gastrointestinal symptoms time, that lead to protect against mucosal damages that induced by parasites. In addition, they can reduce the *G. duodenalis* proportion load by directly targeting the parasite. They can produce some anti-giardial factors that feature destroy the parasite's cellular architecture and suppress the parasite's proliferation and growth [64, 65].

3.3 Effect of probiotics on Eimeria

Eimeria is an apicomplexan parasite responsible for formed coccidiosis found in poultry, cattle, rabbits, dogs, and cats mainly small animals. A primary parasitic ailment in poultry is avian coccidiosis, with a major economic importance worldwide impact [66]. When the chickens ingest oocysts, it is become inflamed and eventually exocyst to shape sporozoites within the lumen of the top gut. Those sporozoites migrate to their preferred sites of development. They then invade villi enterocytes and undergo a first asexual multiplication, the schizogony, leading to the discharge of numerous merozoites that initiate a 2d schizogony via infecting new epithelial cells. Macro- and microgametes are finally produced, starting up the sexual phase that yields environmental resistant oocysts which might be shed within the feces [67]. Two main ways to control this parasite are by drugs, such as amprolium, halofuginone, and monensin lasalocid, or live vaccines. But stay vaccines against coccidiosis are incredibly effective, primarily based on non-attenuated and attenuated lines.

Probiotic supplementation can enhance performance and help alleviate the negative effects of a mixed *Eimeria* infection. The study by Ritzi et al. [68] evaluated the effects of probiotics on birds and resistance to a mixed *Eimeria* infection in commercial broilers. Using treatments, including negative control (non-infected, NEG), positive control (*Eimeria*-infected, PoS), anticoccidial control (0.01% salinomycin, SAL), irregular high-dose water-applied probiotic (WPI), irregular low-dose water-applied probiotic (WPC), and feed-supplemented probiotic (FSP). On day 15 of the experiment, all birds except those in NEG were treated with a mixed dose of *Eimeria acervulina*, *Eimeria maxima*, and *Eimeria tenella*. Samples of birds feces were collected from day 20 to 24 for counts of the oocyst and evaluated the lesion scores were at day 21. The probiotic groups were comparable with the birds for SAL-treated, except during the 6 days immediately following the *Eimeria* species challenge, where the SAL birds displayed well performance. The lower duodenal and jejunal lesion scores were found for WPC birds, signifying a healthier intestine and improving the resistance to *Eimeria* species in comparison with the positive control (PoS). Also, fewer oocysts in the feces were recorded for birds in the WPI treatment, although this was not a trend for all of the probiotic treatment groups. The addition of probiotic secretion compounds containing *Pediococcus acidilactici* in the ration of the birds before experimental infection with *E. tenella* resulted in mild improvement in the performance parameters, a slight reduction in lesion score, and in the oocysts count when compared with the birds treated with anticoccidial drugs, but that picture was better than the infected non-treated group. The addition of compounds containing natural microflora (especially those producing lactic acid) to the poultry feed or water to overcome coccidial infection especially [69]. Also, chickens fed on *Lactobacillus*-based ration showed reduced oocysts output compared to controls after challenge with *E. acervulina* [70].

Another effect of probiotics was observed on malaria as the recent study by Elli et al. [71] investigated the use of probiotic *L. casei* in treating malaria in mice with chloroquine. Probiotics in combination with chloroquine showed complete suppression in the parasitemia rate. The data were established by histological observation of two major organs, the liver and spleen. Interestingly, further suppression of parasitemia and hemosiderosis was observed when probiotic was given along with chloroquine. Another author Oliveira-Sequeira et al. [72] have shown a reduction in the number of *Strongyloides venezuelensis* in infected mice about 33% and egg output upon feeding with probiotic *Bifidobacterium animalis*, and probiotics was improved the immune responses. A new study has linked the microbiome of the human gut with immunity against malaria infections. Gut probiotics represent innovative tools for malaria prevention and lead the way to novel types of vaccination strategies [73, 74].

Conflict of interest

All authors have no conflicts of interest to disclose.

Author details

Osama M. Darwesh[1]* and Hoda Samir El-Sayed[2]

1 Department of Agricultural Microbiology, Environmental Biotechnology and Nanotechnology group, National Research Centre, Cairo, Egypt

2 Department of Dairy Science, National Research Centre, Giza, Egypt

*Address all correspondence to: darweshosama@yahoo.com

References

[1] Goldsmid John. 2005. Zoonotic infections–an overview. Chapter 14, 14.1-14.14. Available at: http://www.tropmed.org/primer/chapter14

[2] El-Baz FK, Mahmoud K, El-Senousy WM, Darwesh OM, El Gohary AE. Antiviral – Antimicrobial and Schistosomicidal activities of Eucalyptus camaldulensis essential oils. International Journal of Pharmaceutical Sciences Review and Research. 2015;**31**(1):262-268

[3] Torgerson PR, Devleesschauwer B, Praet N, Speybroeck N, Willingham AL, Kasuga F, et al. World health organization estimates of the global and regional disease burden of 11 foodborne parasitic diseases, 2010: A data synthesis. PLoS Medicine. 2015;**12**:e1001920. DOI: 10.1371/journal.pmed.1001920

[4] Mohamed AA, Ali SI, Darwesh OM, El-Hallouty SM, Sameeh MY. Chemical compositions, potential cytotoxic and antimicrobial activities of Nitraria retusa Methanolic extract sub-fractions. International Journal of Toxicological and Pharmacological Research. 2015;7(4):204-212

[5] Bogitsh BJ, Carter CE, Oeltmann TN. Human parasitology. 5th ed. Cambridge, MA: Academic Press; 2019

[6] Darwesh OM, El-Hawary AS, El Kelany US, El-Sherbiny GM. Nematicidal activity of thermostable alkaline protease produced by Saccharomonospora viridis strain Hw G550. Biotechnology Reports. 2019;**24**:e00386. DOI: 10.1016/j.btre.2019.e00386

[7] Robinson MW, Dalton JP. Zoonotic helminth infections with particular emphasis on fasciolosis and other trematodiases. Philosophical Transactions of the Royal Society B. 2009;**364**(1530):2763-2776

[8] Darwesh OM, El-Maraghy SH, Abdel-Rahman HM, Zaghloul RA. Improvement of paper wastes conversion to bioethanol using novel cellulose degrading fungal isolate. Fuel. 2020;**262**:116518. DOI: 10.1016/j.fuel.2019.116518

[9] McCarthy J, Moore TA. Emerging helminth zoonoses. International Journal for Parasitology. 2000;**12-13**:1351-1360

[10] Abdelhameed RM, El-Sayed HA, El-Shahat M, El-Sayed AA, Darwesh OM. Novel Triazolothiadiazole and Triazolothiadiazine derivatives containing pyridine moiety: Design, synthesis, bactericidal and fungicidal activities. Current Bioactive Compounds. 2018;**14**(2):169-179. DOI: 10.2174/1573407213666170127095158

[11] Ali SI, Mohamed AA, Sameeh MY, Darwesh OM, Abd El-Razik TM. Gamma-irradiation affects volatile oil constituents, fatty acid composition and antimicrobial activity of fennel (Foeniculum vulgare) seeds extract. Research Journal of Pharmaceutical, Biological and Chemical Sciences. 2016;**7**(1):524-532

[12] Caradonna T, Marangi M, Del Chierico F, Ferrari N, Reddel S, Bracaglia G, et al. Detection and prevalence of protozoan parasites in ready-to-eat packaged salads on sale in Italy. Food Microbiology. 2017;**67**:67-75. DOI: 10.1016/j.fm.2017.06.006

[13] Sultan YY, Ali MA, Darwesh OM, Embaby MA, Marrez DA. Influence of nitrogen source in culture media on antimicrobial activity of Microcoleus

lacustris and Oscillatoria rubescens. Research Journal of Pharmaceutical, Biological and Chemical Sciences. 2016;7(2):1444-1452

[14] FAO/WHO. FAO/WHO Multicriteria-Based Ranking for Risk Management of Foodborne Parasites. Report of a Joint FAO/WHO Expert Meeting, 3-7 September 2012. Rome, Italy: FAO Headquarters; 2014. ISBN 978 92 4 156470 0(WHO); ISBN 978-92-5-108199-0 (print) (FAO); E-ISBN 978-92-5-108200-3(PDF) (FAO); ISSN 1726-5274

[15] Youssef AI, Uga S. Review of parasitic zoonoses in Egypt. Tropical Medicine and Health. 2013;**42**(1):3-14

[16] Abdel-Monem RA, Khalil AM, Darwesh OM, Hashim AI, Rabie ST. Antibacterial properties of carboxymethyl chitosan Schiff-base nanocomposites loaded with silver nanoparticles. Journal of Macromolecular Science, Part A. 2020;**57**(2):145-155. DOI: 10.1080/10601325.2019.1674666

[17] Darwesh OM, Eida MF, Matter IA. Isolation, screening and optimization of L-asparaginase producing bacterial strains inhabiting agricultural soils. Bioscience Research. 2018;**15**(3):2802-2812

[18] Darwesh OM, Sultan YY, Seif MM, Marrez DA. Bio-evaluation of crustacean and fungal nano-chitosan for applying as food ingredient. Toxicology Reports. 2018;**5**:348-356. DOI: 10.1016/j.toxrep.2018.03.002

[19] Hill C, Guarner F, Reid G, Gibson GR, Merenstein DJ, Pot B, et al. Expert consensus document: The international scientific Association for Probiotics and Prebiotics consensus statement on the scope and appropriate use of the term probiotic. Nature Reviews Gastroenterology & Hepatology. 2014;**11**:506-514

[20] Marrez DA, Shahy EM, El-Sayed HS, Sultan YY. Detoxification of aflatoxin B1 in milk using lactic acid bacteria. Journal of Biological Sciences. 2018;**18**(3): 144-151

[21] Sadek ZI, Abdel-Rahman MA, Azab MS, Darwesh OM, Hassan MS. Microbiological evaluation of infant foods quality and molecular detection of Bacillus cereus toxins relating genes. Toxicology Reports. 2018;**5**:871-877. DOI: 10.1016/j.toxrep.2018.08.013

[22] Berrilli F, Di Cave D, Cavallero S, D'Amelio S. Interactions between parasites and microbial communities in the human gut. Frontiers in Cellular and Infection Microbiology. 2012;**2**:141

[23] Gupta V, Garg R. Probiotics. Indian Journal of Medical Microbiology. 2009;**27**(3):202-209

[24] Kheiralla ZH, Hewedy MA, Mohammed HR, Darwesh OM. Isolation of pigment producing actinomycetes from rhizosphere soil and application it in textiles dyeing. Research Journal of Pharmaceutical, Biological and Chemical Sciences. 2016;7(5):2128-2136

[25] Oelschlaeger TA. Mechanisms of probiotic actions–a review. International Journal of Medical Microbiology. 2010;**300**(1):57-62

[26] Mourad R, Helaly F, Darwesh OM, Sawy SE. Antimicrobial and physicomechanical natures of silver nanoparticles incorporated into silicone-hydrogel films. Contact Lens & Anterior Eye. 2019;**42**:325-333. DOI: 10.1016/j.clae.2019.02.007

[27] Wohlgemuth S, Loh G, Blaut M. Recent developments and perspectives

in the investigation of probiotic effects. International Journal of Medical Microbiology. 2010;**300**(1):3-10

[28] Kuehbacher T, Ott SJ, Helwig U, Mimura T, Rizzello F, Kleessen B, et al. Bacterial and fungal microbiota in relation to probiotic therapy (VSL# 3) in pouchitis. Gut. 2006;**55**(6):833-841

[29] Mourad RM, Darwesh OM, Abdel-Hakim A. Enhancing physico-mechanical and antibacterial properties of natural rubber using synthesized Ag-SiO2 nanoparticles. International Journal of Biological Macromolecules. 2020;**164**:3243-3249. DOI: 10.1016/j.ijbiomac.2020.08.063

[30] Cleusix V, Lacroix C, Vollenweider S, Le Blay G. Glycerol induces reuterin production and decreases Escherichia coli population in an in vitro model of colonic fermentation with immobilized human feces. FEMS Microbiology Ecology. 2008;**63**(1):56-64

[31] Szajewska H, Kotowska M, Mrukowicz JZ, Arma M, Mikolajczyk W. Efficacy of Lactobacillus GG in prevention of nosocomial diarrhea in infants. The Journal of Pediatrics. 2001;**138**(3):361-365

[32] Perdigon G, Alvarez S, Rachid M, Agüero G, Gobbato N. Immune system stimulation by probiotics. Journal of Dairy Science. 1995;**78**(7):1597-1606

[33] Konstantinov SR, Smidt H, de Vos WM, Bruijns SC, Singh SK, Valence F, et al. S layer protein a of Lactobacillus acidophilus NCFM regulates immature dendritic cell and T cell functions. Proceedings of the National Academy of Sciences. 2008;**105**(49):19474-19479

[34] Arvola T, Laiho K, Torkkeli S, Mykkänen H, Salminen S, Maunula L, et al. Prophylactic lactobacillus GG reduces antibiotic-associated Diarrhea in children with respiratory infections: A randomized study. Pediatrics. 1999;**104**(5):e64-e64

[35] Mazmanian SK, Round JL, Kasper DL. A microbial symbiosis factor prevents intestinal inflammatory disease. Nature. 2008;**453**(7195):620-625

[36] Clark DP. New insights into human cryptosporidiosis. Clinical Microbiology Reviews. 1999;**12**(4):554-563

[37] Darwesh OM, Barakat KM, Mattar MZ, Sabae SZ, Hassan SH. Production of antimicrobial blue green pigment Pyocyanin by marine Pseudomonas aeruginosa. Biointerface Research in Applied Chemistry. 2019;**9**(5):4334-4339. DOI: 10.33263/BRIAC95.334339

[38] Gargala G. Drug treatment and novel drug target against Cryptosporidium. Parasite. 2008;**15**(3):275-281

[39] Alak JI, Wolf BW, Mdurvwa EG, Pimentel-Smith GE, Adeyemo O. Effect of Lactobacillus reuteri on intestinal resistance to Cryptosporidium parvum infection in a murine model of acquired immunodeficiency syndrome. Journal of Infectious Diseases. 1997;**175**(1):218-221

[40] Alak JI, Wolf BW, Mdurvwa EG, Pimentel-Smith GE, Kolavala S, Abdelrahman H, et al. Supplementation with Lactobacillus reuteri or L. acidophilus reduced intestinal shedding of cryptosporidium parvum oocysts in immunodeficient C57BL/6 mice. Cellular and Molecular Biology. 1999;**45**(6):855-863

[41] Waters WR, Harp JA, Wannemuehler MJ, Carbajal NY, CASAS I. Effects of Lactobacillus reuteri on Cryptosporidium parvum infection of gnotobiotic TCR-alpha-deficient mice.

Journal of Eukaryotic Microbiology. 1999;**46**(5):60S-61S

[42] Glass MD, Courtney PD, LeJeune JT, Ward LA. Effects of Lactobacillus acidophilus and Lactobacillus reuteri cell-free supernatants on Cryptosporidium viability and infectivity in vitro. Food Microbiology. 2004;**21**(4):423-429

[43] Foster JC, Glass MD, Courtney PD, Ward LA. Effect of Lactobacillus and Bifidobacterium on Cryptosporidium parvum oocyst viability. Food Microbiology. 2003;**20**(3):351-357

[44] Deng M, Nuanualsuwan S, Cliver DO. Inactivation of Cryptosporidium parvum oocysts by bacterial strains. Journal of Eukaryotic Microbiology. 2001;**48**:37s-39s

[45] Darwesh OM, Matter IA, Eida MF, Moawad H, Oh Y. Influence of nitrogen source and growth phase on extracellular biosynthesis of silver nanoparticles using cultural filtrates of Scenedesmus obliquus. Applied Sciences. 2019;**9**:1465. DOI: 10.3390/app9071465

[46] Pickerd N, Tuthill D. Resolution of cryptosporidiosis with probiotic treatment. Postgraduate Medical Journal. 2004;**80**(940):112-113

[47] Sanad MM, Al-Malki JS, Al-Ghabban AG. Control of cryptosporidiosis by probiotic bacteria. In: International Conference on Agricultural, Ecological and Medical Sciences (AEMS-2015). 2015. pp. 7-8

[48] Del Coco VF, Sparo MD, Sidoti A, Santín M, Basualdo JA, Córdoba MA. Effects of Enterococcus faecalis CECT 7121 on Cryptosporidium parvum infection in mice. Parasitology Research. 2016;**115**(8):3239-3244

[49] Khalifa EA. Probiotics as a promising treatment of experimental cryptosporidiosis in an immuno suppressed mouse model. International Journal of Current Microbiology and Applied Sciences. 2016;**5**(3):97-106

[50] Guitard J, Menotti J, Desveaux A, Alimardani P, Porcher R, Derouin F, et al. Experimental study of the effects of probiotics on Cryptosporidium parvum infection in neonatal rats. Parasitology Research. 2006;**99**(5):522-527

[51] Szajewska H, Mrukowicz JZ. Probiotics in the treatment and prevention of acute infectious diarrhea in infants and children: A systematic review of published randomized, double-blind, placebo-controlled trials. Journal of Pediatric Gastroenterology and Nutrition. 2001;**33**:S17-S25

[52] Santos JDFM, Vasconcelos J, Souza JRD, Coutinho EDM, Montenegro SML, Azevedo-Ximenes E. The effect of Zymomonas mobilis culture on experimental Schistosoma mansoni infection. Revista da Sociedade Brasileira de Medicina Tropical. 2004;**37**:502-504

[53] Benyacoub J, Perez PF, Rochat F, Saudan KY, Reuteler G, Antille N, et al. Enterococcus faecium SF68 enhances the immune response to Giardia intestinalis in mice. The Journal of Nutrition. 2005;**135**(5):1171-1176

[54] Humen MA, De Antoni GL, Benyacoub J, Costas ME, Cardozo MI, Kozubsky L, et al. Lactobacillus johnsonii La1 antagonizes Giardia intestinalis in vivo. Infection and Immunity. 2005;**73**(2):1265-1269

[55] Darwesh OM, Matter IA, Almoallim HS, Alharbi SA, Oh YK. Isolation and optimization of Monascus ruber OMNRC45 for red pigment production and evaluation of the

pigment as a food colorant. Applied Sciences. 2020;**10**:8867. DOI: 10.3390/app10248867

[56] Ankarklev J, Jerlström-Hultqvist J, Ringqvist E, Troell K, Svärd SG. Behind the smile: Cell biology and disease mechanisms of Giardia species. Nature Reviews Microbiology. 2010;**8**(6):413-422

[57] Shukla G, Devi P, Sehgal R. Effect of Lactobacillus casei as a probiotic on modulation of giardiasis. Digestive Diseases and Sciences. 2008;**53**(10):2671-2679

[58] Shukla G, Sidhu RK. Lactobacillus casei as a probiotic in malnourished Giardia lamblia-infected mice: A biochemical and histopathological study. Canadian Journal of Microbiology. 2011;**57**(2):127-135

[59] Darwesh OM, Elshahawy IE. Silver nanoparticles inactivate sclerotial formation in controlling white rot disease in onion and garlic caused by the soil borne fungus Stromatinia cepivora. European Journal of Plant Pathology. 2021;**160**:917-934. DOI: 10.1007/s10658-021-02296-7

[60] Shukla G, Sharma G, Goyal N. Probiotic characterization of lactobacilli and yeast strains isolated from whey beverage and therapeutic potential of Lactobacillus yoghurtin murine giardiasis. American Journal of Biomedical Sciences. 2010;**2**(3):248-261

[61] Goyal N, Tiwari RP, Shukla G. Lactobacillus rhamnosus GG as an effective probiotic for murine giardiasis. Interdisciplinary Perspectives on Infectious Diseases. 2011;**2011**:795219

[62] Amer EI, Mossallam SF, Mahrous H. Therapeutic enhancement of newly derived bacteriocins against Giardia lamblia. Experimental Parasitology. 2014;**146**:52-63

[63] Abd AL-Khaliq, I. M. Effect of Bifidobacterium probiotic in the treatment of giardiasis infection in mice. Baghdad Science Journal. 2019;**16**(4):0849-0849

[64] Dashti N, Zarebavani M. Probiotics in the management of Giardia duodenalis: An update on potential mechanisms and outcomes. Naunyn-Schmiedeberg's Archives of Pharmacology. 2021;**394**(9):1869-1878

[65] Ventura LLA, Oliveira DRD, Gomes MA, Torres MRF. Effect of probiotics on giardiasis. Where are we? Brazilian Journal of Pharmaceutical Sciences. 2018;**54**:e17360

[66] Lee SH, Lillehoj HS, Dalloul RA, Park DW, Hong YH, Lin JJ. Influence of Pediococcus-based probiotic on coccidiosis in broiler chickens. Poultry Science. 2007;**86**(1):63-66

[67] Shirley MW, Smith AL, Tomley FM. The biology of avian Eimeria with an emphasis on their control by vaccination. Advances in Parasitology. 2005;**60**:285-330

[68] Ritzi MM, Abdelrahman W, Mohnl M, Dalloul RA. Effects of probiotics and application methods on performance and response of broiler chickens to an Eimeria challenge. Poultry Science. 2014;**93**(11):2772-2778

[69] Abo EL-Ghany WA, Amer MK, Abd EL-Gaied SS, Amer MM. Comparative study on the effect of a probiotic different anti coccidial drugs against Eimeria tenella infection in broilers chickens. Veterinary Medical Journal. 2007;**55**(1):245

[70] Dalloul RA, Lillehoj HS, Shellem TA, Doerr JA. Enhanced mucosal immunity against Eimeria acervulina in broilers fed a Lactobacillus-based probiotic. Poultry Science. 2003;**82**(1):62-66

[71] Elli M, Zink R, Rytz A, Reniero R, Morelli L. Iron requirement of Lactobacillus spp. in completely chemically defined growth media. Journal of Applied Microbiology. 2000;**88**(4):695-703

[72] Oliveira-Sequeira TCG, David ÉB, Ribeiro C, Guimarães S, Masseno APB, Katagiri S, et al. Effect of Bifidobacterium animalis on mice infected with Strongyloides venezuelensis. Revista do Instituto de Medicina Tropical de São Paulo. 2014;**56**:105-109

[73] Ngwa CJ, Pradel G. Coming soon: Probiotics-based malaria vaccines. Trends in Parasitology. 2015;**31**(1):2-4

[74] Villarino NF, LeCleir GR, Denny JE, Dearth SP, Harding CL, Sloan SS, et al. Composition of the gut microbiota modulates the severity of malaria. Proceedings of the National Academy of Sciences. 2016;**113**(8):2235-2240

Chapter 5

New Uses for Old Drugs and Their Application in Helminthology

Victor Hugo Del Río-Araiza, Romel Hernandéz-Bello and Jorge Morales-Montor

Abstract

Parasitic infection research, performed on both humans and domestic animals, has been mostly focused on vaccines, diagnostic methods, epidemiology, and the evolutionary origins of parasites, thanks to the emergence of genomics and proteomics. However, the basic biology of the host-parasite interactions of several medical or veterinary important parasites has not been fully studied. Limited information has been obtained on the intricate neuroimmunoendocrine effects of host-parasite interplay in particular; therefore, the consequences of these interactions, and their possible therapeutic applications, are in need of thorough research. The current manuscript attempts to review the available literature regarding the host-parasite neuroimmunoendocrine network and to discuss how this basic research can be used to design new treatments using hormones, antihormones, and hormone analogs as a novel therapy against parasitic diseases. In addition, these studies may also contribute in identifying alternative treatments for parasitic diseases in the future. The complex immune-endocrine network may also help in explaining the frequently conflicting results observed in infections with regards to host sex and age and offer helpful insight into other research avenues besides parasite treatment and control strategies. Finally, several natural products isolated from plants, used in traditional medicine, offer an alternative approach for natural products in the preparation of inexpensive and effective antiparasitic drugs.

Keywords: drugs, parasitic diseases, parasitology, parasite, parasite infection treatment

1. Introduction

Parasitic infections rank amongst the most significant causes of morbidity and mortality in the world, yet economic and other factors have contributed to a lack of innovation in treating these diseases. Nitazoxanide (NTZ), a pyruvate ferredoxin oxidoreductase inhibitor, is a new antiparasitic drug notable for its activity in treating common intestinal helminths. The availability of a product with this spectrum of activity raises interesting new possibilities for treating intestinal parasitic infections [1]. Recent studies have shown that NTZ inhibits pyruvate ferredoxin oxidoreductase (PFOR), a vital enzyme of central intermediary metabolism in protozoan. In contrast to the nitroimidazoles, NTZ appears to interact directly with PFOR (i.e., NTZ is not

IntechOpen

dependent on reduced ferredoxin), and the products of NTZ activation do not induce mutations in DNA. This distinct mechanism of action is important in explaining the therapeutic efficacy of this drug against organisms displaying high level of resistance to metronidazole [2].

The use of hormones, or hormone antagonists, as immunoregulators or as agents to prevent colonization, growth, or reproduction of parasites, may be potentially useful in the treatment of a large variety of parasitic diseases, particularly those in which hormones are known to have a strong controlling effect. The discovery of new antiparasitic drugs is a very expensive process that has resulted in few drugs being commercialized over an extended period of time (**Figure 1**).

Since new drugs must be targeted against parasite survival interactions and be selective and unimpaired by known resistance mechanisms, the knowledge gained by studying physiological regulation of the host-parasite interaction could make it less expensive and faster, to produce antiparasitic drugs. Recent advances in genomic technology offer us the opportunity to identify, validate, and develop constructs of parasite key molecules that could be regulated by hormones, for testing drugs such as tamoxifen, RU-486, fadrozole, or flutamide (all of them hormone agonists) that could result in the identification of antiparasitic drug targets. This would also give new uses to old drugs that are already on the market. Understanding how the host's neuroimmunoendocrine system can, under certain circumstances, favor the colonization of a parasite and how the characterization of the parasite's hormone receptors involved might assist the design of hormonal analogs and drugs that affect the parasite exclusively [3]. Most of the current research on parasitic infections that affect humans and domestic animals has been focused on vaccines, diagnostic methods, epidemiology, new drug design, and recently, with the advancement of genomics and proteomics, on the evolutionary origins of parasites. However, the design of new treatments using hormones, antihormones, and hormone analogs as a possible novel therapy during parasitic diseases has been recently proposed. The pharmaceutical industry is now currently investing a higher sum of resources in the development of new antiparasitic

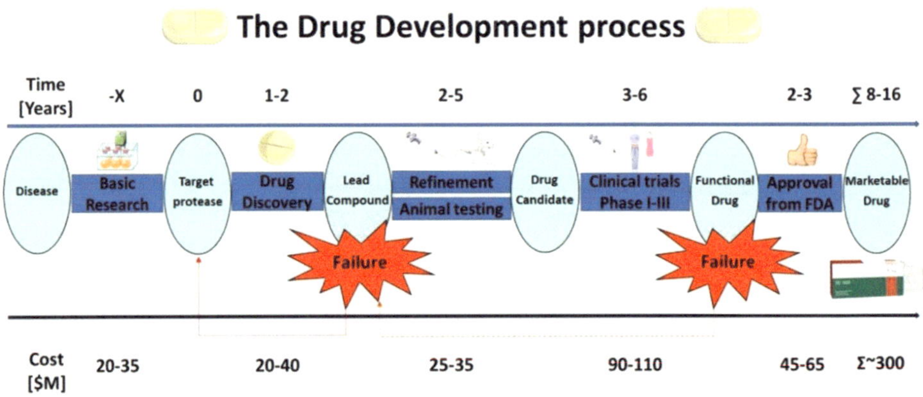

Figure 1.
The cost and time of the drug development process. It does start with targeting the disease. Then it goes throughout the basic research until it gets the lead compound. If there is a failure, and the compound is not promissory, then it goes back. Then the process continues until a marketable drug is obtained. The accumulated cost is around 300 million dollars to get to the final product. Today, these costs are being greatly decreased. The time since the basic compound is found in the marketable drug is around 20 years. However, it may be more if there are failures in the development of the same. In the case of helminthology, few compounds are being discovered since praziquantel, mebendazole, and albendazole were discovered.

drugs. We and other research groups (focusing mainly on sex-associated susceptibility to infection, the direct effects of adrenal and sex steroids as well as the study of parasite genomes) have suggested the study of known drugs, whose formulae have been redesigned, to test possible antiparasitic function. In this respect, animal models are highly convenient in the study of infectious diseases and the design and test of new drugs. It is desirable that these drugs are also tested in *in vitro* systems, where parasite growth, reproduction, and viability can be evaluated in response to pharmacological treatment [3]. An *in vitro* approach is convenient when seeking to define the molecular mechanisms by which a drug affects a parasite without including host-parasite interaction parameters (**Figure 2**).

In the present manuscript, we highlight the novel use of known drugs (currently used in cancer treatment and other proliferative disorders) to treat parasitic infections, i.e., cysticercosis, trichinellosis, ascariasis, schistosomiasis, toxocariasis, onchocerciasis, and others helminthic infections. Parasite fecundity is extremely important in the biological course of infection, therefore, it is worth considering some of the well-described antiproliferative drugs, which may also have inhibitory effects upon parasite reproduction, even if pathogens are inside the host cell. The genome of several parasites is currently being sequenced, which enables the knowledge acquisition on the molecular mechanisms involved in the infectious process, as well as in the design of different transcriptome maps, that could potentially explain the interaction and expression of the involved genes in parasite colonization and reproduction [3]. Hormonal effects are the keystone for parasite development. Experimental evidence, previously obtained by our group, suggests that the scolex evagination of *Taenia solium* cysticerci is stimulated by progesterone, however, other authors refer to the opposite effect for progesterone, which inhibits the reproduction and parasite molting in *Trichinella spiralis* [4, 5]. The target genes for progesterone action remain to be identified, and we must wonder if commercial progestin would inhibit parasite reproduction and differentiation. Although the knowledge of host-parasite interactions has grown over the last few years, there are still many unanswered questions that would allow us to fully unravel these host-parasite events and consider the complex neuroimmunoendocrine network involved in this pathogenic relationship. With this in mind, it is important to understand the biological role of sex steroids and the use of their inhibitors, alongside other drugs, aimed to inhibit cellular proliferation in the parasite. An experimental approach could clarify these points and further contribute

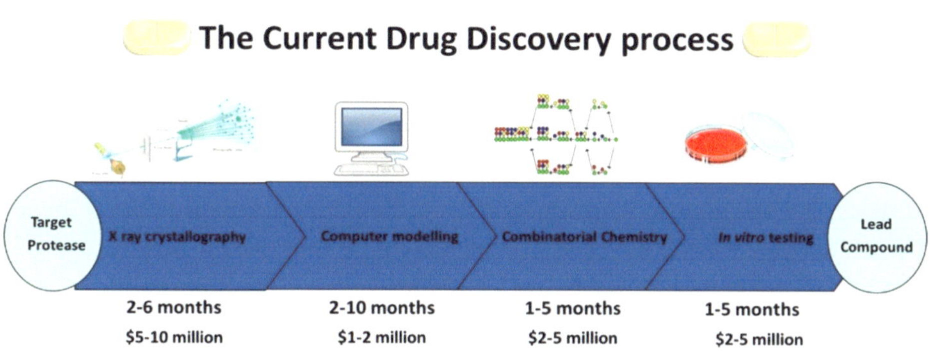

Figure 2.
The current drug discovery process specifically in helminthology. In this case, we focus on proteases as an example. But it is only the step of finding the lead compound. It can take up to 3 years to find the lead compound, and up to 2 million dollars to obtain it. Then, it has to go throughout all the further steps pointed out in **Figure 1**.

to elucidating the host's biological factors that control, or facilitate infection. Research on drugs utilized to treat different diseases could well allow the discovery of their active role in the regulation of parasite gene transcription during proliferation. Only a few novel classes of antiparasitic drugs have emerged over the last few decades thus reflecting the difficulties associated with bringing a safe and effective molecule to the market. Moreover, the screening paradigm has shifted from an empirical whole parasite screening to mechanism-based high-throughput screening. This approach requires a heavy investment in molecular parasitology and in depth understanding of the basic biology of parasites, as well as considerable infrastructure for the screening assays. Add to this the fact that the drug discovery process is interactive with high attrition, and the animal health industry, by necessity, must focus on discovering medicines for diseases that will provide a profit in return. In this regard, the rapid progression of genomics has unlocked a plethora of tools dedicated to target identification, validation, and screening, resulting in revolutionizing mechanism-based screening methods for antiparasitic drug discovery [3]. Therefore, the use of sexual hormones, their analogs, and other immune-regulatory factors are receiving more attention concerning new therapeutic strategies in the prevention and outcome of parasitic diseases. As an example, the treatment with testosterone or dihydrotestosterone in a model of murine cysticercosis, prior to infection, reduced the parasite load by 50% and 70%, respectively. This effect was mediated by significant lymphocyte proliferation recovery and enhanced IL-2 and IFN-γ production in the infected mice [6], suggesting the possible use of androgens to activate the host's immune system and increase resistance against lethal infections [7]. Estrogens and progestins, particularly estradiol and progesterone, contribute to either susceptibility or resistance to parasitic disease during pregnancy [8]. Usually, these sexual hormones are associated with immunosuppression leading to susceptibility to infection, as demonstrated in the murine cysticercosis model [9, 10]. However, parasiticidal activity was observed in murine trichinellosis. *In vitro* and *in vivo* experiments performed on *Trichinella spiralis* newborn larvae (NBL) in pregnant rats showed that progesterone can induce activation of peritoneal cells to destroy NBL in an antibody-independent manner. This observation opened up the possibility for the use of progesterone to treat trichinellosis but not cysticercosis [11, 12]. Sexual hormone precursors, analogs, antagonists, or inhibitors can also be used to modify the immune response induced by specific parasites to affect the outcome of infection. For example, exogenous administration of dehydroepiandrosterone confers resistance to several intracellular metazoan and protozoan parasites [13–15]. Concerning *Taenia crassiceps* in specific, this effect is not mediated through over induction of the Th1 response. Instead, the antiparasitic effect of dehydroepiandrosterone targets the reproduction, growth, viability, and infectivity of the parasite [16]. Regarding sexual steroid analogs, the synthetic androstane steroid 16α-bromoepiandrosterone (HE2000) has shown positive immune effects in experimental infection as malaria and tuberculosis, even infection with human immunodeficiency virus [17], due to its anti-inflammatory properties and the induction of innate and adaptive cellular immunity [13, 17–19].

In other studies, the inhibition of sexual hormones induced the recovery of a specific cellular immune response. Recently, the use of phytoestrogens as antiparasitic drugs has increased. Genistein, an isoflavone isolated from soybean, exhibits significant metacestodicidal activity *in vitro* but also binds to the ER and induces estrogenic effects. Furthermore, modified synthetic genistein derivatives have shown improved metacestodicidal activity [20].

2. Resistance to antihelminthic drugs

The development of resistance to antihelminthic drugs is an increasing problem that compromises livestock productivity and threatens the success of treatment in humans [21]. The intensive use of drugs in the livestock industry has led to widespread resistance to all current antihelminthic drugs [22]. Notably, resistance to antihelminthic drugs occurred rather quickly after their introduction to animals. The first widely administered antihelminthic, phenothiazine, was introduced into the market in the 1940s, and resistant populations were reported by 1957. In 1961, thiabendazole was released by 1964, resistance to this compound had been reported. Similar trends occurred with the release of levamisole in 1968, ivermectin in 1981, and moxidectin in 1991 [21]. Resistance to these was reported in 1979, 1988, and 1995, respectively [23]. Parasite populations are genetically heterogeneous, and this genetic diversity leads to a variable response to drugs. Although the impact of parasitic diseases could be reduced dramatically by improved sanitation for humans and pasture control in domestic animals, such methods are not sufficient to eradicate helminths [21], which are treated with a variety of drugs, i.e., macrocyclic lactones, benzimidazoles, imidazothiazoles, and praziquantel [24].

3. Alternative drugs for parasitology

The fact that hormones have a direct effect upon parasites opens the possibility for designing new strategies for parasitic control and hormonal therapy based on: (1) the knowledge of which hormone has direct restrictive actions on pathogen growth, reproduction, and/or differentiation, independently of the immune system; (2) the design of hormonal analogs that exclusively affect the parasite, diminishing any collateral effects upon the host; and (3) the improvement of drugs that competitively bind to parasite receptors, thus blocking gene expression as well as other important cellular processes of the invading organism.

The pharmaceutical industry invests ~25 million dollars annually for the development of new antiparasitic drugs. However, some of these drugs are being commercialized almost every fifteen years. These new antiparasitic drugs focus on interfering with the parasite's survival; however, they also must be safe for the host and avoid cross-resistance with other existent drugs. Furthermore, the development of new drugs is an expensive and very slow process since these drug candidates must first be tested in experimental animal models where high antiparasitic efficiency and low toxicity for the host must be evaluated before they can be tested in humans. This process takes at least 5–10 years, being the main reason why the pharmaceutical industry and medical research have stopped this task. Presently, the current age of parasite genomics promises to reduce both the cost and time of antiparasitic drug development, again with an impact on the pharmaceutical industry and medical research. However, the genome of several parasites is still being sequenced, and the uses and applications derived from that knowledge are thought to be applicable in at least another five to ten years.

With the results obtained at our laboratory and elsewhere, our research group has sought the possibility of using old drugs (unrelated to parasite infections) with renewed formulae to test their antiparasitic potential in experimental infection models *in vitro* and *in vivo*. In addition, the dire need of developing countries to control or eradicate parasitic infections led us to test certain drugs currently approved by the Food and Drug Administration (FDA) for human use as a strategy to reduce the impact of these parasitic diseases, but also reducing the costs and time in which a new drug is generated.

Considering the fact that parasite reproduction is extremely important in the biological course of the infection, it is possible that some of the well-described antiproliferative drugs could also have inhibitory effects on parasite reproduction (**Table 1**).

The challenge remains, however, to identify novel chemical entities with the required properties to deliver a safe and effective antiparasitic drug. At present, we have data suggesting that steroids can exert a wide spectrum of effects (suppression or induction) on the host's immune system during the course of infection and also affect the viability of metazoan parasites. In this regard, the use of sexual hormones, their analogs, and other immunoregulatory factors is being focused to develop alternative therapeutic strategies to prevent parasitic diseases.

The hypothesis that sex steroids regulate the expression of genes important in either susceptibility or resistance to infection has been explored by testing antihormonal and antiproliferative drugs.

3.1 Dehydroepiandrosterone

We have also shown the protective effects of progesterone on neutered mice infected with *Taenia crassiceps* cysticerci. Neutered male and female mice treated with progesterone were completely protected from the parasite in comparison with untreated-infected, infected Gx, and vehicle-treated infected mice. These results showed higher protective levels than any other reported in the literature yet, including vaccination. Notably, no variation was observed in this experimental system, which otherwise, showed large differences in parasite numbers among mice. The fact that progesterone was being metabolized to DHEA further supports our data indicating that progesterone levels were not as high as expected and, in contrast, DHEA levels were greatly increased. Thus, it seems that the observed effects were the result of adrenal conversion of progesterone metabolism to DHEA. This hypothesis was confirmed when the administration of DHEA prior to infection reduced the parasite load by 50% when compared with untreated mice. Interestingly, this protective effect

Compound	Current status	Possible parasiticidal use	References
DHEA	Complementary health therapy	Schistosomiasis and taeniasis	[14–16, 25–29]
Tamoxifen	Cancer drug	Cysticercosis	[26, 30]
Doxycycline	Antibiotics	Filarial diseases	[31–38]
Amiodarone	For irregular heartbeat treatment	Schistosomiasis	[39–49]
Paclitaxel	Cancer drug	*Echinococcus* protoscoleces and metacestodes	[50, 51]
Docetaxel	Cancer drug	Alveolar echinococcosis	[51]
Cisplatin	Cancer drug	Schistosomiasis	[52]
Genistein	Reduce symptoms of menopause	Metacestodicidal effect	[53–62]

Table 1.
Antiproliferative compounds with parasiticidal effects upon parasites.

was not associated with the host's immune response as there was no effect on the mRNA levels of interleukin (IL)-2, interferon (IFN), IL-4, or IL-10; notably, *in vitro* treatment of *Taenia crassiceps* with DHEA reduced reproduction, motility, and viability in a dose- and time-dependent manner. These results indicate that DHEA has a direct and strong negative modulation effect on murine cysticercosis [16]. DHEA has been demonstrated as a strong parasiticidal molecule in several systems. In another study, exogenous DHEA administration was shown to upregulate the immune system, specifically the cellular immune response, by increasing the number and function of natural killer cells [25]. However, our findings do not support this notion since IL-2 mRNA levels do not change in response to DHEA treatment [16]. The lack of any DHEA effect on cytokine expression, regardless of its dramatic effect on parasite load and reproduction *in vivo* and on survival *in vitro*, supports the hypothesis that DHEA exerts its protective properties by directly affecting the parasite. To the best of our knowledge, this effect is consistent with the known effects of DHEA on the survival of protozoan parasites [14–16].

For example, it has been suggested that in human schistosomiasis, DHEA is the cause of the puberty-associated drop in susceptibility. This idea has been reinforced by experiments in which the treatment of mice with the bloodstream form of DHEA (DHEA-s) protected them from infection with *Schistosoma mansoni* [15].

In this manuscript, we extend these findings on the role of DHEA in protecting mice against *Taenia crassiceps* infection. Our findings of decreased DHEA levels in mice as the infection progresses agree with previous results in a *S. mansoni*-baboon model, in which baboons with primary infections showed decreasing levels of DHEA as the infection progressed, compared with uninfected and re-exposed baboons [63].

Our results showing that DHEA treatment protects mice against *Taenia crassiceps* infection support and extend the notion that androgens are an important factor involved in limiting *Taenia crassiceps* colonization in immunocompetent hosts. Previous immunological experiments have suggested that testosterone and dihydrotestosterone, two potent androgens (such as DHEA), negatively regulate parasite reproduction in mice of both sexes, presumably by interfering with the thymus-dependent cellular immune mechanisms that inhibit parasite growth (Th2) and enhancing those that facilitate it (Th1) [63], but also by directly affecting parasite motility, survival, and reproduction [16].

It has been shown that administration of tamoxifen (an antiestrogen) increases the cellular immune response, which protects against the parasite but also has a direct parasiticidal effect on the parasite's reproduction, motility, and survival. These activities lead to a reduction of 80% and 50% of parasite burden in female and male mice infected with *Taenia crassiceps*, respectively. Also, increased mRNA levels of interleukin (IL)-2 (Th1) and IL-4 (Th2) and a decreased expression of estrogen receptors (ER) (ER-α and ER-β) were observed. In all, these features indicate that the treatment of cysticercosis with tamoxifen could well be a new therapeutic possibility [26]. In other cases, the inhibition of sexual hormones could induce recovery of the specific cellular immune response. In murine cysticercosis, 17β-estradiol (E_2) positively regulates parasite reproduction in hosts of both genders, obstructing the Th1 response and facilitating the Th2 immune response [27, 28]. Administration of fadrozole, an aromatase inhibitor, suppressed the production of 17β-estradiol in males and females interfering with the enzyme P450 aromatase, which converts testosterone to E2 in ovary and testes [29]. This led to a 70% reduction in parasite burden, an increase in IL-6 serum levels, and a shift of the Th2 to the Th1 immune response [9], opening the possibility of a new therapeutic approach against several infections.

3.2 Tamoxifen

Tamoxifen is one of the most prescribed drugs used in cases of estrogen-dependent breast cancer in the world. A selective modulator of estrogen receptors, its mechanism of action is to prevent estrogen binding in cancer cells, thus halting replication and cancer progression. Indicated in the treatment or prevention of breast cancer, it is administered continuously over 5 years with daily doses of 20–40 mg [30]. The use of Tamoxifen in parasitic diseases, such as *Taenia crassiceps*, has also been attempted, showing that tamoxifen administration produced an 80% parasite load reduction in female mice and a weaker effect of 50% in male mice [26]. This protective effect was associated, in both genders, with increased mRNA levels of IL-2 (a cytokine associated with protection against cysticerci) and IL-4 (no effect on infection). *In vitro*, treatment of *Taenia crassiceps* with tamoxifen reduced both reproduction rate and loss of motility. These results indicate that tamoxifen treatment is a new therapeutic possibility in the treatment of cysticercosis because it can act at both ends of the host-parasite interaction, i.e., increasing the protective cellular immune response against the parasite and directly affecting the parasite's reproduction and survival capabilities [26].

3.3 Antibiotics

Antibiotics do not have any antiparasitic effects against helminths; however, different therapeutical approach has been developed in the last two decade for filarial diseases. Filarial nematodes (*Onchocerca volvulus*, *Wuchereria bancrofti* and *Brugia* spp) infect over 138 million individuals worldwide, causing morbidity, disability, and economic hardship and are distributed mainly in tropical and subtropical regions. The majority of infections are caused by *Onchocerca volvulus*, which causes human Onchocerciasis (river blind-ness) in sub-Saharan Africa, Latin America, and the Arabian Peninsula [31, 32]. After Onchocerciasis Control Programme (OCP) (1974–2002) using mainly insecticides for vector control, subsequently the ivermectin, a microfilaricidal drug, was distributed on large scale since 1989 in all communities where onchocerciasis was endemic. The ivermectin mass treatment reduced the burden of parasite infection since it can produce "embryostatic" effect, which temporarily prevents the release of microfilariae and temporary parasites' sterility [33]. Unfortunately, the drug has been administered for years and some *Onchocerca volvulus* populations are less responsive to ivermectin, which could be explained by genetic drift [34].

In the last twenty years, key drug trials have been performed with a new chemotherapeutical approach to antifilarial therapy, targeting the essential *Wolbachia* endosymbiotic bacteria present in many filariae that is important for their viability and fertility [35]. The objectives of the anti-*Wolbachia* (A-WOL) research programmed by the Bill and Melinda Gates Foundation (BMGF) proposed to evaluate antibiotics such as doxycycline, rifampicin, and azithromycin in *Onchocerca volvulus* infected population to find out the most effective dose for large scale use [36]. After extensive research, it was demonstrated that doxycycline had the better larval burden reduction since it affects development embryonic stages as well as the development from L3 into adult worms [37, 38].

3.4 Amiodarone

Amiodarone is an antiarrhythmic medication that affects heartbeat rhythm. This compound has been tested against different protozoan parasites such as *Trypanosoma cruzi* [39–42], *Acanthamoeba castellanii* [43], *Leishmania* spp. [42, 44–46], and *Plasmodium* [47].

In the case of helminth parasites, this compound has been tested against *S. mansoni*. Porto *et al.*, (2021), by electron microscopy analysis, reported that amiodarone affects the viability of schistosomes *in vitro* with effective concentrations of 50% and 90% values ranging from 8 to 50 μM. Also, amiodarone was tested in a murine model of schistosomiasis for both early and chronic *S. mansoni* infections using a single oral dose of 400 mg/kg or 100 mg/kg daily for five consecutive days. They report that Amiodarone had a low efficacy in chronic infection, with the worm and egg burden reduction ranging from 10 to 30%. In contrast, this compound caused a significant reduction in worm and egg burden in early infection (>50%) [48]. Similarly, Talaam *et al.*, (2021), evaluated the possible effect of amiodarone against *S. mansoni*. In this experiment, amiodarone showed complete inhibition of cercaria motility after 18 hours. In the case of schistosomula, after 24 hours with amiodarone, the inhibition of motility was complete. In adult parasites, amiodarone inhibited the motility after 20 hours of incubation was not complete, providing mean motility scores of 0.3 and 1.0 for the male and female, respectively [49]. In *in vivo* experiments, mice were prophylactically treated with amiodarone (50 mg/kg) by 4 days of once-daily intraperitoneal injection, starting 1 day prior to infection, and then euthanized six days postinfection to recover the schistosomula from the lungs. The results show a worm burden reduced to 14.7%. In the case of therapeutic treatment, the mice at week six after infection were treated intraperitoneally with amiodarone (50 mg/kg) for 4 days, and subsequently, they were sacrificed 14 days after the last treatment, the parasite load showed a decrease to 29.2% [49].

3.5 Paclitaxel

Paclitaxel (Taxol) is a drug used in the treatment of breast, ovarian, lung, bladder, prostate, melanoma, esophageal, and other types of solid tumor cancers. It has also been used in Kaposi's sarcoma.

The use of this drug against helminths has been little tested. Pensel *et al.*, (2014), tested the *in vitro* effect of this compound against germinal cells, protoscoleces and cysts of *Echinococcus granulosus*, and parasites responsible for echinococcosis in humans. They report that the use of paclitaxel at a concentration of 1, 5, and 10 μg/ml inhibited the growth of *Echinococcus granulosus* cells in a time-dependent manner. In addition, paclitaxel had a direct effect against protoscoleces in a dose- and time-dependent manner. At 30 days postexposure with 10 and 5 μg/ml paclitaxel, viability of protoscoleces decreased to approximately 60% and the treatment with 1 μg/ml also showed protoscolicidal effect, with 75.3% of parasites remaining viable in culture. Finally, in an *in vitro* cyst incubation it was shown that paclitaxel resulted in dramatic alterations within 3 to 5 days after initiation of treatment [50]. In another experiment, Huang *et al.* (2018) evaluated the effect of paclitaxel on growth and proliferation of *Echinococcus multilocularis* metacestodes. They exposed metacestode tissues *in vitro* to paclitaxel (2, 5, and 10 μM) for one week and, thereafter, were injected into the peritoneum of *Meriones unguiculatus*. After, magnetic resonance imaging and simultaneous positron emission tomography were applied to monitor *in vivo* growth of drug-exposed *Echinococcus multilocularis*. The *in vivo* growth of metacestodes was suppressed until 3 months postinfection, thereafter, parasite tissues enlarged up to 3 cm^3 [51].

3.6 Docetaxel

Docetaxel (taxotere) is a chemotherapeutic drug administered as a treatment for some types of cancer, such as breast, prostate, and non-small cell lung cancer, but it also may be used for many other types of cancers.

The only report where the effect of docetaxel against a helminth has been evaluated was carried out by Huang *et al.* (2018). They report that at three months postinfection, docetaxel (at 10 μM, 5 μM and 2 μM) inhibited *in vivo* growth and proliferation of *Echinococcus multilocularis*, and at 5 months postinfection, only in the 2 μM docetaxel exposure group 0.3 cm^3 of parasite tissue was found [51]. Moreover, in *Meriones* infected with *Echinococcus multilocularis* metacestodes previously exposed to docetaxel, *in vivo* grown parasite tissues weighed 0.2 g and *in vitro* cultured *Echinococcus multilocularis* metacestodes exposed to docetaxel did not produce vesicles until 7 weeks post-drug exposure. With the above, they suggest that the use of this drug can work as an alternative option for the treatment of alveolar echinococcosis [51].

3.7 Cisplatin

Cisplatin is a first-generation platinum-containing drug, used in the treatment of various solid tumors. This drug prevents or inhibits cell maturation and proliferation.

The effect of cisplatin against helminths was tested by Eldeed *et al.*, (2018), in an *in vivo* and *in vitro* experiments where they tested a single dose of cisplatin against *S. mansoni*. In *in vitro* experiments, they report that a single dose of cisplatin (10 to 200 μg/ml) for 24 or 48 hours demonstrated as reduction in viability of the treated worms after 24 hours and, especially, after 48 hours. Moreover, the survival rate of the treated worms decreased gradually in a concentration-dependent manner [52]. On the other hand, in *in vivo* experiments in which female mice were injected subcutaneously with cercariae *of S. mansoni* and administered cisplatin at a dose of 8 mg/kg/day for 3 days beginning on day 42 postinfection, to which samples were collected 2 weeks after the last dose of treatment, they reported that cisplatin significantly reduced the number of living ova, while the number of dead eggs significantly increased. Furthermore, the number of worms recovered was less compared to the control group [52]. The examination for the tegument of adult male *S. mansoni* recovered from infected mice showed erosion, necrosis, and severe damage to the tegument surface, abnormal dropped spines from the tegument surface, vacuolization of the subtegumental cells, and disorganization of muscle layers after treatment with cisplatin [52]. Finally, hepatic histological analysis of *S. mansoni*-infected mice shows that cisplatin treatment decrease granuloma size. In liver function tests, alanine aminotransferase was decreased in infected animals treated with cisplatin compared to their infection control [52].

3.8 Natural products

Recently, the use of phytoestrogens with antiparasitic activity has increased. One of them, genistein, an isoflavone isolated from soybean, exhibits significant metacestodicidal activity *in vitro,* but also binds to the ER and induces estrogenic effects. Furthermore, synthetic genistein derivatives have shown an improved metacestodicidal effect [53].

Parasitic diseases remain a major public health problem affecting hundreds of millions of people, particularly in tropical developing countries. The limited availability and affordability of pharmaceutical medicines mean that the majority of the world's population depends on traditional medical remedies, and it is estimated that some 20,000 species of higher plants are used clinically throughout the world [54]. In medieval times, plants with reputed antihelminthic properties were often mixed with mineral salts (arsenic, copper, etc.) or more esoteric materials (blood, feces, fluids from reptiles, wild animals, etc.) to form quite bizarre and often hazardous concoctions – for both parasites and hosts alike. With time, trial, and error, such preparations were refined in an attempt to at least moderate the undesirable consequences to the host, but with the advent of safer and more effective synthetic antihelminthic compounds, they rapidly disappeared from the veterinary antihelminthic market. Nevertheless, it is of interest to note that the WHO has recently estimated that 80% of the population of developing countries rely on traditional medicine, mostly plant drugs, for their primary health care needs. Higher plants represent a rich source of new molecules with pharmacological properties, which are lead compounds for the development of new drugs. During the last decades, the renewed interest in researching natural products has led to the introduction of several important drugs, such as the anticancer drugs vinblastine and taxol or the antimalarial agent artemisinin. Success in natural products research is conditioned by careful plant selection, based on various criteria such as chemotaxonomic data, information from traditional medicine, field observation, or even random collection. One main strategy in the isolation of new lead compounds consists of so-called bioactivity-guided isolation, in which pharmacological or biological assays are used to target the isolation of bioactive compounds. One major drawback of this strategy is the frequent isolation of known metabolites. The tropical fruit *Carica papaya* and its seeds have proven antihelminthic and anti-amoebic activities [55]. To determine the effectiveness of air-dried *C. papaya* seeds on human intestinal parasitosis, 60 asymptomatic Nigerian children with stool microscopic evidence of intestinal parasites received immediate doses (20 mL) of either an elixir composed of air-dried C. papaya seeds and honey (CPH) or honey alone (placebo) in two randomized treatment groups. Repeat stool microscopic examinations were conducted 7 days post-intervention for intestinal parasites. Significantly more subjects given CPH elixir than those given honey had their stools cleared of parasites [23 of 30 (76.7%) vs. five of 30 (16.7%); $z = 4.40$, $P = .0000109$]. There were no harmful effects. The stool clearance rate for the various types of parasites encountered was between 71.4% and 100% following CPH elixir treatment compared with 0–15.4% with honey. Thus, air-dried C. papaya seeds are efficacious in treating human intestinal parasites and without significant side effects. Their consumption offers a cheap, natural, harmless, readily available monotherapy, and preventive strategy against intestinal parasitosis, especially in tropical communities. Further and large-scale intervention studies to compare *C. papaya* with standard antiparasitic preparations are desirable [55]. For example, schistosomiasis, a widespread helminthic disease whose treatment is chemotherapy based, the drug of choice being praziquantel. Since resistance to praziquantel has been discovered in the exposed parasites, alternative drugs must be considered. Myrrh is an oleo-gum resin from the stem of the plant *Commiphora molmol* [56]. This study was performed on 204 patients with schistosomiasis. The drug was administered at a dose of 10 mg/kg of body weight/day for three days, inducing a cure rate of 91.7%. Re-treatment of cases who did not respond with a dose of 10 mg/kg of body weight/day for six days gave a cure rate of 76.5%, increasing the overall cure rate to 98.09%. The drug was well tolerated, and side effects were mild and transient. Twenty cases provided biopsy samples six months after treatment and none of them showed living ova [56]. Other treatments involve hand infusions and decoctions of the leaves, roots, and inflorescences of the herbaceous shrub *Chenopodium ambrosioides* (American wormseed, goosefoot, epazote, paico); additional related species, indigenous to the New World, have been used for centuries as dietary condiments and as traditional antihelminthics by native peoples in the treatment of intestinal worms [57]. Commercial preparations of *Chenopodium* oil and its active constituent, ascaridol, obtained by steam distillation, have been and continue to be used with considerable success in mass treatment campaigns. Ethnopharmacological studies in a community of Mayan subsistence farmers in Chiapas, Mexico, confirmed that decoctions containing up to 300 mg of dry plant material (kg/body weight) were widely used and traditionally highly regarded in the treatment of ascariasis. However, therapeutic doses of up to 6000 mg (kg/body weight) of powdered, dried plant material had no significant antihelminthic effect on the adults of *Necator, Trichuris,* or *Ascaris*. Gas-liquid chromatographic analyses of plant samples used consistently demonstrated the presence of ascaridol in the expected amounts. Possible origins of subjective belief in the efficacy of *C. ambrosioides* may be related to the positive association of spontaneous or peristalsis-induced passage of senescent worms immediately following a therapeutic episode [57]. It is also possible that, in the past, varieties of the plant containing much more ascaridol were used. The results of these controlled field studies did not sustain any widely held traditional beliefs nor did they support the value of the therapeutic practices regarding this plant. It is, therefore, essential that all indigenous ethnomedical practices be objectively evaluated for efficacy and safety using the appropriate protocols before being considered for their adaptation or promotion in health care programs [57].

Naphthoquinones are naphthalene-derived compounds that can be found in some plants. These products possess antibacterial, antifungal, antitumoral, and antiparasitic properties. Aranda-López *et al.,* (2021), evaluated *in vitro* anti-helminth effect of a pure naphthoquinone (naphthoquinone 4a) in a model of murine cysticercosis caused by *Taenia crassiceps*. Naphthoquinone 4a causes paralysis in the cysticerci membrane from day 3 of the in vitro treatment. Moreover, it induces changes in the shape, size, and appearance of the cysticerci and a decrease in the reproduction rate depending on the duration of the treatment and the concentration of the compound [58]. Wang *et al.,* (2017), evaluated the effect of 1,4 naphthoquinone against *Caenorhabditis elegans* nematodes and eggs and report that 1,4 naphthoquinone kills more than 50% of nematodes and inhibits more than 50% of eggs hatching at a dose of 50 μg/ml. This effect is mediated by stimulating oxidative stress (increase reactive oxygen production, superoxide dismutase activity, and the heat-shock transcription factor (HSF)-1 pathway). In addition, they showed that the lethality caused by naphthoquinone was related to the Insulin/IGF signaling (IIS) pathway, and the effect on IIS pathway-related genes (*age-1, sod-3, mtl-1, ctl-2, daf-12*) indicated that 1,4-naphthoquinone could activate this pathway and suppress the expression of DAF-16 target genes [59]. El-Beshbishi *et al.,* (2019), in an *in vitro* study tested the use of artemisinin-naphthoquinone phosphate combination against *Schistosoma haematobium* and its vector *Bulinus truncates*. They report that naphthoquinone treatment at a dose of 1 μg/ml of *Schistosoma haematobium* worms for 24 hours reduces worm motility, while the dose of 20 μg/ml results in 25–100% mortality of adult flukes within 48–72 hours. Moreover, the incubation of miracidia and cercaria with artemisinin-naphthoquinone phosphate at a concentration of 7.5 μg/ml killed all the free larval stages within 40 and

15 min, respectively. Finally, the exposure of *Bulinus truncatus* adult snails to 20 ppm of the combined regimen caused a mortality rate of 100% within 24 hours [60]. In an experiment realized by Cha *et al.*, (2019), where they evaluated the nematicidal activity of three naphthoquinones (1,4-naphthoquinone, juglone, and plumbagin) against the pine wood nematode (*Bursaphelenchus xylophilus*), showed that lethal concentration 50 (LC_{50}) at 48 hours of exposure was 100 ppm for 1,4 naphthoquinone, 57 ppm for juglone, and 104 ppm for plumbagin. In *in vivo* test, they report that mortality of *Bursaphelenchus xylophilus* was significantly affected by the presence of the three naphthoquinones at concentrations above 62.5 ppm. In the semi-*in vivo* assay, the population of inoculated *Bursaphelenchus xylophilus* was significantly decreased at two weeks after treatment with juglone when compared with the effects of treatment with 1,4-naphthoquinone and plumbagin. The mechanism by which mortality occurs was associated with the generation of reactive oxygen species by naphthoquinones that cause oxidative stress in the parasite [61]. Rufener *et al.*, (2018), tried *in vitro* and *in vivo* buparvaquone (a second-generation naphthoquinone with action on hemoprotozoa) against *Echinococcus multilocularis*. Their results show that buparvaquone has an Inhibitory Concentration 50 (IC_{50}) of 2.87 μM against *in vitro* cultured *Echinococcus multilocularis* metacestodes. Moreover, transmission electron microscopy revealed that treatment with buparvaquone impaired parasite mitochondria early on, and additional tests showed that had a reduced activity under anaerobic conditions. Furthermore, buparvaquone show an inhibition effect of the cytochrome bc_1 complex in *Echinococcus multilocularis* germinal layer cells. On the other hand, in a *in vivo* experiment using mice with secondary alveolar echinococcosis were treated with buparvaquone (100 mg/kg per dose, three doses per week, four weeks of treatment), the treatment failed to reduce the parasite burden [62].

Acknowledgements

Grant IN-209719 from Programa de Apoyo a Proyectos de Innovación Tecnológica (PAPIIT), Dirección General de Asuntos del Personal Académico (DGAPA), Universidad Nacional Autónoma de México (UNAM). Grant FC2016-2125 from Fronteras en la Ciencia, Consejo Nacional de Ciencia y Tecnología (CONACYT), both to Jorge Morales-Montor. Grant IA-206220 and Víctor H del Río Araiza, from PAPIIT, DGAPA, UNAM. Grant CB-2015-2101 from Ciencia Básica, Consejo Nacional de Ciencia y Tecnología (CONACYT) (number: 255173) and grant Programa de Apoyo a la Investigación Científica y Tecnológica (PAICYT) (number: SA211-15) to Romel Hernández-Bello.

Conflict of interest

The authors declare no conflict of interest.

Author details

Victor Hugo Del Río-Araiza[1], Romel Hernandéz-Bello[2] and Jorge Morales-Montor[3]*

1 Faculty of Veterinary Medicine and Zootechnics, Department of Parasitology, National Autonomous University of Mexico, Mexico City, Mexico

2 Faculty of Medicine, Department of Microbiology, Autonomous University of Nuevo León, Monterrey, Nuevo León, Mexico

3 Departmento de Inmunología, Instituto de Investigaciones Biomédicas, Universidad Nacional Autonoma de México, Ciudad de México, México

*Address all correspondence to: jmontor66@biomedicas.unam.mx

References

[1] Gilles HM, Hoffman PS. Treatment of intestinal parasitic infections: A review of nitazoxanide. Trends in Parasitology. 2002;**18**:95-97

[2] Abboud P, Lemée V, Gargala G, Brasseur P, Ballet JJ, Borsa-Lebas F, et al. Successful treatment of metronidazole- and albendazole-resistant giardiasis with nitazoxanide in a patient with acquired immunodeficiency syndrome. Clinical Infectious Diseases. 2001;**32**:1792-1794

[3] Hernández-Bello R, Escobedo G, Guzmán C, Ibarra-Coronado EG, López-Griego L, Morales-Montor J. Immunoendocrine host-parasite interactions during helminth infections: From the basic knowledge to its possible therapeutic applications: Review Article. Parasite Immunology. 2010;**32**:633-643

[4] Aguilar-Díaz H, Nava-Castro KE, Escobedo G, Domínguez-Ramírez L, García-Varela M, Del Río-Araiza VH, et al. A novel progesterone receptor membrane component (PGRMC) in the human and swine parasite Taenia solium: Implications to the host-parasite relationship. Parasites and Vectors. 2018;**11**:1-11

[5] Hernández-Bello R, Ramirez-Nieto R, Muñiz-Hernández S, Nava-Castro K, Pavón L, Sánchez-Acosta AG, et al. Sex Steroids Effects on the Molting Process of the Helminth Human Parasite Trichinella spiralis. Journal of Biomedicine & Biotechnology. 2011;**2011**:1-10

[6] Morales-Montor J, Baig S, Hallal-Calleros C, Damian RT. Taenia crassiceps: Androgen reconstitution of the host leads to protection during cysticercosis. Experimental Parasitology. 2002;**100**:209-216

[7] Loria RM. Immune up-regulation and tumor apoptosis by androstene steroids. Steroids. 2002;**67**:953-966

[8] Vargas-Villavicencio JA, De León-Nava MA, Morales-Montor J. Immunoendocrine mechanisms associated with resistance or susceptibility to parasitic diseases during pregnancy. Neuroimmunomodulation. 2009;**16**:114-121

[9] Morales-Montor J, Baig S, Mitchell R, Deway K, Hallal-Calleros C, Damian RT. Immunoendocrine interactions during chronic cysticercosis determine male mouse feminization: role of IL-6. Journal of Immunology. 2001;**167**:4527-4533

[10] Vargas-Villavicencio JA, Larralde C, De León-Nava MA, Morales-Montor J. Regulation of the immune response to cestode infection by progesterone is due to its metabolism to estradiol. Microbes Infectious Elsevier Masson SAS. 2005;**7**:485-493

[11] Nuñez GG, Costantino SN, Gentile T, Venturiello SM. Immunoparasitological evaluation of Trichinella spiralis infection during human pregnancy: a small case series. Transactions of the Royal Society of Tropical Medicine and Hygiene. 2008;**102**:662-668

[12] Nuñez GG, Gentile T, Costantino SN, Sarchi MI, Venturiello SM. In vitro and in vivo effects of progesterone on Trichinella spiralis newborn larvae. Parasitology. 2005;**131**:255-259

[13] Albright JW, Albright JF. Ageing alters the competence of the immune system to control parasitic infection. Immunology Letters. 1994;**40**:279-285

[14] Carrero JC, Cervantes C, Moreno-Mendoza N, Saavedra E, Morales-Montor J, Laclette JP. Dehydroepiandrosterone decreases while cortisol increases in vitro growth and viability of Entamoeba histolytica. Microbes and Infection. 2006;**8**:323-331

[15] Fallon PG, Richardson EJ, Jones FM, Dunne DW. Dehydroepiandrosterone sulfate treatment of mice modulates infection with Schistosoma mansoni. Clinical and Diagnostic Laboratory Immunology. 1998;**5**:251-253

[16] Vargas-Villavicencio JA, Larralde C, Morales-Montor J. Treatment with dehydroepiandrosterone in vivo and in vitro inhibits reproduction, growth and viability of Taenia crassiceps metacestodes. International Journal of Parasitology. 2008;**38**:775-781

[17] Hernández-Pando R, Aguilar-Leon D, Orozco H, Serrano A, Ahlem C, Trauger R, et al. 16alpha-Bromoepiandrosterone restores T helper cell type 1 activity and accelerates chemotherapy-induced bacterial clearance in a model of progressive pulmonary tuberculosis. Journal of Infectious Diseases. 2005;**191**:299-306

[18] Chikanza IC, Grossman AB. Reciprocal interactions between the neuroendocrine and immune systems during inflammation. Rheumatic Diseases Clinics of North America. 2000;**26**:693-711

[19] Pedersen NC, North TW, Rigg R, Reading C, Higgins J, Leutenegger C, et al. 16alpha-Bromo-epiandrosterone therapy modulates experimental feline immunodeficiency virus viremia: initial enhancement leading to long-term suppression. Veterinary Immunology and Immunopathology. 2003;**94**:133-148

[20] Naguleswaran A, Spicher M, Vonlaufen N, Ortega-Mora LM, Torgerson P, Gottstein B, et al. In vitro metacestodicidal activities of genistein and other isoflavones against Echinococcus multilocularis and Echinococcus granulosus. Antimicrobial Agents and Chemotherapy. 2006;**50**:3770-3778

[21] James CE, Hudson AL, Davey MW. Drug resistance mechanisms in helminths: is it survival of the fittest? Trends in Parasitology. 2009;**25**:328-335

[22] Wolstenholme AJ, Fairweather I, Prichard R, Von Samson-Himmelstjerna G, Sangster NC. Drug resistance in veterinary helminths. Trends in Parasitology. 2004;**20**:469-476

[23] Kaplan RM. Drug resistance in nematodes of veterinary importance: A status report. Trends in Parasitology. 2004;**20**:477-481

[24] McKellar QA, Jackson F. Veterinary anthelmintics: Old and new. Trends in Parasitology. 2004;**20**:456-461

[25] Solerte SB, Fioravanti M, Vignati G, Giustina A, Cravello L, Ferrari E. Dehydroepiandrosterone sulfate enhances natural killer cell cytotoxicity in humans via locally generated immunoreactive insulin-like growth factor I. The Journal of Clinical Endocrinology and Metabolism. 1999;**84**:3260-3267

[26] Vargas-Villavicencio JA, Larralde C, De León-Nava MA, Escobedo G, Morales-Montor J. Tamoxifen treatment induces protection in murine cysticercosis. The Journal of Parasitology. 2007;**93**:1512-1517

[27] Terrazas LI, Bojalil R, Govezensky T, Larraide C. A role for 17-β-estradiol in immunoendocrine regulation of murine cysticercosis (Taenia crassiceps). Journal

of Parasitology American Society of Parasitologists. 1994;**80**:563-568

[28] Morales-Montor J, Escobedo G, Vargas-Villavicencio J, Larralde C. The Neuroimmunoendocrine Network in the Complex Host-Parasite Relationship During Murine Cysticercosis. Current Topics in Medicinal Chemistry. 2008;**8**:400-407

[29] Morales-Montor J, Hallal-Calleros C, Romano MC, Damian RT. Inhibition of P-450 aromatase prevents feminisation and induces protection during cysticercosis. International Journal for Parasitology. 2002;**32**:1379-1387

[30] Vogel VG, Costantino JP, Wickerham DL, Cronin WM, Cecchini RS, Atkins JN, et al. Effects of tamoxifen vs raloxifene on the risk of developing invasive breast cancer and other disease outcomes: the NSABP Study of Tamoxifen and Raloxifene (STAR) P-2 trial. JAMA. 2006;**295**:2727-2741

[31] Onchocerciasis [Internet]. [cited 2022 Feb 18]. Available from: https://www.who.int/news-room/fact-sheets/detail/onchocerciasis

[32] Boatin BA, Richards FO. Control of onchocerciasis. Advances in Parasitology. 2006;**61**:349-394

[33] Basáñez MG, Pion SD, Boakes E, Filipe JA, Churcher TS, Boussinesq M. Effect of single-dose ivermectin on Onchocerca volvulus: a systematic review and meta-analysis. The Lancet Infectious Diseases. 2008;**8**:310-322

[34] Doyle SR, Bourguinat C, Nana-Djeunga HC, Kengne-Ouafo JA, Pion SDS, Bopda J, et al. Genome-wide analysis of ivermectin response by Onchocerca volvulus reveals that genetic drift and soft selective sweeps contribute to loss of drug sensitivity. PLoS Neglected Tropical Diseases. 2017;**11**:1-11

[35] Tamarozzi F, Halliday A, Gentil K, Hoerauf A, Pearlman E, Taylor MJ. Onchocerciasis: The role of Wolbachia bacterial endosymbionts in parasite biology, disease pathogenesis, and treatment. Clinical Microbiology Reviews. 2011;**24**:459-468

[36] Kuesel AC. Research for new drugs for elimination of onchocerciasis in Africa. International Journal for Parasitology: Drugs and Drug Resistance. Elsevier. 2016;**6**:272-286

[37] Debrah AY, Specht S, Klarmann-Schulz U, Batsa L, Mand S, Marfo-Debrekyei Y, et al. Doxycycline Leads to Sterility and Enhanced Killing of Female Onchocerca volvulus Worms in an Area With Persistent Microfilaridermia After Repeated Ivermectin Treatment: A Randomized, Placebo-Controlled, Double-Blind Trial. Clinical Infectious Diseases. 2015;**61**:517-526

[38] Abegunde AT, Ahuja RM, Okafor NJ. Doxycycline plus ivermectin versus ivermectin alone for treatment of patients with onchocerciasis. Cochrane Database of Systematic Reviews. 2016;**2016**

[39] Benaim G, Sanders JM, Garcia-Marchán Y, Colina C, Lira R, Caldera AR, et al. Amiodarone has intrinsic anti-Trypanosoma cruzi activity and acts synergistically with posaconazole. Journal of Medicinal Chemistry. 2006;**49**:892-899

[40] Adesse D, Azzam EM, De Meirelles MNL, Urbina JA, Garzoni LR. Amiodarone inhibits Trypanosoma cruzi infection and promotes cardiac cell recovery with gap junction and cytoskeleton reassembly in

vitro. Antimicrobial Agents and Chemotherapy. 2011;**55**:203-210

[41] Benaim G, Paniz Mondolfi AE. The emerging role of amiodarone and dronedarone in Chagas disease. Nature Reviews. Cardiology Nature Publishing Group. 2012;**9**:605-609

[42] Benaim G, Paniz-Mondolfi AE, Sordillo EM. The Rationale for Use of Amiodarone and its Derivatives for the Treatment of Chagas' Disease and Leishmaniasis. Current Pharmaceutical Design. 2021;**27**:1825-1833

[43] Baig AM, Iqbal J, Khan NA. In vitro efficacies of clinically available drugs against growth and viability of an Acanthamoeba castellanii keratitis isolate belonging to the T4 genotype. Antimicrobial Agents and Chemotherapy. 2013;**57**:3561-3567

[44] Oryan A, Bemani E, Bahrami S. Emerging role of amiodarone and dronedarone, as antiarrhythmic drugs, in treatment of leishmaniasis. Acta TropicalElsevier. 2018;**185**:34-41

[45] Pinto EG, Tempone AG. Activity of the antiarrhythmic drug amiodarone against Leishmania (L.) infantum: an in vitro and in vivo approach. Journal of Venomous Animals and Toxins including Tropical Diseases; 2018;24.

[46] Bahrami S, Oryan A, Bemani E. Efficacy of amiodarone and voriconazole combination therapy in cutaneous leishmaniasis in the mice experimentally infected with Leishmania major. Journal of Infection and Chemotherapy. Elsevier. 2021;**27**:984-990

[47] Bobbala D, Alesutan I, Föller M, Tschan S, Huber SM, Lang F. Protective effect of amiodarone in malaria. Acta Tropica. 2010;**116**:39-44

[48] Porto R, Mengarda AC, Cajas RA, Salvadori MC, Teixeira FS, Arcanjo DDR, et al. Antiparasitic properties of cardiovascular agents against human intravascular parasite schistosoma mansoni. Pharmaceuticals (Basel). 2021;**14**:2-15

[49] Talaam KK, Inaoka DK, Hatta T, Tsubokawa D, Tsuji N, Wada M, et al. Mitochondria as a potential target for the development of prophylactic and therapeutic drugs against schistosoma mansoni infection. Antimicrobial Agents and Chemotherapy. American Society for Microbiology 1752 N St., N.W., Washington, DC. 2021;**65**:1-12

[50] Pensel PE, Albani C, Gamboa GU, Benoit JP, Elissondo MC. In vitro effect of 5-fluorouracil and paclitaxel on Echinococcus granulosus larvae and cells. Acta Tropica. Elsevier B.V. 2014;**140**:1-9

[51] Huang X, Wiehr S, Wild AM, Voßberg P, Hoffmann W, Grüner B, et al. The effects of taxanes, vorinostat and doxorubicin on growth and proliferation of Echinococcus multilocularis metacestodes assessed with magnetic resonance imaging and simultaneous positron emission tomography. Oncotarget. 2018;**9**:9073-9087

[52] Eldeeb E, Fahmy S, Elbakry K, Hyder A. A single dose of the antineoplastics hydroxyurea or cisplatin has praziquantel-like effects on Schistosoma mansoni worms and host mouse liver. Biomedicine & PharmacotherapyElsevier. 2018;**99**:570-575

[53] Gibson TE. Factors influencing the application of anthelmintics in practice. Veterinary Parasitology Elsevier. 1980;**6**:241-254

[54] Queiroz E, Wolfender J-L, Hostettmann K. Modern Approaches in

the Search for New Lead Antiparasitic Compounds from Higher Plants. Current Drug Targets. 2009;**10**:202-211

[55] Okeniyi JAO, Ogunlesi TA, Oyelami OA, Adeyemi LA. Effectiveness of dried Carica papaya seeds against human intestinal parasitosis: A pilot study. Journal of Medicinal Food. 2007;**10**:194-196

[56] Sheir Z, Nasr AA, Massoud A, Salama O, Badra GA, El-Shennawy H, et al. A safe, effective, herbal antischistosomal therapy derived from myrrh. The American Journal of Tropical Medicine and Hygiene. 2001;**65**:700-704

[57] Kliks MM. Studies on the traditional herbal anthelmintic Chenopodium ambrosioides L.: ethnopharmacological evaluation and clinical field trials. Social Science & Medicine. 1985;**21**:879-886

[58] Aranda-López Y, López-López L, Castro KEN, Ponce-Regalado MD, Becerril-Villanueva LE, Girón-Pérez MI, et al. Cysticidal effect of a pure naphthoquinone on Taenia crassiceps cysticerci. Parasitology Research Springer Berlin Heidelberg. 2021;**120**:3783-3794

[59] Wang J, Zeng G, Huang X, Wang Z, Tan N. 1,4-Naphthoquinone Triggers Nematode Lethality by Inducing Oxidative Stress and Activating Insulin/IGF Signaling Pathway in Caenorhabditis elegans. Molecules. Multidisciplinary Digital Publishing Institute. 2017;**22**:1-12

[60] El-Beshbishi SN, El Bardicy S, Tadros M, Ayoub M, Taman A. Biological activity of artemisinin-naphthoquine phosphate on Schistosoma haematobium stages and the vector Bulinus truncatus. Transactions of the Royal Society of Tropical Medicine and Hygiene. 2019;**113**:320-325

[61] Cha DJ, Kim J, Kim DS. Nematicidal activities of three naphthoquinones against the Pine Wood Nematode, Bursaphelenchus xylophilus. Molecules. Multidisciplinary Digital Publishing Institute. 2019;**24**:1-9

[62] Rufener R, Dick L, D'Ascoli L, Ritler D, Hizem A, Wells TNC, et al. Repurposing of an old drug: In vitro and in vivo efficacies of buparvaquone against Echinococcus multilocularis. International Journal for Parasitology: Drugs and Drug ResistanceElsevier. 2018;**8**:440-450

[63] Morales-Montor J, Newhouse E, Mohamed F, Baghdadi A, Damian RT. Altered levels of hypothalamic-pituitary-adrenocortical axis hormones in baboons and mice during the course of infection with Schistosoma mansoni. Journal of Infectious Diseases. 2001;**183**:313-320

Section 2

Advances in the Molecular and Immune Response in Helminth Infection

Chapter 6

Perspective Chapter: Parasitic Platyhelminthes Nuclear Receptors as Molecular Crossroads

Adriana Esteves and Gabriela Alvite

Abstract

Thanks to the increasing availability of the parasitic Platyhelminthes genomes in recent years, several studies have been directed to the identification of the nuclear receptors set expressed by these organisms. Nevertheless, important gaps in our knowledge remain to be addressed, concerning their mechanism of action, ligands, co-regulator proteins, and DNA binding sequences on target genes. The proposed review chapter will be an account of research into the nuclear receptors field of parasitic Platyhelminthes. Several *in vitro* effects of host steroid hormones on Taenia and Echinococcus species were observed, however, the classical mammalian estrogen, androgen, or progesterone receptors could not be identified in databases. Nonetheless, novel nuclear receptors and related proteins and genes, are being identified and characterized. The elucidation of their target genes as well as ligands in parasitic Platyhelminthes could allow discovery of new and specific pathways differing from those of their hosts. In this sense, these parasitic proteins seem to be good putative targets of new drugs.

Keywords: nuclear receptors, parasitic Platyhelminthes, host–parasite relationship

1. Introduction

Since the biochemical identification of the first nuclear receptor (NR) more than 60 years ago [1], the study of these proteins has been increasing. In particular, the cloning of the first NR was a milestone [2], ushering in a new chapter in research into the regulation of cell function and metabolism [3]. NRs are transcription factors that modulate numerous physiological processes such as metabolism, development, reproduction, and inflammation [4–6], through the regulation of target genes transcription by binding to specific DNA response elements [3, 6]. Unlike other transcription factors, the activity of nuclear receptors can be modulated by the binding of specific ligands, these being mainly small lipophilic molecules that easily penetrate biological membranes [7], providing a direct link between the cellular signals and the transcriptional responses of a cell. These lipophilic ligands can be fatty acids, steroids, retinoids, and phospholipids. This protein family also contains "orphan" members for which no ligand has yet been identified [8].

Despite the diversity of functions presented by the different NRs, they share a common modular structure, with various degrees of conservation among their respective domains. A typical nuclear receptor contains an N-terminal domain (NTD or A/B region), a highly conserved DNA binding domain (DBD or C region), a poorly conserved hinge domain (region D), a ligand-binding domain (LBD or E region), and a C-terminal region (F region) [9, 10]. The A/B region is a poorly structured domain that shows a low percentage of conservation at size and sequence level and may not be present in some NRs [6]. This domain is regulated by the interaction with co-regulatory proteins and also contains an autonomous transactivation region 1 (AF-1, Activation Factor 1) independent of ligand binding [11]. The DBD is the most conserved region compared to the other domains [12] and it is responsible for the binding of the NR to specific DNA sequences, named response element (RE) [13]. Structural studies have determined that the DBD has two subdomains that each contain four cysteine residues that coordinate a zinc ion to create the typical DNA-binding zinc finger motif [14–16]. The hinge domain is the region with the lowest sequence conservation and it constitutes a flexible linker between the DBD and the LBD [10], giving the connecting domains some independent mobility [17]. The LBD regulates the receptor activity through ligand binding and direct interaction with co-regulatory proteins [18, 19]. This region contains functionally related interaction surfaces: a dimerization surface, which mediates interaction with another LBD [20]; a hydrophobic ligand-binding pocket (LBP) that interacts with lipophilic small molecules [21]; and an activation function surface called AF-2 (Activation Function-2), essential for the ligand-dependent transcription activation [22, 23]. Finally, the F domain is a poorly conserved region, and even many members of the family lack this domain. However, when this domain is present, its deletion or mutation alters transactivation, dimerization, and the receptor response after ligand binding [24].

More than 900 nuclear receptor genes have been identified throughout the animal kingdom [25, 26]. The NRs have a common ancestral origin and a high conservation rate in all animal taxa and therefore are considered strong phylogenetic markers of animal evolution [27]. This protein group shows an interesting complexity probably driven by gene duplication and gene loss [28], for example, 2 members have been identified from sponges, 48 in mammals and up to more than 250 in nematodes [29–32]. Phylogenetic studies demonstrated that NRs emerged long before the divergence of vertebrates and invertebrates, during the earliest metazoan evolution [33]. The nomenclature currently used to name the NRs is based on phylogenetic relationships, generated from conserved DBD sequence alignment and the construction of phylogenetic trees. This classification, which was approved by the Nuclear Receptor Nomenclature Committee in 1999 [34], subdivides the nuclear receptor family into six subfamilies (NR1-NR6). The subfamily NR0 was added later and includes atypical nuclear receptors that contain only DBD (NR0A, identified in arthropods and nematodes) or only LBD (NR0B, present in some vertebrates) [34]. In the last decades, the existence of a new NR subgroup called 2DBD-NR was evidenced in parasitic Platyhelminthes; whose members present two DBDs and one LBD [35, 36]. This new group has not yet been included in the classification system described by the NR Nomenclature Committee [21, 34]. However, recent publications already classify it as a subfamily NR7 [37]. Furthermore, nuclear receptors can be classified according to their mechanism of action into four types (I-IV). This classification groups the NRs according to the signaling mechanisms, taking into account the subcellular site where NR-ligand binding occurs (cytosol or nucleus) and the mode of DNA binding (homodimer, heterodimer, or monomer) [6]. Briefly, type I NRs reside in the cytosol and upon ligand binding are trafficked into the nucleus where they typically bind to palindromic REs in promoters as a homodimer. Type II NRs are localized in the nucleus and generally form heterodimeric complexes with RXR; in their unliganded state, are inactive and upon ligand binding, they activate by the co-regulators exchange. Type III NRs are similar to Type II, however, these receptors bind to direct repeat REs as homodimers. Type IV NRs have a similar mechanism of action to Type II and III NRs but instead, bind to DNA as a monomer and recognize extended half-sites within RE [6].

Platyhelminthes are a phylum of bilaterian, unsegmented, soft-bodied invertebrates, but also, they are acoelomates and lack specialized circulatory and respiratory organs. These characteristics make these organisms have a flattened shape that allows the exchange of gases and nutrients throughout the body [38]. Platyhelminthes are traditionally divided into four classes: Rhabditophora, Monogenea, Cestoda (tapeworms), and Trematoda (flukes). The class Rhabditophora includes all free-living flatworms, while all members in classes of Monogenea, Trematoda, and Cestoda are parasitic flatworms [39]. The Platyhelminthes or flatworms include more than 20,000 species [40, 41].

Parasitic Platyhelminthes are a large group of parasites that can affect both human and animal health, causing neglected diseases such as Schistosomiasis, Paragonimiasis and Cestodiasis that can be fatal and are difficult to treat. These infections generally lead to pain, physical disabilities, etc., impeding economic development through human disability and billions of dollars of lost production in the livestock industries [42, 43].

In the last decade, the advent of genome projects has allowed the identification of the nuclear receptors expressed in the different parasitic Platyhelminthes [21, 44]. Nevertheless, only a few NRs have been characterized in these organisms and their biological function continues to be unknown. The first parasitic Platyhelminthes NRs were identified in *Schistosoma mansoni* [45–48] and after this, NRs were identified in the genomes of 33 Platyhelminthes species [44, 49]. The number of NRs varies from 15 to 61 in Platyhelminthes, 18–23 NRs are present in Monogenea, 15–20 NRs are present in Cestoda, 21–22 NRs are found in Trematoda, and 27–61 members are identified in Rhabditophora [49]. In this chapter, we performed a systematic review of characteristic and underlying mechanisms of parasitic Platyhelminthes nuclear receptors hoping to provide directions and ideas for future research.

2. Parasitic Platyhelminthes nuclear receptors

2.1 Subfamily 1

The most characterized proteins of this group are SmTRα and SmTRβ from *S. mansoni*. Both proteins share the consensus structure of TR receptors, including a conserved N-terminal signature of TRs in the A/B domain as well as the specific sequence CEGCKGFFRR of the NR1 subfamily. SmTRs can form a heterodimer with RXR (SmRXR1), similarly to vertebrate members of this family [50].

Screening *S. mansoni* female worms using the whole-mount *in situ* hybridization was conducted to the identification of a gene predicted to encode a homolog of the *Drosophila melanogaster* nuclear hormone receptor Ecdysone-Induced protein 78c [51]. A second putative member of this group of nuclear receptors is the Smp_248100, an uncharacterized protein from *S. mansoni* [52]. Primary sequence analysis confirmed that Smp_248100 contains a DBD with high amino acid identity to DBDs from other vertebrates and invertebrate NRs, including HRp6 from *D. melanogaster* and DAF-12 from *Caenorhabditis elegans* [52].

In 2011, Förster and collaborators characterized for the first time a cestode NR, named EmNHR1. The isolated *Echinococcus multilocularis* receptor is homologous to NRs of the DAF-12/HR96 group that regulates cholesterol homeostasis and longevity in metazoans. EmNHR1 gene expression was described in all *E. multilocularis* larval stages that are involved in the infection of the intermediate host. The authors report that EmNHR1 is related with the TGF-beta signaling pathway and that human and bovine host serums contain a ligand that induces homodimerization of EmNHR1 LBD. Since the serum is an important component in all culture media that enables the *E. multilocularis* development *in vitro* [53–56], it was suggested that this NR could play a role in host cross-communication mechanisms during infection [57].

The second NR characterized in cestodes was EgHR3 of *E. granulosus.* This protein contains the typical structure with a DBD and an LBD. The *EgHR3* expression was especially high in the early stage of adult worm development. Immunolocalization revealed that the protein was localized in the parenchyma of protoscoleces and adult worms [58]. The authors suggested that this protein could participate in development-specific responses to ecdysteroid as was described for insects [59]. On the other hand, ecdysteroids and molecules of the ecdysteroid signaling pathway had been identified in protoscoleces of *E. granulosus* [60]. With this input, a genomic search allowed the identification of two sequences coding to the following nuclear receptors: E78 (GenBank accession: CDS17388.1) and FTZ-F1 (GenBank accession: CDS15732.1) [61, 62].

2.2 Subfamily 2

Several members of subfamily 2 nuclear receptors were isolated and characterized in Platyhelminthes: SmTR2/4, SmRXR1, SmRXR, HNF4, and HR78. SmTR2/4 is a protein of 223 kDa with extremely large A/B and hinge domains. It shares sequence identity with the DBD of other members of this group of NRs ranging from 69 to 88%, while with de LBD shares from 16 to 38% of similarity. The corresponding gene is expressed in all *S. mansoni* developmental stages. SmTR2/4 might play a role in the regulation of schistosoma female reproductive development [63].

Homologous proteins of vertebrate retinoid-X-receptor (RXR) were identified in *S. mansoni* being classified as NR2B4-A and NR2B4-B [64–67]. Vertebrate counterparts can heterodimerizate with thyroid hormone receptor, retinoic acid receptor, or vitamin D receptor. They bind to DR1 to D5 response elements with the consensus sequence Pu GGTCA [68]. These receptors contain the general basic structure of the nuclear receptors. DNA binding domain sequence of both receptors shares high identity with mouse and human RXRα, and *Drosophila* USP receptor. Low conservation was observed when ligand-binding domain is analyzed. Long A/B, hinge domains, and C terminal tail (F domain) are characteristics of both *S. mansoni* receptors. Members of this group usually lack the F domain. Sequence differences in ligand-binding signature and AF-2 motif between SmRXR and SmRXR1 suggest that specific cofactors may be necessary for the transactivation activity. A low level of identity was also found comparing the DBD sequences of both receptors, strengthening the idea that these two NRs differ in the recognition of their target genes. In addition, DNA binding properties also differentiate both receptors, while SmRXR1 binds to a DR1 response element, SmRXR fails to bind to direct repeat response elements on its own. SmRXR probably binds to conventional response elements and dimerizes with SmFtz-F1 [69]. A differential regulation expression was observed between both *S. mansoni* receptors since SmRXR transcript is expressed at all life cycle stages with highest levels in miracidia and cercaria and much lower in female worms, while SmRXR1 seems to be constitutive.

Hnf4 expression was detected by a single-cell sequence approach in *S. mansoni* stem cells. *RNAi* experiments indicated that the gene product could be a regulator of intestinal cell proliferation. Further studies indicated that luminal microvilli were altered and the loss of cathepsin proteolytic activity, an enzyme involved in hemoglobin digestion. These results encouraged the authors to initiate *in vivo* trials, to assess the digestive capability of *hnf4* (RNAi) parasites, finding that the treated parasites failed to ingest or digest red blood cells. Finally, mice receiving *hnf4* (RNAi) parasites had morphologically normal livers in contrast to controls infected with native parasites. This key regulator of blood-feeding parasites was proposed as a potential therapeutic target to blunt the pathology caused by adult parasites [70]. Since egg deposition depends on blood digestion, *hnf4* is at least indirectly required for parasite growth and egg-induced pathology *in vivo*.

Four more members of this family were also identified in *S. mansoni* by cDNA cloning of the entire DBD. They are SmTLL, SmPNR, SmDSF, SmCoup-FII [71]. The expression at mRNA level was examined in egg, adult, female, and adult male. Only *SmCoup-TFII* was expressed in all stages at similar levels; *SmTLL* expression was high at the egg stage while *SmPNR* and *SmDSF* had a very low expression compared with the other receptors [71].

Finally, the orthologues of fax-1 and NHR236 receptors were recently identified in free-living and parasitic flatworms, respectively. It is the first time that an orthologue of NHR236 has been shown to exist in parasitic Platyhelminthes [49].

2.3 Subfamily 3

For a long time, it has not been possible to identify subfamily 3 NRs in Platyhelminthes [21, 72], so this class of proteins seems to have been lost in this phylum. However, recent genome sequence analysis studies identified several ERRs (estrogen-related receptor) belonging to subfamily 3 [37, 49].

Several reports strongly indicate that host steroid sex hormones affect the biology, and in particular reproduction and growth, of parasitic flatworms. However, to date, it has not been possible to identify steroid hormone receptors similar to those of mammalian hosts in the available genomes. It was demonstrated through *in vitro* assays that sex steroids act directly on *Taenia crassiceps* (Cestoda) cysticerci proliferation and viability [73]. Host hormones 17-β estradiol (E2) and progesterone (P4) promote parasite reproduction without affecting their viability. On the contrary, testosterone (T4) and dihydrotestosterone (DHT) significantly inhibit parasite proliferation, generating a deleterious effect. When 17-β-estradiol concentrations increased, the number of *T. crassiceps* cysticercus buds also increased, and an opposite behavior was observed when tamoxifen (human alpha estrogen receptor antagonist) was tested in cysticerci culture [73]. However, the existence of a *T. crassiceps* ER-like protein (GenBank: AY596184.1) is controversial since a similar protein could not be identified in any of the published genomes of *Taenia* and *Echinococcus* species which are available in WormBase Parasite (https://parasite.wormbase.org/index.html). Although this *T. crassiceps* protein is not the product of contamination by host cells, functional studies are necessary to demonstrate that it is capable of binding estrogens. Undoubtedly, this parasitic flatworm would have to express one or more proteins responsible for the binding of the hormone and triggering of signaling. Finally, in 2014, two papers showed the inhibition of the survival of *Echinococcus granulosus* protoscoleces and

Echinococcus multilocularis metacestode vesicles after an *in vitro* tamoxifen treatment and a pharmacological screening, respectively [74, 75]. Nevertheless, the parasitic estrogen receptors or other proteins responsible for these effects have not yet been isolated and characterized.

It was *in vitro* demonstrated that *T. solium* cysticerci treatment with P4 increases evagination and growth [76]. The P4 direct effect could be mediated by the presence of a putative progesterone-binding protein in the parasite similar to a nuclear classical progesterone receptor (PR) or a membrane receptor. A nuclear classical progesterone receptor could not be identified in *Taenia spp*. genomes. However, it was reported that *T. solium* cells expressed a P4-binding like protein exclusively located at the cysticercus subtegumental tissue. This protein named as membrane-associated progesterone receptor component (PGRMC) was identified by 2D-electrophoresis and sequencing [77]. Molecular docking showed that PGRMC is potentially able to bind steroid hormones such as progesterone, estradiol, testosterone, and dihydrotestosterone with different affinities, and the binding domain to steroids was localized in the C-terminal region. Moreover, the *T. solium* PGRMC is related to a steroid-binding protein of *Echinococcus granulosus* (GenBank: CDS20257.1). A putative mechanism was proposed where progesterone is captured from the external environment and exerts its action upon cysticerci differentiation involving a progesterone membrane receptor and a nuclear PR-like protein [77]. It should be mentioned that the latter protein has not yet been identified in the available genomes of other taeniid cestodes.

The above-cited scientific papers point to a better understanding of the host–parasite molecular cross-communication, providing new information which could be useful in designing anti-helminthic drugs. The strategy consists in the designing of new drugs specifically directed to inhibit or block key parasite molecules, such as hormone-binding proteins, transduction proteins, transcription factors, or nuclear receptors involved in the parasite establishment, growth, and proliferation in the host. In addition, it is a requirement that the new drug specifically recognize parasite cells with minimal secondary effects to the host, so the search has to be directed toward molecules that are differentially expressed in the parasitic Platyhelminthes.

2.4 Subfamily 4 and 6

NR4A was the only subfamily 4 member identified in parasitic platyhelminths. Phylogenetic analysis suggested that it is orthologue of *Drosophila*, Mollusca, and human NR4A receptor [49]. The relative mRNA expression level of SmNR4A5 from *S. mansoni* was similar in egg, adult female, and adult male [71].

Concerning subfamily 6 of NRs, only one member of subfamily 6 (MlNR6) identified belongs to the free-living flatworm *Macrostomum lignano* [49].

2.5 Subfamily 5

Until now the only two receptors of subfamily 5 characterized in parasitic Platyhelminthes are Ftz-F1 (Fushi Tarazu-factor 1) NRs from *S. mansoni*, one called SmFtz-F1 belonging to the NR5B1 group, and the other named SmFtz-F1α classified in the NR5A3 group [48, 49, 78, 79]. In addition, the previously mentioned sequence identified in *E. granulosus* genome Ftz-F1 (GenBank accession number: CDS15732) also belongs to this subfamily [60–62].

SmFtz-F1 was the first member of this subfamily to be characterized from a lophotrochozoan [48]. Subfamily 5 only contains orphan receptors that bind to their response element as monomers, the most studied members being mammalian SF-1 (steroidogenic factor-1) and LRH-1 (liver receptor homolog-1), both involved in embryonic development. The first member of the subfamily was isolated from *D. melanogaster* [80, 81]. SmFtz-F1 has a deduced amino acid sequence of 731 residues and an apparent molecular mass of 78 kDa (GenBank accession number AF158103), while SmFtz-F1α contains 1892 residues and an apparent mass of 207,402 kDa (GenBank accession number AY665680). The length of these receptors differs from orthologue members of the family, however, both proteins conserved the general structure of the nuclear receptors [48, 78]. The hinge region of SmFtz-F1α is particularly long (1027 amino acids). The DBDs of the two NRs share an identity of 55 to 75% to other members of the family, while LBDs are less conserved but contain the typical LBD signatures of the family as well as a high identity with the AF-2 sequence [48, 78]. Both receptors exhibit the expected monomeric DNA-binding ability since the DBD recognizes an SF1 response element-like sequence. However, SmFtz-F1 recognized this response element with a different binding affinity than SmFtz-F1α. The transactivation mechanism is also different between both receptors [79]. On the other side, as was previously mentioned, it was demonstrated that SmFtz-F1 dimerizes with SmRXR [69].

Although Ftz-F1 protein and mRNA expression are detected during all life cycles, expression levels differed according to the developmental stage. The higher expression of SmFtz-F1 was observed in the larval stages of miracidia, sporocysts, and cercaria, while the protein highest level was found in cercaria, schistosomula, and male adult work suggesting a role during host invasion and adaptation. The transcription behavior of SmFtz-F1α makes a difference between the two NRs since the higher mRNA level was detected in the schistosoma egg stage. A similar gonad distribution was also observed in several Ftz-F1 homologues [82, 83].

Taken together these events, it was hypothesized that target genes of both receptors exert different roles during the parasite development and these two receptors also have different ligands or co-activators. Co-activators characterization could start to decipher the transcriptional regulation complex formed by each nuclear receptor. In this sense, the search of transcription regulators of SmFtz-F1 was performed. The transcription co-activator CREB-binding protein (CBP) homologs from *S. mansoni*, named SmCBP1 and SmCBP2, were characterized. SmCBP1 can interact with SmFtz-F1 and activate the transcription of a reporter gene [84]. On the other side, a specific transcriptional co-repressor protein named SmFIP-1, which interacts with the AF2-AD motif of SmFtz-F1, was identified [85].

Finally, an interesting finding was the identification of the first target gene of SmFtz-F1, the micro-exon gene *meg-8.3* [86]. *meg-8.3* is expressed exclusively in the worm's esophageal gland, an enigmatic tissue that has recently been shown to play a critical role in defending the worm from host attack [87].

2.6 New subfamily 7

A very interesting finding for the biology of parasitic Platyhelminthes was the identification in *S. mansoni* of a new group of NRs that has two tandem DNA-binding domains and one LBD, named 2DBD, lacking in vertebrates [71]. Subsequently, members of this 2DBD subfamily have been identified in some mollusks, in *Echinococcus granulosus,* and other Platyhelminthes [21, 35, 36, 49]. *S. mansoni* expresses three

2DBD (Sm2DBDα, Sm2DBDβ, Sm2DBDγ) and homologous sequences were found in other parasitic Platyhelminthes including Monogenea, Cestoda, and Trematoda [21, 49]. 2DBD-NRs have the same P-box sequence (CEACKK) in the first DBD that is not present in another known NR [35, 71]. This characteristic P-box could determine a new target DNA binding specificity [88]. *In vitro* and *in vivo* studies show that Sm2DBDα could interact as a homodimer, not interacting with SmRXR or SmRXR1. Homodimer formation implies that four P-boxes may be involved in DNA binding. In addition, Wu and collaborators reported that the three Sm2DBDs are regulated during development and may have a differential role in the different stages [35]. Although the databases of *E. granulosus* (WormBase Parasite) report three Eg2DBD, our research group has cloned from protoscoleces of *E. g. sensu lato*, a coding sequence for an Eg2DBDα isoform (GenBank MH092994.2) not reported in existing databases. This transcript was probably originated through mRNA alternative splicing and was named Eg2DBDα.1 [36]. A bioinformatic description of this isoform, including domains structure, putative NLS signals, post-translational modifications, and a 3D model of the two DNA-binding domains, was performed [36].

Recently, molecular docking studies showed that unsaturated long-chain fatty acids, in particular oleic, linoleic, and arachidonic acids, are the Eg2DBDα.1 preferred ligands [89]. It is worth mentioning that this ligand's preference is similar to that of the EgFABP1 protein, previously characterized and studied by our research group [90, 91]. EgFABP1 is a fatty acid-binding protein which was localized in the nuclei of *E. granulosus* protoscoleces cells and other subcellular compartments [92]. Parasitic Platyhelminthes FABPs are considered essential proteins for these organisms since they are not able to synthesize fatty acids *de novo*, so these molecules could participate in host fatty acids uptake and distribution [93]. The interaction between vertebrate FABPs and PPAR nuclear receptors was demonstrated by several reports [94–97]. Taking into account the aforementioned, a model is proposed in **Figure 1**, where

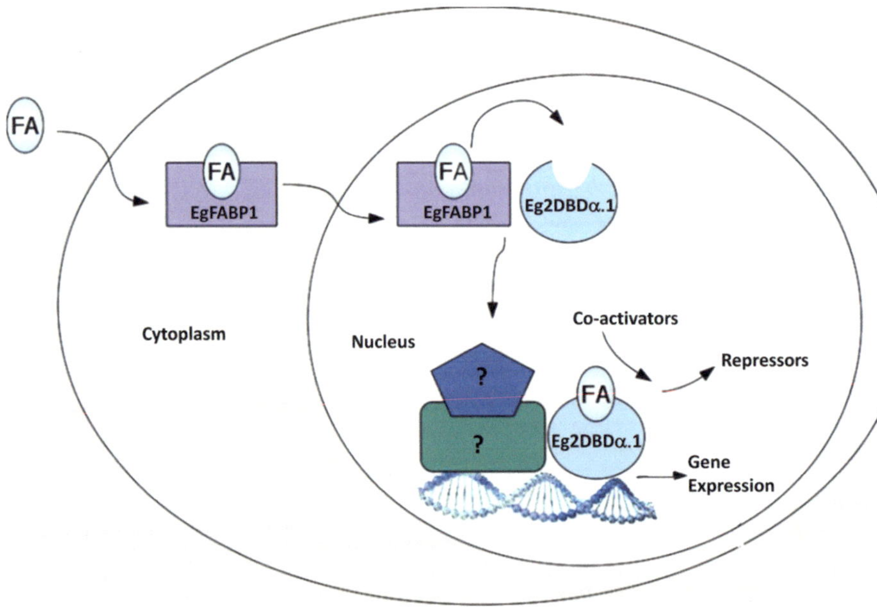

Figure 1.
Schematic model of the putative Eg2DBDα.1 mechanism of action.

EgFABP1 could transport host unsaturated long-chain fatty acids (FA) to the nucleus and transfer its ligand to Eg2DBDα.1. In this way, Eg2DBDα.1 could homodimerize or heterodimerize with other NR and bind to specific DNA response elements to regulate the gene expression of its target genes. Since, these fatty acids are probably acquired from the parasite–host, the signaling mechanism proposed involves a possible host–parasite communication mediated by Eg2DBDα.1 and EgFABP1. In addition, it is possible that co-activator and/or repressor proteins participate as part of the transcriptional regulatory complex.

Acknowledgements

This work was financially supported by the Sectorial Commission for Scientific Research (CSIC, Grants N° C206-348, and N° C112-347) (UdelaR) and the National Agency for Research and Innovation (Grant N° ANII-FCE 2017_1_136527).

Conflict of interest

The authors declare no conflict of interest.

Author details

Adriana Esteves and Gabriela Alvite*
Biochemistry Section, Faculty of Sciences, Universidad de la República, Montevideo, Uruguay

*Address all correspondence to: gabial@fcien.edu.uy

References

[1] Jensen EV. On the mechanism of Estrogen action. Perspectives in Biology and Medicine. 1962;**6**:47-60. DOI: 10.1353/pbm.1963.0005

[2] Govindan MV, Devic M, Green S, Gronemeyer H, Chambon P. Cloning of the human glucocorticoid receptor cDNA. Nucleic Acids Research. 1985;**13**:8293-8304. DOI: 10.1093/nar/13.23.8293

[3] Evans RM, Mangelsdorf DJ. Nuclear receptors, RXR, and the big bang. Cell. 2014;**157**:255-266. DOI: 10.1016/j.cell.2014.03.012

[4] Kininis M, Kraus WL. A global view of transcriptional regulation by nuclear receptors: Gene expression, factor localization, and DNA sequence analysis. Nuclear Receptor Signaling. 2008;**6**:e005. DOI: 10.1621/nrs.06005

[5] Gustafsson JA. Historical overview of nuclear receptors. The Journal of Steroid Biochemistry and Molecular Biology. 2016;**157**:3-6. DOI: 10.1016/j.jsbmb.2015.03.004

[6] Weikum ER, Liu X, Ortlund EA. The nuclear receptor superfamily: A structural perspective. Protein Science. 2018;**27**:1876-1892. DOI: 10.1002/pro.3496

[7] Novac N, Heinzel T. Nuclear receptors: Overview and classification. Current DrugTarget -Inflammation & Allergy. 2004;**3**:335-346. DOI: 10.2174/1568010042634541

[8] Benoit G, Cooney A, Giguere V, Ingraham H, Lazar M, Muscat G, et al. International Union of Pharmacology. LXVI. Orphan Nuclear Receptors. Pharmacological Reviews. 2006;**58**:798-836. DOI: 10.1124/pr.58.4.10

[9] Giguère V, Hollenberg SM, Rosenfeld MG, Evans RM. Functional domains of the human glucocorticoid receptor. Cell. 1986;**46**:645-652. DOI: 10.1016/0092-8674

[10] Pawlak M, Lefebvre P, Staels B. General molecular biology and architecture of nuclear receptors. Current Topics in Medicinal Chemistry. 2012;**12**:486-504. DOI: 10.2174/156802612799436641

[11] Kumar R. Thompson EB, Transactivation functions of the N-terminal domains of nuclear hormone receptors: Protein folding and coactivator interactions. Molecular Endocrinology. 2003;**17**:1-10. DOI: 10.1210/me.2002-0258

[12] Danielsen M. Bioinformatics of nuclear receptors. Methods in Molecular Biology (Clifton, N.J.). 2001;**176**:3-22. DOI: 10.1385/1-59259-115-9:3

[13] Kumar V, Gree S, Staub A, Chambon P. Localisation of the oestradiol-binding and putative DNA-binding domains of the human oestrogen receptor. The EMBO Journal. 1996;**5**:2231-2236. DOI: 10.1002/j.1460-2075.1986.tb04489.x

[14] Luisi BF, Xu WX, Otwinowski Z, Freedman LP, Yamamoto KR, Sigler PB. Crystallographic analysis of the interaction of the glucocorticoid receptor with DNA. Nature. 1991;**352**:497-505. DOI: 10.1038/352497a0

[15] Schwabe JWR, Chapman L, Finch JT, Rhodes D. The crystal structure of theestrogen receptor DNA-binding domain bound to DNA: How receptors discriminate between their response elements. Cell. 1993;**75**:567-578. DOI: 10.1016/0092-8674(93)90390-c

[16] Gronemeyer H, Moras D. How to finger DNA. Nature. 1995;**375**:190-191. DOI: 10.1038/375190a0

[17] Aggarwal P, Bhavesh NS. Hinge like domain motion facilitates human RBMS1 protein binding to proto-oncogene c-myc promoter. Nucleic Acids Research. 2021;**49**:5943-5955. DOI: 10.1093/nar/gkab363

[18] Moras D, Gronemeyer H. The nuclear receptor ligand-binding domain: Structureand function. Current Opinion in Cell Biology. 1998;**10**:384-391. DOI: 10.1016/s0955-0674(98)80015-x

[19] Weatherman RV, Fletterick RJ, Scanlan TS. Nuclear-receptor ligands and ligand-binding domains. Annual Review of Biochemistry. 1999;**68**:559-581. DOI: 10.1146/annurev.biochem.68.1.559

[20] Wurtz JM, Bourguet W, Renaud JP, Vivat V, Chambon P, Moras D, et al. A canonical structure for the ligand-binding domain of nuclear receptors. Nature Structural Biology. 1996;**3**:87-94. DOI: 10.1038/nsb0196-87

[21] Wu W, LoVerde PT. Nuclear hormone receptors in parasitic Platyhelminths. Molecular and Biochemical Parasitology. 2019;**233**:111218. DOI: 10.1016/j.molbiopara.2019.111218

[22] Barettino D, Ruiz MMV, Stunnenberg HG. Characterization of the ligand dependent transactivation domain of thyroid hormone receptor. The EMBO Journal. 1994;**13**:3039-3049. DOI: 10.1002/j.1460-2075.1994.tb06603.x

[23] Bourguet W, Ruff M, Chambon P, Gronemeyer H, Moras D. Crystal structure of the ligand-binding domain of the human nuclear receptor RXR-α. Nature. 1995;**375**:377-382. DOI: 10.1038/375377a0

[24] Patel SR, Skafar DF. Modulation of nuclear receptor activity by the F domain. Molecular and Cellular Endocrinology. 2015;**418**:298-305. DOI: 10.1016/j.mce.2015.07.009

[25] Sladek FM. What are nuclear receptor ligands? Molecular and Cellular Endocrinology. 2022;**334**:3-13. DOI: 10.1016/j.mce.2010.06.018

[26] Mazaira GI, Zgajnar NR, Lotufo CM, Daneri-Becerra C, Sivils JC, Soto OB, et al. The nuclear receptor field: A historical overview and future challenges. Nuclear Receptor Research. 2018;**5**:101320. DOI: 10.11131/2018/101320

[27] Escrivá H, Laudet V, Robinson-Rechavi M. Nuclear receptors are markers of animal genome evolution. Journal of Structural and Functional Genomics. 2003;**3**:177-184. DOI: 10.1023/a:1022638706822

[28] Fonseca E, Machado AM, Vilas-Arrondo N, Gomes-dos-Santos A, Verissimo A, Esteves P, et al. Cartilaginous fishes offer unique insights into the evolution of the nuclear receptor gene repertoire in gnathostomes. General and Comparative Endocrinology. 2020;**295**:113527. DOI: 10.1016/j.ygcen.2020.113527

[29] Bertrand S, Brunet FG, Escriva H, Parmentier G, Laudet V, Robinson-Rechavi M. Evolutionary genomics of nuclear receptors: From twenty-five ancestral genes to derived endocrine systems. Molecular Biology and Evolution. 2004;**21**:1923-1937. DOI: 10.1093/molbev/msh200

[30] Bridgham JT, Eick GN, Larroux C, Deshpande K, Harms MJ, Gauthier MEA, et al. Protein evolution by molecular tinkering: Diversification of the nuclear receptor superfamily from a

ligand-dependent ancestor. PLoS Biology. 2010;**8**:e1000497. DOI: 10.1371/journal.pbio.1000497

[31] Cheng Y-Y, Tao W-J, Chen J-L, Sun L-N, Zhou L-Y, Song Q, et al. Genome-wide identification, evolution and expression analysis of nuclear receptor superfamily in Nile tilapia, Oreochromisniloticus. Gene. 2015;**569**:141-152. DOI: 10.1016/j.gene.2015.05.057

[32] Yang P-J, Chen E-H, Song Z-H, He W, Liu S-H, Dou W, et al. Molecular characterization and expression profiling of nuclear receptor gene families in oriental fruit Fly, Bactrocera Dorsalis (Hendel). Insects. 2020;**11**:126. DOI: 10.3390/insects11020126

[33] Escrivá H, Bertrand S, Laudet V. The evolution of the nuclear receptor superfamily. Essays in Biochemistry. 2004;**40**:11-26. DOI: 10.1042/bse0400011

[34] Laudet V, Auwerx J, Gustafsson J, Wahli WA. Unified nomenclature system for the nuclear receptor superfamily. Cell. 1999;**97**:161-163. DOI: 10.1016/s0092-8674(00)80726-6

[35] Wu W, Niles EG, Hirai H, LoVerde PT. Evolution of a novel subfamily of nuclear receptors with members that each contain two DNA binding domains. BMC Evolutionary Biology. 2007;**7**:27. DOI: 10.1186/1471-2148-7-27

[36] Alvite G, Riera X, Cancela S, Paulino M, Esteves A. Bioinformatic analysis of anovel *Echinococcus granulosus* nuclear receptor with two DNA binding domains. PLoS One. 2019;**14**:e0224703. DOI: 10.1371/journal.pone.0224703

[37] Cheng Y, Chen J, Mukhtar I, Chen J. Genome-wide characterization of the nuclear receptor gene family in *Macrostomum lignano* imply its evolutionary diversification. Frontiers in Marine Science. 2021;**8**:653447. DOI: 10.3389/fmars.2021.653447

[38] Walker JC, Anderson DT. The Platyhelminthes. In: Anderson DT, editor. Invertebrate Zoology. England: Oxford University Press; 2001. pp. 58-80

[39] Norena C, Damborenea C, Brusa F. Phylum Platyhelminthes. Ecology and general biology. In: Thorp JH, Rogers C, editors. Thorp and Covich's Freshwater Invertebrates. 4th ed. Vol. I. Amsterdam: Elsevier Academic Press; 2015. pp. 181-203

[40] Riutort M, Álvarez-Presas M, Lázaro E, Solà E, Paps J. Evolutionary history of the Tricladida and the Platyhelminthes: An up-to-date phylogenetic and systematic account. The International Journal of Developmental Biology. 2012;**56**:5-17. DOI: 10.1387/ijdb.113441mr

[41] Adell T et al. Platyhelminthes. In: Wanninger A, editor. Evolutionary Developmental Biology of Invertebrates 2: Lophotrochozoa (Spiralia). Vienna: Springer Vienna; 2015. pp. 21-40

[42] G.B.D. 2015 Disease and Injury Incidence and Prevalence Collaborators. Global, regional, and national incidence, prevalence, and years lived with disability for 310 diseases and injuries, 1990-2015: A systematic analysis for the global burden of disease study 2015. Lancet. 2016;**388**:1545-1602

[43] International Helminth Genomes Consortium. Comparative genomics of the major parasitic worms. Nature Genetics. 2019;**51**:163-174. DOI: 10.1038/s41588-018-0262-1

[44] Brehm K, Koziol U. Echinococcus–host interactions at cellular and molecular levels. Advances in

Parasitology. 2017;**95**:147-212. DOI: 10.1016/bs.apar.2016.09.001

[45] Freebern WJ, Niles EG, LoVerde PT. RXR-2, a member of the retinoid x receptor family in *Schistosoma mansoni*. Gene. 1999;**233**:33-38. DOI: 10.1016/s0378-1119(99)00161-4

[46] Freebern WJ, Osman A, Niles EG, Christen L, LoVerde PT. Identification of a cDNA encoding a retinoid X receptor homologue from *Schistosoma mansoni*. Evidence for a role in female-specific gene expression. The Journal of Biological Chemistry. 1999;**274**:4577-4585. DOI: 10.1074/jbc.274.8.4577

[47] De Mendonca RL, Escriva H, Bouton D, Zelus D, Vanacker JM, Bonnelye E, et al. Structural and functional divergence of a nuclear receptor of the RXR family from the trematode parasite *Schistosoma mansoni*. European Journal of Biochemistry. 2000;**267**:3208-3219. DOI: 10.1046/j.1432-1327.2000.01344.x

[48] De Mendonca RL, Bouton D, Bertin B, Escrivá H, Noel C, Vanacker JM, et al. A functionally conserved member of the FTZ-F1 nuclear receptor family from *Schistosoma mansoni*. European Journal of Biochemistry. 2002;**269**:5700-5711. DOI: 10.1046/j.1432-1033.2002.03287.x

[49] Wu W, LoVerde PT. Identification and evolution of nuclear receptors in Platyhelminths. PLoS One. 2021;**16**:e0250750. DOI: 10.1371/journal.pone.0250750

[50] Wendt G, Zhao L, Chen R, Liu C, O'Donoghue AJ, Caffrey CR, et al. A single-cell RNA-seq atlas of *Schistosoma mansoni* identifies a key regulator of blood feeding. Science. 2020;**25**(369):1644-1649. DOI: 10.1126/science.abb7709

[51] Wang J, Collins JJ 3rd. Identification of new markers for the *Schistosoma mansoni* vitelline lineage. International Journal for Parasitology. 2016;**46**:405-410. DOI: 10.1016/j.ijpara.2016.03.004

[52] Wang J, Chen R, Collins JJ 3rd. Systematically improved *in vitro* culture conditions reveal new insights into the reproductive biology of the human parasite *Schistosoma mansoni*. PLoS Biology. 2019;**17**:e3000254. DOI: 10.1371/journal.pbio.3000254

[53] Spiliotis M, Brehm K. Axenic *in vitro* cultivation of *Echinococcus multilocularis* metacestode vesicles and the generation of primary cell cultures. Methods in Molecular Biology. 2009;**470**:245-262. DOI: 10.1007/978-1-59745-204-5_17

[54] Spiliotis M, Tappe D, Sesterhenn L, Brehm K. Long-term in vitro cultivation of *Echinococcus multilocularis* metacestodes under axenic conditions. Parasitology Research. 2004;**92**:430-432. DOI: 10.1007/s00436-003-1046-8

[55] Spiliotis M, Lechner S, Tappe D, Krohne G, Brehm K. Transient transfection of *Echinococcus multilocularis* primary cells and complete *in vitro* regeneration of metacestode vesicles. International Journal for Parasitology. 2008;**38**:1025-1039. DOI: 10.1016/j.ijpara.2007.11.002

[56] Spiliotis M, Mizukami C, Oku Y, Kiss F, Brehm K, Gottstein B. *Echinococcus multilocularis* primary cells: Improved isolation, small-scale cultivation and RNA interference. Molecular and Biochemical Parasitology. 2010;**174**:83-87. DOI: 10.1016/j.molbiopara.2010.07.001

[57] Forster S, Gunthel D, Kiss F, Brehm K. Molecular characterisation of a serumresponsive, DAF-12-like nuclear hormone receptor of the fox-tapeworm

Echinococcus multilocularis. Journal of Cellular Biochemistry. 2011;**112**(6):1630-1642. DOI: 10.1002/jcb.23073

[58] Yang M, Li J, Wu J, Wang H, Guo B, Wu C, et al. Cloning and characterization of an *Echinococcus granulosus* ecdysteroid hormone nuclear receptor HR3-like gene. Parasite. 2017;**24**:36. DOI: 10.1051/parasite/2017037

[59] Hoffmann J, Porchet M. Biosynthesis, Metabolism and Mode of Action of Invertebrate Hormones. Berlin: Springer-Verlag; 1984

[60] Mercer JG, Munn AE, Rees HH. *Echinococcus granulosus*: Occurrence of ecdysteroids in protoscoleces and hydatid cyst fluid. Molecular and Biochemical Parasitology. 1987, 1987;**24**:203-214. DOI: 10.1016/0166-6851(87)90107-1

[61] Zheng H, Zhang W, Zhang L, Zhang Z, Li J, Lu G, et al. The genome of the hydatid tapeworm *Echinococcus granulosus*. Nature Genetics. 2013;**45**: 1168-1175. DOI: 10.1038/ng.2757

[62] Tsai IJ, Zarowiecki M, Holroyd N, Garciarrubio A, Sanchez-Flores A, Brooks KL, et al. The genomes of four tapeworm species reveal adaptations to parasitism. Nature. 2013;**496**:57-63. DOI: 10.1038/nature12031

[63] Hu R, Wu W, Niles EG, LoVerde PT. SmTR2/4, a *Schistosoma mansoni* homologue of TR2/TR4 orphan nuclear receptor. International Journal for Parasitology. 2006;**36**:1113-1122. DOI: 10.1016/j.ijpara.2006.06.003

[64] Escrivá H, Safi R, Hänni C, et al. Ligand binding was acquired during evolution of nuclear receptors. Proceedings of the National Academy of Sciences. 1997;**94**:6803-6808. DOI: 10.1073/pnas.94.13.6803

[65] Freebern WJ, Osman A, Niles EG, Christen L, LoVerde PT. Identification of a cDNA encoding a retinoid X receptor homologue from *Schistosoma mansoni*. Evidence for a role in female-specific gene expression. The Journal of Biological Chemistry. 1999;**274**:4577-4585. DOI: 10.1074/jbc.274.8.4577

[66] Mendonça RL, Escrivá H, Vanacker JM, Bouton D, Delannoy S, Pierce RJ, et al. Nuclear hormone receptors and evolution. American Zoologist. 1999;**27**:704-713

[67] Mendonça RL, Escriva H, Bouton D, Zelus D, Vanacker JM, Bonnelye E, et al. Structural and functional divergence of a nuclear receptor of the RXR family from the trematode parasite *Schistosoma mansoni*. European Journal of Biochemistry. 2000;**267**:3208-3219. DOI: 10.1046/j.1432-1327.2000.01344.x

[68] Mangelsdorf DJ, Evans RM. RXR heterodimers and orphan receptors. Cell. 1995;**83**:841-850. DOI: 10.1016/0092-8674(95)90200-7

[69] Bertin B, Caby S, Oger F, Sasorith S, Wurtz JM, Pierce RJ. The monomeric orphan nuclear receptor *Schistosoma mansoni* Ftz-F1 dimerizes specifically and functionally with the schistosome RXR homologue, SmRXR1. Biochemical and Biophysical Research Communications. 2005;**327**:1072-1082. DOI: 10.1016/j.bbrc.2004.12.101

[70] Wendt G, Zhao L, Chen R, Liu C, O'Donoghue AJ, Caffrey CR, et al. A single-cell RNA-seq atlas of Schistosoma mansoniidentifies a key regulator of blood feeding. Science. 2020;**25**(369):1644-1649. DOI: 10.1126/science.abb7709

[71] Wu W, Niles EG, El-Sayed N, Berriman M, LoVerde PT. *Schistosoma mansoni* (Platyhelminthes, Trematoda)

nuclear receptors: Sixteen new members and a novel subfamily. Gene. 2006;**366**:303-315. DOI: 10.1016/j.gene.2005.09.013

[72] Taubenheim J, Kortmann C, Fraune S. Function and evolution of nuclear receptors in environmental-dependent postembryonic development. Frontiers in Cell and Development Biology. 2021 Jun;**10**(9):653792. DOI: 10.3389/fcell.2021.653792

[73] Ibarra-Coronado EG, Escobedo G, Nava-Castro K, Jesús Ramses CR, Hernández-Bello R, García-Varela M, et al. A helminth cestode parasite express an estrogen-binding protein resembling a classic nuclear estrogen receptor. Steroids. 2011;**10-11**:1149-1159. DOI: 10.1016/j.steroids. 2011.05.003

[74] Nicolao MC, Elissondo MC, Denegri GM, Goya AB, Cumino AC. *In vitro* and *in vivo* effects of tamoxifen against larval stage *Echinococcus granulosus*. Antimicrobial Agents and Chemotherapy. 2014;**58**:5146-5154

[75] Stadelmann B, Aeschbacher D, Huber C, Spiliotis M, Muller J, Hemphill A. Profound activity of the anti-cancer drug bortezomib against *Echinococcus multilocularis*metacestodes identifies the proteasome as a novel drug target for cestodes. PLOS Neglected Tropical Diseases. 2014;**8**:e3352

[76] Escobedo G, Camacho-Arroyo I, Hernandez-Hernandez OT, Ostoa-Saloma P, Garcia-Varela M, Morales-Montor J. Progesterone induces scolex evagination of the human parasite *Taeniasolium*: Evolutionary implications to the host-parasite relationship. Journal of Biomedicine & Biotechnology. 2010;**2010**:591079

[77] Aguilar-Díaz H, Nava-Castro KE, Escobedo G, Domínguez-Ramírez L, García-Varela M, Del Río-Araiza VH, et al. A novel progesterone receptor membrane component (PGRMC) in the human and swine parasite *Taeniasolium*: Implications to the host-parasite relationship. Parasites & Vectors. 2018;**11**:161. DOI: 10.1186/s13071-018-2703-1

[78] Lu C, Wu W, Niles EG, LoVerde PT. Identification and characterization of a novel fushitarazu factor-1 (FTZ-F1) nuclear receptor in *Schistosoma mansoni*. Molecular and Biochemical Parasitology. 2006;**150**:25-36

[79] Lu C, Niles EG, LoVerde PT. Characterization of the DNA-binding properties and the transactivation activity of *Schistosoma mansoni* nuclear receptor fushitarazu-factor 1α(SmFTZ-F1α). Molecular and Biochemical Parasitology. 2006;**150**:72-82

[80] Ueda H, Sonoda S, Brown JL, Scott MP, Wu C. Asequence-specific DNA-binding protein that activates fushitarazu segmentation gene expression. Genes & Development. 1990;**4**:624-635.3

[81] Lavorgna G, Ueda H, Clos J, Wu C. FTZ-F1, a steroid hormone receptor-like protein implicated in the activation of *fushitarazu*. Science. 1991;**252**:848-851

[82] Gissendanner CR, Sluder AE. Nhr-25, the *Caenorhabditis elegans*ortholog of ftz-f1, is required for epidermal and somatic gonad development. Developmental Biology. 2000;**221**:259-272

[83] Ramayya MS, Zhou J, Kino T, Segars JH, Bondy CA, Chrousos GP. Steroidogenic factor 1 messenger ribonucleic acid expression in steroidogenic and nonsteroidogenic human tissues: Northern blot and in situ hybridization studies. The Journal of

Clinical Endocrinology and Metabolism. 1997;**82**:1799-1806

[84] Bertin B, Oger F, Cornette J, Caby S, Noel C, Capron M, et al. Schistosoma mansoni CBP/p300 has a conserved domain structure and interacts functionally with the nuclear receptor SmFtz-F1. Molecular and Biochemical Parasitology. 2006;**146**:180-191

[85] Oger F, Bertin B, Caby S, Dalia-Cornette J, Adams M, Vicogne J, et al. Molecular cloning and characterization of *Schistosoma mansoni* Ftz-F1 interacting protein-1 (SmFIP-1), a novel corepressor of the nuclear receptor SmFtz-F1. Molecular and Biochemical Parasitology. 2006;**148**:10-23. DOI: 10.1016/j.molbiopara.2006.02.016

[86] Romero AA, Cobb SA, Collins JNR, Kliewer SA, Mangelsdorf DJ, Collins JJ 3rd. The Schistosoma mansoninuclear receptor FTZ-F1 maintains esophageal gland function via transcriptional regulation ofmeg-8.3. PLOS Pathogens. 2021;**17**:e1010140. DOI: 10.1371/journal.ppat.1010140

[87] Lee J, Chong T, Newmark PA. The esophageal gland mediates host immune evasion by the human parasite *Schistosoma mansoni*. Proceedings of the National Academy of Sciences of the United States of America. 2020;**117**:19299-19309. DOI: 10.1073/pnas.2006553117

[88] Wu W, LoVerde PT. Nuclear hormone receptors in parasitic helminths. Molecular and Cellular Endocrinology. 2011;**334**:56-66. DOI: 10.1016/j.mce.2010.06.011

[89] Cancela S, Esteves A, Alvite G, Paulino M. Modeling, molecular dynamics and docking studies of a full-length *Echinococcus granulosus* 2DBD nuclear receptor. Journal of Biomolecular Structure and Dynamics. 2022:1-10. DOI: 10.1080/07391102.2021.2023641 [Epub ahead of print]

[90] Alvite G, Pietro SMD, Santome JA, Ehrlich R, Esteves A. Binding properties of *Echinococcus granulosus* fatty acid binding protein. Biochim Biophys Acta - Molecular and Cell Biology of Lipids. 2001;**1533**:293-302. DOI: 10.1016/s1388-1981(01)00164-0

[91] Jakobsson E, Alvite G, Bergfors T, Esteves A, Kleywegt GJ. The crystal structure of *Echinococcus granulosus* fatty-acid-binding protein 1. Biochimica et Biophysica Acta. 2003;**1649**:40-50. DOI: 10.1016/s1570-9639(03)00151-1

[92] Alvite G, Esteves A. *Echinococcus granulosus* fatty acid binding proteins subcellular localization. Experimental Parasitology. 2016;**164**:1-4. DOI: 10.1016/j.exppara.2016.02.002

[93] Alvite G, Garrido N, Kun A, Paulino M, Esteves A. Towards an understanding of *Mesocestoides vogae* fatty acid binding proteins' roles. PLoS One. 2014;**9**:e111204. DOI: 10.1371/journal.pone.0111204

[94] Hostetler HA, McIntosh AL, Atshaves BP, Storey SM, Payne HR, Kier AB, et al. L-FABP directly interacts with PPARα in cultured primary hepatocytes. Journal of Lipid Research. 2009;**50**:1663-1675. DOI: 10.1194/jlr.m900058-jlr200

[95] McIntosh AL, Atshaves BP, Hostetler HA, Huang H, Davis J, Lyuksyutova OI, et al. Liver type fatty acid binding protein (L-FABP) gene ablation reduces nuclear ligand distribution and peroxisome proliferator-activated receptor-alpha activity in cultured primary hepatocytes. Archives of Biochemistry and Biophysics. 2009;**485**:160-173. DOI: 10.1016/j.abb.2009.03.004

[96] Wolfrum C, Borrmann CM, Borchers T, Spener F. Fatty acids and hypolipidemic drugs regulate peroxisome proliferator-activated receptors alpha - and gamma-mediated gene expression via liver fatty acid binding protein: A signaling path to the nucleus. Proceedings of the National Academy of Sciences of the United States of America. 2001;**98**:2323-2328. DOI: 10.1073/pnas.051619898

[97] Tan NS, Shaw NS, Vinckenbosch N, Liu P, Yasmin R, Desvergne B, et al. Selective cooperation between fatty acid binding proteins and peroxisome proliferator-activated receptors in regulating transcription. Molecular and Cellular Biology. 2002;**22**:5114-5127. DOI: 10.1128/MCB.22.14.5114-5127.2002

Chapter 7

Perspective Chapter: Molecular Crosstalk and Signal Transduction between Platyhelminths and Their Hosts

Ednilson Hilário Lopes-Junior, Rafaella Pontes Marques, Claudio Romero Bertevello and Katia Cristina Oliveira

Abstract

Parasitic infection is an intimate relationship between host and parasite with exchange of signal and complex signaling systems involved in these organisms' molecular crosstalk. With the advances of knowledge due to the genomic and transcriptomic projects in the last two decades, several genes and the molecular mechanism involved in the biological function of platyhelminths have been described. Cytokines, hormones, and other molecules from the host have influenced the growth, development, and reproduction of platyhelminths. We are going to review the effects of host cytokines (IL-1, IL-4, IL-12, IL-7, TGF-β, TNF-α) and hormones (T4, estrogen, progesterone, and androgens) that directly or indirectly affect parasites' development and reproduction, and the possible associated signaling pathway. These are excellent models for system biology studies, and the generated knowledge may be helpful in the development of new strategies to combat these helminthiases.

Keywords: platyhelminths, signaling pathways, molecular crosstalk, cytokines, hormones

1. Introduction

Parasitism is a complex relationship between two organisms and requires several adaptations at the molecular level to establish successful interactions throughout evolution. Intricate signaling systems are necessary to transduce each signal from host to pathogen and vice versa. These systems or networks are relevant because they capture various signals from the environment in which the parasite lives (host), release stimuli, and send signals between different organs and tissues to regulate complex biological processes.

Many host signals (molecules) modulate the development and growth of parasites and directly or indirectly interfere in the course of parasitic infection. It is as

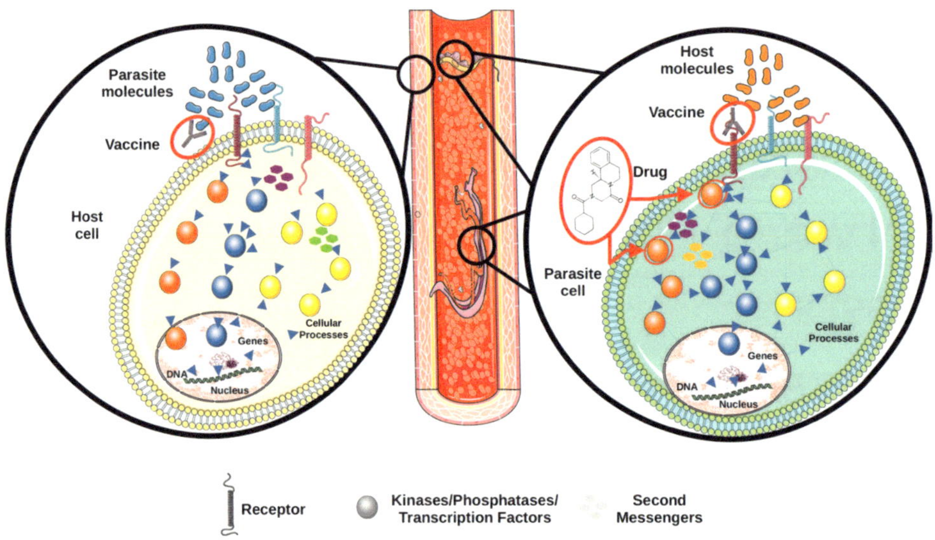

Figure 1.
Molecular cross-talk between parasite and host. Schematic representation of parasite and host cells, signaling pathways, and molecules secreted (potential ligands) by both organisms. The ellipses represent signaling elements as indicated in the figure and the different colors represent distinct signaling pathways; the hexagons represent second messengers, and the arrows indicate the sequential interaction between proteins of the signaling pathways that culminate in the activation of transcription of target genes that will trigger various cellular processes. Potential molecular targets for drugs and vaccines are highlighted in red circles.

important to understand the mechanism of action of these molecules to improve the knowledge of the basic biology of parasitism as the description of the effects itself is necessary.

With the development of sequencing technologies, the difficulties and costs of sequencing a genome or transcriptome have been reduced significantly; consequently, the number of sequences available dramatically increased [1], including the sequences from platyhelminth genomes [2–6] and transcriptomes [7–12]. This data collection allowed the scientific community to perform evolutive studies and investigate the signaling elements such as receptor, kinase and phosphatase proteins, and transcription factors [13–16]. These advances reflect the understanding of the molecular crosstalk mechanism between host and parasites. Studying the signaling elements is essential to comprehend parasitism, parasite development and identify new targets for developing strategies against these diseases (**Figure 1**) [17, 18].

This chapter reviews the host molecules (cytokines and hormones) and their effects and signals transduction pathways in platyhelminths. The most studied model of platyhelminth is *Schistosoma mansoni* (*S. mansoni*) and most of the information available in this chapter refers to this parasite.

2. Host cytokines' effects on platyhelminths

Cytokines are small proteins (5–25 kDa) produced by many cells (especially from the immune system), which exert a signaling effect (at an autocrine, paracrine, or endocrine level) in a broad range of tissues [19]. Generally, cytokine studies focus on the immune system's regulation when faced with an infection; however, we will describe how the host cytokines can modulate platyhelminths' biological/physiological processes and their possible signaling pathways.

2.1 Interleukins (12, 2, 7, 4, and 1)

Interleukin-7 (IL-7) is a cytokine secreted by bone-marrow, endothelial, and epithelial-stromal cells essential in the hematopoietic system for the proliferation, differentiation, and development of B cells [20]. It is also involved in the thymic development of mature T lymphocytes, natural killer (NK), and lymphokine-activated killer (LAK) cells [21].

IL-7 interferes in the development of *S. mansoni* (in murine infection) [22]. Female knockout mice for the IL-7 gene (IL-7−/−) infected with *S. mansoni* showed significant differences in parasite development, egg-induced pathology, and worm recovery rate. It was also observed that fewer eggs were laid *in vivo,* and more dead eggs were detected without IL-7. The decreasing egg burden ameliorated the liver pathology, and morphological differences in the length of male and female worms in the IL-7−/− mice were observed [22].

Studies with radiolabeled IL-7 suggested that this cytokine did not bind directly on the parasite surface; hence, the observed effects of IL-7 deficient mice could be attributed to the cytokine's interactions with the host's immune and or endocrine responses [23, 24].

Interleukin-2 (IL-2) is a cytokine with autocrine and paracrine effects secreted by activated T-CD4 + cells [25]. Further investigations interrogated the modulation of *S. mansoni* development by IL-7 and IL-2 through the influence of these cytokines on CD4+ T (T helper) cells [26]. With the use of knockout mice for IL-7 receptor (IL-7Rα−/−) and IL-2 (IL-2−/−) for *S. mansoni* infection, the morphology of adult worms is affected. In both knockout mice, the infected mice produced smaller male worms than the control group. In the IL-7 receptor knockout mice, the parasite's egg production was drastically reduced [26]. Studies with IL-2 receptor knockout mice (IL-2Rα−/−) infected with *S. mansoni* revealed a similar impact on the parasite's development, using the knockout mice for the cytokine. Thus, it could be concluded that the modulation of IL-7 and IL-2 in *S. mansoni* development (adult growth and egg-laying and granuloma formation) is indirect; the cytokines act on the host's CD4+ T cells [26].

Interleukin-12 (IL-12) and interleukin-4 (IL-4) reciprocally regulate differentiation of naïve CD4+ T lymphocytes and directly promote the development of CD4+ Th1 cells and the CD4+ T-cell differentiation in the Th2 phenotype (which also produces IL-4). In 2012, Cheng et al. [27] used an approach with hybridoma cells injected into different mice groups to evaluate the effect of monoclonal antibodies against IL-12 and IL-4 on parasite infection. The effect of IL-12 and IL-4 on worm development and granuloma formation in a murine infection by *Schistosoma japonicum* (*S. japonicum*) was evaluated. It was observed that, 24 days post-infection, the group of anti-IL-12 had a significant increase in the number of eggs per couple and eggs in the liver. The granuloma size and fibrosis in the liver in the anti-IL-12 mice were significantly more prominent on day 42. The decreasing of T helper 1 (Th1) cytokine expression through the blocking of IL-12 promotes the T helper 2 (Th2) cytokine expression and reduces Interferon-γ (IFN-γ) and Interferon-α (IFN-α) cytokine levels.

The length of worms in the anti-IL-12 group was increased; however, the degree of increase was different in males and females. The female size was higher in anti-IL-12 than in anti-IL-4 and control groups at 28 and 42 days post-infection, while the male size was higher just at 28 days in the anti-IL-12 [27]. The data in this study suggest that IL-12 deficiency benefits *S. japonicum* worm development in the early days of infection, indicating the action of cytokine against the schistosome. At the same time, its effect was reduced at 42 days post-infection, revealing a transitory effect. It is important to note that IL-12 promotes a Th1 response.

Finally, interleukin-1 (IL-1) from *Biomphalaria glabrata* (*B. glabrata*), the intermediate host of *S. mansoni*, also affects the parasite. In the vertebrate's immune system, the cytokine IL-1 mediates cytotoxic, humoral, and inflammatory responses, induces leukocyte recruitment to the inflammation site, and is involved in the cytotoxic reactive oxygen intermediate (ROI) production mechanism in the effector cells [28]. In the immune defense system of the invertebrate *B. glabrata*, molecules with functional homology to the vertebrate IL-1 (SnaIL-1) have been detected and isolated. It was observed that, in response to schistosome infection's primary sporocysts, susceptible snail strains exhibit a decrease in plasmatic SnaIL-1 levels, while the SnaIL-1 cytokine levels rise in resistant strains. Also, when the susceptible snails are treated with a recombinant human Interleukin-1β (rhIL-1β), there is a rapid phagocytosis activation and ROI production at the same levels found in the resistant snail strains [29].

In 1998, Connors et al. [30] investigated if the treatment of two strands of susceptible *B. glabrata* with rhIL-1β had effect on the infection of the invertebrate host (directly or mediating by hemocyte's activity). After 15 days of exposure, the authors observed a significant decrease of 50% in the number of counted miracidia on snails from both treated groups. Histological analysis of snail tentacles performed 3 days after exposure revealed a significantly higher percentage of dead or disrupted parasites compared to the control. *In-vitro* assays using hemocytes-free cultured parasites in contact with the plasma from rhIL-1β -injected snails showed an immediate killing effect on the parasites.

These results imply that the cytokine may stimulate *in-vivo* induction of a cell-free killing mechanism in the *B. glabrata*. Parasites' killing seems to have no connection with the hemocyte's encapsulation of the parasites, suggesting the presence of both a humoral cytotoxic molecule and a cellular signaling mechanism. Injection of the recombinant human IL-1β on the susceptible snails has activated the otherwise reduced cytotoxic capabilities of the snail's immune system; however, other factors such as reduced number of hemocytes compared to resistant strains may limit the killing of the parasites. Further, invertebrates' cytokine-like activity may occur in molecules with substantially different structures from their mammalian counterparts, obviating the need for more analysis of the elements involved in the host-parasite signaling mechanisms.

2.2 Transforming growth factor-β (TGF-β)

TGF-β plays an essential role in wound healing, angiogenesis, immunoregulation, and cancer development. These cytokine's effects are dual-sided, contributing to the differentiation of regulatory (suppressive) T cells (Tr cells) and inflammatory Th17 cells. In mammals, all leukocytes produce at least one isoform of TGF-β [31]. TGF-β is locally produced by the host's immune system cells in response to the presence of helminth parasites.

In the genome of *Taenia solium* (*T. solium*) and *Taenia crassiceps* (*T. crassiceps*, a canine tapeworm), protein-coding genes for the pivotal signaling elements were identified [32]. TsTGFβR1, TsTGFβR2, TGF-β Type I, Bone Morphogenetic Protein (BMP) Type-I receptor Tr-3, and activin (TGF-ligand) were identified and had a high identity with *Echinococcus* sp. The expression of TsTGFβR1, TsTGFβR2 at mRNA, and protein level was detected in *T. solium* and *T. crassiceps* cysticerci. It showed that both TGF receptors are expressed in the parasite's teguments more prominently in the tegument of *T. crassiceps* and the periphery of *T. solium* cysticerci from the brain than in the cysticerci from skeletal muscle of infected pigs. It is interesting because the TGF-β levels in the cerebrospinal fluid are higher than in serum, suggesting that the exposure to the host's molecule could be involved in cysticerci growth and differentiation [32].

It is interesting to note that *T. solium* and *T. crassiceps* cysticerci were *in vitro* exposed to three concentrations of recombinant human TGFβ-1 (0.001, 0.01, and 0.1 ng/mL). The human cytokine caused a significant increment in the size of cysticerci in *T. crassiceps*. In the *T. solium* cysticerci, a considerable improvement in the survival rate was observed with no effect on its size. The parasite could internalize the host's TGF-β via endocytosis as a regulatory event. However, these effects may be mediated by the direct interaction of the host's cytokine with the parasite receptors. The results observed on the parasites in an *in vitro* treatment and the antibody recognition of receptors are lower when TGF- β incubation occurs. The lower antibody recognition of both Type-I and Type-II parasite receptors when cysticerci were cultured with increasing levels of TGF-β suggests that TGF-βcould bind the Type-II receptor (avoiding the recognition of antibody), then the complex TGF-β-TsTGFβR2 receptor would recruit the Type-I receptor, forming a complex which would prevent the bounding of Type-I receptor antibody. These results point to hTGF-β as a factor in cysticerci growth and survival, which could also play a role in the lack of effectiveness of cysticidal treatment of patients.

In *S. mansoni,* several TGF-β signaling pathway elements have been identified and described, including two TGF-β receptors (SmTβR1 and SmTβR2), one homolog gene to Inhinbin/Activin (SmInAct), a homolog to the BMP (SmBMP), Smp300/CBP, Smad2, and Smad4. In female worms, these elements could play a role in vitelline cell development and egg embryogenesis, as these molecules' expression is detected in these organs (reviewed in [33].

Oliveira et al. [34] studied the effects of the human TGF-β (hTGF-β) on the gene expression profile of *S. mansoni* adult worms. Microarray experiments were performed with RNA extracted from adult worms that were *in vitro* treated with the human cytokine. This experiment revealed that changes in the expression influence the pattern of treated worms. With this approach, 381 genes were detected as differentially expressed, with 316 down-regulated and 65 up-regulated. These genes are related to biological functions such as muscular system development and function, tissue morphology, cellular assembly and organization, organ development, tissue development and cellular growth, and proliferation. Some functions, such as contractile fiber and myosin complex, hydrolase activity, and adenyl ribonucleotide binding, are related to the down-regulated genes. It correlates with the already described TGF-β induction of cytoskeleton remodeling through the myosin chain and Rho GTPase [35, 36].

Figure 2 summarizes host cytokines' direct or indirect effect on the parasites.

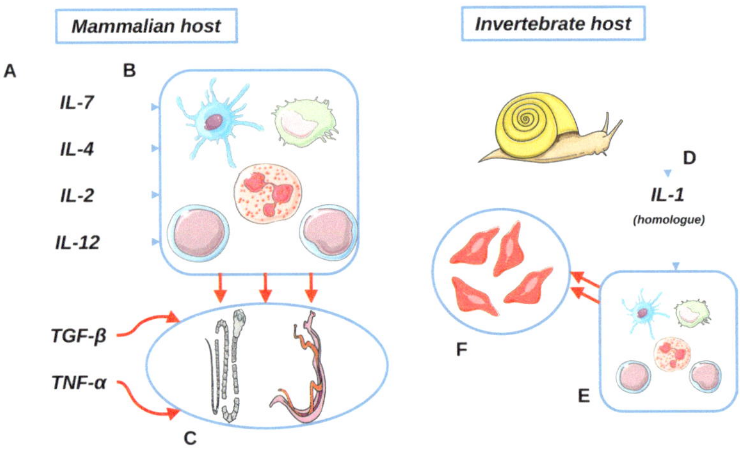

Figure 2.
Influences of mammals and invertebrate host's cytokines on platyhelminths. (A) Cytokines. (B) Vertebrate immune system cells. (C) Platyhelminthes. (D) Cytokine. (E) Invertebrate effector cells. (F) S. mansoni primary sporocysts. Some cytokines (TNF-α and TGF-β) exert direct effects on the parasite; on the other hand, other cytokines (such as interleukins) exert effects on immune system cells and these cells regulate parasites´ biological processes.

2.3 The example of human Tumor Necrosis Factor-α (TNF- α) on *S. mansoni*

Human TNF-α and its effect on *S. mansoni* are excellent examples of how the comprehension of the molecular crosstalk between host and pathogen has increased in the last decades. Some studies have described the influence of the pro-inflammatory cytokine TNF-α on the fecundity and metabolism of the parasite *S. mansoni*. Amiri et al. [37] described that human TNF-α induces the formation of granulomas and causes a positive effect on the parasite's egg-laying. Controversially, it was shown that egg-laying decreases and induces changes in the uptake of tyrosine [38] and methionine [39] on *S. mansoni* in the presence of the human cytokine. It was also documented that parasites' egg-laying and fecundity occurred later when immunodeficient mice (SCID) were used for infection with the parasite [40]. Finally, Davies et al. [41] reported that host TNF-α promotes the parasite survival and the development of adult worms.

In this context, the molecular mechanism started to be elucidated by searching for *S. mansoni* homologous gene to the human TNF-α receptor. A homolog gene was identified and characterized (SmTNFR) [42] and generated a transcript of 1967 nucleotides that encodes a receptor composed of 599 amino acids. The predicted protein has an extracellular portion that contains four TNF-α conserved domains (cysteine-rich domains), the main characteristic of the TNF receptor family. Extracellular domains' modular architecture is similar to the neural growth factor receptor (NGFR). The first analysis of the intracellular portion revealed no conserved domains, which is not expected in a homologous gene to NGFR characterized by Death Domain (DD), which makes it similar to TNF-R2, a non-death domain. The transcript expression level (mRNA) is detected in all developmental stages, but the highest expression level is detected in cercaria [42].

Parallel to the description of SmTNFR, other homolog genes for a possible signaling pathway were also identified. It is interesting to highlight that all elements required and activated by the human TNF-R2 signaling pathway (which does not have DD and, therefore, is not related to the activation of apoptosis) were found [42].

Recently, through *in-silico* analysis, 29 genes of homologous receptors to SmTNFR in other species of parasitic flatworms were identified. The homologs may evidence conservation of the TNF-α signaling pathway in a part of helminths. Additionally, highly conserved homologs of endogenous TNF-α ligands only in free-living flatworms were also identified. This suggests that the loss of the endogenous ligand (observed in parasitic flatworms) and the consequent use of the host's ligand was an event that occurred throughout the evolutionary process, as a cause or consequence of the parasitism [43].

Further, TNFR homologs identified in platyhelminths had conserved DD, which was concluded after the analysis of the secondary structure of intracellular regions. The intracellular portion of all receptors was reanalyzed, and evidence of the presence of DD was found in most SmTNFR homologs in platyhelminths but with different levels of conservation. Generally, cestodes have a more conserved DD than trematodes. This urges us to rethink the possible signaling pathway triggered by SmTNFR, since this receiver was initially classified as without DD [42].

Parallelly, Oliveira et al. [42] investigated the effect of human TNF-α on the gene expression profile in newly transformed schistosomula (NTS) and adult worms. NTSs (3 h after transformation) were treated with human TNF-α for 1 h (at the concentration of 20 ng/mL), and adult worms treated with human TNF-α for 1 h and 24 h. Microarray experiments revealed 548 genes with altered expression in NTSs after treatment with the human cytokine (309 up-regulated and 239 down-regulated). These genes are involved in biological functions related to the regulation of gene expression, cell proliferation and growth, and cell development. Two groups of differentially expressed genes were identified in adult worms treated for 1 h and 24 h. One group had transient changes in expression, that is, an inverse change pattern within 24 h compared to the pattern obtained within 1h. This group comprises 1365 genes, 821 of which have their expression level increased in 1 h of treatment and decreased in 24 h, and 544 have the opposite expression pattern. The second group has sustained changes in its expression level in 1 h and 24 h; this group comprises 492 genes, 337 being with the expression level increased by treatment with human TNF-α and 155 with the expression level decreased. These differentially expressed genes were organized in gene expression networks, and the most significantly enriched network interacts with TNF-α in other organisms. The network suggests that the parasite response to the human cytokine is conserved and similar to the reaction in humans [42]. Interestingly, the enzyme lactate dehydrogenase (responsible for producing lactate) was differentially expressed in schistosomula and adult worms treated with human TNF-α.

Thus, it was described that human TNF-α induces the phosphorylation of different proteins in adult male worms after *in vitro* treatment for 15 min. Differentially phosphorylated proteins were related to muscle contraction, cytoskeletal remodeling, cell signaling, and metabolism. Lactate dehydrogenase and a subunit of ATP synthase are differentially phosphorylated proteins. These results indicate that this enzyme, in the glycolytic pathway of the parasite, is being potentially regulated by the host's TNF-α in its expression level (mRNA) and activity [44].

Since the literature description of egg-laying is contradictory, and lactate dehydrogenase is differentially expressed and phosphorylated, the effect of TNF-α on egg-laying and metabolism was investigated in the adult parasites, in an *in vitro* treatment with doses of the human cytokine (5, 20, and 40 ng/mL) during 5 days [45].

The average number of eggs/couple increased on the second day in the treatment with 40 ng/mL. On the third day, there was a significant decrease in the average of eggs/couple for the treatments with 20 and 40 ng/mL; besides, there was a decrease for the doses of 5 and 40 ng/mL on the fourth day of incubation with the cytokine. The most important observation is that the total number of eggs was not different between treatments and control over the 5 days of treatment. The conclusion is that although egg-laying dynamics were affected, the fecundity was not. The host's TNF-α causes a decrease in the half-life of the egg-laying; therefore, when faced with the stimulus, couples lay eggs more quickly, but not in greater or lesser amounts than the respective negative control [45].

The TNF-α treatment induced significant changes in lactate concentration or possibly the glucose uptake when there was also a change in egg-laying. On the third day of treatment, for example, when lactate production decreased, the number of eggs laid was also reduced, indicating that energy metabolism is a relevant actor regulated by human TNF-α and interferes in the production dynamics and egg-laying [45].

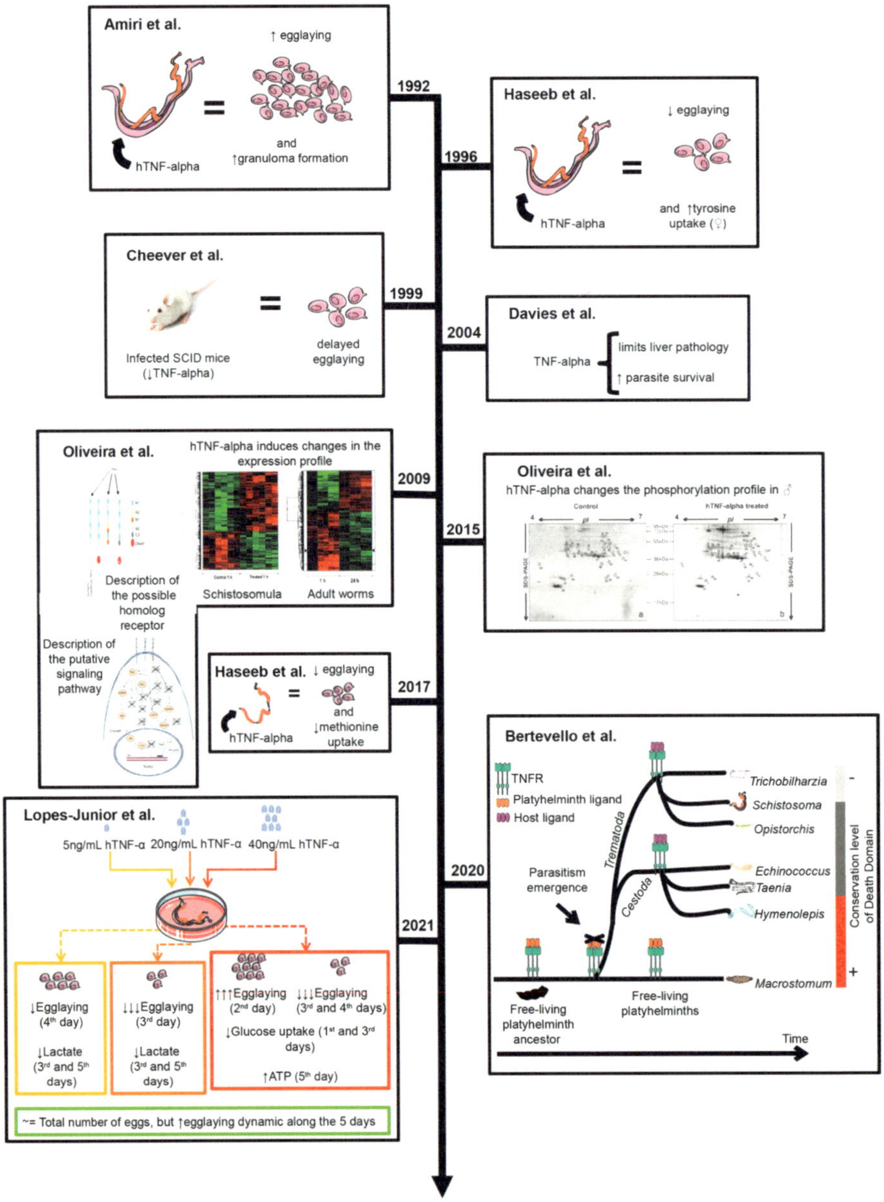

Figure 3.
Timeline of main discoveries described in the literature about host TNF-α and its effects on S. mansoni.

In addition, the increase in the accumulation of adenosine triphosphate (ATP) in adult worms on the fifth day was observed. The compromised egg-laying can explain it at this time: the high demand for ATP is destined for oogenesis and, when not necessary, this molecule can accumulate, especially against the modulation induced by the human cytokine [45]. It is also interesting to note that one subunit of ATP synthase is regulated by human TNF-α [44].

Figure 3 summarizes the history of the characterization of the effects of TNF-α on Schistosoma mansoni. It is an exciting example of how a cytokine effect can be elucidated like a puzzle, piece by piece.

3. Host hormones influences in metabolism, development, and viability of platyhelminths

The interaction between host and parasite depends on the ability of the parasite to successfully adapt to the host's microenvironment, allowing for a complete life cycle and parasite development [46]. That relationship suffers interference from age, sex, and reproductive status of the host and influences the hormonal profile [47]. Hormones, especially sex steroids, are fundamental for many biological processes such as reproduction, growth, development, and immunity. Parasites can evade the immune system. They can also exploit the host's hormones to improve their growth and reproduction, demonstrating that these organisms have mechanisms to interact with the host's molecules [48, 49].

Female supremacy is an older concept that assumes that female mammals suffer less parasitism than males. The statement that supports this paradigm implies that sexual dimorphism to parasite infections is based, principally, on the host immune system and has less interference of direct effects of hormones on parasites. Analysis of literature contests this paradigm, showing that publications represent few host-parasite systems, most of which have a medical bias, exploring, in general, human infections. Furthermore, there is no definition of infection and the immune parameters that contribute to host resistance or susceptibility to parasitism, casting doubt on the protective effect of those immune indicators. There are several exceptions to female supremacy: in malaria, toxoplasmosis, and cysticercosis, females are more affected by parasite infections than males [50].

Another line of discussion focuses on the influence of host sex in the genetic diversity of parasites. In this study of 2006, the researchers showed that independent of sex, schistosomes have more genetic diversity in male hosts. The authors postulated three hypotheses that explain the genetic variability of schistosomes: the relationship between rat-sex and duration of infection by cercaria; a combination of rat sex and specific habitat on host males that can contribute to more genetic diversity in parasites; a host sex bias in immunocompetence that select more diverse clones in male rats [51].

Together, these pieces of evidence raise new questions about the participation of host hormones in the host-parasite relationship. Do differences in concentrations of sex hormones between males and females have a significant role in the susceptibility to parasite infections? Can host hormones directly affect parasite biology? Do the parasites exploit the host hormones for their growth? Here in this topic, we aim to review the interaction between host hormones and platyhelminths, especially in *S. mansoni*, *T. crassiceps*, and *T. solium*.

As previously mentioned, hormones are important for the modulation of immune responses. The influence of host sex on resistance and susceptibility to parasitism in CBAJ/mice infected with *S. mansoni* showed the following results: females and castrated males had the worst survival rates, with 80% dead after 16 weeks of infection, compared to under 40% of infected males that died. In another experiment, investigators revealed that schistosomula grow better in the low testosterone level group, as noticed by the higher recovery rates of adult worms per cercaria. A possible explanation is the differences promoted by testosterone in the decline of infection effects, represented by a more pronounced organomegaly in the liver and spleen in females and castrated males, which are early pre-mortality indicators. These results start a discussion about the relationship between the host sex and differences in the parasite infection [52, 53].

When it comes to cestodes, we also see the effects of hormones on immunity. To test the influence of androgens in the parasite loads, the researchers investigated the effect of testosterone, dihydrotestosterone (DHT), and 17β-estradiol in castrated female and male mice infected with *T. crassiceps*. The castration triplicated the parasite burden in males and had the opposite effect in females, decreasing the number of parasites by 45%. The treatment with testosterone and DHT reduces de parasite loads in both genders, respectively, 60% and 70%. However, estradiol treatment increases the parasite number in female and male mice three times. Another experiment shows that parasite infection in male mice results in a high level of estradiol, a lower 90% testosterone, and a 95% decrease in DHT [54].

The antibodies' and cytokines' production is also affected by the sex steroids levels. In general, testosterone and DHT have no effect on the production of IgG, IL-6, and IL-10 in both sexes. On the other hand, the production of IL-2 and IFN-γ increases significantly in both sexes, and DHT promotes 70% recovery of the cytokines in males. Estradiol increases levels of anti-parasite IgG by 60% and duplicates IL-6 and IL-10 production in males and females. Those results demonstrated that androgens increase the cellular response in *T. crassiceps* infection with a specifically TH1 pattern. Oppositely, estrogens produce a TH2 immune response, which has no value in stopping the parasite's growth [54].

The effect of progesterone is also investigated in *T. crassiceps* and *T. solium* cysticercosis. In *T. crassiceps* treatment with progesterone, the number of parasites increases by three folds in male and two folds in female mice. Estradiol is increased two times in both genders, suggesting that progesterone is metabolized in the gonad. The cytokines, IL-4, IL-6, and IL-10 levels increase under the infection, with no change after progesterone treatment. In addition, IL-2, TNF-α, and IFN-γ concentration in the spleen is not modified with infection and treatment, but IL-2 is undetected in both sexes infected, and IFN-γ and TNF-α are increasing in progesterone-treated mice. Moving to *T. solium*, progesterone treatment decreases tapeworm length and increases IL-4, IL-6, and TNF-α in the duodenum, combined with a polymorphonuclear leukocytes infiltration. Once again, these results show that progesterone modulates TH1 immune response in *T. crassiceps* and improves intestinal mucosal immunity [55, 56].

Host hormones also directly affect the biology of parasites. Previous experiments showed that dehydroepiandrosterone (DHEA) and DHEA-S have a protected effect on mice infected with *S. mansoni* [57]. Another study demonstrated a negative correlation between DHEAS and intensity of parasitism, and this decline of *S. mansoni* infection also correlated to age [58]. Researchers investigated the effects of hypothalamic-pituitary-adrenal axis (HPA) hormones on *S. mansoni*, including DHEA. Cercariae are more affected than schistosomula and adults, with 100% dead after 48 h of culture, showing a concentration- and time-dependence.

Interestingly, males and paired worms are more resistant to the harmful effects of DHEA than females and separated worms. This fact suggests a beneficial effect of the relationship between female and male worms [59]. *T. crassiceps* is negatively affected by DHEA treatment with lower reproduction, motility, and viability [60].

17β-estradiol (E2), progesterone (P4), testosterone (T4), and dihydrotestosterone (DHT) also modulate the parasite physiology. Estrogens stimulated the reproduction and viability of *T. crassiceps*, with E2 being more effective than P4. These hormones are also involved in a high expression of genes c-fos and c-jun of the parasite, correlated to differentiation, reproduction, and apoptosis, showing a relative impact on viability changes. Since this parasite expressed estrogen and androgen receptors (excluding P4), sex steroids can bind these specific receptors and directly affect reproduction [61]. E2 and P4 also increase the expression of actin, tubulin, and myosin, major components of flame cells of the excretory system, benefiting the growth of *T. crassiceps* [62]. Progesterone also affects the development of *T. solium* by promoting evagination, maintaining motility, and inducing growth of the worms by two times [63].

In contrast to the positive effects of estrogens, T4 and DHT have deleterious actions, inhibiting the reproduction and reducing the viability of parasites. Additionally, they reduce the expression of c-fos and c-jun, explaining the changes in reproduction and growth of *T. crassiceps.* This data also agrees that cysticerci grow better in female and castrated males, proposing that the differences in sex steroids' concentrations in males and females are involved [61]. Moreover, T4 and DHT reduce the viability of the parasite by almost 90%, disrupting tegument and changing the structure of flame cells, with direct interaction with actin, tubulin, and myosin, without changes in their expression. This interaction results in the intoxication of the parasite, which explains the significant reduction in viability [64].

These findings improve the critical role of host sex hormones on the host-parasite relationship. Those sex hormones can determine the course of infection by direct effects like modulation in growth, reproduction, and viability or indirect effects such

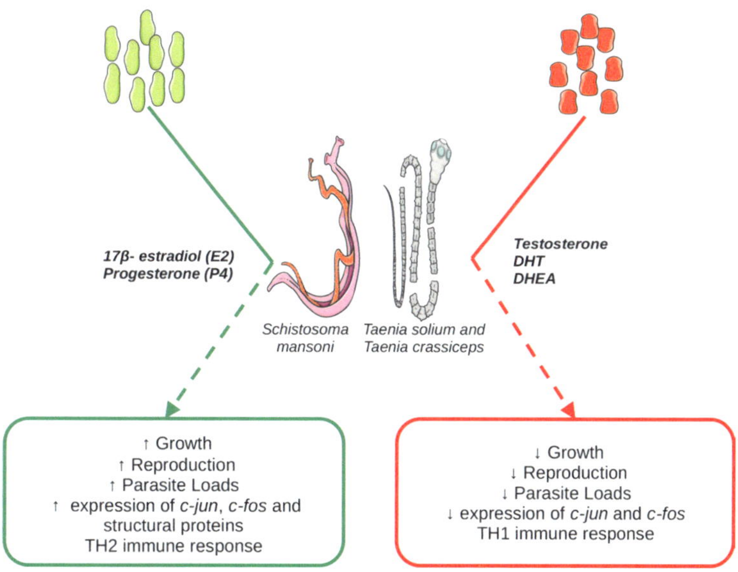

Figure 4.
Effects of sex steroids in parasites S. mansoni, T. crassiceps, and T. solium. Estrogens like E2 and P4 have positive effects on parasites and also modulate the immune response to the Th2 pattern. In contrast, testosterone, dihydrotestosterone (DHT), and dehydroepiandrosterone (DHEA) decrease parasite growth and reproduction and increase Th1 cytokines, which protect the host.

as changes in gene expression and immune system of the host, which sometimes benefit the host and other, permitting the parasite to exploit the microenvironment (**Figure 4**). The knowledge that estrogens and progesterone are related to positive effects on parasites and androgens protecting the host can urge the investigation of the beneficial use of sex steroids as new therapeutic targets to the parasitic infections. It is currently known that taximofen, an antiestrogen, and RU486, a progesterone antagonist, can negatively affect the reproduction and growth of *T. crassiceps* and *T. solium*, respectively [50, 63]. In this way, more discovery of the crosstalk between parasites and sex hormones can change the scenario about antiparasitic drugs, permitting a faster development process with high efficacy and low toxicity [65].

Figure 4 summarizes the effect of host hormones in the platyhelminths.

4. Conclusions and perspectives

We have reviewed some host molecules and their effects on the parasite. It is interesting to note how many distinct molecules produced along with the immune response (cytokines, pro or anti-inflammatory) or regularly produced by the endocrine system (such as sexual hormones) may interfere with parasites' development and fecundity. The study of molecular targets of this signaling is relevant to understanding how the evolution prepares the parasite's genome to respond and adapt to different signals from the environment and the hosts.

These biological models are exciting for system biology sciences and drug and vaccines discoveries; however, for a better understanding, functional genomic approaches must be improved to be applied in platyhelminths models to clarify the contribution of the signaling elements in the transduction and regulation of parasites' biological process.

As technologies have been developed and adapted, much information will be obtained from these particularly complex and challenging biological models. As information increases, new solutions for combating parasitic diseases will be elaborated and applied.

Author details

Ednilson Hilário Lopes-Junior†, Rafaella Pontes Marques†,
Claudio Romero Bertevello† and Katia Cristina Oliveira*,†
Departamento de Microbiologia, Imunologia e Parasitologia, Escola Paulista de Medicina, Universidade Federal de São Paulo, São Paulo, Brazil

*Address all correspondence to: katia.oliveira@unifesp.br

† These authors equally contributed.

References

[1] Human genome at ten: The sequence explosion. Nature. 2010;**464**:670-671. DOI: 10.1038/464670a

[2] Howe KL, Bolt BJ, Shafie M, Kersey P, Berriman M. WormBase ParaSite—A comprehensive resource for helminth genomics. Molecular and Biochemical Parasitology. 2017;**215**:2-10

[3] Tsai IJ, Zarowiecki M, Holroyd N, Garciarrubio A, Sanchez-Flores A, Brooks KL, et al. The genomes of four tapeworm species reveal adaptations to parasitism. Nature. 2013;**496**:57-63

[4] Coghlan A, Tyagi R, Cotton JA, Holroyd N, Rosa BA, Tsai IJ, et al. Comparative genomics of the major parasitic worms. Nature Genetics. 2019;**51**:163-174

[5] Berriman M, Haas BJ, Loverde PT, Wilson RA, Dillon GP, Cerqueira GC, et al. The genome of the blood fluke *Schistosoma mansoni*. Nature. 2009;**460**:352-358

[6] The Schistosoma Japonicum Genome Sequencing and Functional Analysis Consortium. The Schistosoma japonicum genome reveals features of host–parasite interplay. Nature. 2009;**460**:345-351

[7] Verjovski-Almeida S, DeMarco R, Martins EAL, Guimarães PEM, Ojopi EPB, Paquola ACM, et al. Transcriptome analysis of the acoelomate human parasite *Schistosoma mansoni*. Nature Genetics. 2003;**35**:148-157

[8] Chai M, McManus DP, McInnes R, Moertel L, Tran M, Loukas A, et al. Transcriptome profiling of lung schistosomula, in vitro cultured schistosomula and adult *Schistosoma japonicum*. Cellular and Molecular Life Sciences. 2006;**63**:919-929

[9] Anderson L, Amaral MS, Beckedorff F, Silva LF, Dazzani B, Oliveira KC, et al. *Schistosoma mansoni* egg, adult male and female comparative gene expression analysis and identification of novel genes by RNA-Seq. PLoS Neglected Tropical Diseases. 2015;**9**:e0004334

[10] Lu Z, Sessler F, Holroyd N, Hahnel S, et al. Schistosome sex matters: A deep view into gonad-specific and pairing-dependent transcriptomes reveals a complex gender interplay. Scientific Reports. 2016;**6**:31150. DOI: 10.1038/srep31150

[11] Li WH, Yang Y, Zhang NZ, Wang JK, Liu YJ, Li L, et al. Comparative transcriptome analyses of the developmental stages of *Taenia multiceps*. Frontiers in Veterinary Science Frontiers Media SA. 2021;**8**:707

[12] Wu X, Fu Y, Yang D, Zhang R, Zheng W, Nie H, et al. Detailed transcriptome description of the neglected Cestode *Taenia multiceps*. PLoS One. 2012;**7**:e45830

[13] Osman A, Niles EG, Verjovski-Almeida S, LoVerde PT. *Schistosoma mansoni* TGF-β receptor II: Role in host ligand-induced regulation of a schistosome target gene. PLoS Pathogens. 2006;**2**:0536-0550

[14] Avelar LGA, Nahum LA, Andrade LF, Oliveira G. Functional diversity of the *Schistosoma mansoni* tyrosine kinases. Journal of Signal Transduction. 2011;**2011**:1-11

[15] Zhang C, Li J, Aji T, Li L, Bi X, Yang N, et al. Identification of functional MKK3/6 and MEK1/2 homologs from Echinococcus granulosus and investigation of Protoscolecidal activity

of mitogen-activated protein kinase signaling pathway inhibitors *In vitro* and *In vivo*. Antimicrobial Agents and Chemotherapy. 2019;**63**:e01043-e01018

[16] Yang M, Li J, Wu J, Wang H, Guo B, Wu C, et al. Cloning and characterization of an *Echinococcus granulosus* ecdysteroid hormone nuclear receptor HR3-like gene. Parasite. 2017;**24**:36

[17] Salzet M, Capron A, Stefano GB. Molecular crosstalk in host-parasite relationships: Schistosome- and leech-host interactions. Parasitology Today. Parasitol Today. 2000;**16**:536-540

[18] You H, Gobert GN, Jones MK, Zhang W, DP MM. Signalling pathways and the host-parasite relationship: Putative targets for control interventions against schistosomiasis: Signalling pathways and future anti-schistosome therapies. BioEssays. 2011;**33**(3):203-214

[19] Murphy K, Travers P, Walport M, Janeway C. Janeway's Immunobiology. 8th ed. New York: Garland Science; 2012

[20] Cheung LC, Strickland DH, Howlett M, Ford J, Charles AK, Lyons KM, et al. Connective tissue growth factor is expressed in bone marrow stromal cells and promotes interleukin-7-dependent B lymphopoiesis. Haematologica. 2014;**99**:1149-1156

[21] Alderson MR, Sassenfeld HM, Widmer MB. Interleukin 7 enhances cytolytic T lymphocyte generation and induces lymphokine-activated killer cells from human peripheral blood. The Journal of Experimental Medicine. 1990;**172**:577-587

[22] Wolowczuk I, Nutten S, Roye O, Delacre M, Capron M, Murray RM, et al. Infection of mice lacking interleukin-7 (IL-7) reveals an unexpected role for IL-7 in the development of the parasite *Schistosoma mansoni*. Infection and Immunity. 1999;**67**:4183-4190

[23] Abdel Wahab MF, Warren KS, Levy RP. Function of the thyroid and the host-parasite relation in murine *Schistosomiasis mansoni*. The Journal of Infectious Diseases. 1971;**124**:161-171

[24] Saule P, Adriaenssens E, Delacre M, Chassande O, Bossu M, Auriault C, et al. Early variations of host thyroxine and interleukin-7 favor *Schistosoma mansoni* development. The Journal of Parasitology. 2002;**88**:849-855

[25] Yamane H, Zhu J, Paul WE. Independent roles for IL-2 and GATA-3 in stimulating naive CD4+ T cells to generate a Th2-inducing cytokine environment. The Journal of Experimental Medicine. The Rockefeller University Press. 2005;**202**:793-804

[26] Blank RB, Lamb EW, Tocheva AS, Crow ET, Lim KC, McKerrow JH, et al. The common γ chain cytokines interleukin (IL)-2 and IL-7 indirectly modulate blood fluke development via effects on CD4+ T cells. The Journal of Infectious Diseases. 2006;**194**:1609-1616

[27] Cheng YL, Song WJ, Liu WQ, Lei JC, Kong Z, Li YL. The effects of interleukin (IL)-12 and IL-4 deficiency on worm development and granuloma formation in *Schistosoma japonicum*-infected mice. Parasitology Research. 2012;**110**:287-293

[28] Sullivan GW, Carper HT, Sullivan JA, Murata T, Mandell GL. Both recombinant Interleukin-1 (Beta) and purified human monocyte Interleukin-1 prime human neutrophils for increased oxidative activity and promote neutrophil spreading. Journal of Leukocyte Biology. 1989;**45**:389-395

[29] Granath WO, Connors VA, Tarleton RL. Interleukin 1 activity in haemolymph from strains of the snail biomphalaria glabrata varying

in susceptibility to the human blood fluke, *Schistosoma mansoni*: Presence, differential expression, and biological function. Cytokine. 1994;**6**:21-27

[30] Connors VA, de Buron I, Jourdane J, Théron A, Agner A, Granath WO. Recombinant human Interleukin-1-mediated killing of Schistosoma mansoni primary Sporocysts in *Biomphalaria glabrata*. The Journal of Parasitology. 1998;**84**:920-926

[31] Li MO, Wan YY, Sanjabi S, Robertson A-KL, Flavell RA. Transforming growth factor-β regulation of immune resposes. Annual Review of Immunology. 2006;**24**:99-146

[32] Adalid-Peralta L, Rosas G, Arce-Sillas A, Bobes RJ, Cárdenas G, Hernández M, et al. Effect of transforming growth factor-β upon *Taenia solium* and *Taenia crassiceps* cysticerci. Scientific Reports. 2017;7:1-13

[33] LoVerde PT, Osman A, Hinck A. *Schistosoma mansoni*: TGF-β signaling pathways. Experimental Parasitology. 2007;**117**:304

[34] Oliveira KC, Carvalho MLP, Verjovski-Almeida S, Loverde PT. Effect of human TGF-β on the gene expression profile of *Schistosoma mansoni* adult worms. Molecular and Biochemical Parasitology. 2012;**183**:132-139

[35] Birukova AA, Birukov KG, Adyshev D, Usatyuk P, Natarajan V, Garcia JGN, et al. Involvement of microtubules and rho pathway in TGF-β1-induced lung vascular barrier dysfunction. Journal of Cellular Physiology. 2005;**204**:934-947

[36] Edlund S, Landström M, Heldin C-H, Aspenström P. Smad7 is required for TGF-β-induced activation of the small GTPase Cdc42. Journal of Cell Science. 2004;**117**:1835-1847

[37] Amiri P, Locksley RM, Parslow TG, Sadickt M, Rector E, Ritter D, et al. Tumour necrosis factor α restores granulomas and induces parasite egg-laying in schistosome-infected SCID mice. Nature. 1992;**356**:604-607

[38] Haseeb MA, Solomon WB, Palma JF. Schistosoma mansoni: Effect of recombinant tumor necrosis factor α on fecundity and [14C]-tyrosine uptake in females maintained in vitro. Comparative Biochemistry and Physiology Part C: Pharmacology, Toxicology and Endocrinology. 1996;**115**:265-269

[39] Haseeb MA, Agrawal R, Fried B. Reduced [14C]-methionine uptake and fecundity in *Schistosoma mansoni* females treated with recombinant tumor necrosis factor α in vitro. Acta Parasitologica. 2017;**62**:164-170

[40] Cheever AW, Poindexter RW, Wynn TA. Egg laying is delayed but worm fecundity is normal in SCID mice infected with *Schistosoma japonicum* and *S. mansoni* with or without recombinant tumor necrosis factor alpha treatment. Infection and Immunity. 1999;**67**:2201-2208

[41] Davies SJ, Lim KC, Blank RB, Kim JH, Lucas KD, Hernandez DC, et al. Involvement of TNF in limiting liver pathology and promoting parasite survival during schistosome infection. International Journal for Parasitology. 2004;**34**:27-36

[42] Oliveira KC, Carvalho MLP, Venancio TM, Miyasato PA, Kawano T, DeMarco R, et al. Identification of the Schistosoma mansoni TNF-alpha receptor gene and the effect of human TNF-alpha on the parasite gene expression profile. PLoS Neglected Tropical Diseases. 2009;**3**:e556

[43] Bertevello CR, Russo BRA, Tahira AC, Lopes-Junior EH,

Demarco R, Oliveira KC. The evolution of TNF signaling in platyhelminths suggests the cooptation of TNF receptor in the host-parasite interplay. Parasites and Vectors. 2020;**13**:491

[44] Oliveira KC, Carvalho MLP, Bonatto JMC, Schechtman D, Verjovski-Almeida S. Human TNF-α induces differential protein phosphorylation in *Schistosoma mansoni* adult male worms. Parasitology Research. 2016;**115**:817-828

[45] Lopes-Junior EH, Amaral MS, Kanamura CT, Pinto PLS, Krüger RF, Verjovski-Almeida S, et al. Human TNF-α affects the egg-laying dynamics and glucose metabolism of Schistosoma Mansoni adult worms in vitro. Parasites and Vectors. 2022;**15**:176

[46] Beckage NE. Host-parasite hormonal relationships: A common theme? Experimental Parasitology. 1991;**72**:332-338

[47] vom Steeg LG, Klein SL. Sex steroids mediate bidirectional interactions between hosts and microbes. Hormones and Behavior. 2017;**88**:45-51

[48] Escobedo G, Roberts CW, Carrero JC, Morales-Montor J. Parasite regulation by host hormones: An old mechanism of host exploitation? Trends in Parasitology. 2005;**21**:588-593

[49] Hernandez-Bello R, Nava-Castro K, Muniz-Hernandez S, Nava-Luna P, Trejo-Sanchez I, Tiempos-Guzman N, et al. Beyond the reproductive effect of sex steroids: Their role during immunity to helminth parasite infections. Mini-Reviews Medicine Chemistry. 2012;**12**:1071-1080

[50] Morales-Montor J, Chavarria A, De León MA, Del Castillo LI, Escobedo EG, Sánchez EN, et al. Host gender in parasitic infections of mammals: An evaluation of the female host supremacy paradigm. Journal of Parasitology. 2004;**90**(3):531-546. DOI: 101645/GE-113R3

[51] Caillaud D, Prugnolle F, Durand P, Théron A, de Meeûs T. Host sex and parasite genetic diversity. Microbes and Infection. 2006;**8**:2477-2483

[52] Eloi-Santos S, Olsen NJ, Correa-Oliveira R, Colley DG. Schistosoma mansoni: Mortality, pathophysiology, and susceptibility differences in male and female mice. Experimental Parasitology. 1992;**75**:168-175

[53] Nakazawa M, Fantappie MR, Freeman GL, Eloi-Santos S, Olsen NJ, Kovacs WJ, et al. *Schistosoma mansoni*: Susceptibility differences between male and female mice can Be mediated by testosterone during early infection. Experimental Parasitology. 1997;**85**:233-240

[54] Morales-Montor J, Baig S, Hallal-Calleros C, Damian RT. *Taenia crassiceps*: Androgen reconstitution of the host leads to protection during cysticercosis. Experimental Parasitology. 2002;**100**:209-216

[55] Vargas-Villavicencio JA, Larralde C, De León-Nava MA, Morales-Montor J. Regulation of the immune response to cestode infection by progesterone is due to its metabolism to estradiol. Microbes and Infection. 2005;**7**:485-493

[56] Escobedo G, Camacho-Arroyo I, Nava-Luna P, Olivos A, Pérez-Torres A, Leon-Cabrera S, et al. Progesterone induces mucosal immunity in a rodent model of human taeniosis by *Taenia solium*. International Journal of Biological Sciences. 2011;**7**:1443-1456

[57] Fallon PG, Richardson EJ, Jones FM, Dunne DW. Dehydroepiandrosterone sulfate treatment of mice modulates infection with *Schistosoma mansoni*.

Clinical and Diagnostic Laboratory Immunology. 1998;**5**:251-253

[58] Abebe F, Birkeland KI, Gaarder PI, Petros B, Gundersen SG. The relationships between dehydroepiandrosterone sulphate (DHEAS), the intensity of *Schistosoma mansoni* infection and parasite-specific antibody responses. APMIS. 2003;**111**:319-328

[59] Morales-Montor J, Mohamed F, Ghaleb AM, Baig S, Hallal-Callerost C, Damian RT. *In vitro* effects of hypothalamic-pituitary-adrenal axis (HPA) hormones on *Schistosoma mansoni*. The Journal of Parasitology. 2001;**87**:1132-1139

[60] Vargas-Villavicencio JA, Larralde C, Morales-Montor J. Treatment with dehydroepiandrosterone in vivo and in vitro inhibits reproduction, growth and viability of *Taenia crassiceps* metacestodes. International Journal for Parasitology. 2008;**38**:775-781

[61] Escobedo G, Larralde C, Chavarria A, Cerbón MA, Morales-Montor J. Molecular mechanisms involved in the differential effects of sex steroids on the reproduction and infectivity of *Taenia crassiceps*. Journal of Parasitology. 2004;**90**(6):1235-1244

[62] Ambrosio JR, Ostoa-Saloma P, Palacios-Arreola MI, Ruíz-Rosado A, Sánchez-Orellana PL, Reynoso-Ducoing O, et al. Oestradiol and progesterone differentially alter cytoskeletal protein expression and flame cell morphology in *Taenia crassiceps*. International Journal for Parasitology. 2014;**44**:687-696

[63] Escobedo G, Camacho-Arroyo I, Hernández-HernándezOT,Ostoa-SalomaP, García-Varela M, Morales-Montor J. Progesterone induces Scolex Evagination of the human parasite *Taenia solium*: Evolutionary implications to the host-parasite relationship. Journal of Biomedicine & Biotechnology. 2010;**2010**:10. DOI: 10.1155/2010/591079. Article ID 591079

[64] Ambrosio JR, Valverde-Islas L, Nava-Castro KE, Palacios-Arreola MI, Ostoa-Saloma P, Reynoso-Ducoing O, et al. Androgens exert a cysticidal effect upon *Taenia crassiceps* by disrupting flame cell morphology and function. PLoS One. 2015;**10**:e0127928

[65] Hernández-Bello R, Escobedo G, Guzmán C, Ibarra-Coronado EG, López-Griego L, Morales-Montor J. Immunoendocrine host–parasite interactions during helminth infections: From the basic knowledge to its possible therapeutic applications. Parasite Immunology. 2010;**32**:633-643

Chapter 8

Helminths Derived Immune-Modulatory Molecules: Implications in Host-Parasite Interaction

Koushik Das, Shashi Upadhyay and Neeraj Mahindroo

Abstract

The parasitic life cycle of helminths greatly relies on sophisticated manipulation of host environment and successful evasion of host defense. Helminths produce a repertoire of secretory molecules (including, extracellular vesicles and/or exosomes) to invade and generate habitable host-environment, and also to modulate the host immune responses in such a way that ensures their prolonged survival within host. An outline on helminths derived immune-modulatory molecules and their implications in host-parasite crosstalk have been presented. Queries with regard to the new direction of investigation to reveal specific molecular strategies, used by helminths to manipulate the host systems are also discussed.

Keywords: helminthiasis, host parasite interaction, secretory molecules

1. Introduction

Helminth parasites infect their hosts for an extended period, demonstrating their capacity to induce a new immunological and physiological equilibrium, which accommodates the invader [1]. Over parasites have evolved a unique arsenal of finely-tuned biochemical adaptations that control, block, or initiate modification in pathways or distinct host cells in order to maximize the success of parasites through eons of evolutionary time [2, 3]. In this book chapter, we look at some of the most current and intriguing advances in the field of host-parasite interaction with molecular pathways where the parasitic worms are known as helminths that belong to the phyla of round-worms (nematodes) and flatworms (platyhelminthes), which are lower invertebrate's phyla. A vast range of helminth species may colonize a wide range of habitats and host organisms, evading host defense and expulsion systems in each case. Helminths' goal is to regulate and manipulate immunity in order to disarm immunological defenses, resulting in the host failing to eradicate parasites [4]. Helminths fundamentally gain hold by going undetected, primary disabling host recognition techniques that would otherwise trigger an alarm, and then infecting tolerance of parasite antigens by the immune system, as well as suppressing reactions to bystander antigens in allergy or autoimmune [5].

Where, the helminth's soft textured technique has consequences for the manner in which they engage with their hosts and their immune systems, implying that constant dialog is required to preserve the tolerance condition. Because stable populations of long-lived parasites characterize the disease, it is plausible to believe that the products secreted on a regular basis by live parasites that target different immune system components [2]. Supported this notion by the fact that most of the molecular mechanism of helminth infections are reversed after drug-mediated parasite clearance [6–8]. As a result, the antigens of helminths that are "excretory-secretory" (ES) have received a lot of attention, a practical method for collecting combinations of released proteins that have been around for over 60 years [9]. Of course, more recently, the use of mass spectrometry, transcriptomic, and genomics has revolutionized their knowledge to diverse preparations and compound by identifying parasites to release particular molecular components to change their surroundings [2]. Some, products like glycan, nucleic acids, and lipids, including miRNAs, as well as tiny molecules and metabolites, are released in a variety of "packages," one of which being lipid vesicles, as discussed below.

2. Parasite identification by the host system

The first meeting of host and parasite usually breaches the surface (like, epithelium of intestinal or skin) that incites the "alarmin" discharge [10] and is

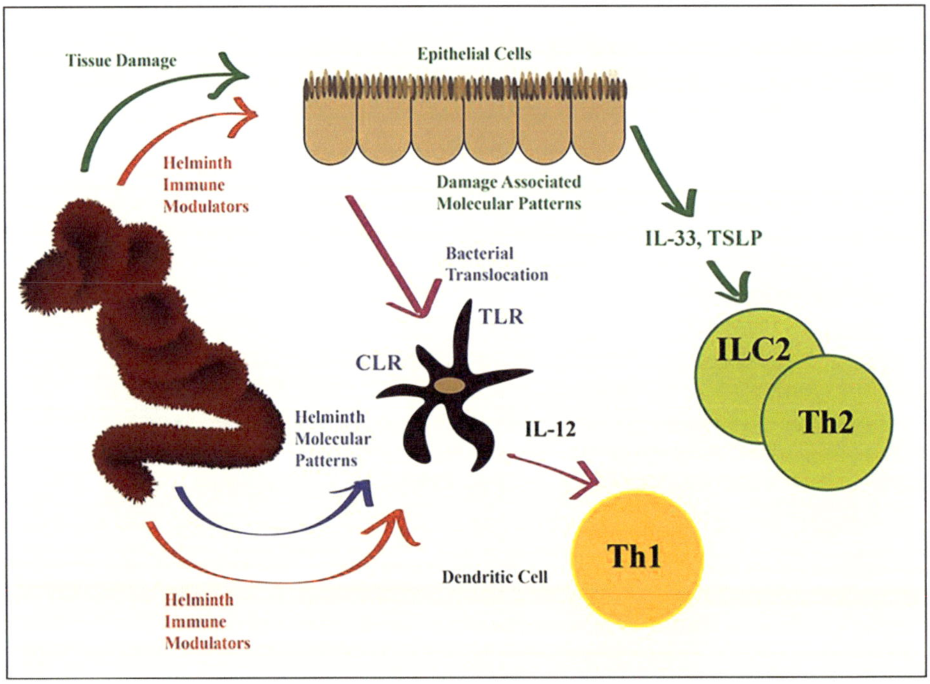

Figure 1.
Recognition of helminth infection by immune system. Innate immune system releases alarmins (IL-33, TSLP) in response to tissue invasion, which might elicit a type 2 immune response; helminth have ability to either inhibit the release of alarmins or block the respective receptors (e.g., IL-33R and ST2). The C-type lectin receptors (CLRs) or Toll-like receptors (TLRs) can recognize pathogen-associated molecular patterns, either presented directly by helminths or by bacteria, moved through damaged epithelium. In the second situation, immune modulators released by helminths suppress the Th1 response, induced by IL-12.

recognized through pattern recognition receptors (PRRs), as an example, Toll-like receptors (TLRs) which initiate the production of inflammatory cytokine. Alarmins such as thymic stromal lymphopoietin (TSLP) and interleukin-33 (IL-33) [11, 12], where together stimulate a Type 2 immune response that is anti-helminth and pro-allergic, are strongly related with helminth-mediated tissue damage. Yet, helminths have option to avoid entirely or partially this warning (**Figure 1**); as an example, *Nippostrongylus brasiliensis* compounds effectively prevent dendritic cells (DCs) from responding to TLR ligation and other helminths, with interleukin-12 (IL-12) production being particularly suppressed [13–17]. While the release of IL-33 from the epithelial cell, is directly obstructed through the released products from *Heligmosmoides polygyrus* [18]. Some of the chemical mediators that prevent innate activation are now being identified, as mentioned in the next section.

The prototypical PRRs respond to microbiological substances like lipoteichoic acid and lipopolysaccharide (LPS) by releasing pro-inflammatory cytokines like IL-12, which promote the Th1 response. The consistent ability of various helminth products to inhibit the release of IL-12 in response to TLR stimulation could be a mechanism aimed not so much at blocking anti-parasite immunity as it is at avoiding collateral inflammation at barrier sites where, for example, bacterial translocation may accompany helminth invasion. While the key role of TLRs in pathogen pattern recognition via the host is now well recognized, it is surprising that no analogous recognition mechanism for Th2-inducing species like helminths has yet been defined. However, helminth TLR ligands have been discovered, including the RNA activating TLR3 [19] and the lysophosphatidylserine glycolipid [20] from *Schistosoma mansoni* (*S. mansoni*), and additional receptor like C-type lectin receptors (CLRs) may fulfill the role of innate detection in different situations [21–23].

3. Host-parasite molecular interaction

In the extracellular environment, simple protein-protein interactions, involving with either exposed receptors or fluid-phase host components on the surfaces of host cells can be considered the first stage communication between the host and the parasite. *H. polygyrus*, secretes a functional mimic of the immunomodulatory cytokine TGF-, which binds to mammalian surface receptors and sends an inhibitory signal to the T cells (Johnston et al. submitted to be published). Space blocks further conversation of the numerous singular proteins currently observed to be associated with have helminth cooperation, yet maybe the most fascinating are individuals' superfamily of the cysteine-rich secretory proteins, antigen 5, and pathogenesis-related 1 proteins (CAP) (Pfam00188) which are significantly extended across all helminth parasite heredities [24, 25], and profoundly addressed in the emitted protein sections [26, 27]. One member of this family, a hookworm named *Necator americanus*, was one among the first to be identified as a potential partner as NIF, an emitted integrin restriction inhibitor that stops neutrophils [28].

While functional roles for members of the CAP gene family other than NIF are sparse, a homolog attaches to a tomato plant innate defense protein, limiting resistance systems, and triggering infection in a plant-parasitic worm [29]. As a result, helminth-released proteins are not limited to cooperating at the host cell surface, but can also play functions inside cells, raising the question of how they enter the cell.

3.1 Helminth derived proteins and their intracellular functions

Two well documented helminth glycoproteins infiltrate the host cells and have immense implications. The *S. mansoni* egg-inferred glycoprotein ω1 is a ribonuclease with Lewis X glycan side chains that bind to the surface lectin of dendritic cells, interfering with take-up into the phone and causing the protein moiety to serve as a protein blend obstructer [30, 31]. DCs treated with ω1 activate the type 2 immune pathway, causing immature T cells to mature into Th2 effector cells. The major secreted glycoprotein of the filarial nematode *Acanthocheilionema viteae* (*A. viteae*) is a distinct mediator of ES-62 could be 62-kDa component with N-linked phosphoryl choline (PC) side chains. Through interaction with ES-62 enters the cell via TLR4 on the surface, and the PC moiety disrupts the downstream signaling of both the B cell receptor and TLR4 within the intracellular milieu, effectively blocking cell activation [32]. Although TLR3 is an intracellular pathogen sensor, and the FheCL1 cysteine protease from *Fasciola hepatica* (*F. hepatica*) kills TLR3 in host macrophages, limiting activation; despite the fact that TLR3 is an intracellular pathogen sensor, FheCL1 can reach the endosome and degrade the receptor in situ [17].

The filarial cystatin molecule CPI-2 is used to target a distinct route. This protein contains two blocking sites that are resistant to cysteine proteases and asparagine endo peptidase (AEP) [33]. Human B cells that have been exposed to CPI-2 from *Brugia malayi* (*B. malayi*) (a human filarial parasite) are no longer able to practice presenting protein antigen to T cells, a process that is dependent on AEP activity in the endosome [33]. Advance research on a closely related cystatin from *A. viteae* show that it is taken up by mouse macrophages and activates ERK and p38 kinases, resulting in the production of immune regulation interleukin-10 (IL-10), which is linked to the activation of the CREB and STAT3 signaling pathways [34].

Although the entrance pathway cannot always be determined, other products have been found to modulate intracellular signaling in host cells. The ALT-2 protein, for example, is generated from a large larval transcript of the filarial parasite *B. malayi*, when this protein was given to macrophages or introduced into macrophages via the intracellular protozoan *Leishmania mexicana* (*L. mexicana*), it induced the signaling proteins GATA3 and SOCS1, which are active to generate type 2 responses and inhibit IFN-dependent intracellular inflammatory signaling [35].

3.2 Identification of exosomes and their implications in host-parasite interactions

Apparently, particularly exosomes and extracellular vesicles appear to play an important role in cellular communication. Exosomes are nano vesicles with a diameter of around 50–100 nm that are secreted by all cells to allow the transfer of specific cargo, primarily lipids, proteins, and RNA species, as well as other phenotypic markers from their cell of origin [36, 37]. Exosomes are formed by the inward budding of multi-vesicular endosomes within a cell, and include components of the original cell, such as RNAs or proteins, that may be trafficked into the same compartment. The extracellular vesicles have been discovered from kinetoplastids growths, and microorganisms' group, the hypothesis that exosome-interceded correspondence could work on a cross-animal categories stage, by which parasite-inferred exosomes could associate with, and conceivably adjust, the host invulnerable framework [38]. Exosomes have just recently been discovered as integral products of extracellular organisms such as helminths [38, 39].

According to the recent research, exosomes are produced by parasitic helminths. The excretory-secretory portions of the trematodes *F. hepatica*, and *Echinostoma caproni*, which contaminate the liver and gastrointestinal system individually, were the first to disclose this [40], as well as the nematode *H. polygyrus*, which contaminates the small intestinal tract [41]. Information derived from the trematode concentrates additional advises that ES inferred exosomes are fit for arriving at the host climate, as they seem, by all accounts, to be discovered unblemished on the para destinations' covering. The capacity of helminth exosomes to cross-phylum communication between mammals, and helminths is further supported by their uptake by host intestinal epithelial cells.

Exosome formation in free-living nematodes was first demonstrated in helminths, with the demonstration that a novel secretion pathway from the apical membrane of *Caenorhabditis elegans* co-secretes multi vesicular bodies containing exosome-like vesicles with peptides that normally promote cuticle growth [42]. Helminths and protozoa exosomes have similarities in various specific markers. In heat-shock protein 70 (HSP70), endosomal sorting components like surface tetraspanins, and *Alix*, including CD63 and CD9 are all found in mammalian exosomes [37]. As an example, when exosomes secreted by macrophages, which are *Leishmania*-infected experience a series of phenotypic alterations followed by infection, and they hold some exosome markers, with CD63, TsG101, and *Alix* [43]. Furthermore, transcriptome investigation of the cestode, *Echinococcus granulosus*, revealed the existence of other CD63-like tetraspanin family members [44]. Tetraspanins have been chosen as a vaccine against *Echinococcus multilocularis*, a tapeworm that causes alveolar echinococcosis, a highly lethal illness that has spread throughout areas of Central Europe, China, and Siberia [45, 46]. This tetraspanin-targeting vaccination is also being investigated as a potential treatment for the human pathogen *S. mansoni* [47, 48].

Earlier, it was seeming that *H. polygyrus*, a mouse gastrointestinal nematode, has previously been demonstrated to release exosomes containing various miRNA types as well as a significant number of proteins, accounting for around 10% of an adult worm's total protein secretion [41]. The enrichment of a number of important components within the exosomes was also established by a proteomic analysis of the released products represented in the soluble and vesicular fractions using ultracentrifugation separation. Interestingly, some of these proteins have previously been found in the region of *C. elegans'* intestinal epithelial apical membrane cells; electron microscopy revealed multi-vesicular bodies in the intestinal tissues of *H. polygyrus* adults, as well as exosome-like structures freed into the lumen [41], strongly implying that the parasite releases exosomes from its alimentary tract (**Figure 2a**).

Exosomes from external helminths were also found to have immunomodulatory properties. Exosomes from *H. polygyrus* dominate the innate immune response to the fungus *Alternaria alternata*, which is linked to respiratory allergies, mostly through modulating type 2 innate lymphoid cells (ILC2s) [41]. Helminths communicate with host systems by releasing a repertoire of molecules, such as proteins, glycan, and extracellular vesicles/exosomes containing miRNA (**Figure 2b**). Both *in-vitro* and *in-vivo*, *H. polygyrus* exosomes demonstrate a lower expression of IL1RL1/ST2 transcript in mouse cell types. This gene encodes the IL-33 receptor, which is essential for ILC2s to trigger the type 2 immune response, which is compatible with exosomes' in vivo protection from allergic inflammation. The role of the IL-33 ligand-receptor axis in anti-parasite responses is also well established [18, 49]. As a result, our findings support the ability of *H. polygyrus* derived exosomes to evade parasite clearance by altering a critical element of the host immune system.

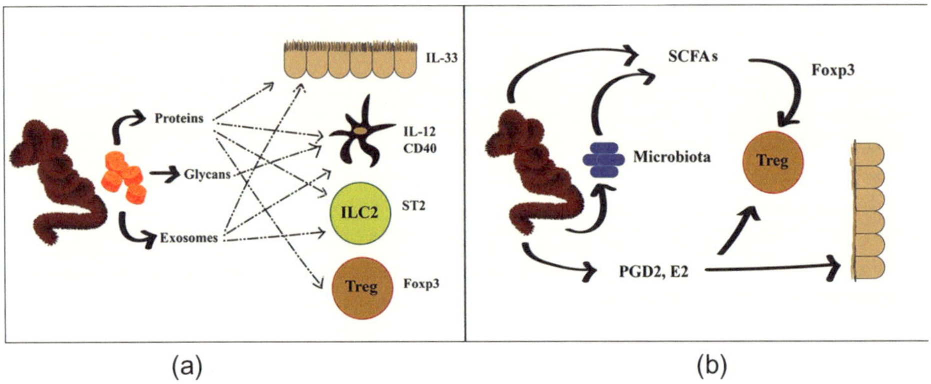

Figure 2.
Host-helminth molecular cross-talk. (a) Helminths communicate with host systems by releasing a repertoire of molecules, such as proteins, glycan, and extracellular vesicles/exosomes containing miRNA. (b) Helminth triggers the Foxp3+ Treg population by producing short-chain fatty acids (SCFAs) and also stimulates the gut-microbes, those secrete SCFAs.

Exosomes were identified in the culture media of the digenean trematode livestock parasite *Dicrocoelium dendriticum*, which included over 80 protein components and at least 30 miRNA species with similarity or near-identity to known sequences [50]. Despite the lack of functional studies, the scientists noted similarities with the key *Schistosoma* miR-3479, miRNAs Bantam, and miR-10, which are visible indicators in the plasma of infected animals [51].

Moreover, Nowacki et al. identified over 200 miRNAs, 20 tRNA-derived short RNAs, and over 100 proteins in 30–100 nm exosome-like vesicles released by *S. mansoni* schistosomula that are enriched in certain non-coding RNAs and proteins [52]. Furthermore, it was discovered that the *B. malayi* L3 infective stage secretes 50–120 nm vesicles rich in miRNA species, as well as a protein complement that includes not only conventional exosome-associated products, but also those that could interfere with host cell responses, like *Cathepsin L* [53]. Importantly, the adult worm stage was shown to produce less exosomes than the infective stage, which is likely due to the demands of converting from vector to host at this point in the life cycle. Adult *S. mansoni* worms also release 50–130 nm-sized exosome vesicles with approximately 80 identifiable proteins, five of which are tetraspanins, and an abundant saposin-like protein, according to Sotillo et al. [54]. It is also shown that a number of recognized schistosome vaccine candidate antigens, including the tetraspanins, are key components of the exosomes, as previously mentioned. Wang et al. reported that adult worms of the similar parasite *S. japonicum* emit 30–100 nm vesicles after being cultivated *in-vitro* for 5 h, which can be detected using ultracentrifugation of the culture solution [55]. Although this work did not identify the protein cargo of the exosomes, these scientists discovered that *S. japonicum* exosomes boosted the production of nitric oxide in the murine macrophage-like cell line RAW264.7, along with other markers of a Type 1 pathway. The presence of many important proteins and RNA species in secreted vesicles emphasizes both the complexity and diversity of cargo within exosomes, as well as the broad range of potential connections between recipient cells [56].

Investigations of the liver fluke *Opisthorchis viverrini*, a trematode common in regions of Southeast Asia and causally connected to cholangiocarcinoma (bile duct cancer) have revealed a larger chance for helminth exosomes. Exosomes (measured 40–180 nm) were found in secretory material from the species mentioned above, along with a similar spectrum of related proteins, including tetraspanins [57]. In the bile fluid of infected hosts, some proteins linked to exosomes were discovered. Anti-tetraspanin antibodies prevented exosomes from entering host cells, implying that this protein is likely to be represented on the vesicular surface in the same way that mammalian exosomes. Suggestively, exosomes from *O. viverrini* were shown to stimulate cell proliferation and induce the generation of the pro-inflammatory cytokine interleukin-6 (IL-6) in a human cholangiocyte cell line in a way that was partially inhibited by an anti-tetraspanin antibody. Taken together, these findings support the theory that *O. viverrini* energies cause tumorigenic alterations in the host bile duct, which could explain the parasite's carcinogenic effects.

3.3 Exosomes contain helminth miRNAs

It's been a while, all around archived that micro-RNAs and non-coding RNAs specifically, move among cells and life forms through their epitome inside exosomes and other vesicles found outside of the cell [58]. Certainly, this gives a piece of machinery for RNA protection from destruction outside the cell, and appears to provide an absorption pathway to transfer RNA to the recipient's proper cellular compartment. Many of the investigations mentioned above, including those from the nematodes *B. malayi* [53] and *H. polygyrus* [41], as well as the trematodes *D. dendriticum* [50] and *S. mansoni*, identified short RNAs within parasite exosomes [52].

We were able to show a collection of RNA species bundled inside exosomes, including miRNAs such as let-7, miR200, and diminutive [41], which may block the mouse phosphatase Dusp1 using a quantitative measure, thanks to *H. polygyrus*. New information differentiating wide miRNA collections in parasitic helminths is rapidly emerging, albeit the circulation of these released conservative exosomes inside parasitic helminths has yet to be established.

Most importantly, definitive proof for helminth-derived miRNAs acting on host genes has yet to be discovered; however, the circumstantial evidence remains enticing; not only are extensive seed sequences shared between helminth and host miRNAs, but the miRNA-rich exosomes (at least of *H. polygyrus*) also contain worm Argonaut protein [41, 59]. Indicating that a functional gene repression package is being delivered to the targeted cells.

4. Host-parasite communications through small molecules

Mechanisms of tiny molecules, hormones, molecular cues, and metabolites, which are closely involved in intercellular communication, draw much attention. As an example, short-chain fatty acids (SCFAs, butyrate, acetate, and propionate), for example, which are commensal derivatives at the level that promote regulatory T cells, are not generated by mammalian organisms [60]; dysbiosis is thus considered harmful for the disruption of this path [61, 62]. Surprisingly, these chemicals can also be produced by helminths [63], implying that commensal bacteria can produce a significant amount of SCFAs [64].

Another tiny molecules produced by filarial parasites *B. malayi* and *Onchocerca volvulus*, as well as skin-invasive cercariae of *S. mansoni*, include prostaglandins D2 and E2 [65–67]. In addition to tiny chemicals and metabolites, helminths change small ligands derived from the host, such as acetylcholine (through acetylcholinesterase) [68], the enormous discussion of platelet-activating factor (PAF hydrolase [69]) and ATP (apyrase [70]), among many others, is beyond the scope of this paper.

5. Microbiome-mediated interactions

In the gastrointestinal system, particularly, helminth parasites contribute their position with numerous microorganisms, predominantly numerous bacterial species recognized as microbiota [71–73]. Remarkably, helminth contamination depend on excessive range on the existence of these parasites: as an illustration, in the lack of caecal bacteria, *Trichuris* eggs do not mature in the gut [74]. The majority of microbiota study in mice infection with gut helminths have discovered important and sometimes comprehensive alterations in species arrangement, mainly within *Lactobacillus* populations and *Bacteroides* [71–73]. Newly, it was declared that BALB/c mice infected with *H. polygyrus* showed enlargement of the *L. taiwanensis* species, and the degree of colonization with this bacterium was found to be positively linked with both adult worm populations and Treg activation [75]. Surprisingly, mice administered *L. taiwanensis* before receiving *H. polygyrus* larvae were shown to be more susceptible to infection, implying that the bacteria and helminth species work together to promote infection.

It has also been suggested that the immune-modulating capabilities of helminth infection could be aided in part by altering the microbiome of the intestine. To date, fascinating research have shown that infected mice's intestinal contents (which comprise bacteria as well as a variety of host and parasite products) can lessen allergy symptoms when transmitted to recipient mice [64]. It will be interesting to investigate this consequence minutely and mostly if *L. taiwanensis*, specific bacteria is responsible.

Considerably, a recent study showed that fecal miRNAs produced from intestinal epithelial cells might influence the microbiome, possibly by interacting directly with bacterial genes [76]. Feasibly these miRNAs could potentially be found in extracellular vesicles, raising the possibility that the helminths and host both might modify the microbiome through this innovative mechanism, and indeed as stated below, that host exosomes might have an impact on the helminth organism, parasitizing the intestinal tract.

6. Host-helminth interaction is bi-directional process

While this analysis has focused on how helminths communicate with the immune system of hosts, there are several enthralling examples of how helminths detection and response towards host immune state. Adult *N. brasiliensis* worms acclimate towards an immunized host through adjusting secreted acetylcholinesterase expression levels and isoforms, according to previous research [77]. All the more as of late, identification of cytokines from host, has been found in schistosomes, which need the existence of TNF from host to develop to laying of egg [78] and filarial parasites reacting towards high IL-5 levels present *in-vivo* by speeding up the development and off-spring formation [79]. Helminth receptor illustration is ready to ligate host cytokine was set up on account of *S. mansoni* TGF-β family receptor [80].

An appealing chance of extracellular vesicles from the host may offer of communications of network, which accelerates the helminth parasites, although it is still not proved that, parasites can directly receptive to vesicle-mediated signals. There are a developing literature representing the how host-derived extra-mobile vesicle effect against defense in opposition of pathogens. As an instance, in recipient infected cells, IFN-α, exosomes derived from stimulated cell could induce the antiviral activity and bound viral replication [81, 82]. Additionally, semen exosomes from human is associated in resistant to HIV-1 resulting their uptake into immature cells by reducing viral fitness [83]. Innate response towards protozoan parasite *Cryptosporidium parvum* is also established as an instance of exosome-mediated host defense. Activation of host epithelium through TLR mediation enhances the secretion of antimicrobial exosomes, which contains peptides that limits infection rate of pathogen in the intestinal environment [84]. The progress of a targeted host exosomes anti-pathogen response has also been examined the usage of a clinical setting, in which host exosomes collected from parasite antigen-primed dendritic cells encourage protection against various protozoan contaminations, counting *Toxoplasma gondii* infection [85] and *Leishmania major* [86].

7. Exploitation of helminth-induced immune modulation as novel therapeutic strategy

With people parasitic, helminths have coevolved with centuries, unpredictably filtering and fostering a variety in instruments to smother or slant the host's invulnerable framework, accordingly advancing their drawn-out endurance. A few helminths, like hookworms, make minimal no obvious pathology when present in unobtrusive numbers and can even give profits to their hosts humans. Clinical studies on helminth infection of humans have been conducted and analyzed for the protection and efficiency of a variety of immune dysfunction to take advantage of this evolutionary phenomenon, with mixed results [87]. It was shown that treatment of live helminth on mice and larger animals resulting excretory/secretory products, having drug-like properties of anti-inflammation, represent an updated pharmacopeia. Such molecules include proteins, glycans, and extracellular vesicles, modifications after the translation process, several metabolites. Helminth-motivated treatments grips guarantee, this adds a test to the medication improvement local area, which is for the most part new to unfamiliar biologics that do not act like antibodies. The identification and characterization of helminth compounds and vesicles, as well as the molecular pathways they target in the host, provides a unique opportunity to produce customized therapeutics stimulated through nature that is safe, efficacious, and immunogenic [88].

8. Conclusions and future perspectives

Throughout evolution, helminths have conveyed a wide variety of host species, emerging sophisticated links, also regulate channels with, and even control of, their hosts' immune systems. In host-parasite biology, there is the fast invention that several helminth species mediate cross-phylum interactions by releasing exosomes which leads to the importance of this pathway. Classification as helminths, how large the extracellular parasites, may be capable to "reach in" into the host cells intracellular mechanism, rebuilding the behavior through every possible way. The absorption of exosomes is not a receptor-dependent process; this is hard for the host to grow countermeasures to inhibit properties of exomes on parasites, whereas this would be easier for the parasite for abusing the tracking exosome for operative interfering particles, from enzymes to small RNAs, proteins and other modifiers of gene expression. Additionally, these vesicles suggest vigorous machinery to the parasites, which might transport their "message" through extracellular spaces present in diverse nature and quite probably through cells and tissues.

More information from exosomes of helminths would lead towards balancing their effects, gaining our prevailing knowledge about immunomodulatory proteins and glycan. If we can produce antibody reactions towards components of the surface membrane, which are needed for cell entry, exosomes could be a good vaccine target. Additionally, new drug aims may appear from elaborating the paths needed for the biogenesis of exosome in helminths, and the cellular events of a host cell, which occurs after helminth exosome uptake. Hereafter, a new opening has unlocked on how helminths overthrow the immunity system and how they deal works by defeating the strategy of the helminth.

Author details

Koushik Das[†], Shashi Upadhyay[†] and Neeraj Mahindroo*
Department of Allied Health Sciences, School of Health Sciences and Technology, University of Petroleum and Energy Studies, Dehradun, India

*Address all correspondence to: nmahindroo@ddn.upes.ac.in

† These authors have contributed equally.

References

[1] Maizels RM et al. Helminth parasites: Masters of regulation. Immunological Reviews. 2004;**201**:89-116

[2] Hewitson JP, Grainger JR, Maizels RM. Helminth immunoregulation: The role of parasite secreted proteins in modulating host immunity. Molecular and Biochemical Parasitology. 2009;**167**:1-11

[3] Allen JE, Maizels RM. Diversity and dialogue in immunity to helminths. Nature Reviews. Immunology. 2011; **11**:375-388

[4] Maizels RM, Hewitson JP, Smith KA. Susceptibility and immunity to helminth parasites. Current Opinion in Immunology. 2012;**25**:459-466

[5] Johnston CJ, McSorley HJ, Anderton SM, Wigmore SJ, Maizels RM. Helminths and immunological tolerance. Transplantation. 2014;**97**(2):127-132

[6] Sartono E et al. Elevated cellular responses and interferon-release after long-term diethylcarbamazine treatment of patients with human lymphatic filariasis. The Journal of Infectious Diseases. 1995;**171**:1683-1687

[7] Grogan JL, Kremsner PG, Deelder AM, Yazdanbakhsh M. Elevated proliferation and interleukin-4 release from $CD4^+$ cells after chemotherapy in human *Schistosoma haematobium* infection. European Journal of Immunology. 1996;**26**:1365-1370

[8] Semnani RT et al. Filaria-induced monocyte dysfunction and its reversal following treatment. Infection and Immunity. 2006;**74**(8):4409-4417

[9] Campbell CH. The antigenic role of the excretions and secretions of *Trichinella spiralis* in the production of immunity in mice. The Journal of Parasitology. 1955;**41**:483-491

[10] Oppenheim JJ, Yang D. Alarmins: Chemotactic activators of immune responses. Current Opinion in Immunology. 2005;**17**(4):359-365

[11] Cayrol C, Girard JP. IL-33: An alarmin cytokine with crucial roles in innate immunity, inflammation and allergy. Current Opinion in Immunology. 2014;**31C**:31-37

[12] Ziegler SF, Artis D. Sensing the outside world: TSLP regulates barrier immunity. Nature Immunology. 2010;**11**(4):289-293

[13] Balic A, Harcus Y, Holland MJ, Maizels RM. Selective maturation of dendritic cells by *Nippostrongylus brasiliensis* secreted proteins drives T helper type 2 immune responses. European Journal of Immunology. 2004;**34**:3047-3059

[14] Cervi L, MacDonald AS, Kane C, Dzierszinski F, Pearce EJ. Dendritic cells copulsed with microbial and helminth antigens undergo modified maturation, segregate the antigens to distinct intracellular compartments, and concurrently induce microbe-specific Th1 and helminth-specific Th2 responses. Journal of Immunology. 2004;**172**(4):2016-2020

[15] Segura M, Su Z, Piccirillo C, Stevenson MM. Impairment of dendritic cell function by excretory-secretory products: A potential mechanism for nematode-induced immunosuppression. European Journal of Immunology. 2007;**37**:1887-1904

[16] Massacand JC et al. Helminth products bypass the need for TSLP in Th2 immune responses by directly modulating dendritic cell function. Proceedings of the National Academy of Sciences of the United States of America. 2009;**106**:13968-13973

[17] Donnelly S et al. Helminth cysteine proteases inhibit TRIF-dependent activation of macrophages via degradation of TLR3. The Journal of Biological Chemistry. 2010;**285**:3383-3392

[18] McSorley HJ, Blair NF, Smith KA, McKenzie ANJ, Maizels RM. Blockade of IL-33 release and suppression of type 2 innate lymphoid cell responses by helminth secreted products in airway allergy. Mucosal Immunology. 2014;7:1068-1078

[19] Aksoy E et al. Double-stranded RNAs from the helminth parasite *Schistosoma* activate TLR3 in dendritic cells. The Journal of Biological Chemistry. 2005;**280**(1):277-283

[20] van der Kleij D et al. A novel host-parasite lipid cross talk: Schistosomal lysophosphatidylserine activates Toll-like receptor 2 and affects immune polarization. The Journal of Biological Chemistry. 2002;**277**:48122-48129

[21] Van Die I et al. The dendritic cell specific C-type lectin DC-SIGN is a receptor for *Schistosoma mansoni* egg antigens and recognizes the glycan antigen Lewis-x. Glycobiology. 2003;**13**:471-478

[22] van Kooyk Y. C-type lectins on dendritic cells: Key modulators for the induction of immune responses. Biochemical Society Transactions. 2008;**36**(Pt 6):1478-1481

[23] Ritter M et al. *Schistosoma mansoni* triggers Dectin-2, which activates the Nlrp3 inflammasome and alters adaptive immune responses. Proceedings of the National Academy of Sciences of the United States of America. 2010;**107**:20459-20464

[24] Cantacessi C et al. A portrait of the SCP/TAPS proteins of eukaryotes—Developing a framework for fundamental research and biotechnological outcomes. Biotechnology Advances. 2009;**27**:376-388

[25] Chalmers IW, Hoffmann KF. Platyhelminth venom allergen-like (VAL) proteins: Revealing structural diversity, class-specific features and biological associations across the phylum. Parasitology. 2012;**139**(10):1231-1245

[26] Hawdon JM, Jones BF, Hoffman DR, Hotez PJ. Cloning and characterization of ancylostoma-secreted protein. A novel protein associated with the transition to parasitism by infective hookworm larvae. Journal of Biological Chemistry. 1996;**271**:6672-6678

[27] Hewitson JP et al. Proteomic analysis of secretory products from the model gastrointestinal nematode *Heligmosomoides polygyrus* reveals dominance of venom allergen-like (VAL) proteins. Journal of Proteomics. 2011;**74**:1573-1594

[28] Moyle M et al. A hookworm glycoprotein that inhibits neutrophil function is a ligand of the integrin CD11b/CD18. The Journal of Biological Chemistry. 1994;**269**:10008-10015

[29] Lozano-Torres JL et al. Dual disease resistance mediated by the immune receptor Cf-2 in tomato requires a common virulence target of a fungus and a nematode. Proceedings of the National Academy of Sciences of the United States of America. 2012;**109**(25):10119-10124

[30] Everts B et al. Schistosome-derived omega-1 drives Th2 polarization by suppressing protein synthesis following internalization by the mannose receptor. The Journal of Experimental Medicine. 2012;**209**(10):1753-1767

[31] Steinfelder S et al. The major component in schistosome eggs responsible for conditioning dendritic cells for Th2 polarization is a T2 ribonuclease (omega-1). The Journal of Experimental Medicine. 2009;**206**(8):1681-1690

[32] Harnett W, Harnett MM. Filarial nematode secreted product ES-62 is an anti-inflammatory agent: Therapeutic potential of small molecule derivatives and ES-62 peptide mimetics. Clinical and Experimental Pharmacology & Physiology. 2006;**33**(5-6):511-518

[33] Manoury B, Gregory WF, Maizels RM, Watts C. Bm-CPI-2, a cystatin homolog secreted by the filarial parasite *Brugia malayi*, inhibits class II MHC-restricted antigen processing. Current Biology. 2001;**11**:447-451

[34] Klotz C et al. A helminth immunomodulator exploits host signaling events to regulate cytokine production in macrophages. PLoS Pathogens. 2011;7(1):e1001248

[35] Gomez-Escobar N et al. Heterologous expression of the filarial nematode alt gene products reveals their potential to inhibit immune function. BMC Biology. 2005;**3**(8):1-16

[36] Colombo M, Raposo G, Thery C. Biogenesis, secretion, and intercellular interactions of exosomes and other extracellular vesicles. Annual Review of Cell and Developmental Biology. 2014;**30**:255-289

[37] Raposo G, Stoorvogel W. Extracellular vesicles: Exosomes, microvesicles, and friends. The Journal of Cell Biology. 2013;**200**(4):373-383

[38] Coakley G, Maizels RM, Buck AH. Exosomes and other extracellular vesicles: The new communicators in parasite infections. Trends in Parasitology. 2015;**31**(10):477-489

[39] Marcilla A et al. Extracellular vesicles in parasitic diseases. Journal of Extracellular Vesicles. 2014;**3**:25040

[40] Marcilla A et al. Extracellular vesicles from parasitic helminths contain specific excretory/secretory proteins and are internalized in intestinal host cells. PLoS One. 2012;**7**(9):e45974

[41] Buck AH et al. Exosomes secreted by a nematode parasite transfer RNA to mammalian cells and regulate genes of the innate immune system. Nature Communications. 2014;**5**:5488

[42] Liegeois S, Benedetto A, Garnier JM, Schwab Y, Labouesse M. The V0-ATPase mediates apical secretion of exosomes containing Hedgehog-related proteins in *Caenorhabditis elegans*. The Journal of Cell Biology. 2006;**173**(6):949-961

[43] Hassani K, Olivier M. Immunomodulatory impact of *Leishmania*-induced macrophage exosomes: A comparative proteomic and functional analysis. PLoS Neglected Tropical Diseases. 2013;**7**(5):e2185

[44] Parkinson J et al. A transcriptomic analysis of *Echinococcus granulosus* larval stages: Implications for parasite biology and host adaptation. PLoS Neglected Tropical Diseases. 2012;**6**(11):e1897

[45] Dang Z et al. A pilot study on developing mucosal vaccine against alveolar echinococcosis (AE) using recombinant tetraspanin 3: Vaccine efficacy and immunology.

PLoS Neglected Tropical Diseases. 2012;**6**(3):e1570

[46] Dang Z et al. Evaluation of *Echinococcus multilocularis* tetraspanins as vaccine candidates against primary alveolar echinococcosis. Vaccine. 2009;**27**(52):7339-7345

[47] Tran MH et al. Tetraspanins on the surface of *Schistosoma mansoni* are protective antigens against schistosomiasis. Nature Medicine. 2006;**12**:835-840

[48] Pinheiro CS et al. A multivalent chimeric vaccine composed of *Schistosoma mansoni* SmTSP-2 and Sm29 was able to induce protection against infection in mice. Parasite Immunology. 2014;**36**(7):303-312

[49] Humphreys NE, Xu D, Hepworth MR, Liew FY, Grencis RK. IL-33, a potent inducer of adaptive immunity to intestinal nematodes. Journal of Immunology. 2008;**180**(4): 2443-2449

[50] Bernal D et al. Surface analysis of *Dicrocoelium dendriticum*. The molecular characterization of exosomes reveals the presence of miRNAs. Journal of Proteomics. 2014;**105**:232-241

[51] Cheng G, Luo R, Hu C, Cao J, Jin Y. Deep sequencing-based identification of pathogen-specific microRNAs in the plasma of rabbits infected with *Schistosoma japonicum*. Parasitology. 2013;**140**(14):1751-1761

[52] Nowacki FC et al. Protein and small non-coding RNA-enriched extracellular vesicles are released by the pathogenic blood fluke *Schistosoma mansoni*. Journal of Extracellular Vesicles. 2015;**4**:28665

[53] Zamanian M et al. Release of small RNA-containing exosome-like vesicles from the human filarial parasite *Brugia malayi*. PLoS Neglected Tropical Diseases. 2015;**9**(9):e0004069

[54] Sotillo J et al. Extracellular vesicles secreted by *Schistosoma mansoni* contain protein vaccine candidates. International Journal for Parasitology. 2016;**46**(1):1-5

[55] Wang L et al. Exosome-like vesicles derived by *Schistosoma japonicum* adult worms mediates M1 type immune-activity of macrophage. Parasitology Research. 2015;**114**(5):1865-1873

[56] Kalra H, Drummen GP, Mathivanan S. Focus on extracellular vesicles: Introducing the next small big thing. International Journal of Molecular Sciences. 2016;**17**(2):170-200

[57] Chaiyadet S et al. Carcinogenic liver fluke secretes extracellular vesicles that promote cholangiocytes to adopt a tumorigenic phenotype. The Journal of Infectious Diseases. 2015;**212**(10):1636-1645

[58] Valadi H et al. Exosome-mediated transfer of mRNAs and microRNAs is a novel mechanism of genetic exchange between cells. Nature Cell Biology. 2007;**9**(6):654-659

[59] Buck AH, Blaxter M. Functional diversification of Argonautes in nematodes: An expanding universe. Biochemical Society Transactions. 2013;**41**(4):881-886

[60] Arpaia N et al. Metabolites produced by commensal bacteria promote peripheral regulatory T-cell generation. Nature. 2013;**504**(7480):451-455

[61] Maslowski KM et al. Regulation of inflammatory responses by gut microbiota and chemoattractant receptor GPR43. Nature. 2009;**461**(7268):1282-1286

[62] Trompette A et al. Gut microbiota metabolism of dietary fiber influences allergic airway disease and hematopoiesis. Nature Medicine. 2014;**20**(2):159-166

[63] Tielens AGM, van Grinsven KWA, Henze K, van Hellemond JJ, Martin W. Acetate formation in the energy metabolism of parasitic helminths and protists. International Journal for Parasitology. 2010;**40**(4):387-397

[64] Zaiss MM, Rapin A, Lebon L, Dubey LK, Mosconi I, Sarter K, et al. The intestinal microbiota contributes to the ability of helminths to modulate allergic inflammation. Immunity. 2015;**43**:998-1010

[65] Liu LX, Buhlmann JE, Weller PF. Release of prostaglandin E_2 by microfilariae of *Wuchereria bancrofti* and *Brugia malayi*. The American Journal of Tropical Medicine and Hygiene. 1992;**46**:520-523

[66] Brattig NW, Schwohl A, Rickert R, Buttner DW. The filarial parasite *Onchocerca volvulus* generates the lipid mediator prostaglandin E(2). Microbes and Infection. 2006;**8**(3):873-879

[67] Ramaswamy K, Kumar P, He YX. A role for parasite-induced PGE2 in IL-10-mediated host immunoregulation by skin stage schistosomula of *Schistosoma mansoni*. Journal of Immunology. 2000;**165**(8):4567-4574

[68] Selkirk ME, Lazari O, Matthews JB. Functional genomics of nematode acetylcholinesterases. Parasitology. 2005;**131**(Suppl):S3-S18

[69] Blackburn CC, Selkirk ME. Inactivation of platelet activating factor by a putative acetylhydrolase from the gastrointestinal nematode parasite *Nippostrongylus brasiliensis*. Immunology. 1992;**75**:41-46

[70] Gounaris K, Selkirk ME, Sadeghi SJ. A nucleotidase with unique catalytic properties is secreted by *Trichinella spiralis*. Molecular and Biochemical Parasitology. 2004;**136**:257-264

[71] Kreisinger J, Bastien G, Hauffe HC, Marchesi J, Perkins SE. Interactions between multiple helminths and the gut microbiota in wild rodents. Philosophical Transactions of Royal Society of London B Biological Science. 2015;**370**(1675):20140295.

[72] Reynolds LA, Finlay BB, Maizels RM. Cohabitation in the intestine: Interactions among helminth parasites, bacterial microbiota, and host immunity. Journal of Immunology. 2015;**195**(9):4059-4066

[73] Zaiss MM, Harris NL. Interactions between the intestinal microbiome and helminth parasites. Parasite Immunology. 2016;**38**(1):5-11

[74] Hayes KS et al. Exploitation of the intestinal microflora by the parasitic nematode *Trichuris muris*. Science. 2010;**328**(5984):1391-1394

[75] Reynolds LA et al. Commensal-pathogen interactions in the intestinal tract: *Lactobacilli* promote infection with, and are promoted by, helminth parasites. Gut Microbes. 2014;**5**:10-19

[76] Liu S et al. The host shapes the gut microbiota via fecal MicroRNA. Cell Host & Microbe. 2016;**19**(1):32-43

[77] Jones VE, Ogilvie BM. Protective immunity to *Nippostrongylus brasiliensis* in the rat III. Modulation of worm acetylcholinesterase by antibodies. Immunology. 1972;**22**:119-129

[78] Amiri P et al. Tumour necrosis factor a restores granulomas and

induces parasite egg-laying in schistosome-infected SCID mice. Nature. 1992;**356**:604-607

[79] Babayan SA, Read AF, Lawrence RA, Bain O, Allen JE. Filarial parasites develop faster and reproduce earlier in response to host immune effectors that determine filarial life expectancy. PLoS Biology. 2010;**8**(10):e1000525

[80] Beall MJ, Pearce EJ. Human transforming growth factor-activates a receptor serine/threonine kinase from the intravascular parasite *Schistosoma mansoni*. The Journal of Biological Chemistry. 2001;**276**:31613-31619

[81] Li J et al. Exosomes mediate the cell-to-cell transmission of IFN-alpha-induced antiviral activity. Nature Immunology. 2013;**14**(8):793-803

[82] Giugliano S et al. Hepatitis C. virus infection induces autocrine interferon signaling by human liver endothelial cells and release of exosomes, which inhibits viral replication. Gastroenterology. 2015;**148**:392, e313-402

[83] Madison MN, Jones PH, Okeoma CM. Exosomes in human semen restrict HIV-1 transmission by vaginal cells and block intravaginal replication of LP-BM5 murine AIDS virus complex. Virology. 2015;**482**:189-201

[84] Hu G et al. Release of luminal exosomes contributes to TLR4-mediated epithelial antimicrobial defense. PLoS Pathogens. 2013;**9**(4):e1003261

[85] Beauvillain C, Ruiz S, Guiton R, Bout D, Dimier-Poisson I. A vaccine based on exosomes secreted by a dendritic cell line confers protection against *T. gondii* infection in syngeneic and allogeneic mice. Microbes and Infection. 2007;**9**(14-15):1614-1622

[86] Schnitzer JK, Berzel S, Fajardo-Moser M, Remer KA, Moll H. Fragments of antigen-loaded dendritic cells (DC) and DC-derived exosomes induce protective immunity against *Leishmania major*. Vaccine. 2010;**28**(36):5785-5793

[87] RyanSM,EichenbergerRM,RuscherR, Giacomin PR, Loukas A. Harnessing helminth-driven immunoregulation in the search for novel therapeutic modalities. PLoS Pathogens. 2020;**16**(5): e1008508. DOI: 10.1371/journal.ppat.1008508

[88] Coakley G, Amy H, Buck AH, Maizels RM. Host parasite communications—Messages from helminths for the immune system: Parasite communication and cell-cell interactions. Molecular and Biochemical Parasitology. 2016;**208**(1):33-40. DOI: 10.1016/j.molbiopara.2016.06.003

Chapter 9

Oxygen and Redox Reactions Contribute to the Protection of Free-Living and Parasite Helminths against Pathogens and/or Host Response

Agustin Plancarte and Gabriela Nava

Abstract

Millions of years ago, the reductive atmosphere environment of Earth was replaced by an oxidative one because of redox reactions. These conditions allowed aerobic organisms to populate the planet and control the toxicity of oxygen. Aerobic organisms began to produce reactive oxygen species (ROS) via oxygen redox reactions and used them for their physiology process. Free-living helminths appeared in the early Paleozoic era and parasite helminths in the late same era. Free-living helminths, such as *Caenorhabditis elegans* and earthworms, have been used as host models to understand their micro pathogen defenses, particularly those associated with ROS. We speculate that the micro pathogens of *C. elegans* are equivalent to the parasite helminth hosts in terms of generating a worm's defense response. Therefore, parasite helminths may share similar defense mechanisms to humans, as in *C. elegans*. This last observation suggests the existence of a conservative pathogen protection process for centuries. This review discusses the evolution of oxygen molecules and redox reactions, as well as of the Earth's atmosphere, and changes over time in the protection of helminths mechanisms. These mechanisms have been so successful that have improved our understanding and have had a positive impact on humans.

Keywords: Earth origins, oxidoreduction, helminths, antioxidant defenses, innate immunity

1. Introduction

There are two types of helminths: free-living and parasitic helminths. For decades, free-living helminths have been used as models in studies on mechanisms used to survive against the pathogenic effects of micro pathogens. Because of the evolutionary link between free-living helminth defenses and human innate immunity, this research is highly relevant to humans [1].

On the other hand, little is known about the micro pathogens that affect animal helminth parasites, particularly in the adult form, despite coexisting with large numbers of microorganisms in the intestine of their host. This gap in our understanding is problematic because of the damage that helminth parasites can inflict on the health of their hosts, including humans and livestock.

Identifying the defense mechanism that helminth parasites use against their micro pathogens, as is known for free-living helminths, would be extremely useful. However, this is technically impossible, despite indirect information suggesting that helminth parasites develop defense mechanisms against micro pathogens as a result of the long periods of time they spend inside the intestine of their hosts [2].

One observation relevant to helminth parasites, in relation to the defense mechanisms used by free-living helminths, is that of aerobic organism conditions. Under these conditions, free-living helminths survive against their micro pathogens using in some situations the toxic capacity of the oxygen molecule to induce oxidative stress [3].

The defense mechanisms of helminths against micro pathogens are important in the study of the evolution of helminths from their ancient origins to the modern day. Understanding these mechanisms will provide insights into oxidative mechanisms and reduction-oxidation reactions (redox) more generally, both of which are chemical events present in the defense mechanisms of any pathogen.

2. The origin of helminths

Helminths are free-living parasitic invertebrate metazoan organisms. They include nematodes (round worms), trematodes (flukes), cestodes (tapeworms), and acanthocephalans (thorny-headed worms). The fossil record provides evidence that ectoparasitic helminths (e.g., worm-like pentastomid arthropods) have existed since the early Paleozoic era (542–444 million years (My)), while endoparasitic helminths (cestodes) arose during, or possibly even before, the late Paleozoic era (416–251 My) [4]. Therefore, the origins of helminths, all from free-living and parasitic organisms, were derived from a world in which the atmospheric conditions were initially reductive before transforming to oxidative [5].

3. The "rusting" of the Earth

The amount of oxygen (O_2) in the atmosphere before the Paleozoic era was at levels <0.001% of those present in the atmosphere today. However, during the Paleozoic and after this era, free oxygen was spawned by cyanobacteria producing land releasing it as a by-product of photosynthesis [6], causing the Great Oxidation Event (GOE), which dramatically changed the composition of the Earth's life forms and led to the near extinction of anaerobic organisms. The GOE is believed to have input sufficient oxygen into the atmosphere to allow for the evolution of animal respiration **Figure 1**.

On the other hand, if cyanobacteria were fundamental for the "rusting" of the Earth, redox reactions (electron transfer mechanism or redox) would still be relevant, in particular for the physiology of aerobic organisms.

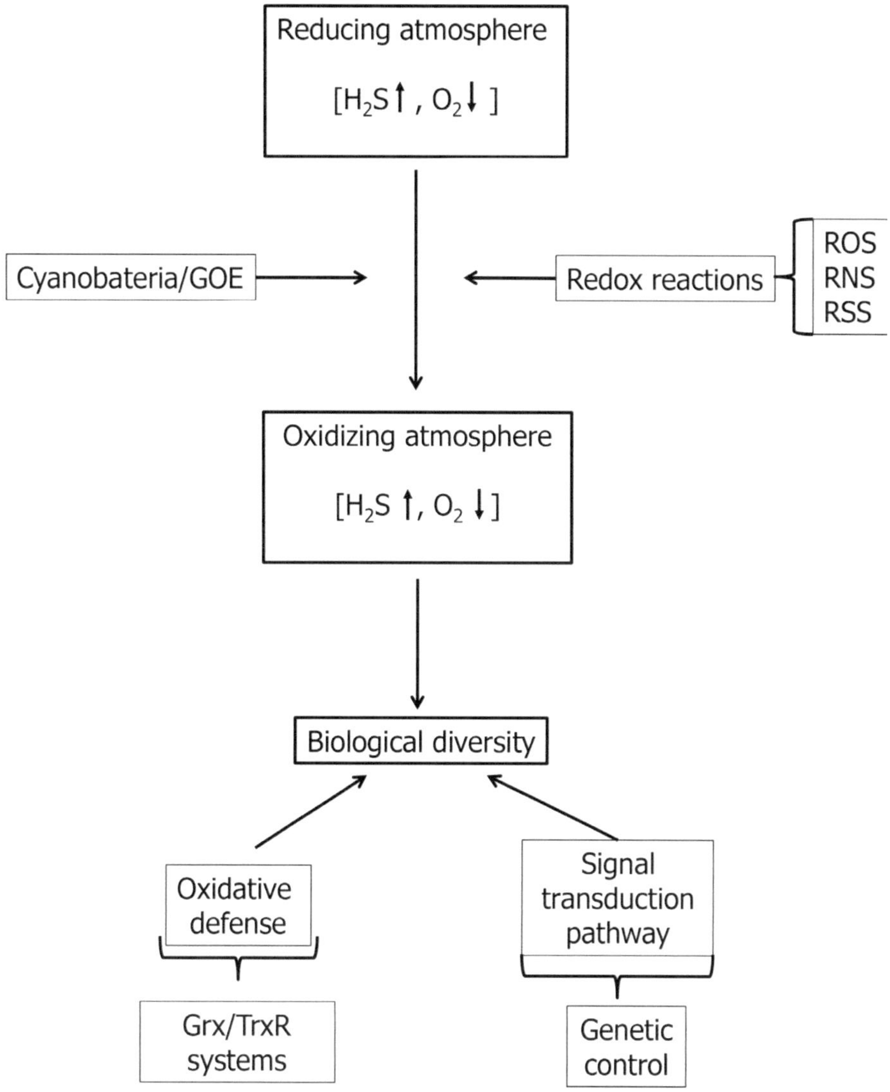

Figure 1.
Earth atmosphere modification and consequences on living organisms. Cyanobacteria are associated with the Great Oxidation Event (GOE) on Earth. Then redox reactions contribute to the development of reactive oxygen, nitrogen, and sulfur species (ROS, RNS, RSS). High concentrations of these are avoided through glutathione (GSH)/thioredoxin (TrxR) systems, but low species concentrations are necessary for signal transduction pathway cells to control gene expressions.

In the Hadean eon (4.6 billion years ago), redox reactions were a response to the large amounts of energy in the primitive Earth resulting from cosmic and geophysical reactions occurring at the time [7].

4. Energy flow theory

The energy flow theory proposed by Harold Morowitz is useful for explaining the origin of life [8]. In the primitive Earth, millions of reduction-oxidation reactions took place, one of which occurred between molecular hydrogen (reductor) and carbon dioxide (oxidant). This redox reaction was not spontaneous. Therefore, primitive organisms, such as helminths, acquired the skills needed to manage this reaction via enzyme catalysis. The citric acid or Krebs cycle is one such example. In addition to the citric acid cycle, aerobic organisms, such as helminths, developed a group of metabolic cycles to obtain their capacity to manage oxygen because of their dual contrasting molecular characteristics **Figure 2**.

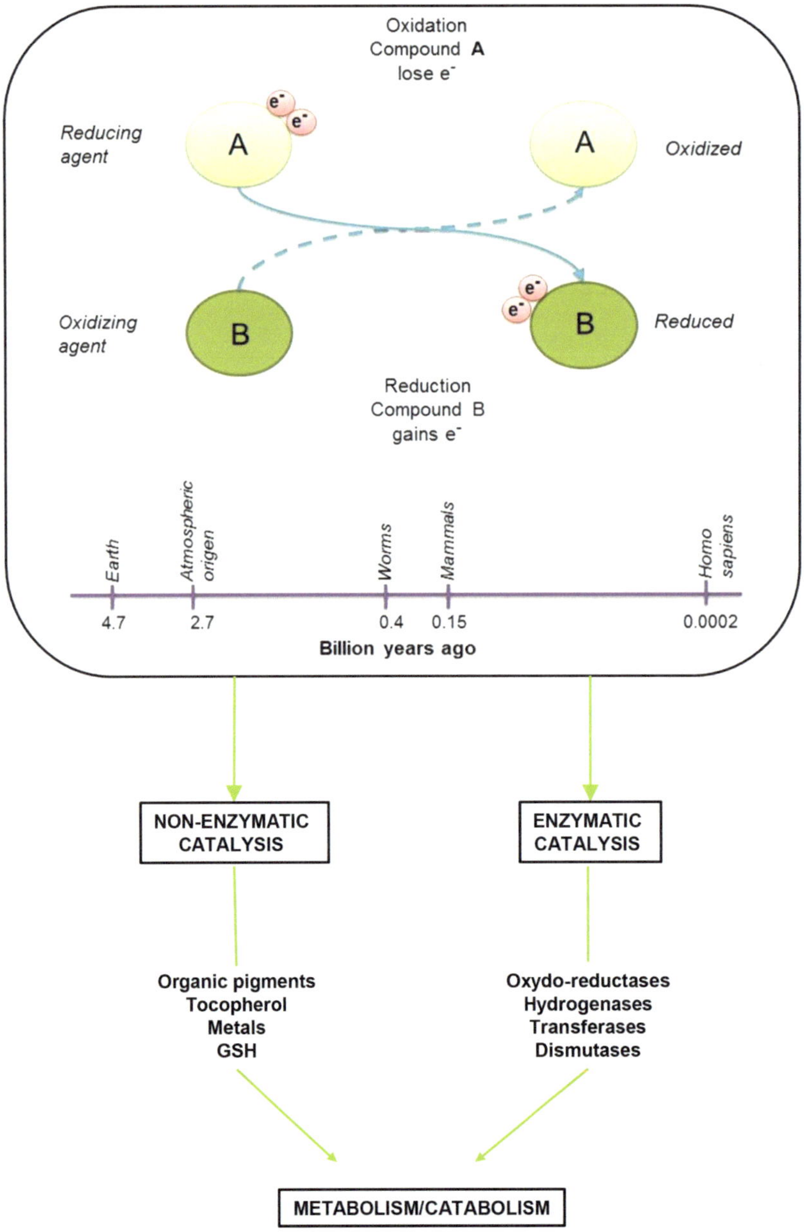

Figure 2.
Redox throughout life's evolution. Two different groups of molecules that originate redox reactions. Principally, metals, in the early Earth contributed to its oxidation. Redox enzymes in organism, including helminths, contributed to their homeostasis.

5. The contrasting oxygen molecule

As described previously, although molecular oxygen is vital for aerobic organisms, it is also a toxic mutagenic gas due to the production of intermediary oxygen molecules and reactive oxygen species (ROS) [9]. The toxicity of oxygen arises from its chemical electron acceptability by redox mechanisms, producing superoxide radicals (O•−), hydrogen peroxide (H_2O_2), hydroxyl radicals (•OH), and singlet oxygen (O_2), also known as reactive oxygen species (ROS). When concentration of ROS exceeds the capacity of the cells' defense systems, this results in the phenomenon of oxidative stress, which is characterized by an increase in the reduction potential or a large decrease in the reducing capacity of the cellular redox couples.

Oxidative stress is associated with damage to biological molecules. ROS can oxidize amino acid chains and cross-link proteins, as well as oxidize protein backbones. The highly reactive hydroxyl radical (•OH) reacts with DNA via the addition of double bonds of DNA bases and by the abstraction of a hydrogen atom from the methyl group of thymine and each of the C−H bonds of 2-deoxyribose. Furthermore, ROS also induces the process of lipid peroxidation in lipoprotein particles or membranes, giving rise to a variety of products, including short chain aldehydes, such as malondialdehyde or 4-hydroxynonenal, alkanes, alkenes, conjugated dienes, and a variety of hydroxides and hydroperoxides.

One way to understand how oxidative stress works in free-living helminths is to appreciate the process by which these organisms can be affected by bacterial virulence. This observation is clear from the studies developed in *C. elegans*, which produced hundreds of mutant worms with enough different genes [10] and mutants for the study of all aspects of this organism. Therefore, this worm is an excellent host model for the study of the evolutionarily conserved mechanisms of microbial pathogens.

Based on this, microbes that cause diseases in mammalian hosts have also been shown to be important for diseases in *C. elegans*, and as a terrestrial microbiome, *C. elegans* can be fed not only with the auxotrophic *Escherichia coli* strain OP50, which is harmless to the worm, but also with a variety of pathogenic bacteria. This means that a way to understand how a worm can get a disease is just to see them without movement in culture in the presence of the pathogen bacteria. Specifically, it was observed that C. elegans was killed when the *Pseudomonas aeruginosa* PA14 strain or another pathogenic microbe was provided as a food source [11].

A historical summary of the major results obtained in the study of the *C. elegans* model is as follows: (a) Sifri et al. [12] identified *C. elegans* as a new, simple, and cheap model organism for the study the pathogenesis of the Gram-negative bacteria *P. aeruginosa* and *Salmonella enterica* serovar *Typhimurium*. (b) Garsin et al. [13] showed that the Gram-positive bacteria *Enterococcus faecalis* and *Streptococcus pneumoniae* kill *C. elegans*. (c) Hodgkin et al. [14] demonstrated that the genetically amenable nematode *C. elegans* is ideally suited to identify host factors. Therefore, the biological complementarity between *C. elegans* and pathogenic microorganisms is well suited for the study of bacterial virulence, not least because of the vast bacterial strains available for this aim.

6. How helminths, particularly *C. elegans*, are killed by pathogens

To answer this question, several research groups have developed nematode bacteria experimental systems. Their results can be grouped into five different mechanisms: (1) Colonization: The worm is killed slowly through an infection-like process, which correlates with the accumulation of bacteria within the worm's intestine [15]. (2) Infection persistence: In this mechanism, contact between the worm and live bacterial cells is necessary as they accumulate in the intestinal tract of the animal host. Additionally, the proliferation of bacterial cells inside the worm intestine is also needed to establish a persistent infection. This mechanism suggests that some bacterial species may adhere to the intestinal receptors in worms [16]. (3) Invasive: Bacterial cells, such as *S. enterica*, use a type III secretion system to invade *C. elegans* [17]. In this worm, there are two major surfaces that act as nutritious bacterial interfaces: the first is at the chemosensory and olfactory neurons of the amphids, and the second is at the apical surface of intestinal cells. (4) Biofilms: These occur when bacteria form an obstructive matrix over the animal pharyngeal opening, which accumulates over time and prevents normal feeding and nutrition [18]. (5) Toxin-mediated killing: Bacterial pathogens kill worms via the production of diffusible toxins. Under these conditions, no bacterial but rather a soluble toxin is necessary to kill the worm [19]. For the first four mechanisms, direct contact with the pathogen microbes is necessary. The fifth mechanism requires that a soluble toxin reaches the worm. These mechanisms indicate that toxin-mediated killing associated with ROS products is feasible, as all redox reactions are developed under soluble conditions. For example, if the *C. elegans* mutants mev-1(kn1) and rad-8(mn163) are fed with the human opportunistic pathogen *P. aeruginosa* strain PA14, they will be killed. This is because *P. aeruginosa* secretes phenazines, and this organic compound exerts its toxic effect on *C. elegans* mutants undergoing redox cycling for ROS production.

7. How helminths defend themselves against pathogens

Although the mechanisms by which different bacteria affect the resistance of worm to pathogens are poorly understood, helminths have developed a number of different procedures to survive: (1) Behavioral defense: In this case, the worm detects olfactory stimuli, recognizes odors, and modifies its behavior by olfactory learning and imprinting [20]. (2) Barrier mechanism: The muscular pharynx grinder provides a physical barrier against pathogens, which protects them by disrupting the engulfed microbes [21]. (3) Production of soluble molecules: Examples of antimicrobial proteins and peptides in response to microbial infection [22]. (4) Direct inhibition of pathogens: Exerts a commensal-mediated protective effect on *C. elegans* [23]. (5) RNA interference: *Orsay* virus (OV) is a natural pathogen of *C. elegans*. The worm develops specific protection against this virus via the antiviral RNAi response. This mechanism not only inhibits vertical OV transmission, but also promotes transgenerational inheritance of antiviral immunity [24]. (6) Innate immunity involving signaling pathways: Specific responses that protect and repair against the collateral damage caused by ROS are critical for a successful attack against pathogens. Thus, there is a connection between the generation of ROS by Ce-Duox1/BLI-3 and the upregulation of a protective transcriptional response by SKN-1 [25]. (7) Oxidative damage: The secretion of ROS by gut epithelia [25]. ROS are known to be involved in tissue damage. This is because of the imbalance between the antioxidizing defenses of the organisms and the oxygen intermediaries produced in cells during aerobic metabolism and/or host inflammatory defenses against some pathogens.

NADPH oxidases, whose biological function lies in electron transport, are also a major source of ROS. These enzymes are multi-pass transmembrane proteins that catalyze the reduction of extracellular or luminal oxygen by intracellular NADPH to generate superoxide anions (O_2•) [26]. NADPH oxidases have been discovered in macrophages as a defense mechanism against pathogens, but today it is known that they are widely distributed in different kingdoms with multiple biological functions. The importance of these enzymes in aerobic organisms has led to the discovery of the NOX/DUOX family of NADPH oxidases, which includes three NOX subfamilies: ancestral type, NOX5-like, and DUOX [27]. DUOX isoforms that presumably developed from the NOX5-like subfamily are known as dual oxidases because they have both a peroxidase homology domain and a gp91phox domain. This last domain is the heme-binding subunit of the superoxide-generating NADPH oxidase, the catalytic moiety; thus, DUOXs produce anion superoxide (O_2•) and hydrogen peroxide (H_2O_2) by transferring one and two electrons, respectively, from intracellular NADPH to extracellular oxygen. DUOX is the only type of NOX present in *C. elegans*. The worm encodes two Duox genes (bli-3 and duox-2) that share an amino acid sequence with 94% identity to each other and approximately 30% to human Duox 1 and 2. It is known that *C. elegans* intestinal cells, like mammalian phagocytes, produce ROS, such as O_2• and H_2O_2, via DUOXs as an antimicrobial response [3].

Therefore, *C. elegans* may be able to exert lipid peroxidation in the lipid membrane of micro pathogens in an effort to kill them, as has been described in prokaryotes and other eukaryote parasite-host relationships in the past.

8. The importance of lipid peroxidation

Lipid peroxidation comprises a chain of reactions involving the oxidative degradation of lipids. It is the process in which free radicals, such as O_2•, "steal" electrons from the lipids in cell membranes, resulting in cell damage. This process evolved from a free radical chain reaction mechanism, which comprised three steps: initiation, propagation, and termination. In the first step, O_2• interacts with polysaturated fatty acids. This O_2• is dismuted by superoxide dismutase, and in addition to hydrogen atoms, it breaks down into ordinary molecular oxygen and H_2O_2. Then, H_2O_2 in the presence of Fe^{2+} produces hydroxyl anions (OH•) via the Fenton reaction. The OH• takes away allylic hydrogens from the polyunsaturated fatty acid chains to obtain a radical carbon (L•). Then, the easy reaction with oxygen molecules by L• gives rise to the peroxyl radical (LOO•). When hydrogens are removed from polyunsaturated fatty acid neighbors, this LOO• results in the formation of lipid hydroperoxide (LOOH). The propagation step occurs when LOO• interacts with other polyunsaturated fatty acids, resulting in the formation of further lipid radicals and H_2O_2. Additionally, the catalysis of H_2O_2 by Fe^{2+} makes results in the formation of alkoxy and peroxy radicals during propagation step, with this secondary free radical production beginning another lipid hydrogen peroxide chain. Termination occurs when two radicals are conjugated, the result of which is a non-radical product.

The *C. elegans* model provides an opportunity to gain insights into how free-living helminths and parasite helminths exert this strategy to protect themselves against oxidative stress, even if the ROS are self-produced, as in *C. elegans*, or by the host response, as in human parasite helminths. In addition, the concept of lipid peroxidation can be explained practically since lipid peroxidation starts with the same oxidative molecules in any organism.

Due the short life of *C. elegans* compared with humans, the exertion of lipid peroxidation against micro pathogens could be considered an acute response, if a short one, as it is sufficient to damage the worm's own tissues. In other words, collateral damage can result from the processes by which worms are trying to kill micro pathogens. In human helminthiasis is a rule to see the development of chronic infections besides lipid peroxidation.

9. DUOX/NADPH oxidases in toxicity and signal transduction

C. elegans is known to express antioxidant genes for protection against its autooxidative response, as described previously [28]. Human helminth parasites may also exert similar procedures for protection against oxidative stress. Therefore, understanding how *C. elegans* resist their own protective oxidative response could provide insights into how helminthiasis chronicity evolved in humans.

In this sense, Hoeven et al. [25] found that aerobic organism evolution works in a balanced dualism. For example, when the Earth's atmosphere became oxidant, living forms, including older forms of free-living helminths, developed an extremely complex cellular signal mechanism to manage oxygen toxicity. This permitted them to kill their adversary while surviving the collateral damage at the same time; this strategy is very clever and clearly observed in *C. elegans*. Upon exposure to *P. aeruginosa* and *E. faecalis*, *C. elegans* uses DUOX/1BLI-3 to kill pathogens by producing ROS. In addition, as DUOX/1BLI-3 is activated to kill pathogens found in the intestine of helminths, SKN-1 (Skinhead family member 1) transcription factor, a member of the Cap'n'collar (CNC) protein family, is simultaneously activated to avoid tissue damage [29].

Transcription factors belonging to this group of proteins play a crucial role in protecting cells against oxidative stress. Under physiological conditions, they remain in the cytoplasm in the inactive form or are degraded. However, under oxidative stress conditions, they are translocated to the nucleus and bind to DNA in the antioxidant response element (ARE) motif. Consequently, genes encoding cytoprotective proteins, such as low-molecular-weight antioxidant proteins (i.e., thioredoxin, ferritin, and metallothionein), responsible for protecting cells against the action of ROS, are transcribed. *C. elegans* SKN-1 has been extensively studied, with studies finding that this transcription factor is orthologous with the nuclear factor erythroid 2 (NFE2)-related factor 2 (Nrf2). They are both members of the CNC subfamily of the basic leucine zipper (bZip) transcription factors [30].

Both transcription factors are highly conserved proteins with functions similar to those of the promoters of oxidative-stress-related genes. In fact, Nrf2 and SKN-1 regulate phase II detoxification genes needed to defend against oxidative stress and electrophilic xenobiotics. With this detoxification system, worms can solubilize lipophilic xenobiotics or endobiotics via cytochrome P450s (CYPs) and short-chain dehydrogenases (SDHs), two classic enzymes of the phase I detoxification step. Reactive products, including ROS originating from the original toxic molecules, are detoxified, either via metabolization or conjugation, by the phase II system using UDP-glucuronosyl/glucosyl transferases (UDP) or glutathione transferases (GSTs), among others. Afterward, conjugated toxins are eliminated from cells by phase III proteins, including ATP-binding cassette (ABC) and other transporters.

Thus, similar to Nrf2, SKN-1 controls many critical detoxification processes directly as glutathione transferase enzymes (GSTs).

10. Glutathione transferases (GST) and their importance in detoxification

From an evolutionary point of view, these enzymes emerged over two billion years ago. Based on structural and functional criteria, they can be grouped into four different families: cytoplasmic, microsomal, mitochondrial, and bacterial.

Glutathione transferases are ubiquitous in prokaryotes and eukaryotes, indicating their protective and functional importance. These transferases are a large superfamily of supergene isoenzymes that play important roles in cell detoxification. These enzymes use electrophiles to catalyze the nucleophilic addition of the thiol of reduced glutathione (L-g-glutamyl-L-cysteinyl-glycine) (GSH) to electrophilic centers in organic compounds. The resulting glutathione conjugates are rendered more water-soluble to facilitate their eventual elimination. A wide variety of endogenous (e.g., by-products of reactive oxygen species activity) and exogenous (e.g., polycyclic aromatic hydrocarbons) electrophilic substrates have been identified. In addition, the detoxification functions of these enzymes have been observed not only in one but two mechanisms: passive detoxification and active detoxification. The former, as mentioned by Kostaropoulos et al. [31], refers to a detoxification mechanism characterized by an absence of catalytic function, such as the binding of potentially toxic non-substrate ligands, including porphyrins and lipid peroxides. In fact, GSTs were originally named "ligandins" due to their passive role in detoxification.

Ligandin activity exhibited by GST isoforms was first suggested as a result of the observed affinity for bilirubin, an azo dye carcinogen, and a metabolite of cortisone. The second mechanism was developed by catalytic activity, as described previously **Table 1**.

Glutathione transferases in cestodes were identified several years ago. Initially, these cestode transferase isoforms were associated with the detoxified procedures in several organisms, including *C. elegans* [32, 33]. However, because almost all GSTs

Ligand	I_{50} (mM)	Ki (mM)	%F (mM)
Mesoporphyrin	00.0012–0.1	15, 30, 45	0.0003–0.014
Prothoporphyrin	0.002–0.064	12, 24, 36	0.0012–0.027
Coproporphyrin	0.0005–0.005	0.0015, 0.0045	0.0002–0.014
Hematin	0.0007–0.012	0.002, 0.004	0.00012–0.003
trans,trans-2,4-hexadienal	0.0001–10	1.5, 3	0.003–1.9
trans,trans-2,4-nonadienal	0.0001–10	0.45, 0.9	0.0016–0.35
trans,trans-2,4-decadienal	0.0001–10	0.01, 0.1	0.0016–2.6
Arachidic acid	0.001–0.25	ND	0.0016–0.2
Palmitic acid	0.0001–1	ND	0.0016–0.27
Cholic acid	0.0001–1	ND	0.003–0.045
Chenodeoxycholic acid	0.0001–0.2	ND	0.001–0.011
Lithocholic acid	0.0001–1	ND	0.025–0 .2

*I_{50}, is a parameter giving the inhibitory concentration causing 50% inhibition; Ki is the inhibition catalytic constant value; %F, is the % of Ts26GST intrinsic fluorescence quenching; ND, not determined. (Exp. Par. 2014;**138**:63-70).*

Table 1.
Conditions for inhibition Ts26GST catalytic activity and spectrofluorometric assays.

have GSH as a nucleophilic substrate, and this is the central redox agent of most aerobic organisms, GST functions encompass other purposes, as reported by Ferguson and Bridge in the *C. elegans* model [34].

11. The redox couples in enzyme functions

As mentioned before, the reduced form of glutathione (GSH) serves as a ubiquitous nucleophile for the conversion of a variety of electrophilic substances under physiological conditions. This is possible when GSH is oxidized to glutathione disulfide (GSSG) by a reaction that involves the transfer of electrons between two species; in other words, when it is affected by the redox reaction.

GSH/GSSG is an example of millions of redox couples that are chemically similar or different, present in cells, organs, tissues, biological fluids, and cell organelles. A considerable number of these redox couples could be linked to each other to form a set of related redox couples, or redox couples that work independently. These reactions are achieved by capturing the energy released via oxidation to build cellular and organismic structures, maintain these structures (some avoid pathogenic action), and provide energy for the processes they support.

The production of a large number of redox couples in aerobic organisms occurs by enzymes and proteins of the glutaredoxin and thioredoxin systems, the former using GSH and the latter thioredoxin (Trx) [35].

12. The glutaredoxin and thioredoxin systems

The glutaredoxin system is composed of glutathione reductase (GR or GSR), glutathione (GSH), and glutaredoxin (Grx), while the thioredoxin system comprises thioredoxin reductase (TrxR) and thioredoxin (Trx). The glutaredoxin and thioredoxin systems are likely to have evolved very early in aerobic organisms. Owing to the cysteine moiety of GSH, the entire system is based on common sulfur biochemistry. Therefore, it requires an electron relay, linking the universal reducing agent NADPH to thiol/disulfide metabolism, and a thiol-containing adapter molecule (GSH, which is considered as a universal adaptor) to transfer electrons to a set of different acceptors, such as flavoproteins, which are widely used as electron relays.

Hence, it is not surprising that the reducing equivalents from NADPH enter the glutathione system either with the help of the FAD-dependent enzyme glutathione reductase (GR) or the thioredoxin reductase/thioredoxin couple (TrxR/Trx).

Glutaredoxin protein (Grx) was first described in crude enzyme preparations from beef liver by Racker [36] in 1955. Grxs are small (12–18 kDa) GSH-disulfide oxidoreductase members of the thioredoxin family, which includes the cytosolic (Grx1) and mitochondrial (Grx2) isoforms. Oxidized Grxs are reduced by GSH. According to its active site domain, Grxs are classified as dithiols (CPY/FC motif) and monothiols (CGFS motif), wherein monothiols can contain single or multiple monothiol Grx domains. Dithiol Grxs regulate the redox state of various proteins by catalyzing the reversible reduction of oxidized disulfides. For this purpose, Grxs use both cysteine residues from their active sites. In contrast, the monothiol Grxs reduce mixtures of disulfides (glutathionylation) formed between GSH and the thiols of proteins or other small compounds, using the cysteine residues from the active sites in their amino terminals.

With regard to the glutaredoxin genes of *C. elegans*, five have been annotated: glrx-3, glrx-5, glrx-10, glrx-21, and glrx-22 [37]. Except for glrx-5, which is predicted to be a mitochondrial glutaredoxin, the other annotated glutaredoxins are expected to be found in the cytosol. Based on phylogenetic analysis, the *C. elegans* GLRX-3 isoform has been postulated to be an ortholog of the mammalian GLRX3 protein kinase C-interacting cousin of thioredoxin (PICOT), suggesting that it exerts a protective mechanism against DNA-damage-inducing agents, such as some micro pathogens, by acting as an upstream positive regulator of ATR-dependent signaling pathways. On the other hand, a recent report demonstrated that *C. elegans* exhibits changes in the protein S-thiolation patterns (i.e., S-glutathionylation and S-cysteinylation) of targeted cysteine residues. This evidence suggests that glutaredoxins may provide an evolutionarily conserved mechanism for the catalysis of the reversal of S-glutathionylation, preventing the irreversible oxidation of protein thiols in *C. elegans* derived from micro pathogens.

Recently, the human and pig helminth parasite, *Taenia solium*, was cloned, expressed, and characterized for the first time as glutaredoxin (r-TsGrx1) [38]. The full-length DNA of the TsGrx1 gene comprised one intron of 39 bp and a single ORF of 315 bp, encoding 105 amino acid residues with an estimated molecular weight of 12,582 Da. Sequence analysis revealed a conserved dithiol C34PYC37 active site, GSH-binding motifs (CXXC, Lys and Gln/Arg, TVP, and CXD), and a conserved Gly-Gly motif. The r-TsGrx1 kinetic constants for glutathione (GSH) and 2-hydroxyethyl disulfide (HED) were determined. Conventional enzymes, such as tioredoxin reductase (TrxR) and glutathione reductases (GR or GSR), do not exist in *Theridion solium*. However, the presence of a protein hybrid tioredoxin glutathione reductase (TGR), with tioredoxin and glutathione reductase activity, as described below, makes it possible for the components of Trx and Grx systems in platyhelminth (flatworms) to work as observed in organisms that have independent enzymes for those functions.

Protein S-glutathionylation by glutaredoxins is a widely distributed posttranslational modification of thiol groups with glutathione, which can function as a redox-sensitive switch to mediate redox regulation and signal transduction. Therefore, the presence of Grxs in *C. elegans* and *T. solium* contributes to our understanding of the micro pathogen activation of redox-regulatory processes in these helminths.

GR (also termed GSR, as mentioned before) is a flavoenzyme of the pyridine nucleotide-disulfide oxidoreductase family (EC 1.6.4.2, now 1.8.1.7). This enzyme recycles reduced GSH from its oxidized form GSSG. However, this function was also developed for the thioredoxin system acting as a backup, a trait that is conserved from bacteria to mammals, highlighting its physiological relevance, including protection against toxicity, in both systems.

Glutathione reductase is a GR-isoform from prokaryote and eukaryotes that form stable homodimers of ~110 kDa. From a structural point of view, each subunit is organized into four domains (FAD binding, NADPH binding, central, and interface) and possesses an N-terminal flexible segment of 18 amino acids with a cysteine residue at position 2.

In *C. elegans*, the gsr-1 gene encodes the GSR enzyme, which produces two protein isoforms (GSR-1a and GSR-1b) [39], and its expression of GSR-1 is modulated by the SKN-1 transcription factor.

The GSR-1 gene is vital in *C. elegans* because it supports its embryonic development, and there is no alternative molecule for this purpose. In many organisms, the thioredoxin system exerts GSSG reduction in the absence of GSR. As described previously, this appears not to be the case for *C. elegans*, even though both systems have been shown to cooperate in other processes, such as worm molting.

Therefore, the *C. elegans* thioredoxin and glutaredoxin systems share common functions but also have specific non-overlapping roles in worm physiology. The thioredoxin system was first recognized in the early 1960s as a reductant of methionine sulfoxide and PAPS (3 H-phos- phoadenosine-5 H-phosphosulfate) in yeast and ribonucleotides in *E. coli*.

Thioredoxin reductase (EC 1.6.4.5) (TrxR) was originally identified in *E. coli* as part of the ribonucleoside diphosphate reductase system. TrxR catalyzes the reversible electron transfer from NADPH to oxidized thioredoxin (thioredoxin-S2), a 12 kDa protein containing a single oxidation-reduction active disulfide bond. The oxidation of NADPH leads to the formation of the reduced form of thioredoxin (thioredoxin SH2), which has a dithiol. TrxR directly reduces not only Trx from different species but also many non-disulfide substrates, such as selenite lipid hydroperoxides, although not glutathione disulfide (GSSG).

The *C. elegans* genome encodes two thioredoxin reductases: thioredoxin reductase-1 (TRXR-1), which is the sole selenoprotein in *C. elegans*, with a UGA-encoded Sec in the C-terminal active site, and thioredoxin reductase (TRXR-2), a homolog of a UGU-encoded cysteine substitution for Sec. TRXR-1, the cytosolic TrxR, is required for the acidification of the lysosomal compartment in the intestine, whereas TRX-2, the mitochondrial TrxR, is critical for producing stress conditions. Interestingly, the gene expression of both TRX-1 and TRX-2 is induced by heat shock, which results in the production of ROS. Both observations suggest the involvement of these TrxRs in protection against micro pathogens found in the intestine of the worm [40].

Tioredoxin (Trx), the major TrxR substrate, as mentioned previously, is a disulfide reductase with a molecular weight of approximately 12 kDa and has two cysteine residues in its consensus sequence (CGPC motif). When chemically reduced, this allows for the transfer of reducing equivalents to a wide variety of substrates, such as H_2O_2. Thus, Trxs can, either directly or via 2-Cys peroxidases, catalyze the reduction of hydrogen peroxide (H_2O_2) to water and lipid hydroperoxides (R−O−O−R) to alcohols in the cell. Trxs can also inhibit and/or activate transcription factors related to immune responses in mammals. For example, the activation of nuclear factor kappa-light-chain-enhancer of activated B cells (NF-kB) is inhibited when TRX1 prevents the release of IkB, an inhibitor of NF-κB.

Although the thioredoxin and glutaredoxin systems are vital for aerobic organisms, in platyhelminths (flatworms), both GR and TrxR are missing in their tissues. Instead of these proteins, some platyhelminths have a GR and TrxR molecular link exhibiting the fusion of glutaredoxin (Grx) and thioredoxin reductase (TrxR) domains into a single protein, a selenocysteine-containing enzyme that acts as a thioredoxin glutathione reductase (TGR) [41, 42].

Thus, TGR plays a central role in thiol-disulfide redox reactions by providing electrons to essential detoxification enzymes, such as GR and Prx. GR reduces the tripeptide GSSG to GSH, which acts as the main reducing agent in the catalytic functions displayed by GSTs [43].

Because conventional TrxR and GR are functional in *C. elegans*, no TGR is found in this worm. However, in platyhelminths, TGRs exert an efficient antioxidant defense against lipid peroxidation metabolites. In addition to the essential detoxification function of TGRs in flatworm parasites, as described above, it is necessary to include the TGR activities associated with the Grx domain, such as the deglutathionylase activity of GSH-protein mixed disulfides (protein-S-SG). Protein glutathionylation is the mechanism by which protein-SH groups form mixed disulfides with glutathione to avoid protein-SH group oxidation. In addition, TGRs play essential roles in redox cell signaling and sensing. Cell signaling transduction is the mechanism by which external stimuli are transferred to their inner compartments, resulting in the activation or inhibition of genes; cell sensing is the oxidative modification of protein cysteines with consequent events, such as changes in its activities and interactions with other biomacromolecules, such as native immunity receptors.

Haemonchus contortus has been used as an excellent model to gain insights into the oxidative defenses of hosts against nematodes [44]. *H. contortus* is a blood-sucking nematode parasite of the abomasum of small ruminants that causes a disease known as haemonchosis, in which the abomasal epithelium and highly toxic heme molecules are released [45]. Free heme catalyzes the formation of cytotoxic lipid peroxides via lipid peroxidation using hydrogen peroxide (H_2O_2) as Fenton reaction.

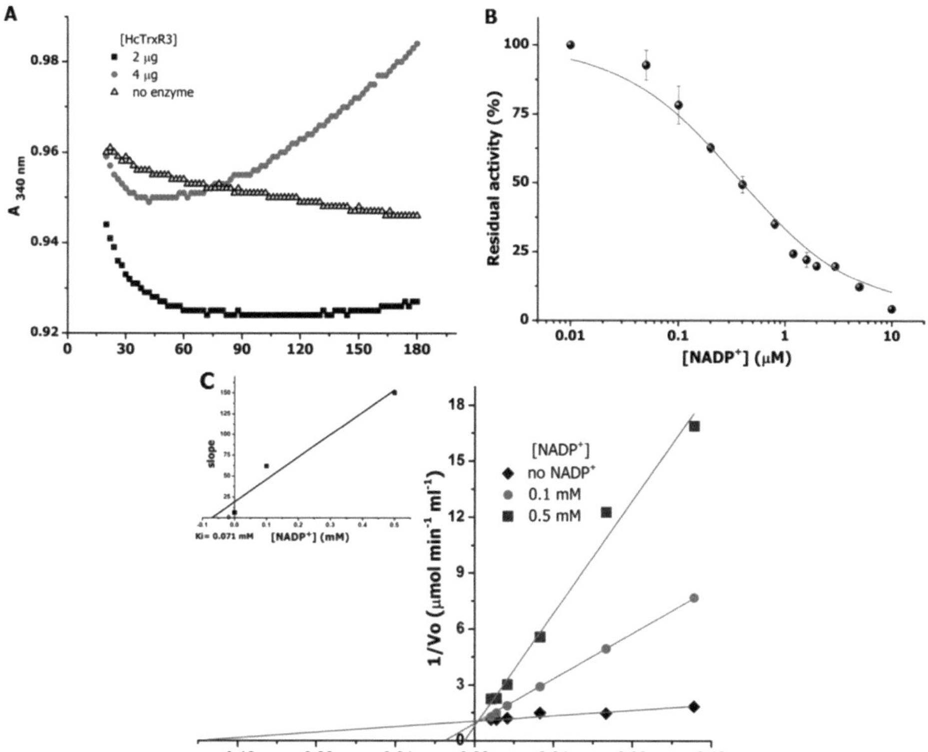

Figure 3.
Kinetic evidences of TR and GR activity from HcTrxR3. (A) Reduction of ebselen by NADPH catalyzed by HcTrxR3 produced ebselen diselenide and ebselen selenol. To 1 ml solutions containing 50 mM Tris-Cl, 1 mM EDTA, pH 7.5, 100 mM NADPH, and 0.1 mM ebselen, 2 μg (■) or 4 μg (•) HcTrxR3, was added, and A_{340} was measured against a blank without ebselen (Δ). Ebselen reduction was shown when absorbance decreased followed by ebselen selenol formation in the highest enzyme concentration. (B) Effect of $NADP^+$ on the glutathione reductase activities of HcTrxR3. IC_{50} plots were obtained; an enzyme aliquot (about 2 μg) was pre-incubated at 25°C in the presence of 100 μM NADPH and different concentrations of $NADP^+$. To start the reaction GSSG at a final concentration of 0.2 mM was added. (C) Show a competitive type inhibition where the 1/v versus 1/[$NADPH^+$] plot of initial velocities HcTrxR3 activity in absence (◆) and the presence of 0.1 mM (•) and 0.5 mM (■) of $NADP^+$ with various concentrations of $NADPH^+$ (0.01–10 μM). Inset shows secondary plot of the slope values derived from the primary 1/v versus 1/[$NADPH^+$] plot versus $NADP^+$ concentration for the determination of Ki [47].

The range of antioxidant enzyme systems available to *H. contortus* for the detoxification of H_2O_2 has been investigated using molecular biology tools. As a result, full-length sequences were obtained for a 2-Cys peroxiredoxin (Prx), a catalase, and a selenium-independent glutathione peroxidase (GPx), indicating that *H. contortus* expresses several antioxidant systems with the potential to detoxify peroxide, most of them within the host's immune response. Other studies identified additional three thioredoxin reductases (TrxRs) (HcTrxR-1, HcTrxR-2, and HcTrxR-3), two mitochondrial thioredoxins (HcTrx-1, HcTrx-5), and one cytosolic (Trx-3) thioredoxin (Trx), increasing the possible mechanisms of *H. contortus* detoxification. All the abovementioned detoxification enzymes and proteins, except catalase, work closely with the two major detoxification and redox systems in animal cells: thioredoxin (Trx) and glutathione (GSH) [46].

Interestingly, for the first time in the study of the TGR system [47], HcTrxR3 was found to catalyze the direct reduction of GSSG, the specific substrate for GR, in the same catalytic range as that of any GR. Its affinity for GSSG, measured as Km value, was higher than that of the 5,5-dithiobis-(2-nitrobenzoic acid) (DTNB) substrate for TrxR, demonstrating its preference for the GSSG substrate. Until now, no TrxR has been identified that is able to directly reduce GSSG.

This GR activity from HcTrxR3 is important not only because the enzyme is a TrxR, but also because information on the presence of GR in the *H. contortus* tissues is lacking thus far **Figure 3**.

13. The models of detoxified and innate immunity in pioneer earthworms

In addition to being essential for soil fertility, earthworms are also an excellent model for the study of the protection mechanisms used by helminths against micro pathogens [48], as in *C. elegans*.

Earthworms are terrestrial invertebrates belonging to the order Oligochaeta, class Chaetopoda, and phylum Annelidae. They range in size from a fraction of a centimeter to exceptional individuals of Megascolides australis, which can measure up to 2.75 m in length and 3 cm in diameter. Approximately 1800 species are distributed all over the world.

Earthworms became a model for comparative immunology in the early 1960s with the publication of results from transplantation experiments that proved the existence of self/non-self-recognition in earthworms. This initiated extensive studies on the immune mechanisms of earthworms, which evolved to prevent invasion by pathogens. In recent decades, important cellular and humoral pathways have been discovered, and numerous biologically active compounds have been characterized and cloned [49].

For example, earthworm coelomocytes (macrophage-like cells) are part of the cellular immune response and are both morphologically and functionally analogous to vertebrate phagocytes. Coelomocyte subpopulations (named as hyaline-, granular amoebocytes, and eleocytes) possess distinct functions, such as phagocytosis, encapsulation, and cellular cytotoxicity.

Additionally, phagocytic defense by the earthworm *Eisenia foetida* against certain pathogenic bacteria has been found to be aided by bacteriostatic or bactericidal substances, which may also play an opsonic role, as in vertebrates. Therefore, given the molecular tools of earthworm coelomocytes, there is a possibility that these organisms also use a functional NOX/DUOX system to eliminate invading micro pathogens via ROS production, as in *C. elegans*.

14. Conclusion

The invertebrate research model has been used to reveal the evolutive link between the oxygen atmosphere and the adaptability of helminths to aggressive environments. These organisms have been found to use oxygen molecules and redox reactions to exert protective effects against micro pathogens. Helminth models have also revealed similarities between the cells, molecules, and mechanisms of helminths and those of human components used against pathogens, highlighting the evolutionary success of these molecules, structures, and biological procedures. Thus, this review shows how understanding the mechanisms by which invertebrates manage their environmental adaptability can provide insights into how humans protect themselves against their own pathogens. Honey bees are another example of this idea, in which individuals are protected against micro pathogens via the concept of social immunity [50].

Acknowledgements

We thank Programa de Apoyo a Proyectos de Investigación e Innovación Tecnológica (PAPIIT), UNAM, IN209819.

Author details

Agustin Plancarte* and Gabriela Nava
Facultad de Medicina, Departamento de Microbiología y Parasitología, Universidad Nacional Autónoma de México, UNAM, México, CDMX, Mexico

*Address all correspondence to: apc@unam.mx

References

[1] Kumar A, Baruah A, Tomioka M, Iino Y, Kalita M, Khan M. *Caenorhabditis elegans*: A model to understand host–microbe interactions. Cellular and Molecular Life Sciences. 2020;**77**:1229-1249. DOI: 10.1007/s00018-019-03319-7

[2] Zakeri A, Hansen EP, Andersen SD, Williams AR, Nejsum P. Immunomodulation by helminths: Intracellular pathways and extracellular vesicles. Frontiers in Immunology. 2018;**8**:2349. DOI: 10.3389/fimmu.2018.02349

[3] Chávez V, Mohri-Shiomi A, Maadani A, Vega LA, Garsin DA. Oxidative stress enzymes are required for DAF-16-mediated immunity due to generation of reactive oxygen species by *Caenorhabditis elegans*. Genetics. 2007;**176**:1567-1577. DOI: 10.1534/genetics.107.072587

[4] Aguinaldo AM, Turbeville JM, Linford LS, Rivera MC, Garey JR, Raff RA, et al. Evidence for a clade of nematodes, arthropods and other moulting animals. Nature. 1997;**387**:489-493. DOI: 10.1038/387489a0

[5] Kendall B, ChT R, Lyons TW, Kaufman AJ, Poulton SW, Anbar DA. Pervasive oxygenation along late Archaean Ocean margins. Nature Geoscience. 2010;**3**:647-652. Available from: https://uwaterloo.ca

[6] Hamilton TL, Bryant DA, Macalady JL. The role of biology in planetary evolution: Cyanobacterial primary production in low-oxygen Proterozoic oceans. Environmental Microbiology. 2016;**18**:325-340. DOI: 10.1111/1462-2920.13118

[7] Harel A, Bromberg Y, Falkowski PG, Bhattacharya D. Evolutionary history of redox metal-binding domains across the tree of life. PNAS. 2014;**111**:7042-7047. DOI: 10.1073/pnas.1403676111

[8] Morowitz HJ. Energy Flow in Biology. Vol. 10. Woodbridge, CT, USA: Ox bow Press; 1968. p. 0125070500

[9] Gerschman R, Gilbert DL, Nye SW, Dwyerand P, Fenn WO. Oxygen poisoning and X-irradiation: A mechanism in common. Science. 1956;**119**:623-626. DOI: 10.1126/science.119.3097.623

[10] Brenner S. The genetic of *Caenorhabditis elegans*. Genetics. 1974;**77**:71-94

[11] Lee SH, Ooi SK, Mahadi NM, Tan MW, Nathan S. Complete killing of *Caenorhabditis elegans* by *Burkholderia pseudomallei* is dependent on prolonged direct association with the viable pathogen. PLoS One. 2011;**6**:e16707. DOI: 10.1371/journal.pone.0016707

[12] Sifri CD, Begun J, Ausubel MF. The worm has turned—Microbial virulence modeled in *Caenorhabditis elegans*. Trends in Microbiology. 2005;**13**:119-127. DOI: 10.1016/j.tim.2005.01.003

[13] Garsin DA, Sifri CD, Mylonakis E, Qin X, Singh KV, Murray BE, et al. A simple model host for identifying Gram-positive virulence factors. Proceedings of the National Academy of Sciences of the United States of America. 2001;**98**:10892-10897. DOI: 10.1073/pnas.191378698

[14] Hodgkin J, Kuwabara PE, Corneliussen B. A novel bacteria pathogen, microbacterium nematophilum, induces morphological change in the nematode *C. elegans*. Current Biology. 2000;**10**:1615-1618. DOI: 10.1016/s0960-9822(00)00867-8

[15] Kurz CL, Chauvet S, Andrès E, Aurouze M, Vallet I, Michel GP, et al. Virulence factors of the human opportunistic pathogen Serratia marcescens identified by in vivo screening. The EMBO Journal. 2003;**22**:1451-1460. DOI: 10.1093/emboj/cdg159

[16] Aballay A, Yorgey P, Ausubel FM. *Salmonella typhimurium* proliferates and establishes a persistent infection in the intestine of *Caenorhabditis elegans*. Current Biology. 2000;**10**:1539-1542. DOI: 10.1016/s0960-9822(00)00830-7

[17] Tenor JL, McCormick BA, Ausubel FM, Aballay A. *Caenorhabditis elegans*-based screen identifies salmonella virulence factors required for conserved host-pathogens interactions. Current Biology. 2004;**14**:1018-1024. DOI: 10.1016/j.cub.2004.05.050

[18] Tan L, Darby C. A movable surface: Formation of *Yersinia* sp. biofilms on motile *Caenorhabditis elegans*. Journal of Bacteriology. 2004;**186**:5087-5092. DOI: 10.1128/JB.186.15.5087-5092.2004

[19] Griffitts JS, Whitacre JL, Stevens DE, Aroian RV. Bt toxin resistance from loss of a putative carbohydrate-modifying enzyme. Science. 2001;**293**:860-864. DOI: 10.1126/science.1062441

[20] Pradel E, Zhang Y, Pujol N, Matsuyama T, Bargmann CI, Ewbank JJ. Detection and avoidance of a natural product from the pathogenic bacterium *Serratia marcescens* by *Caenorhabditis elegans*. Proceedings of the National Academy of Sciences of the United States of America. 2007;**104**:2295-2300. DOI: 10.1073/pnas.0610281104

[21] Labrousse A, Chauvet S, Couillault C, Kurz CL, Ewbank JJ. *Caenorhabditis elegans* is a model host for *Salmonella typhimurium*. Current Biology. 2000;**10**:1543-1545. DOI: 10.1016/s0960-9822(00)00833-2

[22] Roeder T, Stanisak M, Gelhaus C, Bruchhaus I, Grötzinger J, Leippe M. Caenopores are antimicrobial peptides in the nematode *Caenorhabditis elegans* instrumental in nutrition immunology. Developmental and Comparative Immunology. 2010;**34**:203-209. DOI: 10.1016/j.dci.2009.09.010

[23] Iatsenko I, Yim JJ, Schroeder FC, Sommer RJ. *B. subtilis* GS67 protects *C. elegans* from gram-positive pathogens via Fengycin-mediated microbial antagonism. Current Biology. 2014;**24**:2720-2727. DOI: 10.1016/j.cub.2014.09.055

[24] Gammon DB, Ishidate T, Li L, Gu W, Silverman N, Mello CC. The antiviral RNA interference response provides resistance to lethal arbovirus infection and vertical transmission in *Caenorhabditis elegans*. Current Biology. 2017;**27**:795-806. DOI: 10.1016/j.cub.2017.02.004

[25] Hoeven R, McCallum KC, Cruz MR, Garsin DA. Ce-Duox1/BLI-3 generated reactive oxygen species trigger protective SKN-1 activity via p38 MAPK signaling during infection in *C. elegans*. PLoS Pathogens. 2011;7:e1002453. DOI: 10.1371/journal.ppat.1002453

[26] Buvelot H, Jaquet V, Krause K-H. Mammalian NADPH oxidases. In: Knaus UG, Leto TL, editors. NADPH Oxidases, Methods in Molecular Biology. Springer Protocols. New York, USA: Humana Press; 2019. pp. 17-36

[27] Donkó A, Péterfi Z, Sum A, Leto T, Geiszt M. Dual oxidases. Philosophical Transactions of the Royal Society B: Biological Sciences. 2005;**360**:2301-2308. DOI: 10.1098/rstb.2005.1767

[28] Sifri CD, Begun J, Frederick M, Ausubel BJ, Calderwood SB. *Caenorhabditis elegans* as a model host for *Staphylococcus aureus* pathogenesis. Infection and Immunity. 2003;**71**:2208-2217. DOI: 10.1128/IAI.71.4.2208-2217.2003

[29] Inoue H, Hisamoto N, An JH, Oliveira RP, Nishida E, Blackwell TK, et al. The *C. elegans* p38MAPK pathway regulates nuclear localization of the transcription factor SKN-1 in oxidative stress response. Genes & Development. 2005;**19**:2278-2283. DOI: 10.1101/gad.1324805

[30] Blackwell TK, Steinbaugh MJ, Hourihan JM, Ewald CY, Isik M. SKN-1/Nrf, stress responses, and aging in *Caenorhabditis elegans*. Free Radical Biology & Medicine. 2015;**88**:290-301. DOI: 10.1016/j.freeradbiomed.2015.06.008

[31] Kostaropoulos I, Papadopoulos AI, Metaxakis A, Boukouvala E, Papadopoulou-Mourkidou E. Glutathione S-transferase in the defence against pyrethroids in insects. Insect Biochemistry and Molecular Biology. 2001;**31**:313-319. DOI: 10.1016/s0965-1748(00)00123-5

[32] Lindblom TH, Dodd AK. Xenobiotic detoxification in the nematode *Caenorhabditis elegans*. Journal of Experimental Zoology Part A: Comparative Experimental Biology. 2006;**305**:720-730. DOI: 10.1002/Jez.a.324

[33] Nava G, Robert L, Plancarte A. Characterization of *Taenia sodium* cysticerci microsomal glutathione S-transferase activity. Parasitology Research. 2007;**101**:1373-1381. DOI: 10.1007/s00436-007-0655-z

[34] Ferguson GD, Bridge WJ. The glutathione system and the related thiol network in *Caenorhabditis elegans*. Redox Biology. 2019;**24**:101-171. DOI: 10.1016/j.redox.2019.101171

[35] Hanschmann EM, Godoy JR, Berndt C, Hudemann C, Lillig CH. Thioredoxins, glutaredoxins, and peroxiredoxins–molecular mechanisms and health significance: From cofactors to antioxidants to redox signaling. Antioxidants & Redox Signaling. 2013;**19**:1539-1605. DOI: 10.1089/ars.2012.4599

[36] Racker E. Glutathione-Homocystine transhydrogenase. Journal of Biological Chemistry. 1955;**217**:867-874

[37] Morgan KL, Estevez AO, Mueller CL, Cacho-Valadez B, Miranda-Vizuete A, Szewczk NJ, et al. The Glutaredoxin GLRX-21 functions to prevent selenium-induced oxidative stress in *Caenorhabditis elegans*. Toxicological Sciences. 2010;**118**:530-543. DOI: 10.1093/toxsci/kfq273

[38] Nava G, Maldonado G, Plancarte A. Cloning, expression, purification, and kinetic characterization of mitochondrial thioredoxin (TsTrx2), cytosolic thioredoxin (TsTrx1), and glutaredoxin (TsGrx1) from *Taenia solium*. Parasitology Research. 2019;**118**:1785-1797. DOI: 10.1007/s00436-019-06336-4

[39] Mora-Lorca JA, Saenz-Narciso B, Gaffney CJ, Naranjo-Galindo FJ, Pedrajas JR, Guerrero-Gomez D, et al. Glutathione reductase gsr-1 is an essential gene required for *Caenorhabditis elegans* early embryonic development. Free Radical Biology and Medicine. 2016;**96**:446-461. DOI: 10.1016/j.freeradbiomed.2016.04.017

[40] Lacey BM, Hondal RJ. Characterization of mitochondrial thioredoxin reductase from *C. elegans*. Biochemical and Biophysical Research

Communications. 2006;**346**:629-636. DOI: 10.1016/j.bbrc.2006.05.095

[41] Salinas G, Selkirk ME, Chalar C, Maizels RM, Fernandez C. Linked thioredoxin-glutathione systems in platyhelminths. Trends in Parasitology. 2004;**20**:340-346. DOI: 10.1016/j.pt.2004.05.002

[42] Plancarte A, Nava G. Purification and kinetic analysis of cytosolic and mitochondrial thioredoxin glutathione reductase extracted from *Taenia sodium* cysticerci. Experimental Parasitology. 2015;**149**:65-73. DOI: 10.1016/j.exppara.2014.12.009

[43] Mannervik B, Danielson UH. Glutathione transferases, structure and catalytic activity. CRC Critical Reviews in Biochemistry. 1988;**23**:283-337. DOI: 10.3109/10409238809088226

[44] Bagnall NH, Kotze AC. cDNA cloning and expression patterns of a peroxiredoxin, a catalase and a glutathione peroxidase from *Haemonchus contortus*. Parasitology Research. 2004;**94**:283-289. DOI: 10.1007/s00436-004-1204-7

[45] Saleh MA. Erythrocyte oxidative damage in crossbred cattle naturally infected with *Babesis bigeminy*. Research in Veterinary Science. 2009;**86**:43-48. DOI: 10.1016/j.rvsc.2008.05.005

[46] Arnér ES. Focus on mammalian thioredoxin reductases important selenoproteins with versatile functions. Biochimica et Biophysica Acta. 2009;**1790**:495-526. DOI: 10.1016/j.bbagen.2009.01.014

[47] Plancarte A, Nava G, Munguia JA. A new thioredoxin reductase with additional glutathione reductase activity in *Haemonchus contortus*. Experimental Parasitology. 2017;**177**:82-92. DOI: 10.1016/j.exppara.2017.04.006

[48] Edwards CA, Lofty JR, editors. Biology of Earthworms. Dordrecht, Netherlands: Springer Science Business; 1972. p. 283. ISBN: 9781489969125

[49] Engelmann P, Hayashi Y, Bodó K, Molnár L. New aspects of earthworm innate immunity: Novel molecules and old proteins with unexpected functions. In: Ballarin L, Cammarata M, editors. Lessons in Immunity: From Single Cell Organisms to Mammals. Amsterdam, The Netherlands; Cambridge, MA, USA: Elsevier; Academic Press; 2016. pp. 53-66

[50] Harwood G, Salmela H, Freitak D, Amdam G. Social immunity in honey bees: Royal jelly as a vehicle in transferring bacterial pathogen fragments between nestmates. The Journal of Experimental Biology. 2021;**224**:jeb231076. DOI: 10.1242/jeb.231076

Section 3

One Health Approach to Study Helminth Infections

Chapter 10

Toxocariosis: From a One Health Perspective

Fernando Alba-Hurtado and Marco Antonio Muñoz-Guzmán

Abstract

Toxocariosis is a neglected zoonotic infection caused by the nematodes *Toxocara canis* or *Toxocara cati*. The distribution of the disease is worldwide and mainly affects dogs and cats, and its larval stage can cause human infection with serious repercussions on the health of its hosts. The infection causes a delay in the development, digestive disorders, nonspecific nervous manifestations, and occasionally death of some puppies and kittens associated with hyperparasitosis. In humans, the infection produces clinical syndromes known as *visceral larva migrans* (VLM), *ocular larva migrans* (OLM), neurotoxocariosis and covert toxocariosis. The close contact of people with their pets and the environmental conditions that favor the transmission of this diseased place it within the context of one health. The One Health concept is defined as the collaborative efforts of multiple disciplines (medical personnel, veterinarians, researchers, etc.) that work locally, nationally, and globally to achieve optimal health for people, animals, and the environment, from this perspective, toxocariosis is a study model in which classic and recent knowledge of the medical and veterinary area must be combined for its full understanding, with a goal of establishing integrative criteria for its treatment, control, and prevention.

Keywords: *Toxocara*, one health, toxocariosis, zoonosis, visceral larva migrans, ocular larva migrans

1. Introduction

Toxocariosis is a neglected zoonotic disease transmitted from dogs and cats to humans. This is mainly caused by the presence and action of the nematode *Toxocara canis* (*T. canis*) and less frequently by *Toxocara cati* (*T. cati* syn. *T. mystax*). *T. canis* uses canines, mainly puppies, as its definitive host, and *T. cati* uses kittens. In addition, they use a wide variety of paratenic hosts, including pigs, sheep, rabbits, rats, mice, other mammals, chickens, and other birds. In humans, the infection is accidental, and the parasite behaves similarly as it does in paratenic hosts. Some invertebrates, such as earthworms and cockroaches, can also have *Toxocara* larvae in their tissues or their gut [1, 2].

Adult *T. canis* worms live in the small intestine of puppies. The females measure from 10 to 18 cm, and the males measured from 4 to 10 cm. At the anterior end, they have three small lips that do not protrude beyond the diameter of the body.

A dentigerous border can be seen on the inner surface of each lip. Behind the lips are a pair of cervical fins that give the anterior end of the worm an arrowhead appearance. The posterior end in males ends coiled toward the ventral part and has a terminal narrowing in the form of an appendix, and a pair of small and symmetrical spicules (0.75–0.95 mm) are observed. In females, the vulva is located approximately in the middle of the body, and the posterior end ends at a straight, blunt point. *T. cati* adults are very similar to *T. canis*; the cervical fins are broader and convex, giving the anterior end a more marked arrowheaded appearance; males are 3–6 cm long, and females are 4–10 cm long [3].

2. Biological cycle

Embryonated *T. canis* eggs are shed in the feces of puppies. In the environment, a first-stage larva develops inside the egg, which molts twice until it becomes larva 3 (L3). Larvated eggs (passive L3 inside) are the infective stage. Depending on humidity and temperature, the development of the infective stage requires 2–5 weeks in the environment. In susceptible hosts after ingestion of the infective stage, L3 hatches (active L3) in the duodenum and traverses the intestinal wall; the larvae pass into the lymphatic flow or blood capillaries. From this moment on, the development and migration of the larvae vary depending on whether the host is a young dog (<3 months), an adult dog, a pregnant bitch, or a paratenic host (rats, mice, birds, and humans, among others) [4].

In puppies, L3 migrate via blood or lymph to the liver, where they remain for 1 to 2 days. Subsequently, they migrate through blood, pass through the lumen of the atrium and right ventricle of the heart and via the pulmonary artery, reach the lungs, and cross the capillaries to reach the alveoli. The larvae migrate through the lumen of the bronchioles, bronchi, trachea, larynx, and pharynx (tracheal migration), where they are swallowed; during this tracheal migration, the larvae molt to L4. The larvae remain in the stomach for some time (up to Day 10 postinfection), return to the duodenum, and molt to L5 or preadult to finally become adults (19–27 days postinfection). The prepatent period is 4–5 weeks [4].

In paratenic hosts and adult dogs, L3 larvae migrate through the blood and are distributed throughout the body, mainly to the striated muscle, liver, lungs, kidneys, and brain, where they remain for years in a state of latency or dormancy as infective somatic larvae (dormant larvae) until they die and calcify.

In pregnant bitches, on approximately Day 20 of gestation, many of their dormant larvae are reactivated by the influence of progesterone. Between Days 43 and 47 of gestation, under the influence of progesterone and prolactin, the larvae cross the placenta and infect the fetuses. The larvae remain in the fetal liver until birth; later, by blood, they migrate to the lungs where they remain during the first week of life, molting to L4 occurs during this stage or later when the larva arrives in the stomach by tracheal migration. By the end of the third week, the larvae molt at L5 and develop rapidly into adult worms. After copulation, the females produce eggs that are passed in the feces of the pups at 15 days of age. In recently delivered bitches, some reactivated larvae arrive by the influence of prolactin on the mammary gland and are excreted in the colostrum and milk to be ingested by the puppies, constituting another important source of infection for the litter. The larvae ingested in this way molt at L4 and L5 in the intestinal lumen, where they develop into adult worms without tracheal migration [5].

In recently delivered bitches, some larvae may reactivate during gestation migrate to the intestine, molt to L4 and L5 and become adult worms. Bitches can remain up to 60 days passing eggs in feces until the adult worms are eliminated spontaneously. This is one of the ways adult worms can develop in adult dogs [1].

Dormant larvae in the tissues of paratenic hosts can be reactivated when they are predated. If the predator is another paratenic host, the ingested reactivated larvae undergo a new somatic migration and become dormant in this new host. On the other hand, if the predator is an adult dog, the ingested reactivated larvae molt at L4 and L5 and develop into adult worms in the lumen of the small intestine without further somatic migration. In this way, dogs can spend a short time excreting eggs in the feces until the adult worms are eliminated spontaneously. This is another way that adult worms can develop in adult dogs [1].

The life cycle of *T. cati* is similar to that of *T. canis* except that prenatal transplacental infection in this parasite does not occur [6].

3. Epidemiology

3.1 Dogs and cats

T. canis is the most common nematode in dogs in many regions of the world and *T. cati* in cats. In a meta-analysis study where data from more than 13 million dogs from 60 countries were included, the overall prevalence of *Toxocara* infection in dogs was found to be 11.1%. The prevalence was estimated in different World Health Organization regions: Eastern Mediterranean (19.2%), Africa (18.5%), South-East Asia (11.9%), North America (11.1%), South America (10.9%), Europe (10.8%) and Western Pacific (6.4%) [7].

In a second meta-analysis where data from 2,158,069 cats from 51 countries were included, an overall prevalence of *T. cati* of 17% was found. The prevalence was estimated in different World regions: African (43.3%), Eastern Mediterranean (21.6%), North America (18.3%), Europe (17.8%), Western Pacific (17.3%), South-East Asia (14.9%),and South American (12.6%)[8].

Transplacental transmission from bitches to their puppies is the most important form of *T. canis* infection in dogs. Not all somatic larvae in bitches are reactivated during the same gestation; thus, reactivation of larvae occurs in subsequent gestations. In addition, bitches become reinfected by ingesting persistent larvated eggs in an environment contaminated with fecal matter from their puppies. Transplacental transmission does not appear to occur in cats with *T. cati*, making lactogenic infection the most common form of infection in kittens [4, 6].

Puppies are the main source of environmental contamination; they can excrete eggs in feces from 15 days of birth, and the greatest egg shedding occurs between 1 and 3 months of age, when they can eliminate more than a million eggs per day. Gradually, the worm burden in the intestine tends to decrease, and they stop shedding eggs before reaching 6 months of age. In addition, the larvae ingested by the lactogenic route gradually increase the worm burden and the elimination of eggs in the puppies. Puppies under three months of age are the only hosts that can develop adult worms in the intestine by ingesting larvated eggs, although apparently, this is not their main route of infection [9].

Adult *Toxocara* females are very prolific, producing between 25,000 and 85,000 eggs per day, and the presence of many females in the intestine of a puppy can mean the elimination of enormous numbers of eggs in the feces (>100,000/g). In the environment, when eggs are protected from direct sunlight and desiccation, they develop to the infective stage (L3 passive) 2–4 weeks after shedding. In earthen soils, the eggs can remain viable for many months, accumulating in the environment. Therefore, the soil in areas where dogs with toxocariosis commonly defecate is considered a permanent source of infection for animals and humans. In addition, rainwater can carry the eggs to distant places and accumulate them in large concentrations in some places [1]. A study that included 42,797 soil samples in 40 countries showed a global prevalence of *Toxocara* eggs in public places of 21%. The estimated prevalence rates in the different regions ranged from Western Pacific (35%), Africa (27%), South America (25%), South-East Asia (21%), the Middle East and North Africa (18%), Europe (18%) and the North and Central Americas (13%) [10].

Paratenic hosts infected by ingesting larvated eggs present in soil, food or water accumulate L3 in their tissues. If these are predated, they can be a source of infection for adult dogs. If predated by another paratenic host, the larvae can infect the new host, bypassing a definitive host.

3.2 Humans

Due to the great difficulty of identifying the physical presence of somatic larvae, the most common way to identify *Toxocara* infection in humans is by serological tests (ELISA and Western blot). Serologically, it is not possible to distinguish between a *T. canis* infection and a *T. cati* infection, and although *T. canis* infection has generally been considered to be the predominant infection in humans, the seroprevalence of *T. cati* has not been determined, which could have been underestimated [11].

The seroprevalence of *Toxocara* in humans varies in different regions of the world. A meta-analysis carried out in 2019 that included 265,327 participants in 71 countries showed an estimated global *Toxocara* seroprevalence rate of 19.0%. The pooled seroprevalence for regions was as follows: African (37.7%), South-East Asia (34.1%), Western Pacific (24.2%), American regions (22.8%), European regions (10.5%), and Eastern Mediterranean region (8.2%) [12]. Seroprevalence has been associated with different risk factors, such as age, contact with young dogs and kittens, socioeconomic level, consumption of vegetables, and unboiled water, ethnicity, educational level, living in a rural area and pet ownership [13, 14]. The serological differences associated with the different ethnic groups in some countries may be the result of different contextual exposures linked, among other factors, to their socioeconomic level, segregation, and the environmental conditions in which the different ethnic groups live, and not necessarily due to a genetic predisposition [15].

The most common way of infection in humans occurs through the accidental ingestion of *Toxocara* larvated eggs, which can be found on soil in public parks, gardens, dirt floors, sandboxes, and vegetables irrigated with sewage, among others. Although people of any age can be infected, children are more frequently affected due to their habits of playing with pets and dirt, geophagia, and pica, in addition to their commonly poor hygiene habits [16–18]. Infection can also occur through the ingestion of somatic larvae present in raw or undercooked meat and viscera of cattle, pigs, and poultry, among others, which act as paratenic hosts (**Figure 1**) [19–22]. *Blattella germanica* and *Periplaneta americana* cockroaches have recently been shown to be able to ingest and shed larvated *T. canis* eggs in their feces, suggesting that they could carry infective eggs from dog feces to kitchens where human food is prepared [2].

There are multiple reports of the presence of *Toxocara* eggs in the hair of dogs and cats, which is why it has been proposed that they are a source of infection for their

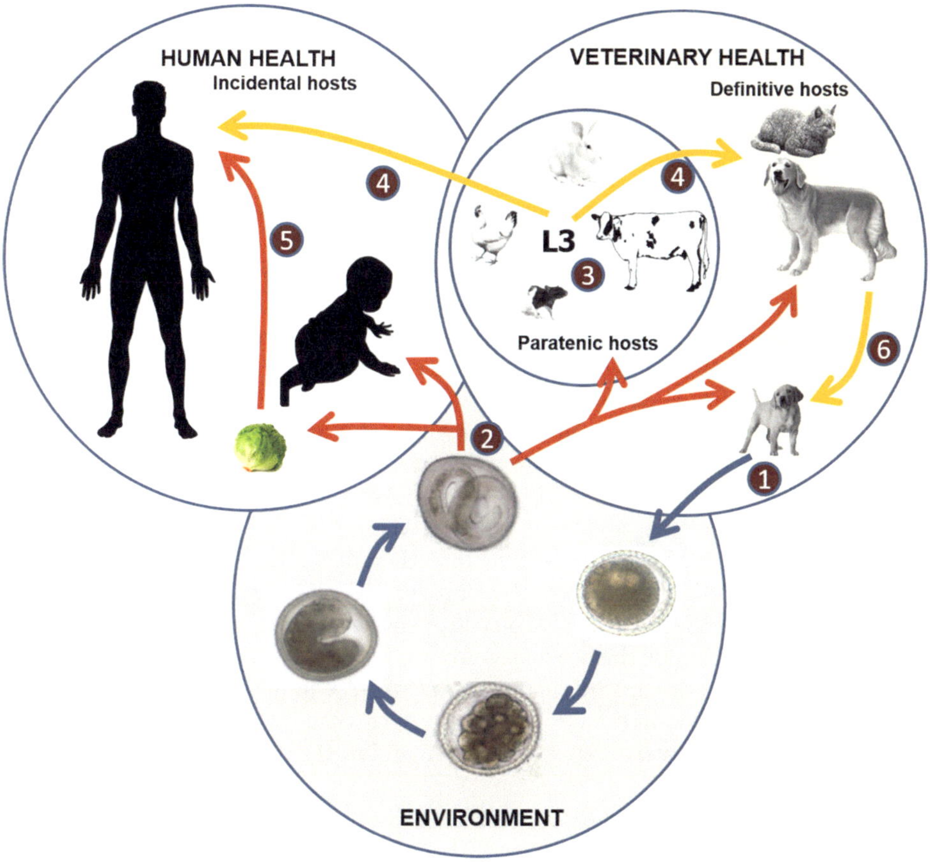

Figure 1.
Epidemiology of toxocariosis from the one health approach. The biological cycle of Toxocara *sp. involves definitive (dogs and cats), paratenic (several species of mammals and birds), and incidental (human) hosts. Puppies are the main eliminators of immature eggs into the environment (1). In optimal environmental conditions of humidity and temperature, passive larvae 3 develop inside the eggs, which are the main infective stage for all hosts (2). Paratenic or incidental hosts that ingest larvated eggs maintain somatic larvae in their tissues (3) that are infective to predators of the infected paratenic host. Human infection occurs mainly by ingestion of larvated eggs or by ingestion of raw animal meat or viscera (chicken, pig, beef) with infective somatic larvae (4). The ingestion of larvated eggs can be facilitated by the consumption of contaminated vegetables (5). Somatic larvae present in the definitive host are transmitted to puppies by transplacental (dog) and lactogenic (dog and cat) routes (6). Blue arrows show the dynamics of egg development in the environment, red arrows show transmission from larvated eggs, and yellow arrows show transmission from somatic larvae.*

owners [23–26]. However, the presence of larvated infective eggs in the hair is very low, probably due to poor temperature and humidity conditions [27], suggesting a low risk of infection for humans when petting the hair of their pets, although the possibility exists.

4. Canine and feline toxocariosis

4.1 Pathogenesis and clinical picture

The adult worms of *T. canis* and *T. cati* feed on intestinal content, compete with the host for nutrients and, depending on the worm burden, can produce different degrees of malnutrition. The presence of adult worms causes intestinal irritation, which induces decreased absorption of nutrients and is responsible for diarrhea and vomiting observed in some young animals. The presence of adult worms in the intestinal lumen exerts a mechanical obstructive action on the normal flow of intestinal content. Microscopically, the presence of adult worms produces mucosal muscular hypertrophy, intestinal villus atrophy, and crypt hyperplasia [1].

Larval migration in mild or moderate infections in puppies generally does not produce obvious clinical signs; however, larval migration in severe infections produces respiratory signs such as tachypnea, cough, and runny nose. Nervous signs such as incoordination or convulsions are occasionally observed in puppies due to the passage of the larvae through the brain. In puppies with intense prenatal infection, the lesions produced by the passage of the larvae in the liver, lungs, or central nervous system can cause the death of the puppies in the first 2 weeks of life [28].

Mild to moderate adult worm infections in puppies are usually asymptomatic or cause mild digestive symptoms and growth retardation. In severe infections, dirty-looking bristly hair, rough skin, painful intestinal distention, vomiting (frequently with adult worms), bulging abdomen (mainly when they have just eaten), presence of large amounts of gas produced by intestinal dysbiosis, alternating periods of constipation and diarrhea with profuse mucus, decreased appetite and growth retardation, can be observed. The blood count shows eosinophilia and anemia. Occasionally, there may be the death of puppies due to aspiration of vomit and intestinal obstruction or rupture. The presence of large numbers of adult worms as a result of massive prenatal infections in puppies can cause complete obstruction of the intestinal lumen, intussusception of the small intestine, and death of the entire litter [9, 29, 30].

In kittens, there is no transplacental transmission; therefore, the development of adult worms occurs until almost 30 days of age and the beginning of the elimination of eggs at approximately 50 days of age. The clinical picture is similar to that described in dogs but less severe, diarrhea, vomiting, and loss of appetite predominate, and deaths are very rare. The highest incidence of *T. cati* in cats occurs between 2 and 6 months of age; in general, the worm burden is lower in kittens than in puppies and occurs when the kittens are older and therefore have a higher degree of development [9, 31].

4.2 Diagnosis of toxocariosis in dogs and cats

Sporadically, shed adult worms can be observed macroscopically in the vomit or feces of puppies. The detection of *Toxocara* eggs in feces is performed by coproparasitoscopic techniques, such as Faust or McMaster; however, this can only be done when there are adult stages in the intestine, mainly in puppies [3]. In the eggs, three external layers are observed, forming the shell; the outermost layer is albuminous, the middle layer is lipoid, and the inner layer chitinous. The shell has depressions on the surface, called pits, which give it an appearance similar to a golf ball. The egg measures 75–85 μm and has a protoplasmic mass that occupies the entire interior.

In adult dogs and paratenic hosts, infection by somatic larvae can be demonstrated by the detection of specific antibodies against excretion-secretion antigens using immunological techniques such as ELISA or Western blot; however, due to their cost, difficulty in obtaining the antigens, and their difficult implementation, these techniques are not widely used in the veterinary field [32].

5. Human toxocariosis

Human toxocariosis is a neglected worldwide zoonosis caused by nematodes of the genus *Toxocara* (*T. canis* and *T. cati*). Current data indicate that toxocariosis is an infection of global distribution whose importance has been significantly underestimated [12, 15, 33, 34]. Human toxocariosis occurs in four clinical forms: *visceral larvae migrans* (VLM) syndrome, *ocular larvae migrans* (OLM) syndrome, neurotoxocariosis and covert toxocariosis.

5.1 VLM syndrome

In the 1950s, second-stage larvae of *T. canis* (now known to be third-stage larvae) were identified in the tissues of several children associated with the presence of clinical signs and a pathology that has since been known as VLM [35]. The associated syndrome in these children was characterized by extensive eosinophilia, hepatomegaly, splenomegaly, hypergammaglobulinemia, and chronic cough with eosinophilic pulmonary infiltration. VLM is more common in children (1–5 years) than in adults because they are more exposed to the infection through the ingestion of larvated eggs of *T. canis*, favored by factors such as living with puppies, poor hygienic habits, and pica [14, 36].

In humans, after ingestion of infective eggs, the larvae hatch in the small intestine and penetrate the intestinal wall, from which they are transported by the blood circulation to various organs, mainly the liver, heart, lungs, brain, muscle, and eyes [37]. In these organs, the larvae actively migrate, aided by proteases with which they cause tissue damage and exert a histophagous spoliating action (traumatic action). The migrating larvae do not continue their development; however, they remain dormant for several years, but they continue to secrete excretion-secretion antigens that induce an inflammatory response in some organs, such as the liver and spleen (hepatosplenomegaly), or are mediators of immunopathological alterations in other organs, such as the lung, where they produce eosinophilic pulmonary infiltration related to cough and persistent secretion [38].

Given the impossibility of carrying out studies in humans, experimental models have been developed in different species of paratenic hosts, such as primates [39], rabbits [40], rats [41], mice [42], and gerbils [43], where the sequence of pathophysiological and immunological events of VML have been studied. In these models, it has been observed that organ injuries can be acute or chronic. The acute phase is characterized by a severe inflammatory response that causes multifocal lesions with necrosis and vacuolization with polymorphonuclear infiltrate, mainly neutrophils with the presence of eosinophils in the liver and lungs. The chronic phase is characterized by the presence of granulomatous lesions with infiltrates of mononuclear cells, fibroblasts, and eosinophils, as well as the presence of fibrosis around the lesion with traces of calcification in the center of the lesions, which in some cases can be extensive. The main organs affected are the liver, lung, kidney, and brain (**Figure 2**). These lesions can be seen with or without the presence of the larva, which suggests the importance of the antigenic excretion-secretion products released by the larva in the tissues.

The clinical picture of VLM includes hyperleukocytosis (30,000–60,000 cells/mm3), eosinophilia (14–90%), abdominal pain, enlargement of lymph nodes, hepatomegaly, splenomegaly, increased ishemagglutinins and liver enzymes, intermittent fever, cough, and bronchospasm, among others [44–47]. The severity of the condition

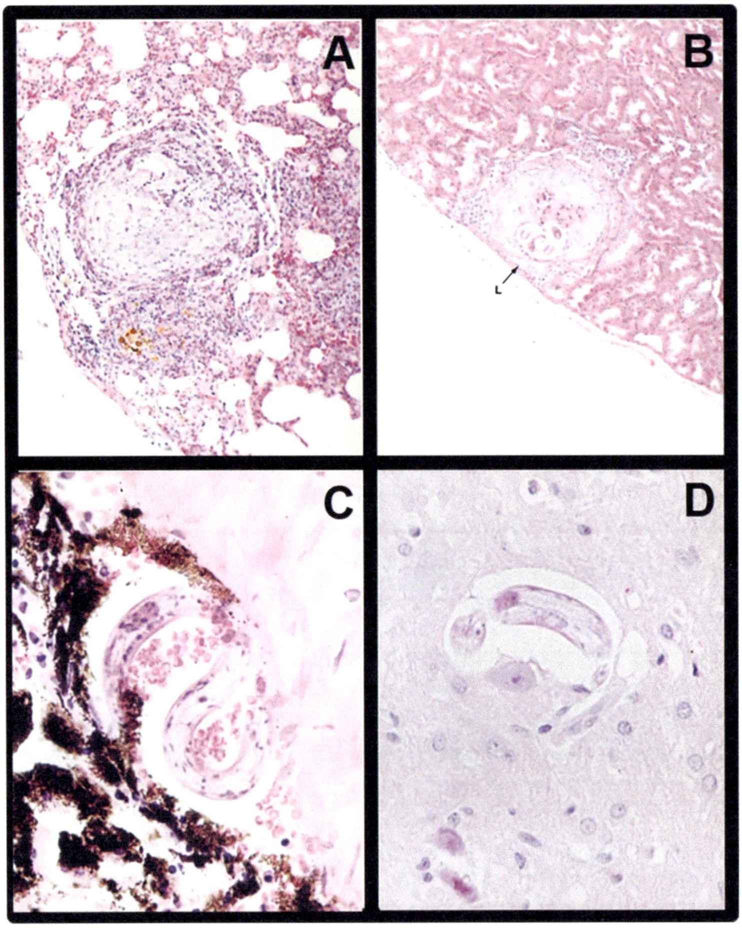

Figure 2.
Lesions produced by Toxocara canis *larvae in Mongolian gerbils (*Meriones unguiculatus*). A: lung with chronic granuloma. B: kidney with chronic granuloma with a larva trapped inside (L). C: larva in the pigmented layer of the retina with rupture of blood capillaries. D: larva the in brain with no apparent tissue reaction (photo credits: Dr. Alba-Hurtado).*

depends on the number of eggs ingested and the presence of larvae in critical places; although most patients recover and the signs subside with anthelmintic treatment, deaths from this infection have been reported [48, 49].

The diagnosis of VLM is based on the initial detection of antibodies against excretion-secretion antigens of *T. canis* by ELISA and its confirmation by Western blot in patients with eosinophilia, with high concentrations of serum IgE or with suggestive clinical manifestations. [50–52]. It has been proposed that the confirmatory diagnosis can be validated with the identification of a larva from a biopsy or by some molecular tests, such as PCR, DNA hybridization and restriction fragment length polymorphism, or sequencing of *Toxocara* ribosomal DNA; however, it is still in the of experimentation in animal models and is not available for humans [53]. Different tools, such as ultrasound (US), contrast-enhanced ultrasound (CEUS), contrast-enhanced computed tomography (ceCT), contrast-enhanced magnetic resonance imaging (ceMRI) and positron emission tomography (PET), are currently used to obtain suggestive images of the main lesions in different human organs [49, 54].

5.2 OLM syndrome

This syndrome was first described by Wilder in 1950, who found nematode larvae (unidentified at the time) in 24 of 46 pseudogliomas in eyes enucleated for endophthalmitis with apparent retinoblastoma [55]. Nichols later identified the larvae as *T. canis* in sections from four out of five of the eyes examined by Wilder [56]. Although, it is currently accepted that *T. canis* larvae are the main etiologic agent of OLM, it has also been shown that T. cati can cause ocular infections in humans [57–59].

OLM is a disease that generally occurs in young patients. In a systematic review and meta-analysis of studies published internationally, it was observed that the highest infection rate was detected in the 1–25 mean age group; within this range, the highest prevalence occurred between 11 and 20 years of age and was higher in men than in women [34]. It has been shown that having contact with dogs, ownership of dogs or cats, exposure to soil, and consuming raw/undercooked meat can be risk factors for OLM [12, 26, 34, 60].

OLM is generally observed in the absence of clinical signs and symptoms of VLM; it is considered to occur in people initially exposed to a small number of larvae, so they do not mount a significant immune response (many patients with a clinical diagnosis of OLM are seronegative to *Toxocara*), and the larvae migrate freely through various organs and accidentally reach the eye [61, 62]. Observations in experimental models and some clinical evidence indicate that *Toxocara* larvae infect the eye by migrating through capillaries or directly from the brain through the optic nerve [63–66].

The lesions detected in the eyes of patients diagnosed with OLM have been granulomas located near the optic disc or intraretinal (see **Figure 2C**), posterior and peripheral retinochoroiditis, panuveitis, optic papillitis, uveitis, retinal deformation or detachment, idiopathic epiretinal membranes, infiltration of inflammatory cells in the humor vitreous, hemorrhagic lesions and neuroretinitis as a sequel to migration of larvae in the retina [60, 67–69]. The main clinical manifestations include poor visual acuity, vision loss, strabismus, leukorrhea, eye irritation, and endophthalmitis [58, 70]. In most cases, lesions occur in only one eye, although there are reports of bilateral conditions [70].

The initial diagnosis of OLM is based on clinical signs and observation of lesions with an ophthalmoscope in the fundus examination. Confirmation of the diagnosis can be made by the detection of antibodies against excretion-secretion antigens of *T. canis* by ELISA in the vitreous humor of the affected eye and the study of the lesions by ultrasound biomicroscopy (UBM) and optical coherence tomography (OCT) [71, 72].

5.3 Neurotoxocariosis

The first report of the presence of an encapsulated larva of *T. canis* in the brain of a child was in 1951; originally, the larva was identified as probably *Ascaris lumbricus* [73]; later, this larva was identified as *T. canis* [74]. The damage produced by *Toxocara* larvae in the central nervous system (CNS) of humans has been widely discussed by many authors. The pathology depends on the number of larvae, the location of the larvae in the nervous system, the time postinfection, the immune response, and some intrinsic factors of the host. Most cases of neuro toxocariosis have been attributed to the presence of *T. canis* and, less frequently, to *T. cati*; however, the latter cannot be ruled out in some neurological infections. In experimental models, a greater tendency for *T. canis* to migrate to the CNS than *T. cati* has been observed [75].

In humans, many *Toxocara* infections in the CNS can go unnoticed and do not produce manifestations; therefore, their frequency is unknown. Some autopsy studies have shown the presence of larvae in the leptomeninges, gray and white matter of the cerebrum, cerebellum, thalamus, and spinal cord, unrelated to previous neurological signs [76].

In experimental models, it has been shown that *T. canis* larvae in the CNS can produce areas of necrosis, loss of Purkinje cells, glial nerve fibers and nerve sheaths, granulomatous lesions, emorrhagic and exudative lesions, vasculitis with eosinophilic and lymphocytic infiltration, gliosis and hemosiderosis. Some larvae can be observed without any response around them (see **Figure 2D**) [76, 77].

The clinical pictures of neurotoxocariosis in humans rarely occur simultaneously with signs of VLM. Most clinical manifestations occur in adult men with an average age of 35–42 years. Clinical signs associated with neurotoxocariosis may be indicators of different neurological disorders, such as myelitis (sensation disorders such as tingling sensation or hypoesthesia to specific dermatomes; motor disorders such as sphincter disturbances and conus medullaris syndrome; autonomic disturbances such as bladder and bowel dysfunction, and erectile failure), encephalitis (focal deficits, confused state, seizure and cognitive disorders) or meningitis (headaches, stiff neck/neck pain, nausea or vomiting, and Kernig's/Brudzinski's sign). Fever may occur on some occasions, although this is not a constant sign [76, 78].

The association between *T. Canis* seropositivity and cognitive development is controversial and has been widely discussed by several authors. Some authors, such as Magnaval et al. [79], found no association between seropositivity and any recognizable neurological syndrome; however, other authors have shown an association between seropositivity and lower cognitive development in children; however, due to incomplete controls and low sample size, the results are not clear [80–83].

In this context, Walsh and Haseeb [84], conducted one of the most conclusive studies; they analyzed a sample of 3,949 children representative of the US child population. Seropositive to *T. canis* children scored significantly lower on the Scale for Children-Revised (WISC-R) and Wide Range Achievement Test-Revised (WRAT-R) than seronegative children. Moreover, this relationship was independent of socioeconomic status, ethnicity, sex, rural residence, cytomegalovirus infection and blood lead levels. These results show another facet of the importance of toxocariosis as a neglected infection.

The diagnosis of neurotoxocariosis is difficult because there is no characteristic clinical syndrome. Due to the lack of confirmatory diagnostic tests and the nonspecific nature of its symptoms, neurotoxocariosis is probably underdiagnosed. As there is no universally accepted criterion for the diagnosis of this syndrome, a comprehensive diagnosis must be considered that must include the broad spectrum of neurological manifestations (signs of meningitis, encephalitis, myelitis, and/or cerebral vasculitis), together with high titers of antibodies against *Toxocara* in cerebrospinal fluid and/or blood, eosinophilia in blood and/or cerebrospinal fluid, suggestive radiological images, the presence of risk factors and clinical and radiological improvement after anthelmintic therapy [54, 78, 85].

5.4 Covert toxocariosis

Taylor et al. [86] proposed the term covert toxocariosis to describe a new clinical entity of human toxocariosis. It is currently considered that covert toxocariosis is characterized by nonspecific symptoms and signs that are not associated with the VLM, OLM,or neurotoxocariosis. Clinical manifestations include asthma, acute bronchitis, pneumonia, wheezing with or without Loeffler's syndrome, chronic urticaria or eczema, lymphadenopathy, myositis, and pseudorheumatoid syndrome, with or without eosinophilia.

The excretion-secretion antigens produced by *T. canis* during migration are strong stimulants of Th2-associated immune responses and the consequent induction of IL-4, IL-5, IL10, and IL-13. This cytokine profile induces an increase in the level of specific IgE-antibodies and eosinophilia, which are effectors to kill some larvae. These same effectors contribute to airway hypersensitivity and inflammation, associating chronic *T. canis* infection with allergic disorders such as asthma, allergic rhinitis, atopic dermatitis, and urticaria [87–89].

Asthma is a lung disease characterized by an exacerbation of the immune response in the airways to a variety of external stimuli, which produces inflammation, bronchospasm, and obstruction of the airways, which are reversible spontaneously or with treatment. Since years ago, several epidemiological and experimental studies have shown a significant relationship between *Toxocara* infection and the development of asthma, mainly in children [90–92]. Meta-analysis studies, where extensive collections of published data were made, have confirmed this association. Li et al. [93] using data from 723 asthmatic patients and 807 controls found a significantly higher prevalence of *T. canis* infection in patients with asthma than in controls (OR 3.36, $P < .001$). Aghaei et al. [87] using data from 872 asthmatics and 4597 non-asthmatics children, found an increased risk for asthma in children with *Toxocara* infection seropositivity (OR, 1.91; 95% CI, 1.47–2.47).

The exact mechanisms by which *Toxocara* infection induces asthma and other allergic disorders remain unclear. *Toxocara* larval migration has been associated with an intense immune response, which causes strong allergic inflammation involving the intestine, muscle, liver, kidney, and lung [43, 94]. An animal model study (mice) showed that previous infection with *T. canis* intensified the ovalbumin-induced allergic airway inflammatory response associated with elevated eosinophil counts and IgE antibody levels in bronchoalveolar fluid and increased expression of IL-4 mRNA in the lung [92]. Several authors have described skin manifestations associated with toxocariosis and the risk of seropositive patients presenting skin lesions [95]. Significant associations have been observed between *Toxocara* seropositivity and pruritus ($OR = 4.1$, $P < 0.1$) and chronic urticaria ($OR = 6.9$, $P < 0.0001$) [96, 97]. Some of these patients presented with symptoms of VLM or OLM; however, the majority had no signs of previous *Toxocara* infection. Similar to neurotoxocariosis, there is no specific diagnosis for the clinical symptoms of cutaneous toxocariosis, so the participation of *T. canis* as a producer of skin alterations has probably been underestimated.

6. Comprehensive control of toxocariosis

The main role in the control of toxocariosis falls on the veterinarian, who is responsible for the diagnosis and deworming programs in dogs and cats, as well as the awareness and health education of pet owners so that they are aware of the threat of this and other infectious diseases from pets to humans. Periodic deworming of dogs and cats is an effective strategy to reduce the worm burden and, therefore, the number of eggs in the environment [98]. Puppies and kittens must be dewormed (piperazine, ivermectin, mebendazole, pyrantel, and febantel, among others) at one month of age, and the treatment should be repeated at least twice in 15 days. In adult dogs, coproparasitoscopic examinations (Faust technique) should be carried out every 6 months, and positive dogs should be dewormed, with special care for dogs with known predatory habits. There are no effective antiparasitic agents against somatic larvae of *Toxocara* sp. In adult female dogs and cats, therefore, to reduce transplacental and/or lactogenic transmission to their puppies, it is necessary to reduce the number of infective eggs in the environment where they live.

The main way of infection in humans is the ingestion of infective eggs (L3 passive) that contaminate their environment. The fecal of dogs and, to a lesser extent, of cats in the soil of public parks, gardens, ridges, and rural areas, among others, is the cause of the gradual accumulation of infective eggs of *Toxocara* sp. in these places. Due to its high resistance, there are no chemical products capable of inactivating these eggs in the soil without seriously affecting other organisms and damaging the ecosystem. Therefore, one of the most important strategies for the control of environmental contamination is the immediate collection of dog feces eliminated during walks and its subsequent disposal in the drainage. It should always be considered that puppies and kittens are the main egg eliminators; however, adult dogs can also eventually eliminate eggs [99].

One of the risk factors most frequently associated with human toxocariosis is ownership of dogs or cats. For this reason, it is necessary to wash the floors daily with soap and water inside the houses or patios where the dogs live and defecate to detach the infective eggs from the surfaces and achieve their mechanical dragging to the drainage, considering that the infective eggs resist most commercial disinfectants. In addition, due to the possible presence of infective eggs attached to pet hair, it is necessary to periodically bathe and brush dogs and cats to avoid the presence of *Toxocara* eggs or other parasites in the hair.

Drainage water contaminated with *Toxocara* eggs can reach places where vegetables are grown or there may be dogs that defecate in these places, so vigorous washing of vegetables with drinking water is essential, especially those that are eaten raw and are grown at ground level (lettuce, cabbage, carrots, and strawberries, among many others) to reduce the risk of ingestion of infective eggs by humans. Another source of infection in humans is the ingestion of raw or undercooked meat or viscera of paratenic hosts infected with somatic larvae (chickens, pigs, cattle, and ducks, among others) in traditional dishes, so it is suggested that this type of dish is cooked with meat from animals raised in conditions free of the parasite. Cooking meat kills somatic larvae. At the government level, it is necessary to implement educational campaigns for the management of pet feces, knowledge of this and other zoonotic diseases, and the control of feral dogs and cats.

7. Health professionals involved

In summary, toxocariosis is a complex disease that, for its comprehensive control from a one health perspective, requires the knowledge of researchers and different health professionals. The veterinarian is the professional responsible for the diagnosis, control, and prevention of toxocariosis in pets that act as definitive hosts of the parasite (dogs and cats), as well as in domestic species that can act as paratenic hosts (chickens, pigs, beef, rabbits, etc.).

From the perspective of human health, the joint work of a very wide variety of health professionals is required to achieve an early and accurate diagnosis of the disease or at least a firm suspicion of the condition. Among these are parasitologists, infectologists, pediatricians, allergists, ophthalmologists, neurologists, dermatologists, imaging specialists, and epidemiologists, who are sensitized and trained to cover the entire clinical spectrum that human toxocariosis can produce. In addition, highly trained laboratory personnel are required for the parasitological, immunological, and molecular diagnosis of toxocariosis in animals and humans.

Acknowledgements

This chapter was funded by grants from PAPIIT/UNAM (No. IN210322 and IN211222). We deeply thank César Cuenca-Verde from FESC-UNAM for their technical assistance.

Conflict of interest

The authors declare no conflict of interest.

Author details

Fernando Alba-Hurtado and Marco Antonio Muñoz-Guzmán*
Facultad de Estudios Superiores Cuautitlán, Department of Biological Sciences, National Autonomous University of Mexico, Cuautitlán Izcalli, Mexico

*Address all correspondence to: mmunoz74@hotmail.com

References

[1] Deplazes P, Eckert J, Mathis A, Samson-Himmelstjerna GV, Zahner H. Parasitology in Veterinary Medicine. Wageningen Academic Publishers: Wageningen; 2016. p. 652

[2] González-García T, Muñoz-Guzmán MA, Sánchez-Arroyo H, Prado-Ochoa MG, Cuéllar-Ordaz JA, Alba-Hurtado F. Experimental transmission of *Toxocara canis* from *Blattella germanica* and *Periplaneta americana* cockroaches to a paratenic host. Veterinary Parasitology. 2017;**246**:5-10

[3] Alba-Hurtado F. Parasitología Veterinaria. Ciudad de México: UNAM; 2020. p. 184

[4] Schnieder T, Laabs EM, Welz C. Larval development of *Toxocara canis* in dogs. Veterinary Parasitology. 2011;**175**:193-206

[5] Muñoz-Guzmán MA, Alba-Hurtado F. Progesterone and prolactin: Hormones important for the reactivation of *Toxocara canis* larvae in bitches. Advances in Neuroimmune Biology. 2018;**7**:67-78

[6] Coati N, Schnieder T, Epe C. Vertical transmission of *Toxocara cati* Schrank 1788 (Anisakidae) in the cat. Parasitology Research. 2004;**92**:142-146

[7] Rostami A, Riahi SM, Hofmann A, Ma G, Wang T, Behniafar H, et al. Global prevalence of *Toxocara* infection in dogs. Advances in Parasitology. 2020;**109**:561-583

[8] Rostami A, Sepidarkish M, Ma G, Wang T, Ebrahimi M, Fakhri Y, et al. Global prevalence of *Toxocara* infection in cats. Advances in Parasitology. 2020;**109**:615-639

[9] Overgaauw PA, Nederland V. Aspects of *Toxocara* epidemiology: Toxocarosis in dogs and cats. Critical Reviews in Microbiology. 1997;**23**:233-251

[10] Fakhri Y, Gasser RB, Rostami A, Fan CK, Ghasemi SM, Javanian M, et al. *Toxocara* eggs in public places worldwide-A systematic review and meta-analysis. Environmental Pollution. 2018;**242**:1467-1475

[11] Fisher M. *Toxocara cati*: An underestimated zoonotic agent. Trends in Parasitology. 2003;**19**:167-170

[12] Rostami A, Riahi SM, Holland CV, Taghipour A, Khalili-Fomeshi M, Fakhri Y, et al. Seroprevalence estimates for toxocariasis in people worldwide: A systematic review and metaanalysis. PLoS Neglected Tropical Diseases. 2019;**13**:e0007809

[13] Gyang PV, Akinwale OP, Lee YL, Chuang TW, Orok AB, Ajibaye O, et al. Seroprevalence, disease awareness, and risk factors for *Toxocara canis* infection among primary schoolchildren in Makoko, an urban slum community in Nigeria. Acta Tropica. 2015;**46**:135-140

[14] Holland CV. Knowledge gaps in the epidemiology of *Toxocara*: The enigma remains. Parasitology. 2017;**144**:81-94

[15] Hotez PJ, Wilkins PP. Toxocariasis: America's most common neglected infection of poverty and a helminthiasis of global importance? PLoS Neglected Tropical Diseases. 2009;**3**:e400

[16] Manini MP, Marchioro AA, Colli CM, Nishi L, Falavigna-Guilherme AL. Association between contamination of public squares and seropositivity for *Toxocara* spp. in children. Veterinary Parasitology. 2012;**188**:48-52

[17] Hernández SA, Gabrie JA, Rodríguez CA, Matamoros G, Rueda MM, Canales M, et al. An integrated study of *Toxocara* infection in Honduran children: Human seroepidemiology and environmental contamination in a coastal community. Tropical Medicine and Infectious Disease. 2020;**5**:135

[18] Wang S, Li H, Yao Z, Li P, Wang D, Zhang H, et al. *Toxocara* infection: Seroprevalence and associated risk factors among primary school children in central China. Parasite. 2020;**27**:30. DOI: 10.1051/parasite/2020028

[19] Hoffmeister B, Glaeser S, Flick H, Pornschlegel S, Suttorp N, Bergmann F. Cerebral toxocariasis after consumption of raw duck liver. The American Journal of Tropical Medicine and Hygiene. 2007;**76**:600-602. DOI: 10.1.1.318.4997&rep=rep1&type=pdf

[20] Yoshikawa M, Nishiofuku M, Moriya K, Ouji Y, Ishizaka S, Kasahara K, et al. A familial case of visceral toxocariasis due to consumption of raw bovine liver. Parasitology International. 2008;**57**:525-529

[21] Choi D, Lim JH, Choi DC, Lee KS, Paik SW, Kim SH, et al. Transmission of *Toxocara canis* via ingestion of raw cow liver: A cross-sectional study in healthy adults. The Korean Journal of Parasitology. 2012;**50**:23-27. DOI: 10.3347/kjp.2012.50.1.23

[22] Karaca I, Menteş J, Nalçacı S. *Toxocara* neuroretinitis associated with raw meat consumption. Turkish Journal of Ophthalmology. 2018;**48**:258. DOI: 10.4274/tjo.27085

[23] Roddie G, Holland C, Stafford P, Wolfe A. Contamination of fox hair with eggs of *Toxocara canis*. Journal of Helminthology. 2008;**82**:293-296

[24] da Cunha-Amaral HL, Rassier GL, Pepe MS, Gallina T, Villela MM, de Oliveira-Nobre M, et al. Presence of *Toxocara canis* eggs on the hair of dogs: A risk factor for visceral larva migrans. Veterinary Parasitology. 2010;**174**:115-118

[25] Bakhshani A, Maleki M, Haghparast A, Shirvan SP, Borji H. A survey on *Toxocara cati* eggs on the hair of stray cats: A potential risk factor for human toxocariasis in Northeastern Iran. Comparative Immunology, Microbiology and Infectious Diseases. 2019;**64**:10-13

[26] Maurelli MP, Santaniello A, Fioretti A, Cringoli G, Rinaldi L, Menna LF. The presence of *Toxocara* eggs on dog's fur as potential zoonotic risk in animal-assisted interventions: A systematic review. Animals. 2019;**9**:827. DOI: 10.3390/ani9100827

[27] Keegan JD, Holland CV. A comparison of *Toxocara canis* embryonation under controlled conditions in soil and hair. Journal of Helminthology. 2013;**87**:78-84

[28] Miller AD. Pathology of larvae and adults in dogs and cats. Advances in Parasitology. 2020;**109**:537-544

[29] Parsons JC. Ascarid infections of cats and dogs. The Veterinary Clinics of North America: Small Animal Practice. 1987;**17**:1307-1339

[30] Epe C. Intestinal nematodes: Biology and control. Veterinary Clinics of North America: Small Animal Practice. 2009;**39**:1091-1107. DOI: 10.1016/j.cvsm.2009.07.002

[31] Ursache AL, Györke A, Mircean V, Dumitrache MO, Codea AR, Cozma V. *Toxocara cati* and other parasitic enteropathogens: More commonly found in owned cats with gastrointestinal signs than in clinically healthy ones. Pathogens. 2021;**10**:198

[32] Muñoz-Guzmán MA, Alba-Hurtado F. Secretory-excretory antigens of *Toxocara canis* recognized by puppies of the Mexico City metropolitan area. Vet Méx. 2010;**41**:59-64

[33] Ma G, Holland CV, Wang T, Hofmann A, Fan CK, Maizels RM, et al. Human toxocariasis. The Lancet Infectious Diseases. 2018;**18**:14-24

[34] Badri M, Eslahi AV, Olfatifar M, Dalvand S, Houshmand E, Abdoli A, et al. Keys to unlock the enigma of ocular toxocariasis: A systematic review and meta-analysis. Ocular Immunology and Inflammation. 2021;**29**:1-12

[35] Beaver PC, Snyder CH, Carrera GM, Dent JH, Lafferty JW. Chronic eosinophilia due to visceral larva migrans: Report of three cases. Pediatrics. 1952;**9**:7-19

[36] Carvalho EA, Rocha RL. Toxocariasis: Visceral larva migrans in children. The Journal of Pediatrics. 2012;**87**:100-110

[37] Lim JH. Toxocariasis of the liver: Visceral larva migrans. Abdominal Imaging. 2008;**33**:151-156

[38] Morsy TA. Toxocariasis: Visceral and ocular larva migrans. Journal of the Egyptian Society of Parasitology. 2020;**50**:41-48

[39] Aljeboori TI, Ivey MH. *Toxocara canis* infection in baboons. The American Journal of Tropical Medicine and Hygiene. 1970;**19**:249-254

[40] Morales OL, Lopez MC, Nicholls RS, Agudelo C. Identification of *Toxocara canis* antigens by Western blot in experimentally infected rabbits. Revista do Instituto de Medicina Tropical de São Paulo. 2002;**44**:213-216

[41] Del Río-Araiza VH, Nava-Castro KE, Alba-Hurtado F, Quintanar-Stephano A, Muñoz-Guzmán MA, Cuenca-Micò O, et al. Endocrine immune interactions during chronic toxocariasis caused by *Toxocara canis* in a murine model: New insights into the pathophysiology of an old infection. Veterinary Parasitology. 2018;**252**:173-179

[42] Kavitha KT, Sreekumar C, Latha BR, Gowri AM, Nagarajan B, Azhahianambi P, et al. Migratory behaviour and pathological changes of *Toxocara canis* in organs and tissues of experimentally infected Balb/c mice. J Entomol Zool St. 2018;**6**:2388-2392

[43] Alba-Hurtado F, Muñoz-Guzmán MA, Valdivia-Anda G, Tórtora JL, Ortega-Pierres MG. *Toxocara canis*: Larval migration dynamics, detection of antibody reactivity to larval excretory–secretory antigens and clinical findings during experimental infection of gerbils (*Meriones unguiculatus*). Experimental Parasitology. 2009;**122**:1-5

[44] Snyder CH. Visceral larva migrans Ten years'experience. Pediatrics. 1961;**28**:85-91

[45] Baldisserotto M, Conchin CF, Soares MDG, Araujo MA, Kramer B. Ultrasound findings in children with toxocariasis: Report on 18 cases. Pediatric Radiology. 1999;**29**:316-319. DOI: 10.1007/s002470050596.pdf

[46] Wiśniewska-Ligier M, Woźniakowska-Gęsicka T, Sobolewska-Dryjańska J, Markiewicz-Jóźwiak A, Wieczorek M. Analysis of the course and treatment of toxocariasis in children-a long-term observation. Parasitology Research. 2012;**110**:2363-2371. DOI: 10.1007/s00436-011-2772-y

[47] Desai SN, Pargewar SS, Agrawal N, Bihari C, Rajesh S. Hepatic visceral larva

migrans with atypical manifestations: A report of three cases. Tropical Gastroenterology. 2020;**39**:211-221. DOI: 10.7869/tg.507

[48] Rugiero E, Cabera ME, Ducach G, Noemi I, Viovy A. Systemic toxocariasis in the adult patient. Revista Médica de Chile. 1995;**40**:1097-1099

[49] Kuenzli E, Neumayr A, Chaney M, Blum J. Toxocariasis-associated cardiac diseases—A systematic review of the literature. Acta Tropica. 2016;**154**:107-120

[50] Mohamad S, Azmi N, Noordin R. Development and evaluation of a sensitive and specific assay for diagnosis of human toxocariasis by use of three recombinant antigens (TES-26, TES-30USM, and TES-120). Journal of Clinical Microbiology. 2009;**47**:1712-1717. DOI: 10.1128/JCM.00001-09

[51] Fillaux J, Magnaval JF. Laboratory diagnosis of human toxocariasis. Veterinary Parasitology. 2013;**193**: 327-336

[52] Mazur-Melewska K, Mania A, Sluzewski W, Figlerowicz M. Clinical pathology of larval toxocariasis. Advances in Parasitology. 2020; **109**:153-163

[53] Özbakış G, Doğanay A. Visceral larva migrans detection using PCR–RFLP in BALB/c mice infected with *Toxocara canis*. Journal of Helminthology. 2020;**94**:1-8

[54] Dietrich CF, Cretu C, Dong Y. Imaging of toxocariasis. Advances in Parasitology. 2020;**109**:165-187

[55] Wilder HC. Nematode endophthalmitis. Transactions of the American Academy of Ophthalmology and Otolaryngology. 1950;**55**:99-109

[56] Nichols RL. The etiology of visceral larva migrans: I. Diagnostic morphology of infective second-stage *Toxocara* larvae. Journal of Parasitology. 1956;**42**:349. DOI: 10.2307/3274518

[57] MRH T. Ocular toxocariasis. In: Holland CV, Smith HV, editors. Toxocara: The Enigmatic Parasite. Pondicherry: Cromwell Press Ltd; 2006. pp. 127-144

[58] Pivetti-Pezzi P. Ocular toxocariasis. International Journal of Medical Sciences. 2009;**6**:129-130. DOI: 10.7150/ijms.6.129

[59] Zibaei M, Sadjjadi SM, Jahadi-Hosseini SH. *Toxocara cati* larvae in the eye of a child: A case report. Asian Pacific Journal of Tropical Biomedicine. 2014;**4**:S53-S55. DOI: 10.12980/APJTB.4.2014C1281

[60] Ahn SJ, Woo SJ, Jin Y, Jin Y, Chang YS, Kim TW, et al. Clinical features and course of ocular Toxocariasis in adults. PLoS Neglected Tropical Diseases. 2014;**8**:e2938. DOI: 10.1371/journal.pntd.0002938

[61] Sharkey JA, McKay PS. Ocular toxocariasis in a patient with repeatedly negative ELISA titre to *Toxocara canis*. The British Journal of Ophthalmology. 1993;**77**:253-254. DOI: 10.1136/bjo.77.4.253

[62] Fata A, Hosseini SM, Woo SJ, Zibaei M, Berenji F, Farash BRH, et al. Frequency of *Toxocara* antibodies in patients clinically suspected to ocular toxocariasis in the northeast of Iran. Iranian Journal of Parasitology. 2020;**16**:305-311

[63] Alba-Hurtado F, Tortora PJL, Tsutsumi V, Ortega-Pierres MG. Histopathological investigation of experimental ocular toxocariasis

in gerbils. International Journal for Parasitology. 2000;**30**:143-147

[64] Taylor MRH. The epidemiology of ocular toxocariasis. Journal of Helminthology. 2001;**75**:109-118

[65] Hayashi E, Akao N, Fujita K. Evidence for the involvement of the optic nerve as a migration route for larvae in ocular toxocariasis of *Mongolian gerbils*. Journal of Helminthology. 2003;**77**:311-315

[66] Choi KD, Choi JH, Choi SY, Jung JH. *Toxocara* optic neuropathy: Clinical features and ocular findings. International Journal of Ophthalmology. 2018;**11**:520-523

[67] Yokoi K, Goto H, Sakai JI, Usui M. Clinical features of ocular toxocariasis in Japan. Ocular Immunology and Inflammation. 2003;**11**:269-275

[68] Stewart JM, Cubillan LD, Cunningham JR, Emmett T. Prevalence, clinical features, and causes of vision loss among patients with ocular toxocariasis. Retina. 2005;**25**:1005-1013. DOI: 10.1097/00006982-200512000-00009

[69] Bae KW, Ahn SJ, Park KH, Woo SJ. Diagnostic value of the serum anti-toxocara IgG titer for ocular toxocariasis in patients with uveitis at a tertiary hospital in Korea. Korean Journal of Ophthalmology. 2016;**30**:258-264

[70] Shields JA. Ocular toxocariasis. A review. Survey of Ophthalmology. 1984;**28**:361-381

[71] Campbell JP, Wilkinson CP. Imaging in the diagnosis and management of ocular toxocariasis. International Ophthalmology Clinics. 2012;**52**:145-153

[72] Inchauspe S, Echandi LV, Dodds EM. Diagnosis of ocular toxocariasis by detecting antibodies in the vitreous humor. Archivos de la Sociedad Española de Oftalmología. 2018;**93**:220-224

[73] Beautyman W, Woolf AL. An *Ascaris* larva in the brain in association with acute anterior poliomyelitis. The Journal of Pathology and Bacteriology. 1951;**63**:635-647

[74] Beautyman W, Beaver PC, Buckley JJ, Woolf AL. Review of a case previously reported as showing an ascarid larva in the brain. The Journal of Pathology and Bacteriology. 1966;**91**:271-273

[75] Springer A, Heuer L, Janecek-Erfurth E, Beineke A, Strube C. Histopathological characterization of *Toxocara canis*-and *T. cati*-induced neurotoxocarosis in the mouse model. Parasitology Research. 2019;**118**:2591-2600

[76] Meliou M, Mavridis IN, Pyrgelis ES, Agapiou E. Toxocariasis of the nervous system. Acta Parasitologica. 2020;**65**:291-299

[77] Cardillo N, Rosa A, Ribicich M, López C, Sommerfelt I. Experimental infection with *Toxocara cati* in BALB/c mice, migratory behaviour and pathological changes. Zoonoses and Public Health. 2009;**56**:198-205

[78] Deshayes S, Bonhomme J, de La Blanchardière A. Neurotoxocariasis: A systematic literature review. Infection. 2016;**44**:565-574. DOI: 10.1007/s15010-016-0889-8

[79] Magnaval JF, Galindo V, Glickman LT, Clanet M. Human *Toxocara* infection of the central nervous system and neurological disorders: A case control study. Parasitology. 1997;**115**:537-543

[80] Worley G, Green JA, Frothingham TE, Sturner RA, Walls KW, Pakalnis VA, et al. *Toxocara* canis infection: Clinical and epidemiological associations with seropositivity in kindergarten children. The Journal of Infectious Diseases. 1984;**149**:591-597

[81] Jarosz W, Mizgajska-Wiktor H, Kirwan P, Konarski J, Rychlicki W, Wawrzyniak G. Developmental age, physical fitness and *Toxocara* seroprevalence amongst lower secondary students living in rural areas contaminated with *Toxocara* eggs. Parasitology. 2010;**137**:53-63

[82] Marmor M, Glickman L, Shofer F, Faich LA, Rosenberg C, Cornblatt B, et al. *Toxocara canis* infection of children: Epidemiologic and neuropsychologic findings. American Journal of Public Health. 1987;**77**:554-559. DOI: 10.2105/AJPH.77.5.554

[83] Nelson S, Greene T, Ernhart CB. *Toxocara canis* infection in preschool age children: Risk factors and the cognitive development of preschool children. Neurotoxicology and Teratology. 1996;**18**:167-174

[84] Walsh MG, Haseeb MA. Reduced cognitive function in children with toxocariosis in a nationally representative sample of the United States. International Journal for Parasitology. 2012;**42**:1159-1163

[85] Fan CK. Pathogenesis of cerebral toxocariasis and neurodegenerative diseases. Advances in Parasitology. 2020;**109**:233-259

[86] Taylor MR, Keane CT, O'connor P, Girdwood ARW, Smith H. Clinical features of covert toxocariasis. Scandinavian Journal of Infectious Diseases. 1987;**19**:693-696

[87] Aghaei S, Riahi SM, Rostami A, Mohammadzadeh I, Javanian M, Tohidi E, et al. *Toxocara* spp. infection and risk of childhood asthma: A systematic review and meta-analysis. Acta Tropica. 2018;**182**:298-304

[88] Maizels RM. *Toxocara canis*: Molecular basis of immune recognition and evasion. Veterinary Parasitology. 2013;**193**:365-374

[89] Mazur-Melewska K, Figlerowicz M, Cwalińska A, Mikoś H, Jończyk-Potoczna K, Lewandowska-Stachowiak M, et al. Production of interleukins 4 and 10 in children with hepatic involvement in the course of *Toxocara* spp. infection. Parasite Immunology. 2016;**38**:101-107. DOI: 10.1111/pim.12303

[90] Hakim SL, Thadasavanth M, Shamilah RR, Yogeswari S. Prevalence of *Toxocara canis* antibody among children with bronchial asthma in Klang Hospital, Malaysia. Transactions of the Royal Society of Tropical Medical and Hygiene. 1997;**91**:528-528

[91] Muñoz-Guzmán MA, del Río-Navarro BE, Valdivia-Anda G, Alba-Hurtado F. The increase in seroprevalence to *Toxocara canis* in asthmatic children is related to cross-reaction with *Ascaris suum* antigens. Allergologia et Immunopathologia. 2010;**38**:115-121

[92] Pinelli E, Brandes S, Dormans J, Gremmer E, Van Loveren H. Infection with the roundworm *Toxocara canis* leads to exacerbation of experimental allergic airway inflammation. Clinical and Experimental Allergy. 2008;**38**:649-658

[93] Li L, Gao W, Yang X, Wu D, Bi H, Zhang S, et al. Asthma and toxocariasis. Annals of Allergy, Asthma & Immunology. 2014;**113**:187-192

[94] Cooper PJ. *Toxocara canis* infection: An important and neglected

environmental risk factor for asthma? Clinical and Experimental Allergy. 2008;**38**:551-553

[95] Gavignet B, Piarroux R, Aubin F. Millon L, Humbert P. Cutaneous manifestations of human toxocariasis. Journal of the American Academy of Dermatology 2008;59:1031-1042

[96] Wolfrom E, Chene G, Boisseau H, Beylot C, Geniaux M, Taieb A. Chronic urticaria and *Toxocara canis*. Lancet. 1995;**345**:196

[97] Wolfrom E, Chene G, Lejoly-Boisseau H, Beylot C, Geniaux M, Taieb A. Chronic urticaria and toxocara canis infection. A case-control study. Annales de Dermatologie et de Venereologie. 1996, January;**123**(4):240-246

[98] Palmer CS, Thompson RA, Traub RJ, Rees R, Robertson ID. National study of the gastrointestinal parasites of dogs and cats in Australia. Veterinary Parasitology. 2008;**151**:181-190

[99] Lee AC, Schantz PM, Kazacos KR, Montgomery SP, Bowman DD. Epidemiologic and zoonotic aspects of ascarid infections in dogs and cats. Trends in Parasitology. 2010;**26**:155-161

Chapter 11

Schistosoma Hybridizations and Risk of Emerging Zoonosis in Africa: Time to Think of a One Health Approach for Sustainable Schistosomiasis Control and Elimination

Abdallah Zacharia, Anne H. Outwater, Eliza Lupenza, Alex J. Mujuni and Twilumba Makene

Abstract

Current control of human schistosomiasis in Africa is based on preventive chemotherapy, whereby populations are mass-treated with an anthelminthic medication, praziquantel. The World Health Organization has set a goal of eliminating schistosomiasis as a public health problem and, ultimately, eliminating transmission in all countries where schistosomiasis is endemic by 2030. However, recurrent hybridization between *Schistosoma* species is an emerging public health concern that has a major impact on the distribution of the disease and ultimately may derail elimination efforts. The One Health approach recognizes interconnections between the health of humans, animals and the environment, and encourages collaborative efforts toward the best outcomes. This chapter explains how the One Health approach can accelerate the control and elimination of schistosomiasis in Africa.

Keywords: Africa, hybridization, introgression, One Health, *Schistosoma*, schistosomiasis, zoonoses

1. Introduction

The World Health Organization (WHO) considers schistosomiasis the most important water-based disease in the world. The disease is caused by infection with trematodes of the genus *Schistosoma* species. These parasitic worms have a complicated life cycle (**Figure 1**). When an egg is passed in the feces or urine, it contains a fully developed miracidium. In freshwater, eggs hatch to miracidia, which swims in the water to find a suitable snail host. Upon finding a host, they penetrate its skin. The

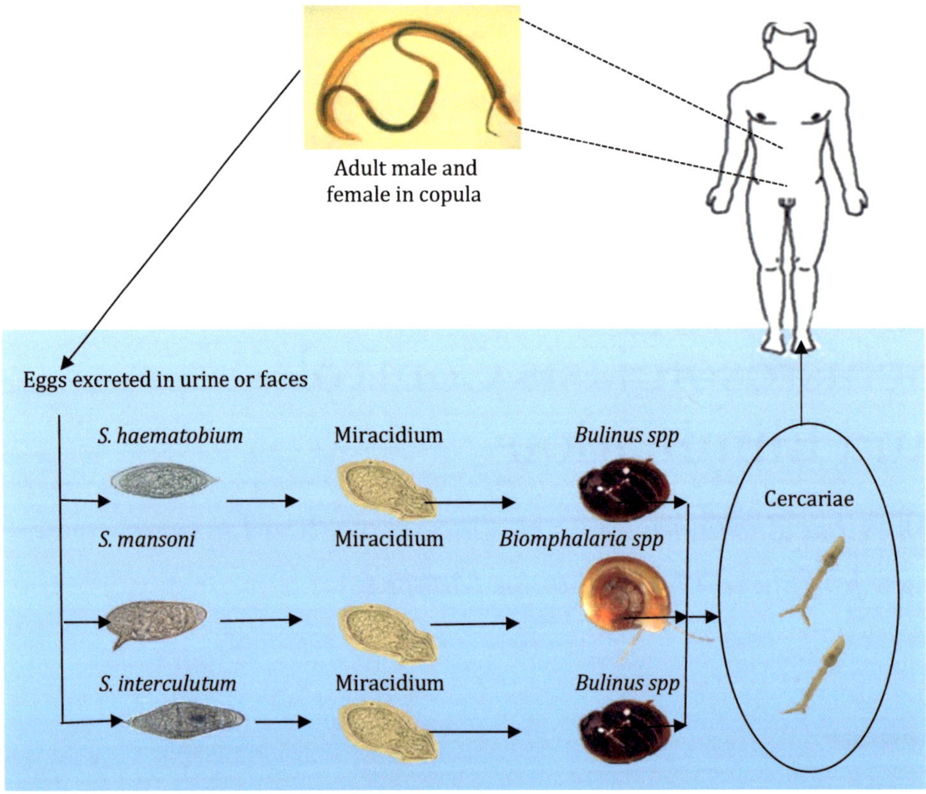

Figure 1.
The life cycle of the most important human Schistosoma *in Africa.*

miracidia then transform into primary-stage sporocysts and migrate to the liver of the snail, where they start asexual reproduction to produce daughter sporocysts. The daughter sporocysts develop into cercariae, which are shed into the water. Then the cercariae swim until they find a susceptible vertebrate host, and penetrate its skin. Once the fluke is inside, it drops its tail, and becomes a schistomulae; upon reaching a blood vessel, the schistomulae enters and starts its journey to the lungs, becoming longer and slenderer and losing its middle spines but retaining its end spines. The parasite reaches the lungs six to eight days after infection and begins to feed. The fluke leaves the lungs through pulmonary veins to the liver. By week four, the adult fluke emerges, and it starts pairing about week five. The paired flukes migrate from the portal vein to the respective blood vessels and start to lay eggs. Using their spines, the eggs penetrate through blood vessels to the intestine or urinary bladder [1, 2].

The damage caused by schistosomiasis results from the movement of eggs through host tissue, which triggers an inflammatory response and acute, chronic disease. Schistosomes (as members of the genus *Schistosoma* (*S.*) are commonly known) have an average lifespan of 3 to 10 years, but can live up to 40 years in their vertebrate hosts [3].

Due to increased human population growth, anthropogenic environmental changes, and global movements of humans and animals, there are increasing reports of hybridization events among *Schistosoma* species across Africa. Since these events involve species that infect both humans and animals (domestic and wild), researchers have raised concerns about the emergence of potential schistosomiasis zoonosis [4]. This chapter explains how the anthropocentric or disjointed sectoral approach to controlling human schistosomiasis requires a paradigm shift that entails a multisectoral (i.e., One Health) approach to preventing zoonotic transmission of schistosomiasis in Africa.

2. Burden of schistosomiasis in Africa

2.1 Human schistosomiasis in Africa

The two major *Schistosoma* species infecting humans in Africa are *Schistosoma haematobium* (*S. haematobium*), which causes urogenital schistosomiasis, and *Schistosoma mansoni* (*S. mansoni*), the causative agent of intestinal schistosomiasis. *Schistosoma guineensis* (*S. guineensis*) also causes intestinal schistosomiasis but is less prevalent. In Africa, *S. mansoni* is found in all countries while *S. haematobium* is found in all but four countries (Eritrea, Burundi, Mauritius, and Rwanda). The less common *S. guineensis* (also called *Schistosoma intercalatum* (*S. intercalatum*)) has been identified in the rain forest areas of western and central Africa. Schistosomiasis transmission has been interrupted in Equatorial Guinea, Morocco, Tunisia, Algeria, Djibouti and Lesotho [2].

The number of deaths attributable to schistosomiasis is difficult to estimate because of hidden pathologies such as liver and kidney failure, bladder cancer and ectopic pregnancies; in addition, the death rate may have decreased over the past decade due to the implementation of large-scale preventive chemotherapy campaigns [3].

The most prevalent species in Africa, *S. haematobium* causes approximately 112 million cases per year. It is estimated that 71 million of these infected individuals experience hematuria (blood in the urine), half of whom have dysuria, and about 18 million suffer from urinary bladder pathology. The current best estimate is that kidney failure due to *S. haematobium* infection is responsible for about 150,000 deaths annually in Africa. More than 54 million individuals are estimated to become infected with *S. mansoni*, with around 4 million people experiencing diarrhea and 8.5 million hepatomegaly; hematemesis-associated deaths are estimated to total about 130,000 annually [2].

Chronic disability is far more common than death. Intestinal schistosomiasis can result in abdominal pain, diarrhea, and blood in the stool. Liver enlargement is common in advanced cases, and is frequently associated with an accumulation of fluid in the peritoneal cavity and hypertension of the abdominal blood vessels. In such cases, there may also be enlargement of the spleen. Hematuria is the classic sign of urogenital schistosomiasis. Fibrosis of the bladder and ureter, bladder cancer, and kidney damage are sometimes diagnosed in advanced cases. In women, urogenital schistosomiasis may present with genital lesions, vaginal bleeding, pain during sexual intercourse, and nodules in the vulva. In men, urogenital schistosomiasis can induce pathology of the seminal vesicles, prostate, and other organs. This disease can also have other long-term irreversible consequences, including infertility. In children, schistosomiasis can cause anemia, stunting and a reduced ability to learn (although the effects are usually reversible with treatment). Praziquantel is the drug of choice for the treatment of schistosomiasis. The drug is recommended for the treatment of all forms of schistosomiasis. Despite that reinfection may occur after treatment, the risk of developing the severe disease is reduced after initiation of treatment [3].

The prevalence of human schistosomiasis in Africa is estimated to be 192 million, which is 93% of the total global prevalence of the disease. About 29 million people are infected by this disease in Nigeria, 19 million in Tanzania, and 15 million each in the Democratic Republic of Congo and Ghana, while Mozambique, with 13 million cases, completes the list of five countries with the greatest prevalence in Africa [5]. The heavy burden of schistosomiasis in Africa is attributed to limited access to clean water, poor sanitation and inadequate health services [2].

2.2 Animal schistosomiasis in Africa

In Africa, animal schistosomiasis is a common parasitic infection among cattle, although it rarely infects other domestic animals such as goats and sheep; nor does it appear to trouble wild rodents and primates [6]. It is estimated that 165 million domestic cattle are affected by schistosomiasis worldwide. The disease is of veterinary and economic significance [7]. In China, 1.5 million cattle suffer from schistosomiasis, and more than 5 million are at risk of infection [8]. Schistosomiasis among livestock does not show clinical effects in most cases. However, if the infection persists for a long time, it can cause enteritis and anemia, as well as emaciation leading to significantly reduced productivity and growth, and even death [9]. Schistosomiasis in animals is caused by several *Schistosoma* species. For example, *Schistosoma japonicum* (*S. japonicum*) (which infects human beings) has been reported to infect more than forty mammal species, including wildlife such as water buffaloes, camels and rats, and domestic animals such as cattle, sheep, pigs, dogs, donkeys, cats and goats [8, 10]. *S. mansoni*, which causes human intestinal schistosomiasis, has been reported to infect at least nine other members of the Primate order, such as monkeys and apes [10].

The three species with significant animal health impact in Africa are *Schistosoma bovis* (*S. bovis*), *Schistosoma curassoni* (*S. curassoni*) and *Schistosoma mattheei* (*S. mattheei*) [2, 7]. The latter two species are known solely from domestic animals [11]. *S. mattheei* is found in southeastern Africa, from South Africa northward to Tanzania and Zambia. *S. bovis* is most common in northern Zambia and northern Senegal [12, 13]. *S. curassoni* has been found in livestock (cattle, sheep and goats) in West African countries [2].

The distribution of *Schistosoma* species is governed by the intermediate host habitat—freshwater bodies such as lakes, dams and rivers. A recent study showed that *S. bovis* can cause high levels of infection among cattle in Côte d'Ivoire, where prevalence rates of up to 53.3% have been recorded [13]. Factors such as age and breed are significantly associated with different rates of schistosome infection. For example, cattle aged 4 years and above have higher rates of *S. bovis* infection than younger ones. "Zebu" and "Taurin" breeds are less likely to have *S. bovis* infections than "Taurin x Zebu" [13]. Livestock management systems in Tanzania have been shown to influence trematode distribution. The highest rates of trematode infection in cattle are found in traditional management systems in which animals are grazed and watered on communal land during the day and housed around the households in open bomas (livestock enclosures) at night. Rates of trematode infection are moderate in large-scale dairy systems and lowest in small-scale dairy systems [14].

Like a human, animals are treated for schistosomiasis through the administration of praziquantel. Effective treatment requires two rounds 3 to 5 weeks apart. However, unlike human schistosomiasis, which is frequently controlled by preventive praziquantel chemotherapy in areas where the infection is endemic [15], schistosomiasis in domestic animals is rarely treated in Africa, probably because little attention has been given by scientists to its zoonotic potential.

3. *Schistosoma* hybridization and risk of emerging zoonosis in Africa

3.1 Schistosoma hybridization in Africa

Environmental and ecological changes due to natural phenomena and anthropogenic activities break species isolation barriers and increase the possibility of acquiring new infections of both human and animal origin. This can lead to the occurrence of multiple infectious species and strains within a single host [4]. Multiple infections of two or more genetically distinct agent species may permit heterospecific (between-species or between-lineage) mate pairings, resulting in the production of a new offspring (species) that can be either infertile or fertile. This process is called *hybridization* [4, 16]. During this process, unidirectional and/or bidirectional allelic exchange occurs among gene pools of the two sympatric interbreeding species to produce offspring organisms with hybrid genomes [17]. The produced hybrid offspring may introduce a single gene or chromosomal region of one of its parent species to the genome of the second (divergent) parent species through repeated backcrossing, a process known as *introgression* or *introgressive hybridization* [18, 19]. Due to the advance in diagnostic technology, there are an increasing number of reported findings of fertile hybridization and introgression events across humans, animals, and eukaryotic parasites. Hybridization and introgression among parasites, particularly those with zoonotic potential, is an emerging public and veterinary health concern at the interface of evolution, epidemiology, ecology, and control [4]. They are characterized by heterotic alterations, speciations, neo-functionalization, and adaptations, called hybrid vigor [16]. Hybrid vigor may increase parasite virulence, transmission potential, resistance, pathology, host use and can lead to the emergence of new diseases [17, 18]. Moreover, hybridization can influence parasite acquisition of novel genotypes, potentially expanding their geographical and host range and leading to novel ecological adaptations detrimental to human and animal populations [17, 20].

Trematode worms of the genus *Schistosoma* are among the parasites known to undergo hybridization and/or introgression. Hybridization and/or introgression of two or more phylogenetically related *Schistosoma* species and/or strains occur when multiple distinct species or strain and their susceptible snail hosts cohabit an area. Cohabitation may be seen as a result of selective pressure imposed by climatic changes and human activities. Activities such as hydraulic projects, road construction and the introduction of new agriculture practices create new water bodies shared by humans and livestock, increasing opportunities for mixing of and subsequent exposure to different *Schistosoma* species [21]. In addition, increases in human and livestock migration facilitate the introduction of *Schistosoma* species and strains into new areas, resulting in novel host–parasite and parasite–parasite interactions [22].

Evidence of the potential occurrence of natural hybridization within and between human and animal *Schistosoma* species was first reported in the 1940s in Zimbabwe (then known as Southern Rhodesia). The evidence was based on the suspicious morphological appearance of *Schistosoma* eggs recovered from human urine with morphological features intermediate between those of *S. haematobium* and *S. mattheei* [23]. Several other studies reported similar morphological changes in other areas; in most cases, the observations were considered, or even dismissed, as misleading identifications [18]. **Figure 2** presents examples of typical eggs of two distinctive *Schistosoma* species and those with intermediate morphological features suspected to be of hybrid schistosomes.

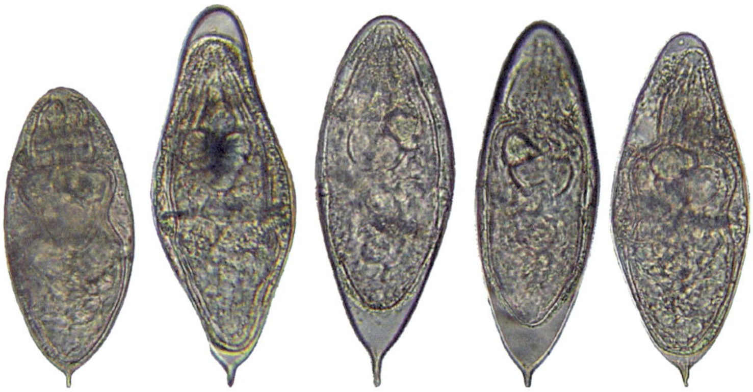

Figure 2.
Typical morphologies of S. haematobium *egg (a),* S. guineensis *egg (b) and intemediate morphologies of suspected* S. hameatobium-guineensis *hybrids eggs (c1.c2 and c3). Picture adapted and modified from Moné et al. [20].*

It was not until 1980, after the invention of biochemical marker technology, that the detection of previously suspected *Schistosoma* hybrids was confirmed to be a result of hybridization between *S. haematobium* and *S. mattheei*. The study was conducted in South Africa [24]. The technology was then used to reveal other hybridizations between different *Schistosoma* species in different parts of the world, especially in Africa [18].

The number of reported *Schistosoma* hybridization and introgression events has grown significantly due to the increased use of modern molecular technology in parasitological research. The use of molecular markers (such as internal transcribed spacer [ITS 1 + 2] and mitochondrial cytochrome c oxidase subunit 1 [cox 1]) and microsatellite markers (such as ribosomal DNA and mitochondrial DNA) have confirmed that *Schistosoma* hybridization occurs in nature, in which viable, fertile hybrid offspring can be produced through first- or successive-generation backcrosses [22, 25]. In addition, these molecular markers have shown that *Schistosoma* hybridization can be either unidirectional or bidirectional. For example, a study in Kenya using microsatellite markers revealed unidirectional gene transfer between two distinct *Schistosoma* species [25], while studies conducted in Senegal, using sequence data of nuclear ITS1 + 2 and mitochondria cox1 loci, reported bidirectional hybridization between several *Schistosoma* species [22, 26].

Several *Schistosoma* species hybrids have been reported based on findings of either molecular, biochemical or morphological (phenotypic) techniques, or combinations of two or all of these techniques. The hybrids have been detected in the snail, domestic and wildlife animals, and human hosts. Moreover, these heterospecific crosses are between human schistosome species (e.g., *S. guineensis* with *S. haematobium* [20]), animal schistosome species (e.g., *S. bovis* with *S. curassoni* [12]), and, perhaps most importantly and interestingly, epidemiologically and clinically, between human schistosome species and animal schistosome species (e.g., *S. haematobium* with *S. bovis* [12]).

There is geographic overlapping between different *Schistosoma* species in different parts of the world, such as Asia (*S. japonicum* and *Schistosoma mekongi* (*S. mekongi*) [27]) and Africa (two or more of the following species: *S. bovis*, *S. curassoni*, *S. guineensis*, *S. haematobium*, *S. intercalatum*, *Schistosoma mansoni*, *Schistosoma rodhaini* (*Sirthenea rodhaini*) and *S. mattheei* [12, 20, 21, 24–26]). However, to date, no evidence of naturally occurring *Schistosoma* hybrids has been detected in Asia, although experimental crossing of the two overlapping species has been achieved [27]. Potential natural schistosome hybrids have been reported across much of Africa, predominantly in West Africa [18]. The evidence of natural hybridization events documented in Africa between human *Schistosoma* species is for that between *S. haematobium* and *S. mansoni*, and *S. haematobium* and *S. intercalatum* or *guineensis*. *S. haematobium* and *S. mansoni* are phylogenetically distant species. However, *S. haematobium-mansoni* hybrids may be suspected if ectopic *S. haematobium* and *S. mansoni* eggs are recovered from, respectively, human stool and urine samples [16]. Elimination of ectopic *S. haematobium* and *S. mansoni* eggs has been suggested to be due to interspecific interactions and heterospecific mating between *S. haematobium* and *S. mansoni*, resulting in males of *S. haematobium* carrying *S. mansoni* females to bladder veins, where the females lay hybrid *S. mansoni* eggs that are passed in the urine. Inversely, *S. mansoni* males carry *S. haematobium* females to mesenteric veins, a process that results in hybrid *S. haematobium* eggs in the feces [28]. In Africa, ectopic *S. haematobium* and/or *S. mansoni* eggs have been widely reported to have been found in human stool and/or urine samples in many countries, including Senegal, Egypt, Tunisia, the Democratic Republic of Congo, Tanzania (formally Tanganyika), Zimbabwe, Sudan, Ethiopia, Côte d'Ivoire and Cameroon [28–30]. Bidirectional *S. haematobium-mansoni* hybridization has been confirmed by molecular analysis of eggs and miracidia collected from people living or traveling in coendemic areas of Senegal and Côte d'Ivoire. However, there is no evidence on whether these people were infected by hybrid cercariae or if mating of male *S. haematobium* and female *S. mansoni* and/or male *S. mansoni* and female *S. haematobium* occurred in these people's bodies [29, 30].

Natural introgressive hybridization between *S. haematobium* and the Lower Guinea strain of *S. guineensis* (which had been previously identified as *S. intercalatum*) has been recorded in Cameroon and Benin [20, 31]. Hybridization between *S. haematobium* and *S. guineensis* has been associated with the replacement of *S. guineensis* by S. *haematobium* in a *S. guineensis* hyperendemic area of Cameroon. This hybridization has been linked to the superiority of male *S. haematobium* to male *S. guineensis* in mating competitiveness [31]. In addition, natural hybridization was reported between *S. haematobium* and *S. intercalatum* (Zaire strain) in the Democratic Republic of Congo (formerly Zaire) resulting in the decline in the transmission of the pure *S. intercalatum* [32].

The natural hybridization events documented between animal (livestock) *Schistosoma species* in Africa are those between *S. bovis* and *S. curassoni*. The *S. bovis-curassoni* hybrids have been identified in cattle, sheep and goats in Senegal [12]. Despite the demonstration that neither *S. bovis* nor *S. curassoni,* as single pure species, can fully develop in humans or nonhuman primates in the field or under experimental laboratory conditions, there is evidence that a child in Niger was infected by the hybrid of the two species [21].

The most important and interesting schistosome hybridization is that between human and animal schistosome species (e.g., *S. haematobium* with *S. bovis* or *S. curassoni* [12, 26] or *S. mattheei* [24] and *S. mansoni* with *S. rodhaini* [25]). Even though it is unable to be maintained in humans, *S. bovis* is capable of mate-pairing with *S. haematobium* in humans to produce viable hybrids. *S. haematobium-bovis* hybrids are the most frequently and widely recovered schistosome hybrids across many African countries. The majority of *S. haematobium-bovis* hybrids have been found in human and snail hosts in West Africa: in Mali, Niger (introgressive hybridization), Senegal (bidirectional hybridization), Cameroon, Benin, Nigeria and Côte d'Ivoire [7, 16]. To date, few studies have reported the presence of a *S. haematobium-bovis* hybrid parasite in a nonhuman vertebrate host (a mouse species, *Mastomys huberti* and cattle) [7, 33]. The *S. haematobium-bovis* hybrid detected in this mouse was a female found paired with a pure male *S. mansoni* [33]. Other heterospecific crosses of human and animal schistosomes detected in Africa are those due to hybridization between *S. mansoni* and *S. rodhaini* [25] and *S. haematobium* and *S. curassoni* [12] or *S. mattheei* [24]. At **Figure 3** is a map showing the distribution of different types of schistosome hybridization events reported across Africa as summarized by Panzner and Boissier [16].

3.2 Current status of Schistosoma zoonosis in Africa

Zoonotic diseases (also known as zoonoses) are those diseases caused by viruses, bacteria, fungi or parasites that are naturally transmitted between humans and other vertebrate animals [18, 34]. Currently, six main species of *Schistosoma* infect humans: *S. mansoni, S. haematobium, S. intercalatum, S. guineensis, S. mekongi* and *S. japonicum.*

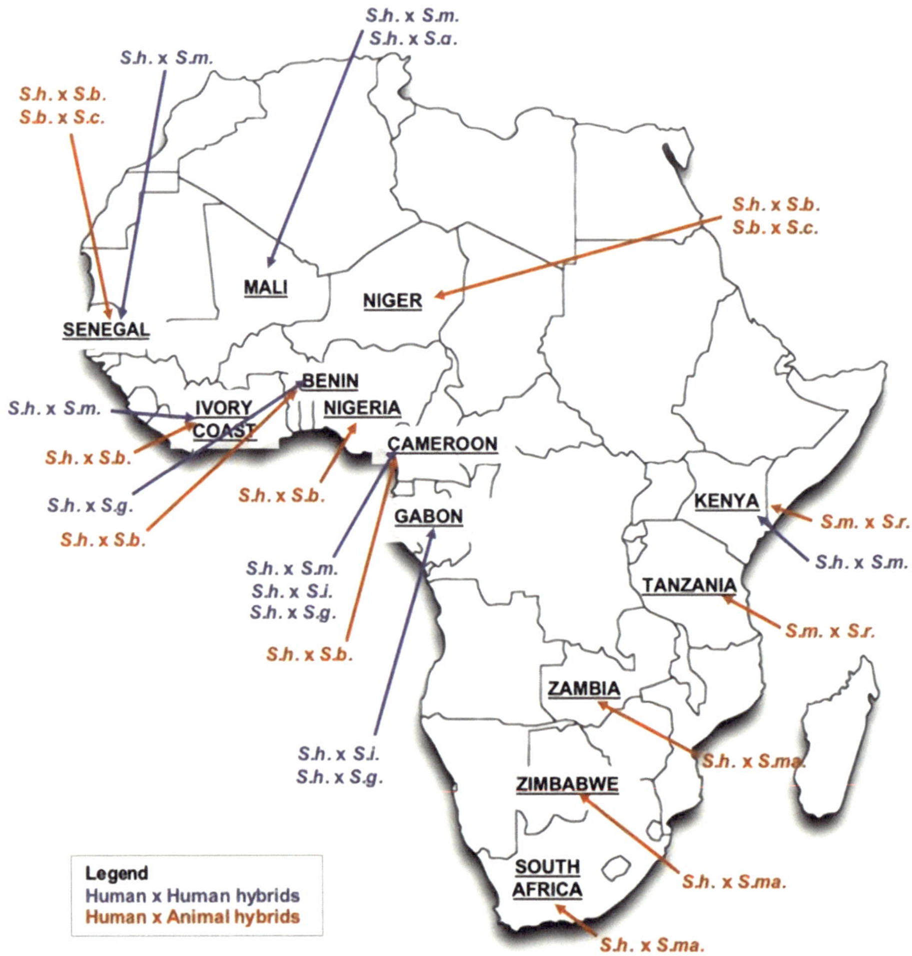

Figure 3.
Distribution of Schistosoma *hybrids across Africa. Notes: S.h.* = S. haematobium; *S.m.* = Schistosoma mansoni; *S.g.* = S. guineensis; *S.i.* = S. intercalatum; *S.b.* = S. bovis; *S.c.* = S. curassoni; *S.r.* = Sirthenea rodhaini; *S.ma.* = S. mattheei. *Figure adapted from Panzner and Boissier [16].*

The latter two species are acknowledged zoonoses, as they are capable of naturally infecting multiple species of mammalian hosts (human, livestock and wildlife) [18]. *S. japonicum* and *S. mekongi* are the major *Schistosoma* species in Asia, geographically distributed across the central and middle areas of the continent. Unlike other animal schistosomes, *S. japonicum* and *S. mekongi* are unique among zoonotic helminths in that they can be transmitted between humans and other animals and maintained by all host species [35]. In Africa, only human *Schistosoma* species are considered to be of public health significance [9]. In addition, wild animals such as rodents are known to be the main reservoir hosts of *S. mansoni* in the Caribbean and South America. Even though *S. mansoni* is one of the two *Schistosoma* species of public health importance in Africa, its magnitude in animals and the contribution of animals to the perpetuation of *S. mansoni* transmission in the African continent is not well established [36], because very few studies have been conducted on livestock or wildlife schistosomiasis [9].

Recent studies have reported evidence of some unique schistosomiasis transmission events in Africa. It had been believed that *S. haematobium* as a single pure species was solely capable of infecting humans. However, a study conducted in Benin showed that pure *S. haematobium* may infect livestock (i.e., cattle) as well [7]. Moreover, the female *S. haematobium-bovis* hybrid previously detected in humans and snail hosts, though never in animal (livestock and wildlife) hosts, has been found in a pair with pure *S. mansoni* in a mouse [33]. In addition, *S. bovis*, *S. curassoni* and *S. mattheei* are known to infect a wide variety of animals including cattle, sheep and goats. Though *S. mattheei* has been detected at high rates of prevalence in humans in one area in South Africa [37], the other two species have never been detected in human as a single pure species. Detection of hybrids of *S. haematobium* with either one of these species was thought by scientists to be evidence of possible human infection with the two animal (livestock) *Schistosoma* species. Human infections with *S. bovis* and *S. curassoni* were suggested to occur through zoonotic spillover; hence, it was believed that the infection could not persist, as these parasites cannot be maintained in the human body [38]. However, some researchers suggest that *S. haematobium-bovis* hybrids could be a result of an ancient introgression event between *S. haematobium* and *S. bovis* that resulted in the introgression of some *S. bovis* genomic tracts into several *S. haematobium* lineages [39].

3.3 Risk of emerging *Schistosoma* zoonosis in Africa

The magnitude of *Schistosoma* zoonotic transmission in which both livestock and wildlife are active participants is yet to be determined in endemic countries across Africa [36]. It has been explained that natural and anthropogenic changes (**Figure 4**) have created opportunities for mixing of and subsequent exposure to both human and animal (livestock and wildlife) schistosomes. The coexistence of multiple *Schistosoma* species and their hosts—both vertebrates (human and animals) and snails—has increased the potential for the emergence and establishment of novel zoonotic *Schistosoma* hybrids [21]. Sporadic studies have revealed several hybrids with potential zoonotic effects that naturally infect humans and animals (livestock and wildlife) across several African countries. Examples of natural *Schistosoma* hybrids with potential zoonotic effects identified in Africa include *S. haematobium-bovis*, *S. haematobium-curassoni*, *S. bovis-curassoni*, *S. haematobium-mattheei* and *S. mansoni-rodhaini* [16].

The ongoing emergence (or discovery) of potential zoonotic *Schistosoma* hybrids has caught the attention of many researchers and scientists, due to possible implications for schistosomiasis transmission and control. Zoonotic *Schistosoma* hybrids are thought to have a wide definitive host range and an increased range of intermediate snail hosts

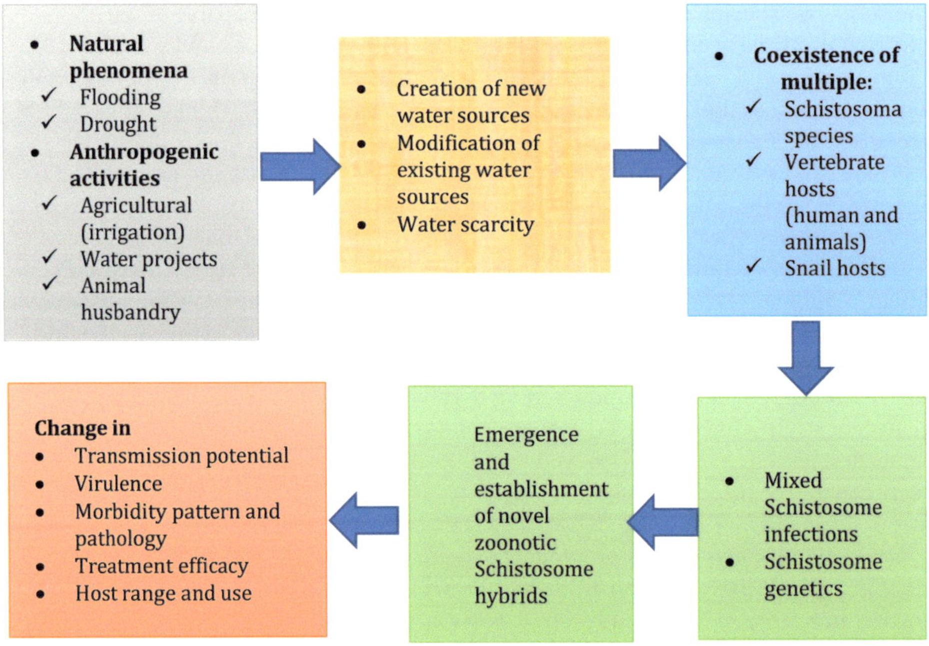

Figure 4.
Schematic presentation of the causes and consequences of schistosome hybridization.

relative to their pure "parent" single species, which may also enable a wider geographic range for hybrid schistosome infections. In addition, zoonotic *Schistosoma* hybrids are capable of establishing themselves in areas where their parental single/pure species are absent (e.g., *S. haematobium-bovis* hybrids on the French island of Corsica). Moreover, experimental studies (on *S. haematobium-bovis* and *S. haematobium-mattheei* hybrids) have revealed that these hybrids have greater virulence than the two parental species, as well as increased adult worm fecundity and increased cercarial shedding rates in snails [9, 39]. Field research (on *S. haematobium-bovis* hybrids) has revealed some indicators of altered patient morbidity patterns and reduced treatment response with praziquantel [4]. Also, researchers have expressed concern that hybridization could accelerate the evolution of drug resistance by allowing drug-resistance genes to be introgressed into new populations. On the other hand, hybridization may lead to the development of refugia for drug-susceptible genotypes and thus potentially help maintain drug susceptibility [9]. Therefore, it is important to understand the transmission dynamics of potential zoonotic *Schistosoma* hybrids [21].

4. Schistosomiasis control and elimination in Africa

4.1 Current strategies for schistosomiasis control and elimination

Recent years have witnessed an increased interest in the control and, finally, elimination of Neglected Tropical Diseases (NTDs), and today the control of schistosomiasis has again become a priority on the agenda of many governments, donors, pharmaceutical companies and international agencies [40]. WHO has developed several road maps for NTDs, and many African countries have made significant progress by rolling out national action plans and programs targeting schistosomiasis control and elimination [41, 42]. Preventive chemotherapy is the main strategy for schistosomiasis control in Africa, supplemented with water, sanitation and hygiene (WASH) interventions in some regions [43].

4.1.1 Preventive chemotherapy

4.1.1.1 An overview of preventive chemotherapy: Praziquantel

Current control of human schistosomiasis in Africa is based on preventive chemotherapy, whereby populations are mass-treated with anthelminthic praziquantel administered in the standard single oral dose of 40 mg/kg body weight. Treatment with praziquantel is currently the strategy of choice and is endorsed by WHO [41, 43]. The ambitious goals of control and eventual elimination are underpinned by targets that require countries to reach at least 75% treatment coverage of school-age children and at-risk adults, with mass drug administration schedules and the designation of target groups depending on schistosomiasis endemicity [43]. This coverage goal is endorsed for schistosomiasis and soil-transmitted helminths in the 2012–2020 WHO road map for NTDs, in which preventive chemotherapy was identified as a key strategy for tackling NTDs [42, 44].

Over the past decade, significant progress has been made on large-scale treatments through integrated control of schistosomiasis and other NTDs. It is estimated that at least 236.6 million people required preventive treatment for schistosomiasis in 2019, of which more than 105.4 million (about 45%) were reported to have been treated [45]. In Africa, 17 countries out of the 40 that require preventive chemotherapy had not achieved the 75% treatment coverage target for school-age children during 2018, when a total of 69.1 million school-age children were treated, representing overall coverage of 62.9% [46]. In general, annual mass drug administration of preventive chemotherapy has had a significant effect on infection prevalence, intensity and associated morbidity among school-age children [47–49]. However, disease reoccurrence and persistent transmission suggest a need for more intense control measures to achieve the goal of schistosomiasis elimination.

Since the adoption of the World Health Assembly Resolution WHA 65.21 and NTDs road map 2021–2030, schistosomiasis control programs have shifted from morbidity control to disease elimination [41]. However, gaps continue to be observed in the implementation of control programs in Africa. Mass drug administration programs commonly overlook large numbers of preschool-age children, adolescents and adults, thus increasing health inequality and the risk of reinfections of previously treated groups [50]. Schistosomiasis cannot be eliminated in communities where mass drug administration is not ongoing. In the past, a key bottleneck to the implementation of preventive chemotherapy for control of schistosomiasis in Africa was the limited access to praziquantel [51]. Though there is now growing access to this medication for schistosomiasis control in Africa, it is not at the level that is projected to be necessary to reach all people who are at risk or who require treatment [52]. Analysis of data reported on treatment coverage for schistosomiasis shows that utilization of available praziquantel by NTD programs is not yet optimal in many countries [46, 52].

4.1.1.2 Strengths and weaknesses of preventive chemotherapy

Praziquantel is the drug of choice for the treatment of schistosomiasis, as it is considered cost-effective, relatively safe, inexpensive and efficacious; also, donor organizations are willing to provide the drug [53]. Despite increased efforts to control schistosomiasis using preventive chemotherapy, several challenges still exist in reaching the target populations. Until recently, preschool-age children, as well as at-risk adults such as fishery workers, have not been included in many mass drug administration programs despite the evidence of schistosomiasis infection among these populations [54, 55]. This increases health inequality and the accumulation of potentially irreversible morbidities due to prolonged infection [56].

A major challenge now lies in the unavailability of a child-size formulation of praziquantel [56, 57]. The currently available formulation presents several limitations: (a) It is a large tablet, which is difficult for young children and infants to swallow and thus must be broken and crushed to allow for safe uptake. (b) It has a very bitter taste, and so is often mixed with a sweetener to make it palatable to young children. (c) The current formulation of 600 mg does not allow for flexible-dose adjustments for this age group.

4.1.2 Water, sanitation and hygiene (WASH) interventions

Clean water provision, sanitation and hygiene are critical components of the global NTD roadmap [41]. For schistosomiasis, improved sanitation across the entire community to prevent contaminated feces and urine from reaching surface water can reduce or eliminate transmission, by stopping worm eggs in feces and urine from entering water sources, which are the snail habitat [58]. The aim of United Nations Sustainable Development Goal 6 (SDG 6) is to ensure the availability and sustainable management of water and sanitation for all by 2030. WASH interventions are among the most important measures used to control water-related diseases in Africa. However, sanitation, hygienic practices, and access to clean water are inadequate in large parts of Africa where schistosomiasis is endemic [59]. According to the United Nations Children's Fund, in 2020 more than two-thirds of the African population did not have basic sanitation services and about 18% practiced open defecation. Ethiopia, Uganda, Kenya and Tanzania had the largest numbers of people in the continent without access to basic sanitation services, while Eritrea, South Sudan and Ethiopia had the largest proportions and numbers of people practicing open defecation [60]. Furthermore, in Eastern and Southern Africa, about 50 million (over 27%) of school-age children had no access to sanitation services, while 117 million (62%) had no access to hand-washing facilities at school [60]. It has also been reported that nearly half of Africans do not have access to clean water and two-thirds lack access to sewage infrastructure [61]. A systematic review and meta-analysis of the relationship between safe water, adequate sanitation, good hygiene and schistosomiasis found that people with access to safe water were significantly less likely to acquire a *Schistosoma* infection than those who, while they had access to adequate sanitation, did not have safe water access [62].

4.2 A different approach to schistosomiasis control: one health

4.2.1 The concept of one health and the one health disease control approach

The Centers for Disease Control and Prevention define One Health as a collaborative, multispectral transdisciplinary approach applied at the local, regional, national and global levels, with the goal of achieving optimal health outcomes that recognize the interconnection among people, animals, plants and their shared environment

[63]. The One Health approach is a collaborative effort between the human health, animal health and environmental sectors to attain optimal health for people, animals and the environment. Over 60% of emerging, re-emerging and endemic human diseases have their origins in animals [64]. Humans are at increased risk of contracting diseases of animal origin because of a wide range of interconnected variables, including mass urbanization, large-scale livestock production and increased travel [64]. Therefore, efforts to unite the sectors working to protect humans and animals and the ecosystem are of paramount significance.

4.2.2 Schistosomiasis control and elimination under the one health approach

The recurrent hybridization between *Schistosoma* species in nature increases the distribution of schistosomiasis and ultimately challenges current elimination efforts. Animal reservoirs can maintain transmission with zoonotic parasites even while the disease they cause in humans seems to be effectively controlled [65]. To be successful, schistosomiasis elimination programs cannot ignore the animal reservoirs of infection in Africa; this requirement demonstrates the need to consider control measures within a One Health framework [40]. The rapid occurrence of reinfection with schistosomiasis further highlights the need for a One Health approach. An anthropocentric or disjointed sectoral approach to controlling human schistosomiasis in Africa, such as the NTD intervention strategies applied alone, may be insufficient to eliminate schistosomiasis. For example, in the Mekong subregion of Southeast Asia, relying solely on deworming to prevent schistosomiasis did not prevent reinfection, but required parallel activities within the One Health framework [66]. Measures should focus on health aspects of the environment, animals and humans. They should also involve state-of-the-art approaches to schistosomiasis diagnosis and surveillance that encompass the environment (water and snails), animals (both domestic fauna and wildlife) and humans to enable an understanding of transmission ecology and the evolution of schistosomiasis across all hosts (**Figure 5**) [6].

4.2.2.1 Environmental health measures

Schistosoma species depend entirely on the presence of freshwater environments harboring susceptible snails to complete their life cycle. Control measures should therefore focus on preventing excreta (fecal or urine) contamination of freshwater sources. The following control measures are ideal for preventing excreta contamination of freshwater sources:

1. *Provision of improved sanitation as it has been explained above*. Provision and proper use of improved sanitation facilities will prevent excreta containing *Schistosoma* eggs from entering freshwater sources containing snail hosts and thus will prevent subsequent snail infections [58]

2. *Preventing direct contact with infested freshwater by human and animals*. Prevention of direct human or animal contact will reduce the chances of excreta contamination and prevent transmission. It may be accomplished through ring-fencing of the contaminated water bodies [67].

3. *Reducing snail populations*. Reinforcing snail control is a part of the WHO strategic approach to eliminating schistosomiasis [68].

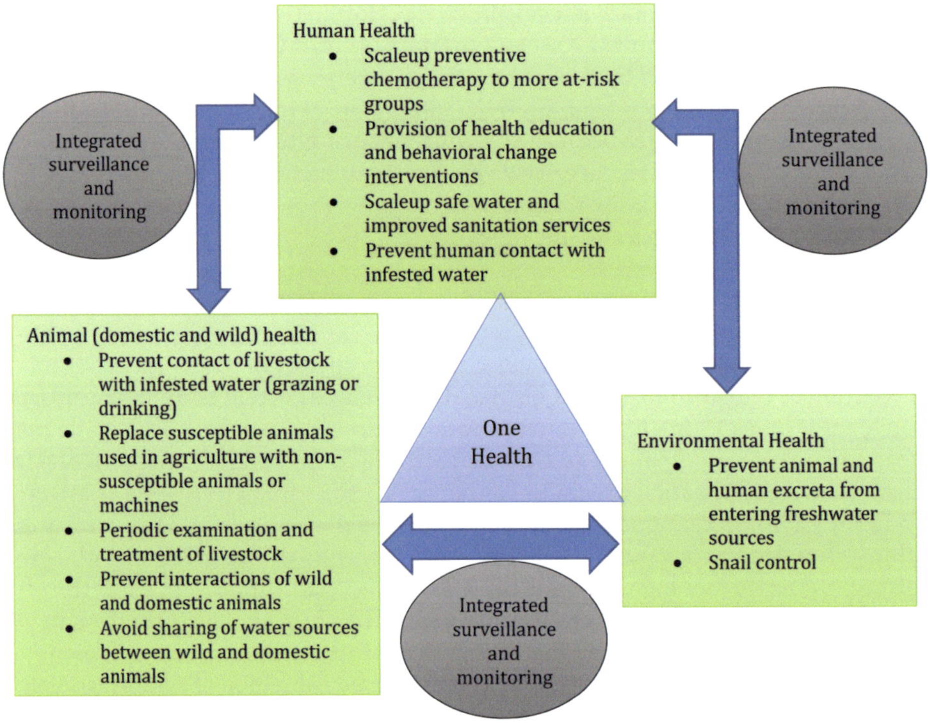

Figure 5.
Schematic presentation of the proposed one health framework for controlling zoonotic schistosomiasis in Africa.

Snail control can be attempted through snail habitat modifications such as altering flow rate and water levels so as to disturb snail habitat and disrupt snails' food sources. Such modifications include constructing V-shaped banks in irrigation channels, removing vegetation and draining water sources that serve no special purpose for humans, wildlife or livestock [67]. Biological control of snails using nonsusceptible competitor snails has been reported to be successful in the Caribbean region [69], although it is important not to run the risk of importing potentially invasive snails. Snail control may also be accomplished through molluscicide application; however, since molluscicides have not been notably effective in past efforts, and may cause damage to other organisms [70], the application should be targeted, and carefully monitored rather than widespread [67].

4.2.2.2 Human health measures

As part of ongoing mass drug administration campaigns, other human interventions should be considered. Therefore, WASH providers must prioritize the reduction of inequality to align with the Sustainable Development Goals agenda, as developed in the recent WASH strategy to accelerate and sustain progress on NTDs [71]. Water scarcity can result in the sharing of water sources between people and animals, which can increase the risk of zoonotic diseases. Improving access to clean water by supplying tap water or wells at homes [65], accompanied by behavioral changes such as avoiding swimming, wading, washing or bathing in contaminated ponds, rivers and lakes, would help to prevent human contact with *Schistosoma*-infested waters. It is safest to consider all freshwater bodies in endemic areas as potential transmission sites [67]. Furthermore, while safe water is unlikely to contain cercariae, its provision often will not prevent all human contact with infested water. In some settings, such as fishing communities, it is important to account for considerable occupational water contact that the availability of safe water supplies would not prevent [72]. Hence, periodic examination and treatment of workers and people at constant risk of infection may be the most feasible approach to controlling schistosomiasis [67]. Interventions to reduce the contamination of water bodies with *Schistosoma* eggs could reduce the potential for disease transmission in both humans and animals [65]. Stakeholders should scale up the provision of improved sanitation services through the construction of latrines (including aboard boats). Also, public toilets along river basins in schistosomiasis-endemic areas must be provided to stop human excrement from entering freshwater sources [67]. In addition, interventions such as the construction of big systems like sewage treatment ponds and constructed wetlands, or home-based smaller systems, would help prevent contamination of water sources. Basically, if the urine and feces of people and animals could be kept from entering water bodies, there would be no more schistosomiasis transmission. This can be seen in two highly infested bodies of water, Lake Victoria and Lake Malawi, where, thanks to local initiatives, there are actually 'safe beaches' with no schistosomiasis [1].

4.2.2.3 Animal health measures

The most effective way of controlling zoonotic schistosomiasis in livestock is also through keeping susceptible domestic animals from coming into contact with infested water. This can be achieved by preventing livestock grazing in infested wetlands, fencing infested water sources and supplying drinking water to the animals in troughs [73]. Apart from reducing the risk of infections to the animals, these measures will also prevent contaminated excreta from livestock from entering freshwater sources. Susceptible animals used in wetland areas for agriculture purposes should be replaced with nonsusceptible species or with farm machinery if the purpose of animals' use is mechanical management. Periodic examination and treatment of susceptible livestock should be conducted. However, reinfection may occur quickly if the source of contamination is left uncontrolled. Regarding wild animals, high-density populations of susceptible wildlife increase the potential for disease transmission. Interaction between livestock and wildlife should be prevented wherever possible, and supplementary feeding of wild animals close to water sources should be avoided. Lastly, scientists and funders should invest in finding *Schistosoma* vaccines for animals and humans [67].

4.2.3 Implementation of the one health approach in Africa under current socioeconomic and political conditions

Strong social, economic and political commitments are key elements in successful schistosomiasis control, which requires persistent efforts and a systematic step-by-step approach with increasingly ambitious targets to reach elimination [35]. The disease context is complex, with the interplay of social, economic, political and cultural factors [20, 27] that may affect the attainment of the goals of the NTD 2021–2030 road map [28]. Concurrent treatment of zoonotic *Schistosoma* reservoirs, at least in terms of livestock hosts in Africa, is likely to be imperative for successful disruption of the transmission of human disease [15]. However, a key problem for the treatment of many zoonotic infections in livestock reservoirs is that, while the costs of treatment fall largely on the agricultural sector, the benefits of reduced transmission to humans are felt largely by the public health and medical sectors [15]. Therefore, motivating the sustainable involvement of livestock authorities and producers, who may have other disease priorities, could be difficult.

Given the potential impact of schistosomiasis on animal health and productivity, a One Health economic evaluation of extending treatment to animal hosts in Africa appears warranted, and requires data to be gathered on the costs and benefits to both the animal and human health sectors. To assess the economics of One Health interventions, the impacts on both sectors need to be integrated so that decision-makers in both sectors can assess and interpret outcomes in a way that is meaningful both to their sector and to society [74]. In light of these challenges, there is a need to revisit the current approach to schistosomiasis control among African countries irrespective of the level of endemicity.

5. Conclusion

Since the novel zoonotic *Schistosoma* hybrid species potentially may play a role in maintaining and exacerbating schistosome transmission in humans and animals, no single strategy will reduce transmission everywhere. What worked well in one place or time can be ineffective or inappropriate in another. The recent approach used to control schistosomiasis in Africa is designed to focus on treatment coverage, the use of vertical programs, and dependence on external supports and donors. The consequences of the approach are the predominance of preventive chemotherapy over other prevention and control strategies and the lack of cross-sector collaboration. Deploying multiple strategies across multiple sectors may help to balance the control portfolio. Therefore, control strategies may have to be adjusted within a jointed One Health framework. This could be facilitated by a successful understanding of the transmission ecology and evolution of zoonotic schistosomiasis across all hosts, both animal and human, as well as the freshwater environment.

Conflicts of interest

The authors declare that there are no conflicts of interest.

Author details

Abdallah Zacharia[1*], Anne H. Outwater[2], Eliza Lupenza[1], Alex J. Mujuni[3] and Twilumba Makene[1]

1 Department of Parasitology and Medical Entomology, Muhimbili University of Health and Allied Sciences, Dar es Salaam, Tanzania

2 Department of Community Health Nursing, Muhimbili University of Health and Allied Sciences, Dar es Salaam, Tanzania

3 Department of Zoology and Wildlife Conservation, College of Natural and Applied Sciences, University of Dar es Salaam, Dar es Salaam, Tanzania

*Address all correspondence to: naayz@ymail.com

References

[1] Outwater AH, Mpangala E. Schistosomiasis and US Peace Corps volunteers in Tanzania. Journal of Travel Medicine. 2005;**12**(5):265-269. DOI: 10.2310/7060.2005.12505

[2] Aula OP, McManus DP, Jones MK, Gordon CA. Schistosomiasis with a focus on Africa. Tropical Medicine and Infectious Diseases. 2021;**6**(3):1-40. DOI: 10.3390/tropicalmed6030109

[3] World Health Organization, Schistosomiasis. 2021. Available from: www.who.int/news-room/fact-sheets/detail/schistosomiasis

[4] Fall CB et al. Hybridized zoonotic Schistosoma infections result in hybridized morbidity profiles: A clinical morbidity study amongst co-infected human populations of Senegal. Microorganisms. 2021;**9**(8):1-18. DOI: 10.3390/microorganisms9081776

[5] Adenowo AF, Oyinloye BE, Ogunyinka BI, Kappo AP. Impact of human schistosomiasis in sub-Saharan Africa. The Brazilian Journal of Infectious Diseases. 2015;**19**(2):196-205. DOI: 10.1016/j.bjid.2014.11.004

[6] Webster JP, Gower CM, Knowles SCL, Molyneux DH, Fenton A. One health—An ecological and evolutionary framework for tackling Neglected Zoonotic Diseases. Evolutionary Applications. 2016;**9**(2):313-333. DOI: 10.1111/eva.12341

[7] Savassi BAES et al. Cattle as natural host for Schistosoma haematobium (Bilharz, 1852) Weinland, 1858 x Schistosoma bovis Sonsino, 1876 interactions, with new cercarial emergence and genetic patterns. Parasitology Research. 2020;**119**(7):2189-2205. DOI: 10.1007/s00436-020-06709-0

[8] Cao ZG, Zhao YE, Lee Willingham A, Wang TP. Towards the elimination of schistosomiasis japonica through control of the disease in domestic animals in the People's Republic of China: A tale of over 60 years. Advances in Parasitology. 2016;**92**:269-306. DOI: 10.1016/bs.apar.2016.03.001

[9] Borlase A, Webster JP, Rudge JW. Opportunities and challenges for modelling epidemiological and evolutionary dynamics in a multihost, multiparasite system: Zoonotic hybrid schistosomiasis in West Africa. Evolutionary Applications. 2018;**11**(4):501-515. DOI: 10.1111/eva.12529

[10] Richards L, Erko B, Ponpetch K, Ryan SJ, Liang S. Assessing the nonhuman primate reservoir of *Schistosoma mansoni* in Africa: A systematic review. Infectious Diseases of Poverty. 2019;**8**(32):1-11

[11] Southgate VR. Schistosomiasis in the Senegal River Basin: Before and after the construction of the dams at Diama, Senegal, and Manantali, Mali, and future prospects. Journal of Helminthology. 1997;**71**(2):125-132. DOI: 10.1017/s0022149x00015790

[12] Léger E et al. Prevalence and distribution of schistosomiasis in human, livestock, and snail populations in northern Senegal: A One Health epidemiological study of a multi-host system. Lancet Planetary Health. 2021;**4**(8):e330-e342. DOI: 10.1016/S2542-5196(20)30129-7

[13] Kouadio JN et al. Prevalence and distribution of livestock schistosomiasis

and fascioliasis in Côte d'Ivoire: Results from a cross-sectional survey. BMC Veterinary Research. 2020;**16**(1):1-13. DOI: 10.1186/s12917-020-02667-y

[14] Keyyu JD, Monrad J, Kyvsgaard NC, Kassuku AA. Epidemiology of *Fasciola gigantica* and Amphistomes in cattle on traditional, small-scale dairy and large-scale dairy farms in the southern highlands of Tanzania. Tropical Animal Health and Production. 2005;**37**(4):303-314. DOI: 10.1007/s11250-005-5688-7

[15] Gower CM, Vince L, Webster JP. Should we be treating animal schistosomiasis in Africa? The need for a One Health economic evaluation of schistosomiasis control in people and their livestock. Transactions of the Royal Society of Tropical Medicine and Hygiene. 2017;**111**:244-247. DOI: 10.1093/trstmh/trx047

[16] Panzner U, Boissier J. Natural intra- and interclade human hybrid schistosomes in Africa with considerations on prevention through vaccination. Microorganisms. 2021;**9**(1465):1-19. DOI: 10.3390/microorganisms9071465

[17] King KC, Stelkens RB, Webster JP, Smith DF, Brockhurst MA. Hybridization in parasites: Consequences for adaptive evolution, pathogenesis, and public health in a changing world. PLoS Pathogens. 2015;**11**(9):1-12. DOI: 10.1371/journal.ppat.1005098

[18] Leger E, Webster JP. Hybridizations within the genus Schistosoma: Implications for evolution, epidemiology and control. Parasitology. 2017;**144**(1): 65-80. DOI: 10.1017/S0031182016001190

[19] Harrison R, Larson E. Hybridization, introgression, and the nature of species boundaries. The Journal of Heredity. 2014;**105**(1982):795-809. DOI: 10.1093/jhered/esu033

[20] Moné H, Minguez S, Ibikounlé M, Allienne JF, Massougbodji A, Mouahid G. Natural interactions between *S. haematobium* and *S. guineensis* in the Republic of Benin. Science World Journal. 2012:793420. DOI: 10.1100/2012/793420

[21] Léger E et al. Introgressed animal schistosomes *Schistosoma curassoni* and *S. bovis* naturallly infecting human. Emerging Infectious Diseases. 2016;**22**(12):2212-2214. DOI: 10.3201/eid2212.1606

[22] Huyse T, Webster BL, Geldof S, Stothard JR, Diaw OT, Rollinson D. Bidirectional introgressive hybridization between a cattle and human schistosome species. PLoS Pathogenesis. 2009;**45**(9):1-9. DOI: 10.1371/journal.ppat.1000571

[23] Alves W. Observations on S. mattheei and S. haematobium. Adults and eggs from experimental animals and man. Transactions of the Royal Society of Tropical Medicine and Hygiene. 1948;**41**(4):430-431. Available from: https://www.cabdirect.org/cabdirect/abstract/19480800853

[24] Wright C, Ross G. Hybrids between *Schistosoma haematobium* and *S. mattheei* identification by isoelectric focusing of enzymes. Transactions of the Royal Society of Tropical Medicine and Hygiene. 1980;**74**(3):326-332. DOI: 10.1016/0035-9203(80)90091-7

[25] Steinauer ML et al. Introgressive hybridization of human and rodent schistosome parasites in western Kenya. Molecular Ecology. 2008;**17**(23):5062-5074. DOI: 10.1111/j.1365-294X.2008.03957.x

[26] Webster BL, Diaw OT, Seye MM, Webster JP, Rollinson D. Introgressive hybridization of *Schistosoma haematobium* group species in Senegal:

Species barrier break down between ruminant and human schistosomes. PLoS Neglectd Tropical Diseases. 2013;**7**(4):1-9. DOI: 10.1371/journal.pntd.0002110

[27] Kruatrachue M, Upatham ES, Sahaphong S, Tongthong T, Khunborivan V. Scanning electron microscopic study of the tegumental surface of the hybrid schistosome between *Schistosoma mekongi* and *S. japonicum*-like (Malaysian). The Southeast Asian Journal of Tropical Medicine and Public Health. 1987;**18**(4):453-466

[28] Cunin P, Tchuem Tchuenté L, Poste B, Djibrilla K, Martin PMV. Interactions between *Schistosoma haematobium* and *Schistosoma mansoni* in humans in north Cameroon. Tropical Medicine & International Health. 2003;**8**(12):1110-1117. DOI: 10.1046/j.1360-2276.2003.01139.x

[29] Huyse T, Van Den Broeck F, Hellemans B, Volckaert FAM, Polman K. Hybridisation between the two major African schistosome species of humans. International Journal for Parasitology. 2013;**43**(8):687-689. DOI: 10.1016/j.ijpara.2013.04.001

[30] Depaquit J, Akhoundi M, Haouchine D, Mantelet S, Izri A. No limit in interspecific hybridization in schistosomes: Observation from a case report. Parasite. 2019;**26**(10):1-5

[31] Tchuem Tchuenté LA, Southgate V, Njiokou F, Njine T, Kouemeni L, Jourdane J. The evolution of schistosomiasis at Loum, Cameroon: Replacement of Schistosoma intercalatum by *S. haematobium* through introgressive hybridization. Transactions of the Royal Society of Tropical Medicine and Hygiene. 1997;**91**:664-665. DOI: 10.1016/s0035-9203(97)90513-7

[32] Cosgrove CL, Southgate VR. Interactions between *Schistosoma intercalatum* (Zaire strain) and *S. mansoni*. Journal of Helminthology. 2003;**77**(3):209-218. DOI: 10.1079/JOH2002165

[33] Catalano S et al. Rodents as natural hosts of zoonotic schistosoma species and hybrids: An epidemiological and evolutionary perspective from West Africa. The Journal of Infectious Diseases. 2018;**218**(3):429-433. DOI: 10.1093/infdis/jiy029

[34] Centers for Disease Control and Prevention, Zoonotic diseases. One Health. 2021. Available from: https://www.cdc.gov/onehealth/basics/zoonotic-diseases.html

[35] Carabin H et al. Zoonotic schistosomosis (schistosomiasis). In: Palmer S, Soulsby L, Torgerson P, Brown DWG, editors. Oxford Textbook of Zoonoses: Biology, Clinical Practice and Public Health. 2nd ed. London: Oxford University Press; 2011

[36] Catalano S et al. Multihost transmission of *Schistosoma mansoni* in Senegal, 2015-2018. Emerging Infectious Diseases. 2020;**26**(6):2015-2018

[37] Van Wyk JA. The importance of animals in human schistosomiasis in South Africa. South African Medical Journal. 1983;**63**(6):201-204

[38] Borlase A, Rudge JW, Léger E, Diouf ND, Fall CB, Diop SD. Spillover, hybridization, and persistence in schistosome transmission dynamics at the human–animal interface. PNAS. 2021;**118**(41):1-11. DOI: 10.1073/pnas.2110711118

[39] Rey O et al. Diverging patterns of introgression from *Schistosoma bovis* across *S. haematobium* African lineages. PLoS Pathogens. 2021;**17**(2):1-20. DOI: 10.1371/JOURNAL.PPAT.1009313

[40] Tchuem Tchuenté LA, Rollinson D, Stothard JR, Molyneux D. Moving from

control to elimination of schistosomiasis in sub-Saharan Africa: Time to change and adapt strategies. Infectious Diseases of Poverty. 2017;**6**(1):1-14. DOI: 10.1186/s40249-017-0256-8

[41] World Health Organization. Ending the Neglect to Attain the Sustainable Development Goals: A Road Map for Neglected Tropical Diseases 2021-2030. Geneva, Switzerland: WHO; 2021

[42] World Health Organization. Schistosomiasis: Progress Report 2001-2011 and Strategic Plan 2012-2020. Geneva, Switzerland: WHO; 2010

[43] WHO Expert Committee. Prevention and Control of Schistosomiasis and Soil Transmitted Helminthiasis. Geneva, Switzerland: WHO; 2002

[44] World Health Organization. World Health Assembly Resolution WHA 65.21: Elimination of Schistosomiasis. Geneva, Switzerland: WHO; 2012

[45] World Health Organization, Schistosomiasis fact sheet. 2021. Available from: https://www.who.int/news-room/fact-sheets/detail/schistosomiasis [Accessed: December 23, 2021]

[46] World Health Organization. Schistosomiasis and soil-transmitted helminthiases: Numbers of people treated in 2018. Weekly Epidemiological Record. 2020;**96**:601-612

[47] Geleta S, Alemu A, Getie S, Mekonnen Z, Erko B. Prevalence of urinary schistosomiasis and associated risk factors among Abobo Primary School children in Gambella Regional State, southwestern Ethiopia: A cross-sectional study. Parasite Vectors. 2015;**8**(215):1-9. DOI: 10.1186/s13071-015-0822-5

[48] Bakuza J. Demographic factors driving schistosomiasis and soil-transmitted helminthiases in Milola Ward, Lindi District, Tanzania: A useful guide for launching intervention. East African Health Research. 2018;**2**:156-167

[49] Mugono M, Konje E, Kuhn S, Mpogoro FJ, Morona D, Mazigo HD. Intestinal schistosomiasis and geohelminths of Ukara Island, North-Western Tanzania: Prevalence, intensity of infection and associated risk factors among school children. Parasites & Vectors. 2014;**7**(1):1-9. DOI: 10.1186/s13071-014-0612-5

[50] Kalinda C, Mindu T, Chimbari MJ. A systematic review and meta-analysis quantifying schistosomiasis infection burden in pre-school aged children (PreSAC) in sub-Saharan Africa for the period 2000-2020. PLoS One. 2020;**15**(12):1-16. DOI: 10.1371/journal.pone.0244695

[51] Hotez PJ, Engels D, Fenwick A, Savioloi L. Africa is desperate for praziquantel. Lancet. 2010;**376**(9740):496-498. DOI: 10.1016/S0140-6736(10)60879-3

[52] World Health Organization. Schistosomiasis and soil-transmitted helminthiases: Numbers of people treated in 2019. Weekly Epidemiological Record. 2019;**95**:629-640

[53] Tesfie A et al. Praziquantel is an effective drug for the treatment of *Schistosoma Mansoni* infection among school-aged children in Northwest Ethiopia. Tropical Medicine Health. 2020;**48**(1):1-8

[54] Faust CL et al. Schistosomiasis control: Leave no age group behind. Trends in Parasitology. 2020;**36**(7):582-591. DOI: 10.1016/j.pt.2020.04.012

[55] Mang'ara R. Prevalence of *Schistosoma mansoni* Infection and

Associated Factors among Fishery Workers. Dar es Salaam, Tanzania: Department of Parasitology and Medical Entomology; 2020

[56] Osakunor DNM, Woolhouse MEJ, Mutapi F. Paediatric schistosomiasis: What we know and what we need to know. PLoS Neglected Tropical Diseases. 2018;**12**(2):1-16. DOI: 10.1371/journal.pntd.0006144

[57] Mduluza T, Mutapi F. Putting the treatment of paediatric schistosomiasis into context. Infectious Diseases of Poverty. 2017;**6**(1):1-6

[58] Grimes JET, Croll D, Harrison WE, Utzinger J, Freeman MC, Templeton MR. The roles of water, sanitation and hygiene in reducing schistosomiasis: A review. Parasites & Vectors. 2015;**8**(156):1-16

[59] World Health Organization/United Nations Children's Fund, WHO/UNICEF joint monitoring program for water supply, sanitation and hygiene (JMP)—Progress on household drinking water, sanitation and hygiene 2000-2020. 2021. Available from: https://www.unwater.org/publications

[60] United Nations Children's Fund. Eastern and southern Africa: Ssanitation and hygiene. Available from: https://www.unicef.org/esa/sanitation-and-hygiene [Accessed: December 23, 2021]

[61] Walker C. Lack of safe water, sanitation spurs growing dissatisfaction with government performance. Afrobarometer. 2016;(76):1-23

[62] Freeman MC, Grimes JET, Croll D, Harrison WE, Templeton MR. The relationship between water, sanitation and schistosomiasis: A systematic review and meta-analysis. PLoS Neglected Tropical Diseases. 2014;**8**(12):e3296. DOI: 10.1371/journal.pntd.0003296

[63] Centers for Disease Control and Prevention, One Health. 2021. Available from: https://www.cdc.gov/onehealth/index.html

[64] Kate PD, Jones E, Patel NG, Levy MA, Storeygard A, Balk D, et al. Global trends in emerging infectious diseases. Nature. 2008;**451**(7181):990-993

[65] Stauffer JR, Madsen H. A One Health approach to reducing schistosomiasis transmission in Lake Malawi. Preventive Medicine and Community Health. 2018;**1**(3):1-4. DOI: 10.15761/PMCH.1000115

[66] World Health Organization. NTD, WASH, Animal Health, Nutrition and Education are Joining Forces to Eliminate Schistosomiasis in Mekong Region. WHO: Geneva, Switzerland; 2018

[67] Cromie RL et al., Ramsar wetland disease manual: Guidelines for assessment, monitoring and management of animal disease in wetlands (Ramsar Technical Report no. 7). Gland, Switzerland: Ramsar Convention Secretariat. 2012

[68] World Health Organization, Schistosomiasis elimination: Refocusing on snail control to sustain progress. 2020. Available from: https://www.who.int/news/item/25-03-2020-schistosomiasis-elimination-refocusing-on-snail-control-to-sustain-progress

[69] Sokolow SH et al. To reduce the global burden of human schistosomiasis, use 'old fashioned' snail control. Trends in Parasitology. 2017;**34**(1):23-40. DOI: 10.1016/j.pt.2017.10.002

[70] Coelho PMZ, Caldeira RJ. Critical analysis of molluscide application in schistosomiasis control programs in Brazil. Infectious Diseases of Poverty. 2016;**5**:57. DOI: 10.1186/s40249-016-0153-6

[71] World Health Organization, Water, sanitation and hygiene for accelerating and sustaining progress on Neglected Tropical Diseases. 2016. Available from: https://www.who.int/publications/i/item/WHO-FWC-WSH-15.12

[72] Omondi I, Odiere MR, Rawago F, Mwinzi PN, Campbell C, Musuva R. Socioeconomic determinants of *Schistosoma mansoni* infection using multiple correspondence analysis among rural western Kenyan communities: Evidence from a household-based study. PLoS One. 2021;**16**(6):1-16. DOI: 10.1371/journal.pone.0253041

[73] De Bont J, Vercruysse J. The epidemiology and control of cattle schistosomiasis. Parasitology Today. 1997;**13**(7):255-262

[74] Shaw APM, Rushton J, Roth F, Torgerson PR. DALYs, dollars and dogs: How best to analyse the economics of controlling zoonoses. Revue Scientifique et Technique. 2017;**36**(1):147-161. DOI: 10.20506/rst.36.1.2618

Chapter 12

Dancing in a Cycle: Global Health Agenda and *Schistosomiasis* Control in Africa

Adetayo Olorunlana

Abstract

Schistosomiasis and other Neglected Tropical diseases (NTDs) affect about 2 billion people globally. Africa shares approximately 90% of the global burden of *schistosomiasis* disease. Despite, World Health Organization (WHO) effort to control the disease, it remains neglected in most African countries. Historically, *schistosomiasis* is as long as 4,000 years in Africa, but lack accurate data and commitment to combat the disease. Control programs exclude adults in Mass Drug Administration (MDAs), and water, sanitation, and hygiene (WASH) as Praziquantel drug is used for the treatment. However, migratory patterns of the neglected population and the interplay of social, economic, political, and cultural factors introduce the disease into previously eliminated or/and new areas. The question is would Africa be able to achieve the new goals of the WHO NTDs 2021–2030 Roadmap, for schistosomiasis elimination? The chapter argued for and against if Africa changes the current top-down approach to *schistosomiasis* control and incorporates a dynamic approach. Or if the previous pattern of late implementation, dependent on only one drug and shifting focus to other diseases of relevance continues. If a new approach is not adopted the dance in the cycle has just begun.

Keywords: Africa, control programme, neglected tropical disease (NTDs), *Praziquantel*, *Schistosomiasis*

1. Introduction

Schistosomiasis is among the Neglected Tropical Diseases (NTDs), and the main challenge is the control of the disease [1]. *Schistosomiasis* transmission has been reported from 78 countries with over 65% in Africa with estimated 800 million people at risk of the disease [2, 3]. Literature affirmed that *Schistosomiasis* is the third-highest burden among parasitic NTDs, 2019 estimation of the World Health Organization peg the infection at over 140 million people and at least 236.6 million people required preventive treatment and it remains among the major global health threats [4–6]. Consequently, *schistosomiasis* is still highly endemic in several countries especially in Sub-Saharan Africa [5–9].

Scientifically, *schistosomiasis* could be a mild, acute, and chronic parasitic disease caused by blood flukes (trematode worms) of the genus *Schistosoma* [2, 6].

Countries	Estimated number requiring preventive chemotherapy for *Schistosomiasis* annually	Estimated number of school-age children requiring preventive chemotherapy for *Schistosomiasis* annually
Algeria	No PC required	No PC required
Angola	5,034,807	3,258,115
Benin	2,300,011	1,367,350
Botswana	1,395,735	366,693
Burkina Faso	4,737,998	4,285,046
Burundi	1,701,480	1,633,550
Cabo Verde	5,674,510	3,835,446
Cameroon	5,670,713	3,329,839
Central African Republic (CAR)	1,216,727	477,715
Chad	3,990,275	2,378,434
Comoros	Non-endemic	Non-endemic
Congo, Democratic Republic	15,977,680	11,521,955
Congo, Republic	421,246	225,225
Djibouti	No PC required	No PC required
Egypt	2,932,815	1,464,425
Equatorial Guinea	62,864	32,196
Eritrea	286,629	243,835
Eswatini	402,727	282,396
Ethiopia	14,979,339	7,774,638
Gabon	180,080	160,0The 42
The Gambia	180,080	160,042
Ghana	10,685,201	4,369,206
Guinea	4,435,048	1,864,900
Guinea-Bissau	160,922	108,416
Kenya	3,519,321	1,924,082
Lesotho	Non-endemic	Non-endemic
Liberia	875,416	447,595
Libya	No PC required	No PC required
Madagascar	9,914,996	4,438,987
Malawi	8,861,768	3,735,144
Mali	6,276,715	3,518,177
Mauritania	844,271	390,854
Mauritius	No PC required	No PC required
Morocco	No PC required	No PC required
Mozambique	16,564,136	6,264,395
Namibia	486,997	203,961

Countries	Estimated number requiring preventive chemotherapy for *Schistosomiasis* annually	Estimated number of school-age children requiring preventive chemotherapy for *Schistosomiasis* annually
Niger	10,249,620	4,553,187
Nigeria	26,289,931	17,444,157
Rwanda	2,784,935	1,685,462
Sao Tome and Principe	39,698	24,126
Senegal	2,614,816	1,340,844
Seychelles	Non-endemic	Non-endemic
Sierra Leone	3,002,879	1,309,396
Somalia	2,847,592	2,549,993
South Africa	4,628,843	3,807,757
South Sudan	2,841,584	1,324,002
Sudan	8,080,706	4,515,705
Tanzania	16,495,074	6,750,656
Togo	3,051,913	1,740,023
Tunisia	No PC required	No PC required
Uganda	12,305,791	5,628,177
Zambia	4,268,909	2,338,006
Zimbabwe	3,413,154	2,021,614

Source: Compiled by Author 2021; extracted from WHO [33].

Table 1.
Status of Schistosomiasis *in 54 African countries showing the estimated number of people and school-age children that required preventive chemotherapy (PC) in the year 2020.*

Africa shares not less than 90% of the global burden of *schistosomiasis* disease necessitating her need for preventive chemotherapy (see **Table 1**) in about 51 endemic countries with moderate-to-high transmission [6]. There are five different types of species causing *schistosomiasis* infection: *Schistosoma haematobium* affecting the urinary tract; *Schistosoma mansoni*, *Schistosoma japonicum*, *Schistosoma intercalatum*, and *Schistosoma mekongi* affecting the intestine. *S. haematobium* and *S. mansoni* infections are common in Africa [9, 10].

In Sub-Saharan Africa (SSA), *S. mansoni* (intestinal *schistosomiasis*) and *S. haematobium* (urogenital *schistosomiasis*) (**Table 2**), transmitted through feces and urine, has been identified as the main species causing human *schistosomiasis* [11]. Research shows that *S. mansoni* is widely distributed across the tropics and subtropics especially in the vast poverty-stricken but environmentally and climatically friendly sub-Saharan Africa [12, 13]. Some reported that S. *haematobium* is the most prevalent parasite in Nigeria, with an estimated population of 30 million people annually [8, 14]. Also, *S. haematobium* is affirmed to be more endemic because of the agricultural activities such as fishing, subsistence farming, and washing among others that forces the rural people to interact with freshwater [15, 16].

Subsequently, the population experiences *schistosomiasis* symptoms like anemia, fever, genital lesions, stunting, and sometimes irreversible organ damage [17].

	Species	Geographical distribution
Intestinal schistosomiasis	*Schistosoma mansoni*	Africa, the Middle East, the Caribbean, Brazil, Venezuela, and Suriname
	Schistosoma japonicum	China, Indonesia, the Philippines
	Schistosoma mekongi	Several districts of Cambodia and the Lao People's Democratic Republic
	Schistosoma guineensis and related *S. intercalatum*	Rain forest areas of central Africa
Urogenital schistosomiasis	*Schistosoma haematobium*	Africa, the Middle East, Corsica (France)
Source: WHO [33].		

Table 2.
Parasite species and geographical distribution of schistosomiasis.

This was the rationale behind the preventive chemotherapy (PC) and the recommendation of *Praziquantel* by WHO as a notable strategy to control schistosomiasis by targeting the school-aged children (SAC) from aged 5–15 years because they were most infected and can be reached successfully through schools [5]. "The PC strategy is indicated by prevalence (estimated by initial parasitological assessment) at implementation unit level, usually, district, the prevalence of infection less than 10% requires triennial PC, 10% to 49% biennial treatment, and 50% or greater annual treatment" [5].

Although some countries recorded success of morbidity control, the narrative is different in most African countries. If some countries were able to eliminate *schistosomiasis*, some scholars have asked the question why not Africa [18]. Could it be argued that the COVID-19 Pandemic hinders the WHO set goals for the control and elimination of *schistosomiasis* in 2020? Or could we measure the progress so far and project that the WHO will achieve the goal of elimination of *Schistosomiasis* as a public health problem in all endemic countries by 2025 or 2030? Complete interruption of transmission is a target in selected regions by 2025 [19–23]. Although strategic plans exist on how the WHO guidance on how *schistosomiasis* can be controlled and scale up to elimination [18, 20], but is yet uncertain if such goals can be achieved with the little time left [23]. The current review traced the historical analysis of *schistosomiasis*, exposed the neglected nature of the disease as a possible reason for persistent transmission, ex-rayed the burden and the challenge of elimination, explained the use of preventive chemotherapy and the proposition for African traditional medication, finally concluded with the global health agenda and *schistosomiasis* control campaign in Africa.

2. Historical analysis of *Schistosomiasis* in Africa

Historically, scholars assumed that *schistosomiasis* in Africa must have originated from Egypt during the Egyptian mummies of the twentieth dynasty around 1250–1000 B.C. because of the symptoms characteristic of urinary *schistosomiasis* which were first described in early Egyptian papyri and the eggs of *S. haematobium* identified in the urinary tracts approximately around 4000 years ago [23, 24].

According to Di Bella, there were reports of persistent *haematuria* recorded by members of Napoleon's army in Egypt in 1798 [24], and in forces involved in the

Boer war (1899–1902). In the Eastern Cape of South Africa, *schistosomiasis* was first recorded in 1863, after Dr. J Harley diagnosed endemic *haematuria* with unknown cause in residents which cause was only known 11 years after. Although *schistosomiasis* affects all age categories but was more common in children in South Africa between 1864 and 1899 this was associated with contact with freshwater [23, 25]. Although certain studies claimed that women and girls were considered to be less affected as they had little contact with "natural" water but other studies claimed they are more likely to be affected because they have more contact with freshwater [2, 25].

The name *schistosomiasis* was given by a German physician called Theodore Bilharz as he was the first to identify the parasite causing *schistosomiasis* in 1851. In his study he recovered two distinct species from autopsies of dead soldiers in Egypt and first named the parasite *Distomum haematobium* and also described hatching of eggs, linking the existence of the parasite to clinical symptoms– primarily *haematuria*– attributed to the disease [23]. Bilharzia was later adopted as the generic term for the *schistosomiasis* parasites after the German physician Theodore Bilharz.

In Africa, cultural interference influenced the way *schistosomiasis* symptoms are described. For example in Nigeria among Song people in the North, schistosomiasis is a sign of manhood; among the Yewa people in Southwestern, is called "*Atosiaja*" as a result of urinating where dogs urinated, while Anambra people in the Eastern part of Nigeria called it "*ogbodu*" meaning red urine, as a sign of venereal disease; a sign of maturity or a result of a curse, malaria fever, witchcraft or dirtiness [26]. In north Cameroon, the Fulbe people relate red urine to "*cille naange*" (sun urine), in Upper Egypt, is seen as "*harzia*", a serious disease that weakens people, eats the liver, and causes blood loss, bladder stones, calcium disease and other afflictions [26]. In most of the African descriptions of *Schistosomiasis*, water contacts or snails were not mentioned. General knowledge of the disease causation and the perceived severity may influence people a little toward the disease.

3. Factors promoting the neglect of *Schistosomiasis* and reasons for persistent transmissions

Author and colleagues [2], emphasize the place of human culture in the persistent transmission of *schistosomiasis*, in Nigeria. Their emphasis was based on human behavior related to occupation, recreation, and daily house chore that necessitate the people to have contact with freshwater bodies that carries the snail with the *schistosomiasis* lava. Notably, *schistosomiasis* is one of the 20 NTDs, is a water-based parasitic disease of public health importance [27].

The NTDs in the early 2000s was categorized as 17 conditions in the WHO portfolio [1, 28], there was a varied group of communicable diseases caused by bacteria, *helminths*, *protozoa*, or viruses, such as *Buruli ulcer*, *Chagas* disease, *dengue*, *dracunculiasis* (guinea worm disease), *echinococcosis*, *foodborne trematodiasis*, human African *trypanosomiasis* (sleeping sickness), *leishmaniasis*, leprosy, *lymphatic filariasis* (elephantiasis), *onchocerciasis* (river blindness), rabies, *schistosomiasis* (snail fever), soil-transmitted *helminthiasis* (intestinal worms), *taeniasis/cysticercosis* (pork tapeworm), blinding *trachoma*, and yaws [1, 28]. Since 2016, this list was expanded with three groups of diseases to currently include 20 NTDs or groups of NTDs. Those new NTDs include *mycetoma*, *chromoblastomycosis*, and other deep *mycoses*; *scabies* and other *ectoparasites*; and snakebite *envenoming* [1].

Generally, Africa lacks accurate data on the NTDs, moreover, the constant contact with water containing S. *haematobium cercariae* released from the *Bulinus* snail, often occurs regularly, resulting in re-infection with the disease [27], this also affects the data on the prevalence of *schistosomiasis* in Africa. Using documented evidence in data gathering, research shows that adult worms could live in humans for as long as 30 years [29]. When humans host the worm for such long a time in endemic areas it becomes possible for infection or/and re-infection at some point in their life [27], leading to a vicious cycle within the communities irrespective of preventive chemotherapy. For example, statistics affirmed that the highest *schistosomiasis* disease burden globally can be found in Nigeria (see **Table 1**), however, Nigeria does not have accurate national data on *schistosomiasis* prevalence. Although, she sometimes embark on a large-scale deworming implementation exercise for SAC in endemic areas with *praziquantel* [30], neglecting the adults and out-of-children as they were not covered by mass administration of *praziquantel* would be a challenge to the control of the disease.

Sometimes, the affected communities and individuals affected by *schistosomiasis* tend to neglect the symptoms, depending on the stage of the infection, because of the wide range of clinical symptoms that may occur, many of which are hard to distinguish from several other diseases [15]. It was also argued from the perspectives of the medical sociologist as perceived by the people as a disease but not an illness [26]. From that argument, the affected community does not see *schistosomiasis* as a serious ailment since they can go about their daily business without being bed riding. However, a study shows that schistosomiasis causes morbidity with many infected persons experiencing *hematuria*, *dysuria*, bladder-wall pathology, and *hydronephrosis* [27]. But because these conditions are not peculiar to *schistosomiasis* alone it tends to be neglected.

From the Nigeria scenario as related to other sub-Sahara Africa, is the cost for diagnosis and tool kits that inform the diseases being neglected. Nigeria did tackle *schistosomiasis* through a 2-step approach: case management and a control program [31]. According to Isere and colleagues, in the case management approach, cases are diagnosed at the primary care level. While for the control program, school-aged children are given *praziquantel* for the treatment of *schistosomiasis*. Sturrock [32], affirmed that *schistosomiasis* is common among children with the highest intensity of infection found in children between ages 5 and 15 years. However, the study also revealed that women and men carry a high risk of urinary *schistosomiasis* due to social and occupational activities such as farming and washing, especially in areas with poor water, and sanitation services [2]. Water-related domestic activities such as washing clothes and fetching water, as well as recreational water activities also increase the risk of infection for women and children [33]. It is also more common in fishing and agriculture dominant communities where direct interactions with water increase the risk of contracting the disease.

Other concerns for *schistosomiasis* being tag neglected disease include missed diagnosis, need for more sensitive, accurate, cheaper, and easy to use devices for the diagnosis and control of *schistosomiasis*. Study shows that several persons do not pass bloody urine which is characteristic of the disease [34]. Notably, most of the control program does not include adults in MDAs [30], meaning that adults with schistosomiasis infections are not being treated. "*Schistosomiasis haematobium* infection is mainly diagnosed using microscopy to detect parasite eggs in urine specimens which are not sensitive in detecting light infections of <50 eggs per 10mls of urine; while labor-intensive, and sensitivity of diagnosis depends on the skill of the laboratory personnel" [35]. "Also, egg excretion in urine varies daily and can be complicated by interaction between the host and the parasite" [36]. There are other tests for the detection of *S. haematobium* infection, but they are contested for their poor specificity and high cost for endemic countries [37].

Although some of the tests are useful they are at the stage of *schistosomiasis* elimination, a phase that the majority of the African countries are yet to reach [17]. From the various range of factors and the tendencies for continuous transmission, it is certain, that the challenge and burden of the *schistosomiasis* will be burdensome.

4. *Schistosomiasis* burden and the challenge of eliminating the disease in Africa

Schistosomiasis disease burden is high in Sub-Saharan Africa [38]. This is because Sub-Saharan Africa accounts for not less than 93% of the world's burden of diseases. As of 2015, there were about 207 million *schistosomiasis* cases, with the highest prevalence found in Nigeria, Tanzania, Ghana, Mozambique, and the Democratic Republic of Congo, these 5 countries account for 78 million cases [39]. In this region, after Nigeria, Tanzania was the second country having the highest cases of *schistosomiasis* and approximately 51.5% of the Tanzanian populations were either exposed or live in areas with a high risk of exposure [40], in current data [6] Mozambique has slightly overtaken Tanzanian (See, **Table 1**).

To combat *schistosomiasis*, WHO did develop numerous roadmaps for NTDs, and significant progress has been made by many sub-Saharan African countries by rolling out national action plans and programs targeting *schistosomiasis* control and elimination [7]. Considering all these efforts, we are tempted to ask why is it that *schistosomiasis* still remains a huge problem in sub-Saharan Africa? With such an unmet need for the treatment [5]. Conversely, over 150 000 deaths are attributable to chronic infection with *S. haematobium* in Africa [41]. Researchers affirm that *schistosomiasis* commonly affects the poor, the majority of them living in rural, underprivileged urban, or peri-urban settings with limited access to clean water, inadequate sanitation, and lack hygienic services [42]. *Schistosomiasis* burden is beyond health impact it also has social and economic implications for communities [39].

Children are at a greater risk of acquiring the infection as well as reinfection [43]. *Schistosomiasis* is known to cause anemia, growth stunting, and reduced productivity; and accounts for between 1.6 and 4.2 million disability-adjusted life years (DALYs) lost annually in sub-Saharan Africa [42, 44, 45]. New data show a reduction of an estimated 1.43 million DALYs lost to *schistosomiasis* in 2016 globally [46]. However, in aggregate *schistosomiasis* with other NTDs were estimated to affect close to 2 billion people at the turn of the millennium, with a collective DALYs burden that was equivalent to HIV/AIDS, tuberculosis, or malaria [47]. There exist indirect consequences of NTDs, which are beyond condemning affected people to live long years with disability and stigma, it was noted that it keeps children out of school, adults out of work, burden households with considerable costs to seek health care, trap communities in endless cycles of poverty and cost developing economies billions of dollars every year [48].

5. Mass drug administration and its inadequacy to control *Schistosomiasis* in Africa

Schistosomiasis control and elimination involve several strategies ranging from disease treatment to managing complications and controlling disease transmission with a combination of preventive chemotherapy dispersed through MDAs, and water, sanitation, and hygiene (WASH) programs [7, 19, 49, 50]. The focus of the WHO plan for *schistosomiasis* control and elimination is on preventive chemotherapy, particularly MDAs in sub-Saharan Africa [51]. Although some progress has been made such as partnerships with donor foundations, interventions of international organizations like Merck the producer of *praziquantel,* and the exercise of large-scale treatments [7, 52]. There is because *Praziquantel* has been considered cost-effective, relatively safe, inexpensive, and effective; with donor organizations willing to provide the drug at no cost making it the only viable choice for the treatment of *schistosomiasis* [19].

Praziquantel is the key bullet for *schistosomiasis* control and elimination, however, Onasanya and colleagues [51], observed that in practice is reactive instead of proactive and is an unavoidable consequence of a one-size-fits-all approach. According to them, this reactive approach is limiting for several reasons. They stated that firstly, despite the "efforts at making *praziquantel* available to those in need and Merck KGaA's commitment to *praziquantel* donations, targets for MDAs coverage have still not reached all people at risk who require treatment" [51, 53]. This they said, "may indicate an under-representation or undercount of cases based on low-level awareness" [8, 12, 54], the disease may be introduced to new or previously eliminated areas due to our migratory patterns [4, 55, 56], it is safe to assume that the similarity of the disease makes its transmission easy across different tropical regions and countries. For example, countries like Nigeria have prioritized *praziquantel* for SAC but leave out adults and preschool children during MDAs [54]. In this context, it implies that *schistosomiasis* cannot be effectively eliminated in communities where MDAs treatment is on-ongoing.

Secondly, it was noted that, although there is a commitment to the donation of *praziquantel*, there is a high chance of recrudescence of disease to pre-MDAs levels once donations reduce or cease, or even during MDAs programs [57, 58]. Thirdly, "*praziquantel* itself has not demonstrated 100% curative ability in both single-dose and multi-dose regimens in various settings, implying that relying only on *praziquantel* treatment use during MDAs is not an effective strategy for control and elimination of this disease" [59–61]. Fourthly, "given the neglected nature of the disease in most healthcare systems in sub-Saharan Africa, there is currently inadequate funding for the disease from the national governments which is likely to persist or worsen in the future once the current external funding and support are reduced. They also noted that there is also a potential for donor fatigue as current gains in treatment to be reversed when donation stops because countries do not have sustainable strategies to own and incorporate programs within their current healthcare systems" [62].

Lastly, Onasayan and colleagues submitted that the disease context is complex with an interplay of social, economic, political, and cultural factors that may affect achieving the goals of the NTD 2021–2030 Roadmap [56, 63, 64]. Affirming that in light of the daunting challenges, there is a need to revisit the current top-down approach to *schistosomiasis* control among sub-Saharan African countries irrespective of the level of the endemicity. From the angle of WHO, there have been several resolutions over time toward the control and elimination of *schistosomiasis*, including renewing interest, addressing partnerships, for example in 2012, the need to attach importance to both preventative and control strategies by developing applicable plans with progressive targets was initiated [20]. Moreover, "in 2013, the WHA66.12 resolution on NTDs focused on advocating for continuous country ownership of programs for NTD prevention, control, elimination, and eradication" [7, 49]. "The current roadmap for 2021–2030 for NTDs also reiterates the importance of community-based and applied research for effective NTD programs, it highlights the need to integrate mainstream approaches into national healthcare systems, coordinate action across sectors, and close coordination and multi-sectoral action across all sectors" [50].

We may wonder if enough literature has not been done on *schistosomiasis* control. But Mazigo and colleagues [65], simply noted that planning and implementation of *schistosomiasis* control activities requires an understanding of the prevalence, intensity of infection, and geographical distribution of the disease in different epidemiological settings. It is safe to assume that the reasons why preventive chemotherapy strategy for *schistosomiasis* fails sometimes are the lack of understanding of the geographical distribution of the disease and the infection level in endemic communities living in different geographical settings [65]. For effectiveness, therefore, Mazigo and colleagues [65], pointed out the importance of identifying areas where infections have continued to be a public health problem despite repeated rounds of MDAs. Noting that this will allow the development of focused integrated control measures. Generalizing from Tanzania research, they affirmed that in many of the *schistosomiasis* endemic countries, there is inadequate attention given to research on the geographical distribution of *schistosomiasis* in other areas outside the historically known and highly researched areas.

5.1 Use of preventive chemotherapy and proposition for Africa traditional medication to control *Schistosomiasis*

If *schistosomiasis* affects the intestine and is not attended to in the time it can become complex and lead to critical organ failure [66, 67]. To prevent this, the single dose of *praziquantel* (PZQ) has been prescribed as a first-line treatment since 2005 with the remarkable success achieved against *schistosomiasis* through targeted mass chemotherapy [52]. According to Moon [68], PZQ was discovered in the 1970s and approved for human use in the United States of America in 1982. For effectiveness and in pursuant of elimination of *schistosomiasis*, preventive treatment should be repeated over several years, to reduce and prevent morbidity [6].

Some progress has been recorded by the World Health Organization (WHO), in 2017 for example, it was estimated that out of at least 290.8 million infected people, and about 98.7 million were treated for *schistosomiasis* [69]. The statistics account for less than 30% of the infected population receiving treatment. What possible factors could be responsible for the low coverage? Hotez, and colleagues [70] attributed the inadequate coverage to cost. Other scholars argued that PZQ has its limitations. For instance, it has the property that reduced *prophylactic* effect at the recommended doses against immature stages [71, 72]. Others claimed that there is little data on PZQ safety and efficacy in preschool children leading to the exclusion of this age group from chemotherapy preventive control programs [73], and others said that there is no oral formulation for infants and preschool children [74]. It was even concluded that the drug has no effect if the liver and spleen are seriously affected [33].

A report from Nigeria shows treatment once annually with *praziquantel* for *schistosomiasis* infections, which is said to be effective for the treatment of all species of *schistosomiasis* [39]. According to some scholars [75], this program was said to have been achieved through school-based deworming (SBD) carried out by the State Ministries of Health in collaboration with the Federal Ministry of Health Nigeria (FMoH), WHO, and other nongovernmental organizations (NGOs). This program according to research [30], offers treatment of all school children in the country. However, due to the poor environment as well as poor hygiene behavior by individuals, reinfection occurs rapidly after treatment.

Though PZQ appears safe and effective against all adult *Schistosomiasis* species in general [76], further research is needed to understand the efficacy and safety of various doses for different *Schistosoma* species. "Some studies reported PZQ therapeutic failure up to 40%" [77, 78]. What should be the main concern? First is the heavy reliance on the single available drug, which studies show has been in use for the past 40 years. Secondly, is the tendencies for drug resistance which is an eventual scenario for any drug, and PZQ cannot be an exception [79]. Hence, there is a need to search for novel drugs against all *schistosomiasis* lifecycle, (see **Figure 1**) and the stages of the parasite with considerations for both pediatric and adult use.

Onasanya and colleagues seem confused because of the lack of clarity on how sub-Saharan African countries would achieve the targets beyond the desire for easy wins through the use of *praziquantel* as a reactive way to achieve the aims of control and elimination of *schistosomiasis* [51]. They stated that if *schistosomiasis* control is to be attained, then it will require a dynamic approach that incorporates more proactive and holistic strategies beyond the current top-down approach. Affirming that such an approach most of the necessity incorporates the socio-cultural, epidemiological, economic, and geographical dynamics within each country to create a mix-set of feasible strategies for *schistosomiasis* control.

Consequently, the WHO calls for the need to eliminate *schistosomiasis* by 2030, and proposed the development of new intervention tools and alternative drugs to PZQ [52].

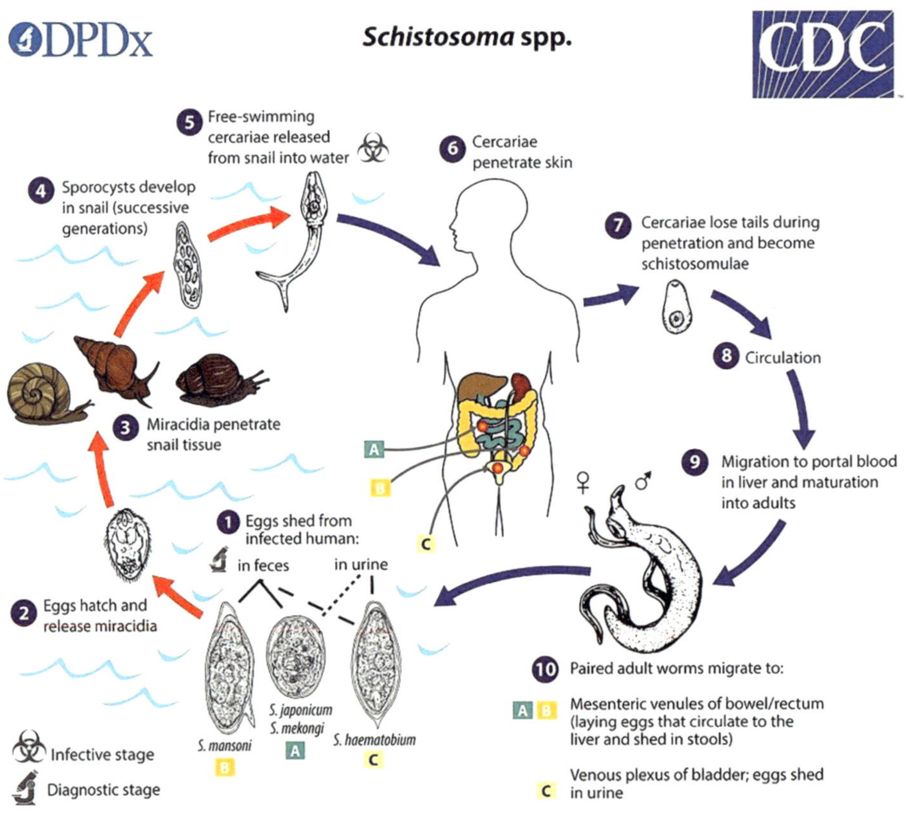

Figure 1.
Schistosomiasis life cycle. Sources: CDC [10]. Available at: https://www.cdc.gov/parasites/schistosomiasis/biology.html.

Scholars are of the view that most modern drugs have their root in traditional medicine, as noted that nearly 30% or more of the modern pharmacological drugs are derived directly or indirectly from plants [80, 81]. Notably, African people are majorly from low-income countries relying heavily on traditional medicine for the treatment of all forms of ailment including *schistosomiasis* and other parasitic diseases [26]. In Ethiopia a large number of communities, particularly in rural areas, rely on traditional medicinal plants to fight several diseases including *schistosomiasis* [82, 83], this is not different from Ghana, Nigeria, Mali, Senegal, and other African countries. One scholar argued that the reasons why people practice traditional medicine are the high cost of modern drugs, paucity and inaccessibility of modern health services, and cultural acceptability of traditional medicine [82]. However, observation shows that in health pathways some African combine both modern and traditional medicine in health help-seeking behavior. Some participants in Nigeria affirmed that there are medicinal plants that have already shown therapeutic efficiency against *schistosomiasis* infection [26]. When will the goal of total elimination of *schistosomiasis* be achieved?

6. Global Health Agenda and *Schistosomiasis* control campaign in Africa

The global health agenda can be traced to the World Health Organization and the World Health Assembly (WHA) in 1975, when the Executive Board called for an international conference to address the conspicuous inequalities in health and health services between countries [84, 85]. In the said conference WHA adopted the call to scale up efforts in drug development, proper engineering design of water management projects, and mobilization of partners for *schistosomiasis* control [86]. In the following year, in 1976, a resolution was passed on the need to consider the epidemiological aspects of the disease during the planning and implementation of water management schemes in endemic countries [23]. The resolution considered the need to implement measures to prevent the spread of *schistosomiasis* to new geographical locations [87]. In 1977, WHA specified that the central social goal of WHO was the level of "acceptable" health that would allow a "socially and economically productive life" for all people by 2000 and called on nation-states to work toward this goal [85]. To pursue this agenda, the primary health care framework was formulated at the Alma-Ata conference in 1978 [88]. The purpose of the Alma-Ata Declaration was to influence strategies, policies, and programs of national and global communities for the next two decades. The declaration emphasized the need to provide "Health for All" by adequate collaboration between biomedical and traditional sectors, in order to encourage encompasses approaches to health care that incorporated community development and community participation [85].

Oyeyemi and colleagues noted that while these efforts recorded some positive outcomes in some countries, the situations in sub-Saharan African countries were rather the same [23]. Another research confirmed the lack of interest in the *schistosomiasis* control campaign in sub-Saharan Africa as other diseases were given more priority in the region's health agenda [89]. Little or no efforts were recorded between the 1970s after the Agenda to the year 2001 when significant results were expected. For example, Oyeyemi and colleagues said there was no single record of an epidemiological study on *schistosomiasis* in some Nigerian States [23]. They, however, agreed that most of the notable *schistosomiasis* control strategies in Nigeria started in the late 2000s.

Over the years, several resolutions aimed toward improvement on *schistosomiasis* control have been made with great commitment but little or no achievement, portraying the African countries like a dancer, dancing around in a cycle. However, there seems to be a resurgent in recent years, as the control of *schistosomiasis* and other NTDs started to have some level of awareness and taken the priority list of some African governments, international organizations, and donors among others [7]. The resurgent can be traced to the WHA 54.19 resolution on *schistosomiasis* and soil-transmitted helminths on attaining at least 75% regular treatment benchmark of all school-aged children in endemic communities by 2010, endorsed in 2001 by the WHO member states [23, 90]. But it took more than a decade for some countries to come up with a national action plan for the control of NTDs. For example, a well-organized control implementation for the *schistosomiasis* program was only supported after the year 2010 by the Nigerian government [23]. As of January 2012, when WHO published NTDs Roadmap, it described the strategic approach to fast-track work to overcome the global impact of NTDs, targeting the period of 2012–2020 [91]. These resolutions received the overwhelming support of donors, member states, and other stakeholders who pledged their support for the WHO Roadmap and its 2020 target [51, 91], in the same 2012, the WHA 65.21 resolution on the elimination of *schistosomiasis* was endorsed [92].

Consequently, all affected regions (See, **Figure 2** and **Table 3**) are to strengthen the control interventions and surveillance and embark on *schistosomiasis* elimination where possible [19]. So, in the year 2013 WHA 66.12 resolution on NTDs, member states were to take ownership of NTDs' various control programs [49]. Then, between

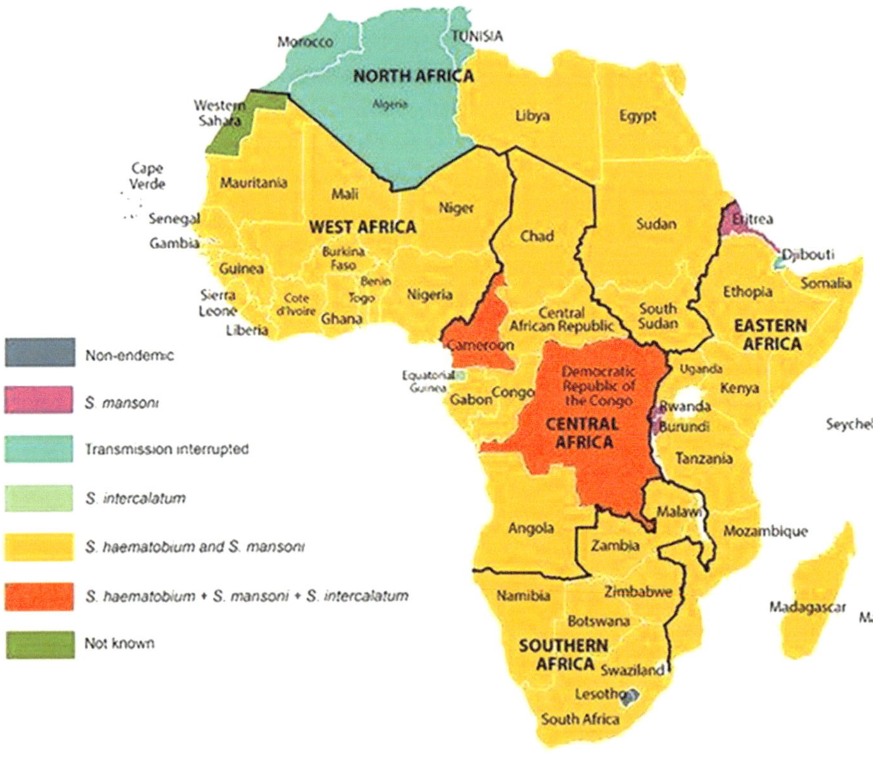

Figure 2.
Principal places affected by Schistosomiasis in Africa. Sources: MDPI [93]. Available at: https://www.mdpi.com/2414-6366/6/3/109.

Name	Value
Africa	218,779,749
Americas	2,252,917
Eastern Mediterranean	17,275,612
European	Not applicable
South-East Asia	24,179
Western Pacific	2,937,454
Global	241,269,911

Source: WHO [33].

Table 3.
Schistosomiasis global statistics.

the years 2015 and 2020, three time-bound goals for control of *schistosomiasis* were set by the WHO NTD Roadmap for the Mediterranean Region, Americas, Western Pacific, and sub-Saharan African countries [7, 23]. Oyeyemi and colleagues, assert that although the WHO NTDs Roadmap envisaged the potential elimination of *schistosomiasis* in some countries in the sub-Saharan region by 2020, it was certain that this feat was unachievable by the end of 2020 [23]. They assumed that conflict in the Nigerian communities might have contributed to the non-realization of the control of *schistosomiasis*. They also alluded to the COVID-19 pandemic as a possible impediment to *schistosomiasis* control implementation programs in Nigeria. The question is, would the WHO NTDs 2020 target have been realized in the absence of conflict and the current pandemic? The answer is possibly a no, going by the previous patterns of attention given to previous resolutions. It was, however, affirmed that epidemiological evidence suggests that the country has a long way to go and a new WHO NTDs Roadmap for control or elimination of *schistosomiasis* is inevitable [23], now that there is a new roadmap for 2021–2030 [52]. Following the previous pattern of late implementation, the presence of other diseases of priority such as COVID-19 and incessant conflict in Africa, are we not going to be singing the same song of a long way to go? We may need time to tell, since the new resolution just began, it may be too early to judge if it will succeed or fail.

7. Conclusion

Historically *schistosomiasis* in Africa can be traced to the Egyptian mummies of the twentieth dynasty, it has spread over the continents with the highest global burden in the world. Despite several efforts brought forth to combat the disease is still categorized among the neglected tropical diseases for several reasons. It is not all affected populations that are treated during MDAs, also certain symptoms look like that of other diseases, mode of transmission also are associated with the people social and occupational activities, sometimes *schistosomiasis* is missed diagnosis and devices for the diagnosis are expensive. The high cost of logistics and the exclusion of adults and out-of-school children during mass drug administration are possible factors that promote continuous transmission of *schistosomiasis* in Africa. *Schistosomiasis* and other NTDs affect close to 2 billion people with other indirect consequences such as disability, stigma, truancy, abscond from duty, poverty, and economic loss. With all the concerted effort of government, donors, and WHO, the MDAs is still inadequate to control *schistosomiasis* in Africa. Maybe because of the inadequate attention is given to research on the geographical distribution of schistosomiasis in other areas outside the researched areas. There is current advocacy for the use of traditional medicine as an additional effort to combat schistosomiasis in Africa. This is because several declarations and roadmap for the control and elimination program have failed, we hope that the 2030 target will be a success.

Conflict of interest

The authors declare no conflict of interest.

Note

I deeply appreciate my wife and children, for their understanding, when I was supposed to have time for them during the Christmas holiday, they allowed me to concentrate on the write-up, love you dearly.

Author details

Adetayo Olorunlana
Caleb University, Imota-Lagos, Nigeria

*Address all correspondence to: adetayo.olorunlana@calebuniversity.edu.ng

References

[1] Engels D, Zhou X. Neglected tropical diseases: An effective global response to local poverty-related disease priorities. Infectious Diseases of Poverty. 2020;**9**:10. DOI: 10.1186/s40249-020-0630-9

[2] Olorunlana A, Jegede AS, Morenikeji O, Hassan A, Nwuba R, Anumudu C, et al. Persistent Transmission of *Schistosomiasis* in Southwest Nigeria: Contexts of culture and contact with infected River Water. World Health & Population. 2016;**16**(3):31-38

[3] WHO. Schistosomiasis Fact Sheet. World Health Organization; 2020 Available from: https://www.who.int/news-room/fact-sheets/detail/schistosomiasis [Accessed: December 9, 2021]

[4] Olorunlana A. European migrant crisis: Health and policy implications. *Irinkerindo:* African Journal of Migration. 2019;**10**:52-80

[5] WHO. Schistosomiasis. 2019. Available from: https://www.who.int/news-room/fact-sheets/detail/schistosomiasis [Accessed: December 9, 2021]

[6] WHO. Schistosomiasis. 2012. Available from: https://www.who.int/news-room/fact-sheets/detail/schistosomiasis [Accessed: December 9, 2021]

[7] Tchuem-Tchuenté LA, Rollinson D, Stothard JR, Molyneux D. Moving from control to elimination of schistosomiasis in sub-Saharan Africa: Time to change and adapt strategies. Infectious Diseases of Poverty. 2017;**6**:42. DOI: 10.1186/s40249-017-0256-8

[8] Ezeh CO, Onyekwelu KC, Akinwale OP, Shan L, Wei H. Urinary schistosomiasis in Nigeria: A 50-year review of prevalence, distribution and disease burden. Parasite. 2019;**26**:19. DOI: 10.1051/parasite/2019020

[9] Chitsulo L, Engels D, Montresor A, Savioli L. The global status of schistosomiasis and its control. Acta Tropica. 2000;**77**:41-51. DOI: 10.1016/S0001-706X(00)00122-4

[10] CDC. Schistosomiasis. Centers for Disease Control and Prevention. 2019. Available from: https://www.cdc. gov/dpdx/schistosomiasis/index.html

[11] WHO. Schistosomiasis: Number of people treated worldwide. Weekly Epidemiological Record. 2018;**93**:681-692 World Health Organization, Geneva, Switzerland

[12] King CH. Parasites and poverty: The case of schistosomiasis. Acta Tropica. 2010;**113**(2):95-104. DOI: 10.1016/j.actatropica.11.012

[13] Lai YS, Biedermann P, Ekpo UF, et al. Spatial distribution of schistosomiasis and treatment needs in sub-Saharan Africa: A systematic review and geostatistical analysis. The Lancet Infectious Diseases. 2015;**15**(8):927-940

[14] Nebe OJ, Anagbogu IN, Ngige EN, Isiyaku S, Adamani WEMA, Nwobi BC. Epidemiological mapping of schistosomiasis and soil-transmitted helminthiasis in 19 states and the federal capital territory (FCT), Nigeria. The American Journal of Tropical Medicine and Hygiene. 2017;**95**(5):559. DOI: 10.4269/ajtmh.abstract2016

[15] LoVerde PT. Schistosomiasis. In: Toledo R, Bernard F, editors. Digenetic

Trematodes. 2nd ed. New York, NY: Springer-Verlag; 2019. pp. 45-70

[16] Ajibola O, Gulumbe B, Eze A, Obishakin E. Tools for detection of schistosomiasis in resource-limited settings. Medical Science. 2018;**6**:39. DOI: 10.3390/medsci6020039

[17] Le L, Hsieh MH. Diagnosing urogenital schistosomiasis: Dealing with diminishing returns. Trends in Parasitology. 2017;**33**:378-387. DOI: 10.1016/j.pt.2016.12.009

[18] Olorunlana A. Government health policies: Scaling up from control to elimination of *schistosomiasis* in Nigeria. In Proceedings of Nigeria Anthropological and Sociological Association NASA Annual Conference 3-5 November 2014; LASU, Lagos: NASA, 216-224. 2014

[19] WHO. Accelerating Work to Overcome the Global Impact of Neglected Tropical Diseases: A Roadmap for Implementation. 2012; Available from: https://www.who.int/neglected_diseases/en [Accessed: December 25, 2021]

[20] WHO. Schistosomiasis: Progress Report 2001-2011, Strategic Plan 2012-2020, World Health Organization, GEN. 2013. Available from: https://apps .who.int/iris/handle/10665/78074 [Accessed: December 13, 2021]

[21] Stothard JR, Campbell SJ, Osei-Atweneboana MY, et al. Towards interruption of schistosomiasis transmission in sub-Saharan Africa: Developing an appropriate environmental surveillance framework to guide and to support "end game" interventions. Infectious Diseases of Poverty. 2017;**6**(1):2253-2264

[22] Deol AK, Fleming FM, Calvo-Urbano B, Walker M, Bucumi V, GnandouI, etal. Schistosomiasis: Assessing progress towards the 2020 and 2025 global goals. New England Journal of Medicine. 2019;**381**(26):2519-2528

[23] Oyeyemi OT, Jeremias WD, Grenfell RFQ. Schistosomiasis in Nigeria: Gleaning from the past to improve current efforts towards control. Elsevier One Health. 2020. DOI: 10.1016/j.onehlt.2020.100183

[24] Di Bella S, Riccardi N, Giacobbe DR, Luzzati R. History of schistosomiasis (bilharziasis) in humans: From Egyptian medical papyri to molecular biology on mummies. Pathogens and Global Health. 2018;**112**:268-273

[25] Appleton CC, Naidoo I. Why did schistosomiasis disappear from the southern part of the Eastern Cape? South African Journal of Science. 2012;**108**:1-11

[26] Olorunlana A. Perception of health-risk and Control of Schistosomiasis in Yewa North, Ogun State, Nigeria [thesis]. Department of Sociology, Faculty of the Social Sciences, University of Ibadan; 2016

[27] Onasanya A, Keshinro M, Oladepo O, Van Engelen J, Diehl JC. A stakeholder analysis of Schistosomiasis diagnostic landscape in South-West Nigeria: Insights for diagnostics co-creation. Frontiers in Public Health. 2020;**8**:564381. DOI: 10.3389/fpubh.2020.564381

[28] WHO. Working to Overcome the Global Impact of Neglected Tropical Diseases. First WHO report on Neglected Tropical Diseases. Geneva: Word Health Organization; 2010. Available from: https://www.who.int/neglected_diseases/resources/9789241564090/en/ [Accessed: December 9, 2021]

[29] Markel SF, LoVerde PT, Britt EM. Prolonged latent schistosomiasis. Journal

of the American Medical Association. 1978;**240**:1746-1747

[30] GiveWell. School-Based Deworming in Cross River State, Nigeria. 2018. Available from: https://www.givewell.org/files/DWDA%202009/DtWI/Deworm_the_World_Cross_River_State_PMCV_report_October_2018.pdf [Accessed: December 13, 2021].

[31] Isere E, Fatiregun A, Ajayi I. An overview of disease surveillance and notification system in Nigeria and the roles of clinicians in disease outbreak prevention and control. Nigerian Medical Journal. 2015;**56**:161-168. DOI: 10.4103/0300-1652.160347

[32] Sturrock RF. Guidelines for the evaluation of soil-transmitted helminthiasis and schistosomiasis at the community level: A guide for managers of control programs. Transactions of the Royal Society of Tropical Medicine and Hygiene. 1998;**92**:470-471

[33] WHO. Control of Neglected Tropical Diseases. Pretoria South Africa: World Health Organisation; 2021. Available from: https://www.who.int/team/control-of-neglected-tropical-diseases/schistosomiasis/epidemiology [Accessed: December 25, 2021]

[34] Uchendu O, Oladoyin V, Idowu M, Adeyera O, Olabisi O, Oluwatosin O, et al. Urinary schistosomiasis among vulnerable children in a rehabilitation home in Ibadan, Oyo State, Nigeria. BMC Infectious Diseases. 2017;**17**:487. DOI: 10.1186/s12879-017-2591-6

[35] Braun-Munzinger RA, Southgate BA. Repeatability and reproducibility of egg counts of Schistosoma haematobium in urine. Tropical Medicine and Parasitology. 1992;**43**:149-154

[36] Weber MD, Blair DM, Clark VV. The pattern of schistosome egg distribution in a micturition flow. The Central African Journal of Medicine. 1967;**13**:75-88

[37] Worrell CM, Bartoces M, Karanja DMS, Ochola EA, Matete DO, Mwinzi PNM, et al. Cost analysis of tests for the detection of Schistosoma mansoni infection in children in western Kenya. The American Journal of Tropical Medicine and Hygiene. 2015;**92**:1233-1239. DOI: 10.4269/ajtmh.14-0644

[38] Steinmann P, Keiser J, Bos R, Tanner M, Utzinger J. Schistosomiasis and water resources development: Systematic review, meta-analysis, and estimates of people at risk. The Lancet Infectious Diseases. 2006;**6**:411-425. DOI: 10.1016/S1473-3099(06)70521-7

[39] Adenowo AF, Oyinloye BE, Ogunyinka BI, Kappo AP. Impact of human schistosomiasis in sub-Saharan Africa. The Brazilian Journal of Infectious Diseases. 2015;**19**:196-205. DOI: 10.1016/j.bjid.2014.11.004

[40] Rollinson D et al. Time to set the agenda for schistosomiasis elimination. Acta Tropica. 2012;**128**:423-440

[41] Senghor B, Diaw OT, Doucoure S, Seye M, Diallo A, Talla I, et al. Impact of annual praziquantel treatment on urogenital schistosomiasis in seasonal transmission focus in central Senegal. PLoS Neglected Tropical Diseases. 2016;**10**(3):e0004557

[42] Hotez PJ, Fenwick A, Savioli L, Molyneux DH. Rescuing the bottom billion through control of neglected tropical diseases. Lancet. 2009;**373**:1570-1575. DOI: 10.1016/S0140-6736(09)60233-6

[43] Ndassi VD, Anchang-Kimbi JK, Sumbele IUN, Wepnje GB, Kimbi HK. Prevalence and risk factors associated with S.haematobium egg excretion

during the dry season, six months following mass distribution of praziquantel (PZQ) in 2017 in the Bafia Health Area, South West Region Cameroon: A cross-sectional study. Journal of Parasitology Research. 2019;**2019**(19):4397263

[44] Green AE, Anchang-Kimbi JK, Wepnje GB, Ndassi VD, Kimbi HK. Distribution and factors associated with urogenital schistosomiasis in the Tiko Health District, a semi-urban setting, South West Region, Cameroon. BMC Infectious Disease of Poverty. 2021;**10**:49. DOI: 10.1186/s40249-021-00827-2

[45] Umeh JC, Amali O, Umeh EU. The socio-economic effects of tropical diseases in Nigeria. Economics and Human Biology. 2004;**2**:245-263. DOI: 10.1016/j.ehb.2004.04.001

[46] GBD. DALYs and HALE Collaborators. Global, regional, and national disability-adjusted life-years (DALYs) for 333 diseases and injuries and healthy life expectancy (HALE) for 195 countries and territories, 1990-2016: A systematic analysis for the Global Burden of Disease Study. Lancet. 2016;**390**:1260-1344

[47] Hotez PJ, Molyneux DH, Fenwick A, Kumaresan J, Sachs SE, Sachs JD, et al. Control of neglected tropical diseases. The New England Journal of Medicine. 2007;**357**(10):1018-1027. DOI: 10.1056/NEJMra064142

[48] Rees CA, Hotez PJ, Monuteaux MC, Niescierenko M, Bourgeois FT. Neglected tropical diseases in children: An assessment of gaps in research prioritization. PLoS Neglected Tropical Diseases. 2019;**13**(1):e0007111

[49] WHO. World Health Organization. World Health Assembly Resolution WHA 66.12 Neglected Tropical Diseases. Geneva: World Health Organization; Report No.:WHA 2013;66.12

[50] WHO. Schistosomiasis Status of Schistosomiasis endemic countries 2020, 2020. Available from: https://apps.who.int/neglected-diseases/ntddata/sch/sch.html [Accessed: December 13, 2021]

[51] Onasanya A, Bengtson M, Oladepo O, Van Engelen J Diehl JC. Rethinking the top-down approach to Schistosomiasis control and elimination in Sub-Saharan Africa. Frontiers in Public Health. 2021;**9**:622809. DOI: 10.3389/fpubh.2021.622809

[52] WHO. Ending the Neglect to Attain the Sustainable Development Goals: A Road Map for Neglected Tropical Diseases 2021-2030. Geneva, Switzerland: World Health Organization; 2020

[53] WHO. World Health Organization. Schistosomiasis: Number of people treated worldwide in 2018. Weekly Epidemiological Record= Relevé épidémiologique hebdomadaire. 2019;**94**:601-612. Available from: https://www.who.int/wer/2019/wer9450/en/ [Accessed: December 13, 2021]

[54] Van GY, Onasanya A, Van Engelen J, Oladepo O, Diehl JC. Improving access to diagnostics for schistosomiasis case management in Oyo State, Nigeria: Barriers and opportunities. Diagnostics. 2020;**10**:328. DOI: 10.3390/diagnostics10050328

[55] Marchese V, Beltrame A, Angheben A, Monteiro GB, Giorgi G, Prandin F, et al. Schistosomiasis in immigrants, refugees and travelers in an Italian referral centre for tropical diseases. Infectious Diseases of Poverty. 2018;**7**:55. DOI: 10.1186/s40249-018-0440-5

[56] Parker M, Allen T. Does mass drug administration for the integrated treatment of neglected tropical diseases really work? Assessing evidence for the control of schistosomiasis and soil-transmitted helminths in Uganda. Health Res Policy Syst. 2011;**9**:3. DOI: 10.1186/1478-4505-9-3

[57] Kittur N, Binder S, Campbell CH, King CH, Kinung'hi S, Olsen A, et al. Defining persistent hotspots: Areas that fail to decrease meaningfully in prevalence after multiple years of mass drug administration with praziquantel for control of schistosomiasis. The American Journal of Tropical Medicine and Hygiene. 2017;**97**:1810-1817. DOI: 10.4269/ajtmh.17-0368

[58] Wiegand RE, Mwinzi PNM, Montgomery SP, Chan YL, Andiego K, Olmedo M, et al. A persistent hotspot of Schistosoma mansoni infection in a five-year randomized trial of praziquantel preventative chemotherapy strategies. The Journal of Infectious Diseases. 2017;**216**:1425-1433. DOI: 10.1093/infdis/jix496

[59] El Ridi RAF, Tallima HA-M. Novel therapeutic and prevention approaches for schistosomiasis: Review. Journal of Advanced Research. 2013;**4**:467-478. DOI: 10.1016/j.jare.2012.05.002

[60] Hoekstra PT, Casacuberta Partal M, Amoah AS, van Lieshout L, Corstjens PLAM, Tsonaka S, et al. Repeated doses of praziquantel in schistosomiasis treatment (RePST): Single versus multiple praziquantel treatments in school-aged children in Côte d'Ivoire: A study protocol for an open-label, randomised controlled trial. BMC Infectious Diseases. 2018;**18**:662. DOI: 10.1186/s12879-018-3554-2

[61] Munisi DZ, Buza J, Mpolya EA, Angelo T, Kinung'hi SM. The efficacy of single-dose versus double-dose praziquantel treatments on Schistosoma mansoni infections: Its implication on undernutrition and anaemia among primary school children in two on-shore communities, Northwestern Tanzania. BioMed Research International. 2017. DOI: 10.1155/2017/7035025

[62] Glenn J, Kamara K, Umar ZA, Chahine T, Daulaire N, Bossert T. Applied systems thinking: A viable approach to identify leverage points for accelerating progress towards ending neglected tropical diseases. Health Research Policy and Systems. 2020;**18**:56. DOI: 10.1186/s12961-020-00570-4

[63] Parker M, Polman K, Allen T. Neglected tropical diseases in biosocial perspective. Journal of Biosocial Science. 2016;**48**:S1-S15. DOI: 10.1017/S0021932016000274

[64] Mwanga JR, Kinung'hi SM, Mosha J, Angelo T, Maganga J, Campbell C. Village response to mass drug administration for schistosomiasis in Mwanza region, Northwestern Tanzania: Are we missing socioeconomic, cultural, and political dimensions? The American Journal of Tropical Medicine and Hygiene. 2020;**103**:1969-1977. DOI: 10.4269/ajtmh.19-0843

[65] Mazigo HD, Uisso C, Kazyoba P, Nshala A, Mwingira UJ. Prevalence, infection intensity and geographical distribution of schistosomiasis among pre-school and school-aged children in villages surrounding Lake Nyasa, Tanzania. Scientific Report: Nature Research. 2021;**11**:295. DOI: 10.1038/s41598-020-80317-x

[66] Costain AH, MacDonald AS, Smits HH. Schistosome egg migration: Mechanisms, pathogenesis, and host immune responses. Frontiers in Immunology. 2018;**9**:3042

[67] Schwartz C, Fallon PG. Schistosoma "eggs-iting" the host: Granuloma formation and egg excretion. Frontiers in Immunology. 2018;**9**:2492

[68] Moon, A. History of Praziquantel. 2006. Available from: http://www.stanford.edu/group/parasites/ParaSites2006/Praziquantel/history.html [Accessed: December 13, 2021]

[69] WHO. Schistosomiasis. World Health Organization; 2018. Available from: https://www.who.int/schistosomiasis/en/ [Accessed: December 13, 2021]

[70] Hotez PJ, Engels D, Fenwick A, Savioli L. Africa is desperate for praziquantel, 2010. Lancet. 2010;**376**(9740):496-498

[71] Silva LM, Menezes R, Oliveira SA, Andrade ZA. Chemotherapeutic effects on larval stages of *Schistosoma mansoni* during infection and re-infection of mice, 2003. Revista da Sociedade Brasileira de Medicina Tropical. 2003;**36**(3):335-341

[72] Pica-Mattoccia L, Cioli D. Sex- and stage-related sensitivity of Schistosoma mansoni to in vivo and in vitro praziquantel treatment. International Journal for Parasitology. 2004;**34**(4):527-533

[73] Keiser J, Ingram-Sieber K, Utzinger J. Antiparasitic drugs for pediatrics: Systematic review, formulations, pharmacokinetics, safety, efficacy and implications for control. Parasitology. 2011;**138**:1620-1632

[74] Stothard JR, Gabrielli AF. Schistosomiasis in African infants and preschool children: To treat or not to treat? African infants and preschool children: to treat or not to treat? Trends in Parasitology. 2007;**23**(3):83-86

[75] Opara KN, Wilson EU, Yaro CA, Alkazmi L, Udoidung NI, Chikezie FM, et al. Prevalence, risk factors, and coinfection of urogenital Schistosomiasis and soil-transmitted helminthiasis among Primary School Children in Biase, Southern Nigeria. Hindawi Journal of Parasitology Research. 2021;**12**:6618394. DOI: 10.1155/2021/6618394

[76] Zwang J, Olliaro PL. Clinical efficacy and tolerability of praziquantel for intestinal and urinary schistosomiasis: A meta-analysis of comparative and non-comparative clinical trials. PLoS Neglected Tropical Diseases. 2014;**8**:11

[77] Ismail MM, Farghaly AM, Dyab AK, Afify HA, el-Shafei MA. Resistance to praziquantel, effect of drug pressure and stability test. Journal of the Egyptian Society of Parasitology. 2002;**32**:589-600

[78] Elmasry A, Aladeeb NM, Elkaref A, Aboulfotouh N. Simvastatin exerts antifibrotic effect and potentiates the antischistosomal effects of praziquantel in a murine model: Role of IL10. Biomedicine & Pharmacotherapy. 2017;**96**:215-221

[79] Cioli D, Pica-Mattoccia L, Basso A. Schistosomiasis control: Praziquantel forever? Molecular and Biochemical Parasitology. 2014;**195**(1):23-29

[80] Fabricant DS, Farnsworth NR. The value of plants used in traditional medicine for drug discovery. Environmental Health Perspectives. 2011;**109**:69-75

[81] WHO. Traditional Medicine Strategy 2002-2005. Geneva, Switzerland: World Health Organization; 2002. Available from: https://apps.who.int/iris/handle/10665/67163 [Accessed: December 13, 2021]

[82] Fullas F. The role of indigenous medicinal plants in Ethiopian healthcare. African Renaissance. 2007;**4**(1):76-80

[83] Wondimu T, Asfaw Z, Kelbessa E. Ethnobotanical study of medicinal plants around 'Dheeraa' town, Arsi Zone, Ethiopia. Journal of Ethnopharmacology. 2007;**112**(1):152-161

[84] WHO. From Alma-Ata to the Year 2000; Reflections at the Midpoint. Geneva: World Health Organization; 1988

[85] Olorunlana A. Community participation and disease control: A case of schistosomiasis in Nigeria and other Tropical region. In: Ijadeniyi OA, Oluwadere CT, editors. Sociology of Health in 21st Century Africa. Akure: Omaluka Enterprises; 2017. pp. 386-411

[86] WHO. World Health Assembly Resolution WHA 28.53 Schistosomiasis. Geneva: World Health Organization; 1975. Available from: http://www.who.int/neglected_diseases/mediacentre/WHA_28.53_Eng.pdf?ua=1 [Accessed: December 13, 2021]

[87] WHO. World Health Assembly Resolution WHA 29.58 Schistosomiasis, World Health Organization, Geneva, 1976. Available from: http://www.who.in t/entity/neglected_diseases/mediacentre/WHA_29.58_Eng.pdf?ua=1 [Accessed: December 13, 2021]

[88] WHO. Primary Health Care. Geneva: World Health Organization, (Health for All series); 1978

[89] Tchuem-Tchuente LA. Control of schistosomiasis and soil-transmitted helminthiasis in sub-Saharan Africa: Challenges and prospects. In: Rodrigues A, Morales AJ, editors. Current Topics in Tropical Medicine. 2012. pp. 359-376

[90] WHO. World Health Assembly Resolution WHA 54.19, Elimination of Schistosomiasis. 2001. Available from: http://www.who.int/entity/neglected_diseases/mediacentre/WHA_54.19_Eng.pdf?ua=1 [Accessed: December 13, 2021]

[91] WHO. The London Declaration on Neglected Tropical Diseases. 2012. Available from: http://www.who.int/neglected_diseases/London_Declaration_NTDs.pdf [Accessed: December 13, 2021]

[92] WHO. World Health Assembly Resolution WHA 65.21 Elimination of Schistosomiasis. Geneva: World Health Organization; 2012

[93] MDPI. Schistosomiasis with a focus on Africa. 2021. Available from: https://www.mdpi.com/2414-6366/6/3/109. [Accessed: 2022-02-08]

Section 4

Management, Biology and Control Strategies in Helminth Infections

Chapter 13

Perspective Chapter: Integrated Root-Knot Nematodes (*Meloidogyne*) Management Approaches

Sarir Ahmad, Mehrab Khan and Ikram Ullah

Abstract

Meloidogyne genus contains the most prevalent and harmful worms formally known as root-knot nematode species. They attack a wide range of plants belonging to different plant families. The infective second stage juveniles (J-II) feed on the roots and as a result, the host plant roots become swollen/produce galls. The attack plant shows stunted growth and in extreme cases, the death of the plant occurs. An integrated pest management (IPM) approach is required to tackle these harmful nematodes spp. The integrated tactics include cultural/agronomic practices, biological and chemical control. A sole management method is not enough to deal with the root-knot nematode. Therefore, a proper IPM package is required for the farmer to gain good health for the crops.

Keywords: root-knot nematode, *Meloidogyne*, integrated pest management, parasites, endophytic-nematodes

1. Introduction

Root knot nematodes (RKN) are sedentary internal plant parasites and belong to the genus *Meloidogyne*. The word *Meloidogyne* is originating from Greek that means a cup-shaped female of RKN (**Figure 1**). They cause huge economic losses due to diverse host range and adaptation to vast climatic conditions. Reverend Miles Joseph Berkeley (clergyman) for the first time discovered galls on the cucumber roots in 1855 [1]. The finest work of Chitwood even remains accurate until now; he classified *Meloidogyne* from Heterodera. That is why the current name of Chitwood is used as intermingled for RKN [2]. Most of the species are pathogenic that may reproduce sexually mainly but in certain cases, they may reproduce through asexual means (facultative pathogenesis) [3]. The worm-like males are short-lived and die after matting with a cup-shaped female (**Figure 1**) that is long-lived and penetrates the root tissues to lay about 500 eggs in a sheet formally known as an egg sac (gelatinous sheet). The amateur stages are juvenile (J) I, II, III, and IV. The first two (I and II) are worm-like and only J-II (**Figure 2**) actively feed and move [4]. The biology of RKN is given in **Figure 3**.

IntechOpen

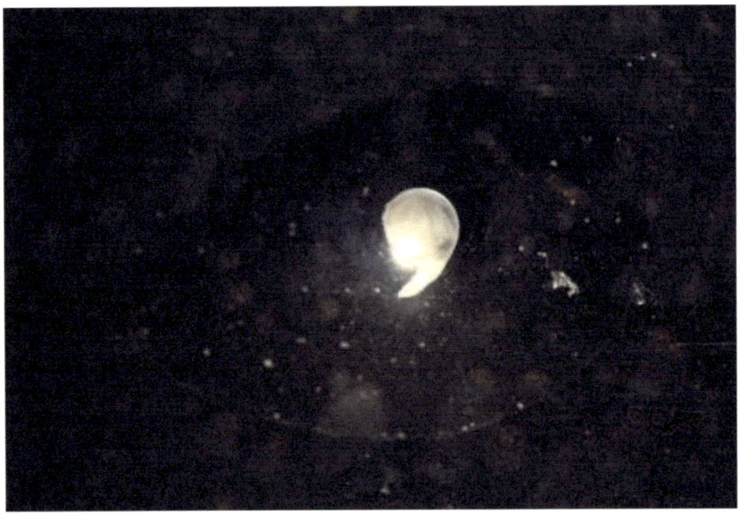

Figure 1.
Adult female of root-knot nematode (microscope view).

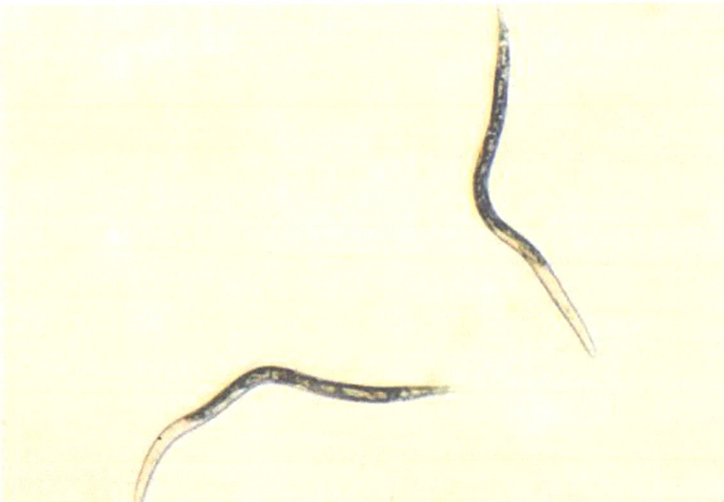

Figure 2.
Juvenile-II female of root-knot nematode (microscope view).

The RKN lacks any rigid skeletal form and thus utilizes the turgor-pressure (TP) for sustaining the bodily shape and locomotion [5]. They possess tiny stylet-like insects that are injected into the plant roots for taking nutrients. The adult female releases secretary proteins that induce the captured cells and cells to become multi-nucleated (with no cell wall formation). This process release protein that is ingested by the RKN through a feeding tube that filters the sap from plant roots. Because of this feeding behavior and cell divisions, the neighboring cells also grow bigger and causing swelling in the roots that ultimately leads to gall formation (**Figure 4**) in the roots [6].

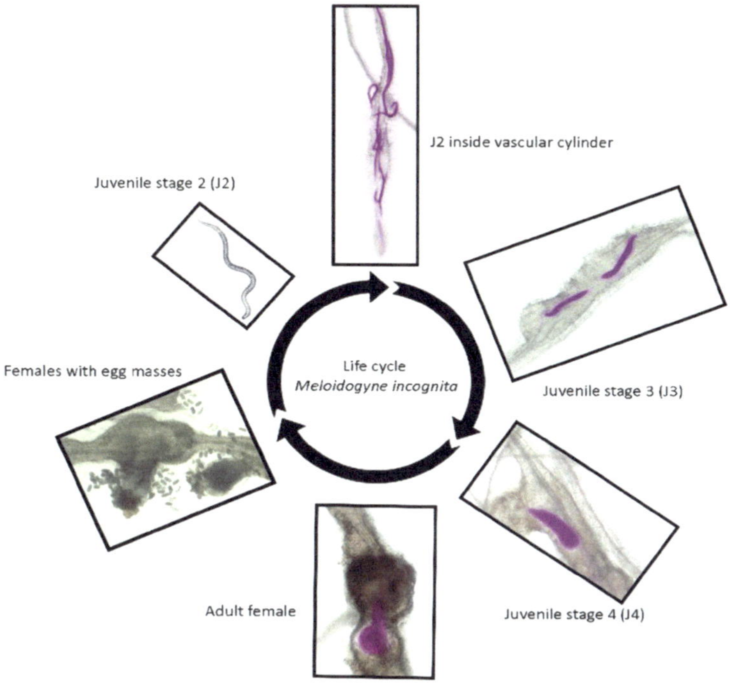

Figure 3.
Lifecycle of root-knot nematode.

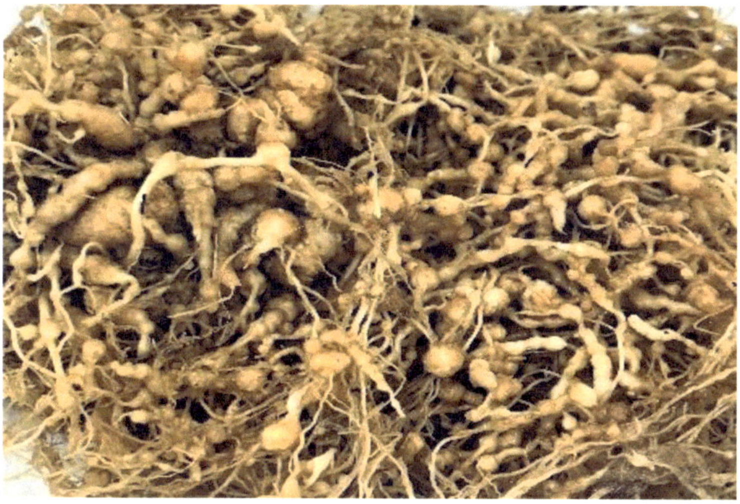

Figure 4.
Galls on infected roots of root-knot nematode.

2. Diversity of root-knot nematode

RKN are among the most successful parasites because of the huge range of hosts and flexible behavior in adapting to a variety of environmental conditions [7]. The

Meloidogyne genus has almost 100 species [8]. However, the four species are of prime significance including *Meloidogyne javanica*, *Meloidogyne arenaria*, *Meloidogyne incognita*, and *M. hapla*) [9].

3. Damages of root-knot nematode

RKN poses a severe danger to the quantity and quality of numerous economic crops around the world. Only the top 20 life-sustaining crops are predicted to suffer an annual crop loss of 12.6% (equivalent to $215.77 billion) due to these worms [10].

The RKN dislodges the vascular system of the host plant and the attacked plant tends to exhibit stunted growth and, death of the seedlings. The RKN infection leaves the plant vulnerable to the attack of other pathogens. The yield declined drastically and in certain cases, the losses may reach up to 90–100% if no management practices are initiated [4].

4. Host range of root-knot nematode

RKN attack a diverse range of plants belonging to different families. The host range is surpassing 5500 plant species. They attack shrubs, trees, ornamental plants, vegetables, and field crops [11].

5. The microbiome of RKN in soil with roots and other microorganisms

The bacterial genera, *Bacillus micrococcus*, *Sphingomonas*, *Rhizobium*, *Methylobacterium*, and *Bosea* exhibit a dominance against J-II of *Meloidogyne hapla*. The fungal genera *Davidiella*, *Rhizophydium*, *Plectosphaerella*, *Lectera*, *Gibellulopsis*, and *Malassezia* suppress J-II of *Meloidogyne incognita*. According to Topalovic et al. [12] that in soil, *Bacillus thuringiensis* and *Plectosphaerella cucumerina* were shown to be associated with *Megalaima incognita* J-II. *B. thuringiensis* produces proteinaceous protoxin crystals {also known as crystal protein or cry protein (CP)} that cause intestinal lysis that leads to nematode death.

Plants have devised a mechanism in which hostile microorganisms in the rhizosphere are selectively stimulated and enriched [13]. The ability of plants to recruit antagonists under various soil management approaches will improve the foundation for new profitable and sustainable microbiome-based crop production systems [14]. Most horticulture growers use harmful chemicals to combat soil-borne infections, whereas organic farmers use conservative practices that preserve soil biodiversity and encourage the RKN antagonistic microbiota. Researchers recently discovered differences in the rhizosphere microbiome under various crop techniques, including impressively low levels of plant pathogens under long-term organic-farming (OF) [15]. Furthermore, microbial shifts in rhizospheres after RKN inoculation suggest that soil can be managed to attract beneficial microorganisms. RKN performance on plant roots should be reduced by the recruitment of microorganisms.

6. Morphometric markers identification of root-knot nematode

Since proper identification of *Meloidogyne* spp. is critical for crop management, a more precise procedure of identification is required. To address this issue, a biochemical procedure of identification was quickly created as a supplement to the morphological way of identification [16]. body width, Body length, stylet length, anal body width, head end to excretory pore, dorsal gland opening, head end to metacorpus valve, esophagus length, hyaline tail length, and tail length are some of the most common morphometric markers used to identify nematodes [17]. Eisenback [18] developed a perennial pattern, head anatomy, and stylet of females to identify *Meloidogyne hapla*, *M. javanica*, *Megalaima incognita*, and *M. arenaria* by using light microscopy (LM) and scanning electron microscopy (SEM). Eisenback [18] distinguished *M. hapla*, *M. javanica*, *M. incognita*, and *M. arenaria* based on stylet morphology and head shape of the males using LM and SEM; produced a visual key based on morphological traits to distinguish *M. hapla*, *M. javanica*, *M. incognita*, and *M. arenaria*. Eisenback [19] successfully distinguished J-II of *Myrmecina graminicola*, *M. nassi*, and *M. javanica* using tail morphology. Furthermore, Eisenback [19] used more comprehensive morphology to identify numerous *Meloidogyne* spp. Identification of nematodes using morphometric data is very simple up to the genus level, but it becomes a difficult task once you get down to the species level. It's not uncommon for major descriptive characteristics from different species to overlap, which can lead to misidentification [17].

7. Molecular techniques for the identification of root-knot nematode

Many fungi, bacteria, and plant-parasitic nematodes have been speciating via polymerase chain reaction (PCR). PCR is a technique that uses a set of primers to amplify a specific region of the genome. PCR can be used to compare genetic similarity or variability between and among species when combined with restriction fragment length polymorphism (RFLP) or sequencing [17]. Powers [20] used the example of a protein-coding 600 nucleotide piece of DNA being able to identify 10 million species based on the variability present on that segment to demonstrate the value of researching DNA that codes for genes. This example illustrates how beneficial PCR may be in differentiating specimens because it amplifies a section of the genome. Denaturation, annealing, and extension are the three processes that make up PCR. To allow the primers to attach to a specific region of single-stranded DNA, double-stranded DNA is de-naturated at a high temperature (90–95°C). Annealing, or the binding of oligonucleotide primers to the target area, takes place at a lower temperature (45–60°C). As the primers attach to the target site, the temperature is raised slightly (70–74°C) to allow the primers to extend on the template DNA with the help of DNA polymerase, a process called extension. To achieve a million-fold amplification of the target location, this technique is routinely performed 30–40 times [17].

8. Root-knot nematode integrated pest management

Integrated pest management (IPM) was defined by Prokopy [21] as "a decision-making procedure involving coordinated employment of numerous methods for maximizing the control of different types of pests (diseases, insects, vertebrates, and weeds) in a way that is both environmentally and economically beneficial. Nematode management is challenging. Preventive approaches, such as sanitation and plant variety selection, are the most reliable. Present infestations can be decreased by following, rotation of crop, and soil solarization. These approaches, however, only work for about a year since they diminish nematodes in the upper foot or soil. They're best used for annual plants or to aid the establishment of young woody plants. If nematodes have infested a crop or an area, struggle to limit infection by shifting dates of the plant to cooler seasons when worms are less active and to make plants more resistant to nematode infection, try to create optimal circumstances for plant growth, such as adequate watering and soil additives [22]. In IPM of root-knot nematode, there are some methods used such as cultural control (crop rotation, sanitation, host plant resistance, solarization, planting, and harvesting dates and irrigation and soil amendments) biological control, and chemical control.

8.1 Cultural control

8.1.1 Management of plant parasite root-knot nematode through crop rotation

The herbivore behavior of RKN has given two good options that can be carried out with crop rotation and change farming methods [23]. In plasticulture systems, control measures such as rotations to non-host crops are restricted because two or more crops vegetables are frequently produced each year on the same land, limiting cycles of rotation. Furthermore, some commercially marketed vegetable types resist nematode [24]. Crop rotation, which involves cultivating non-host crops or resistant types, aims to keep nematode populations below the tolerance limit. By adding non-hosts between sensitive crops, the number of life cycles is reduced significantly, and the nematode population is reduced to a significant level. Crop rotation's effectiveness in reducing the build-up of some plant-parasitic nematodes in cropping systems has been well reported [25]. There is some example such as the rotation of maize with alfalfa or oat it is a non-host crop that can reduce the populations of RKN. Because various species have distinct host ranges, identifying the specific species in the field before relying on crop rotation as a management method is always a good idea [26]. Green manure plants were also tested for their efficiency as crops rotation with beans to reduce RKN. They also explored as basic additions in the control of nematode [27]. *Meloidogyne graminicola*, the rice root-knot nematode, has gained widespread attention due to its ability to cause significant harm in rice-wheat cropping systems. It has emerged as an issue in nurseries and upland rice, as well as its widespread prevalence in deep water and irrigated rice in Southeast Asia's various countries. So the crop rotation of rice with marigold (Tagetes sp.) plays an important role in lowering RKN populations because of its nematicidal properties [28].

8.1.2 Sanitation

Infested soil or plants are commonly used to transfer nematodes into new locations. Use only plants that are free from nematodes acquired from reputable nurseries to keep nematodes out of your garden. Prevent placing plants and soil from affected areas of the garden to control the spread of nematodes. Irrigation water from around infested plants should not be allowed to flow off, as this will propagate nematodes [29].

8.1.3 Resistant or tolerant varieties and rootstocks

Using nematode-resistant vegetable types and fruit tree rootstocks is one of the most effective strategies to manage nematodes. Tomato varieties resistant to nematode species with the code Fusarium, Verticillium, Nematodes (FVN) on the seed packet should be cultivated. Tomatoes that resist nematode produced about six times high tomatoes than a variety susceptible in recent vegetable garden-type studies on root-knot nematode soil [30].

8.1.4 Solarization

Solarization is used to reduce temporarily nematode populations in the upper 12 inches of soil, allowing for the shallow-rooted annual crops production and the establishment of early-stage plants before worm populations rise. Fruit trees, vines, and woody ornamental plants, on the other hand, will not benefit from solarization in the long run. For maximum solarization, moist the soil and cover it with a clear plastic sheet. During the warmest portion of the summer, the sheet should be left in place for 4–6 weeks. When the soil temperature reaches 125°F for 30 min or 130°F for 5 min, RKN, including eggs, die [31].

8.1.5 Planting and harvesting dates

Many nematode species are prevalent during the summer season, and an average temperature below 64°F prevents them from penetrating roots. As a result, farmers could avoid nematode damage to fall-planted crops like carrots, lettuce, spinach, and peas by waiting until soil temperatures drop below 64°F [29].

8.1.6 Irrigation and soil amendments

To lessen the impact of nematodes on crop plants, the soil can be treated using a variety of organic amendments. Manure, peat, and composts are among the amendments that can help increase the water and nutrient-holding capacity of the soil, particularly on sandy soils. Because nematodes are most likely to injure plants that are water-surface, boosting the capacity of soil to grasp water can reduce nematode damage. Similarly, more frequent irrigation can aid in the reduction of nematode damage. You'll have the same number of nematodes in the soil in either situation, but they'll do minimum injure [29].

8.2 Management of plant parasite root-knot nematode through biological control

Many approaches have been made to control plant-parasitic nematodes with varying degrees of success. This includes biological control via soil-borne microbes. Soil suppressiveness is the inability of pathogens to survive and establish in diverse soils, or the ability to establish but not cause disease to a significant amount. Soil biotic suppressiveness can be general, where multiple diseases are suppressed by complex ecological interactions, or specialized, where one or a few organisms fight a specific pathogen [12].

Biological control is a non-lethal method of eliminating pests and pathogens. Antagonists and nematophagous microorganisms are the highest potentials than chemical nematicides. Various forms of nematicides are used to control nematodes, which can be harmful to the environment. As a result, finding new techniques to reduce RKN that aren't hazardous chemical nematicides could be beneficial [32]. Therefore bio-agents can use against different pathogens. In RKN management, only a few nematophagous bacteria and fungi are commercially accessible [10].

Among biocontrol agents, fungi have different suitable strategies for controlling root-knot nematode. They may grab nematodes via constricting and non-constricting rings, adhesive tendrils, and colonies their body parts or produce toxic compounds to destroy them [33]. Many soil-dwelling fungi have been proven to be efficient biological control agents, especially *Paecilomyces lilacinus*, *Trichoderma harzianum*, *Fusarium* spp., *Pochonia* spp., *Chlamydosporium*, and *Penicillium* spp. These fungi have been discovered to be effective at killing worm eggs, juveniles, and female nematodes, as well as reducing parasitic root-knot nematode concentrations in soil [34].

Fungi that belong to the genera *Penicillium*, *Pochonia*, and *Aspergillus* have been identified as nematophagous or antagonistic to RKNs that operate directly by parasitizing eggs, as well as indirectly by stimulating plant defense mechanisms or to produce nematicidal metabolites [35].

Cultural filtrates of fungi were tested for their nematicidal action toward RKN in various plants. For example *Aspergillus* spp. decreased *M. incognita* egg production and were very toxic to juveniles. Soil drench action of *Aspergillus* spp. culture filtrates gave significant seedling growth of *Vigna radiate* and high rate of reduction in nematode population [36]. Sikandar et al. [37] discovered a major reduction in *M. incognita* invading after seed treatment with *Penicillium chrysogenum* cultural filtrates, suggesting *P. chrysogenum* as a possible biological control agent in the case of *M. incognita* in cucumber.

The importance of biological control of pests is growing, As such nematicides represent living systems, several difficulties exist to develop commercial bio-nematicidal products. Problems with their culture and formulation, variable gap between laboratory and field performance, potentially negative effects on non-target or beneficial organisms, and expectations of broad-spectrum activity and quick efficacy based on practice with synthetic chemical nematicides have been addressed in detail by some workers [10]. Bio-products containing antagonists of fungi and bacteria rank high among other bio-nematicides [38]. Rapid progress has been made during the past two decades in different aspects of bio-nematicidal production and use.

8.3 Management of plant parasite root-knot nematode through chemical control

Significant management of plant-parasitic root-knot nematodes in such production systems has relied on the use of chemical nematicides (any substance that is utilized to manage nematode infection in vegetables) as a brief-term control measure, reducing nematode rates in the soil to levels under recognized commercial harm thresholds. Nematode rate must be reduced to under threshold rate to decrease root damage and increase yield in affected fields [39]. Nematicides are chemically manufactured compounds that kill or harm nematodes. The first chemical nematode control trials against *M. incognita* on cantaloupe and tobacco were conducted in southern Italy in 1998. The global market for nematicides is worth around $1 billion per year, with RKN management accounting for 48% of this market. In the case of nematodes, nematicides might have a nemastatic or nematicidal effect. Nematicidal chemicals are extremely poisonous and harm exposed worms, but nemastatic compounds do not kill nematodes but prevent or postpone the hatching of nematode eggs [40].

8.3.1 Types of nematicides

Nematicides are classified as fumigant or non-fumigant based on their soil volatility.

8.3.1.1 Fumigant nematicides

Fumigant nematicides are hazardous chemicals that have a wide range of effects. They may be helpful against a variety of soilborne pests and pathogens in addition to killing plant-parasitic nematodes. In high-value crops like vegetables, fumigants are utilized to clean soil and decrease the risk of yield loss due to soilborne pests. When fumigant compounds are sprayed into the soil, they reach target organisms as a gaseous that passes among soil particles or as a liquid that dissolves into the water film that covers soil particles [41]. Plant-parasitic nematodes can be controlled by fumigant nematicides in a variety of soil, however, they are most successful in rough soils as compared to clay soils. Throughout the United States, including Georgia, soil fumigation has shown better performance in managing root-knot nematodes in vegetable crops production for decades. In Georgia, controlling the species of root-knot nematode such as *Meloidogyne* is critical to the production of vegetables (**Table 1**) [41].

8.3.1.2 Non-fumigant nematicides

Non-fumigant nematicides are non-volatile dangerous substances that can be used before, during, and after planting to lower nematode population densities and protect crops from injury via drenching, drip irrigation, or spraying into crop foliage [41]. These nematicides are divided into two types: contact (which kills nematodes in the soil by direct touch) and systemic (which kills nematodes as they feed on plant roots). Non-fumigant chemicals are distributed by soil water movement after being applied to the soil. Non-fumigants' efficacy is not affected by soil temperature, unlike fumigant nematicides. Due to toxicity and environmental concerns, the many previous non-fumigant nematicides have been taken off the market. Prompting the creation of a new class of chemical molecules that address these issues while still providing effective plant-parasitic nematode management [41]. For usage in vegetable crops, some commercially non-fumigant nematicides are available (**Table 2**).

Trade name	Toxicity	Main ingredient
Chlor-O-Pic	Nematicide/fungicide	96.5–99% chloropicrin
Telone I	Nematicide	1,3 dichloropropene (1,3-D)
Telone C-35	Nematicide/fungicide	65% 1,3-D, 35% chloropicrin
Telone C-17	Nematicide/fungicide	73% 1,3-D, 17% chloropicrin
Telone EC	Nematicide	1,3-D
Dominus	Broad-spectrum	Allyl isothiocyanate
Paladin	Broad-spectrum	Dimethyl disulfide
K-Pam	Broad-spectrum	Metam potassium
Vapam	Broad-spectrum	Metam sodium
PicClor-60	Nematicide/fungicide	40% 1,3-D, 60% chloropicrin
InLine	Nematicide/fungicide	61% 1,3-D, 33% chloropicrin

Table 1.
Currently available chemical fumigant nematicides for use in the production of vegetables.

Trade name	Toxicity	Main ingredient
Salibro	Nematicide	Fluazaindolizine
Counter 20G	Nematicide/insecticide	Terbufos
Movento	Nematicide/insecticide	Spirotetramat
Mocap EC	Nematicide/insecticide	Ethoprop
Mocap 15G	Nematicide/insecticide	Ethoprop
Velum Prime	Nematicide/fungicide	Fluopyram
Nimitz	Nematicide	Fluensulfone
Vydate	Nematicide/insecticide	Oxamy

Table 2.
Currently available non-fumigant nematicides use in vegetable production.

8.4 Plants that inhibit the growth of nematodes

Lesion and root-knot nematodes are suppressed by *Targets* species of marigolds. The most effective marigolds are Petite Blanc, Queen Sophia, Nemagold, and Tangerine (varieties include Petite Blanc, Queen Sophia, Nemagold, and Tangerine). Nematodes will nourish on and generate on *T. signata* or *T. tenuifolia*, *Signet* marigolds. Marigolds are ineffective against the northern root-knot nematode, *M. hapla*, which is found in colder climates. Marigolds provide the best impact when grown as a continuous planting for the full season [42].

The plant extracts effect from *Artemisia absinthium*, *Thymus vulgaris*, *Ricinus communis*, *Citrullus colocynthis*, and *Punica granatum* on the motility of *Meloidogyne incognita*, and *Helicotylenchus dihystera*, as well as the reversibility of the movement inhibition, were investigated by Korayem et al. [43]. *Megalaima incognita*'s egg-hatching inhibition and *H. dihystera*'s acetylcholinesterase (ACHEs) inhibition surprisingly, extracts of *P. granatum*, *A. absinthium*, and *T. vulgaris* and inhibited AChE more than oxamyl, which was previously thought to be a potent AChE inhibitor [44]. Similarly, detailed knowledge on the modes of action of various biological nematicides in terms of nematode acetylcholinesterase inhibition is required [10].

9. Conclusion

Root-knot nematodes are potent silent killers of many plant species belonging to a wide range of plant families. They lower the yield of many economically important crops and decline the quality as well. Many farmers are unaware of their presence due to its concealed behavior under the soil and roots. The second stage juveniles (J-II) feed and reside in the roots that creates galls/knots on the roots which ultimately lead toward the death of the plant. Integrated approaches are advised to the growers to tackle these parasitic worms. The use of resistant varieties, crop rotation, chemical control and utilization of microbiota is necessary to keep their damages below economic threshold level.

Conflict of interest

The authors declare no conflict of interest.

Author details

Sarir Ahmad[1,2]*, Mehrab Khan[2] and Ikram Ullah[2]

1 Department of Plant Protection, The University of Agriculture Peshawar, Peshawar, Pakistan

2 Department of Botany, Abdul Wali Khan University Mardan, Mardan, Pakistan

*Address all correspondence to: sarirplants@gmail.com

References

[1] Groover WL. Integrated Management Strategies for Plant-Parasitic Nematodes on Warm-Season Turfgrass Using Plant Growth-Promoting Rhizobacteria, Chemical Nematicides, and Remote Sensing Technology. Ann Arbor: Auburn University; 2020

[2] Mitkowski NA, Abawi GS. Root-knot nematodes. The Plant Health Instructor. 2003

[3] Yigezu Wendimu G. Biology, taxonomy, and management of the root-knot nematode (*Meloidogyne incognita*) in sweet potato. Advances in Agriculture. 2021. DOI: 10.1155/2021/882021

[4] Forghani F, Hajihassani A. Recent advances in the development of environmentally benign treatments to control root-knot nematodes. Frontiers in Plant Science. 2020;**11**:1125. DOI: 10.3389/fpls.2020.01125

[5] Gheysen G, Mitchum MG. Phytoparasitic nematode control of plant hormone pathways. Plant Physiology. 2019;**179**:1212-1226. DOI: 10.1104/pp.18.01067

[6] Rosso MN, Vieira P, de Almeida-Engler J, Castagnone-Sereno P. Proteins secreted by root-knot nematodes accumulate in the extracellular compartment during root infection. Plant Signaling & Behavior. 2011;**6**(8):1232-1234. DOI: 10.4161/psb.6.8.16290

[7] Archidona-Yuste A, Cantalapiedra-Navarrete C, Liébanas G, Rapoport HF, Castillo P, Palomares-Rius JE. Diversity of root-knot nematodes of the genus *Meloidogyne* Göeldi, 1892 (Nematoda: Meloidogynidae) associated with olive plants and environmental cues regarding their distribution in southern Spain. PloS One. 2018;**13**(6):0198236. DOI: 10.1371/journal.pone.0198236

[8] Singh SK, Ash GJ, Hodda M. Keeping 'one step ahead' of invasive species: Using an integrated framework to screen and target species for detailed biosecurity risk assessment. Biological Invasions. 2015;**17**(4):1069-1086. DOI: 10.1007/s10530-014-0776-0

[9] Philbrick AN, Adhikari TB, Louws FJ, Gorny AM. *Meloidogyne enterolobii*, a major threat to tomato production: Current status and future prospects for its management. Frontiers in Plant Science. 2020;**11**. DOI: 10.3389/fpls.2020.606395

[10] Abd-Elgawad MMM, Askary TH. Fungal and bacterial nematicides in integrated nematode management strategies. Egyptian Journal of Biological Pest Control. 2018;**28**(1). DOI: 10.1186/s41938-018-0080-x

[11] Ahmad S, Hameed A, Safia B, Ali A. Concealed endophytic nematode management in sunflower using plant-based soil amendments. Pure and Applied Biology (PAB). 2020;**9**(3):1763-1772. DOI: 10.19045/bspab.2020.90187

[12] Elhady A, Giné A, Topalovic O, Jacquiod S, Sørensen SJ, Sorribas FJ, et al. Microbiomes associated with infective stages of root-knot and lesion nematodes in soil. PloS One. 2017;**12**(5):0177145. DOI: 10.1371/journal.pone.0177145

[13] Hannula SE, Ma HK, Pérez-Jaramillo JE, Pineda A, Bezemer TM. Structure and ecological function of the soil microbiome affecting plant–soil feedbacks in the presence of a soil-borne pathogen. Environmental Microbiology. 2020;**22**(2):660-676. DOI: 10.1111/1462-2920.14882

[14] Liu H, Brettell LE, Qiu Z, Singh BK. Microbiome-mediated stress resistance in plants. Trends in Plant Science. 2020;**25**(8):733-743. DOI: 10.1016/j.tplants.2020.03.014

[15] Harkes P, Van Steenbrugge JJ, Van Den Elsen SJ, Suleiman AK, De Haan JJ, Holterman MH, et al. Shifts in the active rhizobiome paralleling low *Meloidogyne chitwoodi* densities in fields under prolonged organic soil management. Frontiers in Plant Science. 2020;**10**:1697. DOI: 10.3389/fpls.2019.01697

[16] Hyman BC. Molecular diagnosis of *Meloidogyne* species. Journal of Nematology. 1990;**22**(1):24-30

[17] Churamani K. Identification of Root-Knot Nematodes (*Meloidogyne* spp) of Arkansas using Molecular Diagnostics. 2014. pp. 1-73

[18] Eisenback JD. Morphological comparison of head shape and stylet morphology of second-stage juveniles of *Meloidogyne* species. Journal of Nematology. 1982;**14**:339-343

[19] Aydinli G, Mennan S. Identification of root-knot nematodes (*Meloidogyne* spp.) from greenhouses in the Middle Black Sea Region of Turkey. Turkish Journal of Zoology. 2016;**40**(5):675-685

[20] Powers T. Nematode molecular diagnostics: From bands to barcodes. Annual Review of Phytopathology. 2004;**42**:367-383. DOI: 10.1146/annurev.phyto.42.040803.140348

[21] Prokopy RJ. Two decades of bottom-up, ecologically based pest management in a small commercial apple orchard in Massachusetts. Agricultural Ecosystem and Environment. 2003;**94**:299-309. DOI: 10.1016/S0167-8809(02)00036-1

[22] Barzman M, Bàrberi P, Birch AN, Boonekamp P, Dachbrodt-Saaydeh S, Graf B, et al. Eight principles of integrated pest management. Agronomy for Sustainable Development. 2015;**35**(4):1199-1215. DOI: 10.1007/s13593-015-0327-9

[23] Khanna K, Kohli SK, Ohri P, Bhardwaj R. Plants-nematodes-microbes crosstalk within soil: A trade-off among friends or foes. Microbiological Research. 2021;**248**:126755. DOI: 10.1016/j.micres.2021.126755

[24] Collange B, Navarrete M, Peyre G, Mateille T, Tchamitchian M. Root-knot nematode (*Meloidogyne*) management in vegetable crop production: The challenge of an agronomic system analysis. Crop Protection. 2011;**30**(10):1251-1262. DOI: 10.1016/j.cropro.2011.04.016

[25] Timper P. Conserving and enhancing biological control of nematodes. Journal of Nematology. 2014;**46**(2):75

[26] Dababat AA, Fourie H. Nematode parasites of cereals. In: Plant Parasitic Nematodes in Subtropical and Tropical Agriculture. Wallingford, UK: CAB International; 2018. pp. 163-221

[27] Karuri H. Root and soil health management approaches for control of plant-parasitic nematodes in sub-Saharan Africa. Crop Protection. 2022;**152**:105841. DOI: 10.1016/j.cropro.2021.105841

[28] Dutta TK, Ganguly AK, Gaur HS. Global status of rice root-knot nematode, *Meloidogyne graminicola*. African Journal of Microbiology Research. 2012;**151**:6016-6021

[29] Perry EJ. UC Cooperative Extension, Stanislaus Co., and A. T. Ploeg, Nematology, UC Riverside. University of California Statewide IPM Program. 2013. Available from: http://ipm.ucanr.edu/PMG/PESTNOTES/pn7489.html

[30] Hallmann J, Meressa BH. Nematode parasites of vegetables. In: Plant Parasitic Nematodes in Subtropical and Tropical Agriculture. 2018. p. 346

[31] Flint ML. Pests of the Garden and Small Farm: A Grower's Guide to Using Less Pesticide. UCANR Publications; 2018

[32] Singh A et al. Management of root-knot nematode in different crops using microorganisms. In: Plant Biotic Interactions. Cham: Springer; 2019. pp. 85-99

[33] Poveda J, Abril-Urias P, Escobar C. Biological control of plant-parasitic nematodes by filamentous fungi inducers of resistance: Trichoderma, mycorrhizal and endophytic fungi. Frontiers in Microbiology. 2020;**25**(11):992. DOI: 10.3389/fmicb.2020.00992

[34] Khan RAA, Najeeb S, Mao Z, Ling J, Yang Y, Li Y, et al. Bioactive secondary metabolites from Trichoderma spp. against phytopathogenic bacteria and root-knot nematode. Microorganisms. 2020;**8**:401

[35] Maciá-Vicente JG, Rosso LC, Ciancio A, Jansson HB, Lopez-Llorca LV. Colonisation of barley roots by endophytic *Fusarium equiseti* and *Pochonia chlamydosporia*: Effects on plant growth and disease. Annual Applied Biology. 2009;**155**:391-401. DOI: 10.1111/j.1744-7348.2009.00352.x

[36] Bhat MY, Wani AH. Control of root-knot nematode, *Meloidogyne incognita* by urea coated with Nimin or other natural oils on mung, *Vigna radiata* (L.). R. Wilczek. Journal of Biopesticide. 2012;**5**:255

[37] Sikandar A, Zhang MY, Zhu XF, Wang YY, Ahmed M, Iqbal MF, et al. Efficacy of *Penicillium chrysogenum* strain SNEF1216 against root-knot nematodes (*Meloidogyne incognita*) in cucumber (*Cucumis sativus* L.) under greenhouse conditions. Applied Ecology and Environmental Research. 2019;**17**(5):12451-12464

[38] Wilson MJ, Jackson TA. Progress in the commercialisation of bionematicides. BioControl. 2013;**58**(6):715-722. DOI: 10.1007/s10526-013-9511-5

[39] Reddy PP. Nematode diseases of crop plants: An overview. Nematode Diseases of Crops and their Management. 2021. DOI: 10.1007/978-981-16-3242-6_1

[40] Dutta TK, Khan MR, Phani V. Plant-parasitic nematode management via biofumigation using brassica and non-brassica plants: Current status and future prospects. Current Plant Biology. 2019;**17**:17-32. DOI: 10.1016/j.cpb.2019.02.001

[41] Hajihassani A. Nematology—Vegetable Research, Plant Pathology. 2018. Available from: https://extension.uga.edu/publications/detail.html?number=B1502

[42] Golakiya BB, Delvadiya NA. Biointensive approaches for the management of phytonematodes. Agricultural Science & Green Energy. 2020;**1**(1):7

[43] Korayem AM, Hasabo SA, Ameen HH. Effects and mode of action of some plant extracts on certain plant parasitic nematodes. Anzeiger für Schädlingskunde, Pflanzenschutz, Umweltschutz. 1993;**66**(2):32-36. DOI: 10.1007/BF01909140

[44] Opperman CH, Chang S. Plant-parasitic nematode acetylcholinesterase inhibition by carbamate and organophosphate nematicides. Journal of Nematology. 1990;**22**(4):481-488

Chapter 14

Perspective Chapter: The Potential Role of Nematode Parasites in Wildlife Decline – Evidence from Allegheny Woodrats (*Neotoma magister*), Northern Flying Squirrels (*Glaucomys sabrinus*) and Now the Eurasian Red Squirrel (*Sciurus vulgaris*)

Carolyn Mahan and Michael Steele

Abstract

Climate change and habitat loss alter the landscape for wildlife, resulting in shifts in geographic ranges, occupation of smaller, remnant habitat patches, or use of novel environments. These processes often lead to sympatry between species that historically were non-sympatric. Such interactions increase competition for resources and expose species to novel parasites that reduce a species' fitness leading to wildlife declines. We explore these interactions in species of endangered North American rodents—Northern flying squirrels (*Glaucomys sabrinus*) and Allegheny woodrats (*Neotoma magister*). Northern flying squirrels are declining in the United States due to competition with its congener, southern flying squirrels (*Glaucomys volans*). Evidence indicates that competition is mediated by a shared nematode, *Strongyloides robustus*. Transmission of this nematode to northern flying squirrels is increasing due to forest fragmentation and climate change. We also note the recent discovery of *S. robustus* as a novel parasite and a factor in the decline of the European red squirrel (*Sciurus vulgaris*). Likewise, in Allegheny woodrats, shrinking landscape changes have resulted in increased range overlap with raccoons (*Procyon lotor*) that harbor a nematode fatal to woodrats. The subsequent transmission of this nematode, *Baylisascaris procyonis*, to woodrats is a contributing factor to woodrat decline throughout the Appalachians.

Keywords: Allegheny woodrat, flying squirrels, Eastern gray squirrels, *Baylisascaris*, *Strongyloides*

1. Introduction

Global climate change and human-induced habitat loss alter the landscape for native wildlife, resulting in shifts in geographic ranges, occupation of smaller, remnant habitat patches, or use of novel or new environments. These processes often lead to sympatry between species that historically occupied non-overlapping ranges and habitats. Such interactions may result in increased competition for resources and expose species to novel parasites that adversely affect a species' fitness leading to wildlife declines. For example, if the distribution of a host species shifts, so too will the distribution of its parasites. Therefore, in some ecosystems, invasive and endemic hosts may experience new parasites which may be pathogenic to naïve hosts [1, 2].

Species may shift their distribution as a response to changing climate but some species also may be introduced incidentally or purposefully by human activities – resulting in similar novel host-parasite interactions [3]. For instance, global trade, transport, and the introduction of exotic species likely facilitates parasite-mediated competition between species. These trends may worsen under climate change because new species assemblages may occur, thus creating opportunities for parasite exchange. When previously allopatric host species come into sympatry, novel host–parasite interactions may emerge if parasites are able to successfully infect newly exposed hosts [4]. These parasitic 'co-invaders' may mediate the impacts of biological introductions by potentially amplifying transmission to native species [3]. However, evaluating threats from introduced parasites to native wildlife is difficult due to limited information associated with distribution shifts or introductions [5]. Complicating these interactions, climate change may alter parasite survival, development rates, and periods of transmission between intermediary hosts [2]. We explore these interactions and concurrent species declines in several species of wild rodents demonstrating conservation challenges in a globalizing planet experiencing climate change.

2. *Strongyloides robustus* parasite-mediated competition in squirrels in North American and Europe

Strongyloides robustus is an intestinal nematode reported to occur in several squirrel species (Sciuridae) across at least two continents. Documented hosts include the Eastern gray squirrel (*Sciurus carolinensis*), southern flying squirrels (*Glaucomys volans*), northern flying squirrel (*Glaucomys sabrinus*), and the North American red squirrel (*Tamiasciurus hudsonicus*) in North America as well as the invasive Eastern gray squirrels in Europe and now as a spill-over parasite in Europe's native red squirrel (*Sciurus vulgaris*) [6–9].

Strongyloides robustus exhibits a direct life cycle whereby eggs are shed and hatch, usually within a few days depending on ambient temperature, developing first as a larval (L1) stage, a second, L2 stage (a rhabdidiform larvae) and finally an infective, L3 stage (filariform larvae) [8]. Infection, which results from direct consumption of the L3 larvae, is assumed to occur most often in the nest and may be transmitted from one species to another when nest use overlaps over a relatively short time period [8, 9].

Across North America the two flying squirrel species, in which this nematode occurs, are largely allopatric with *G. sabrinus* occupying mostly coniferous forests (spruce [*Picea* sp.] and fir [*Abies* sp.]) of boreal regions of the United States of America (U.S.A.) and Canada and *G. volans* occurring in hardwood forests of the midwest, east and southeastern U.S.A. However, there are regions in the Appalachian Mountains and areas northward of the eastern U.S.A. where the ranges of the two species exhibit limited sympatry and may compete for nest sites (**Figure 1**). Although both species consume seeds and nuts [7], *G. sabrinus* relies on a steady diet of fungi and lichens throughout most of its range, whereas *G. volans* is generally limited to hardwood stands where it feeds on the nuts of hardwood species. Although these habitat differences and dietary limitations maintain allopatry across much of their range, mixed stands, especially in the east and northeast, often bring the two species together where the edges of each species' range meet. In addition, forest fragmentation due to human-mediated landscape changes has reduced coniferous patches in these regions, permitting *G. volans'* and *G. sabrinus'* ranges to overlap [10]. Furthermore, global climate change has expanded *G. volans'* range northward and increased interactions between these two species [11].

For several decades now, there has been growing circumstantial evidence that *S. robustus* may mediate competitive interactions between the two species of flying squirrels in North America [6, 12]. *G. volans* a common host for *S. robustus* shows no evidence of pathology when infected with this nematode, whereas *G. sabrinus* may be quite negatively affected and even killed by the parasite [6, 13, 14].

Based on these early circumstantial but compelling studies [6, 7], Price et al. [12] included these studies on flying squirrels in their comprehensive examination of parasite-mediated competition between similar pairs of species. They proposed two hypotheses to potentially explain how parasites of one host are likely to negatively impact a

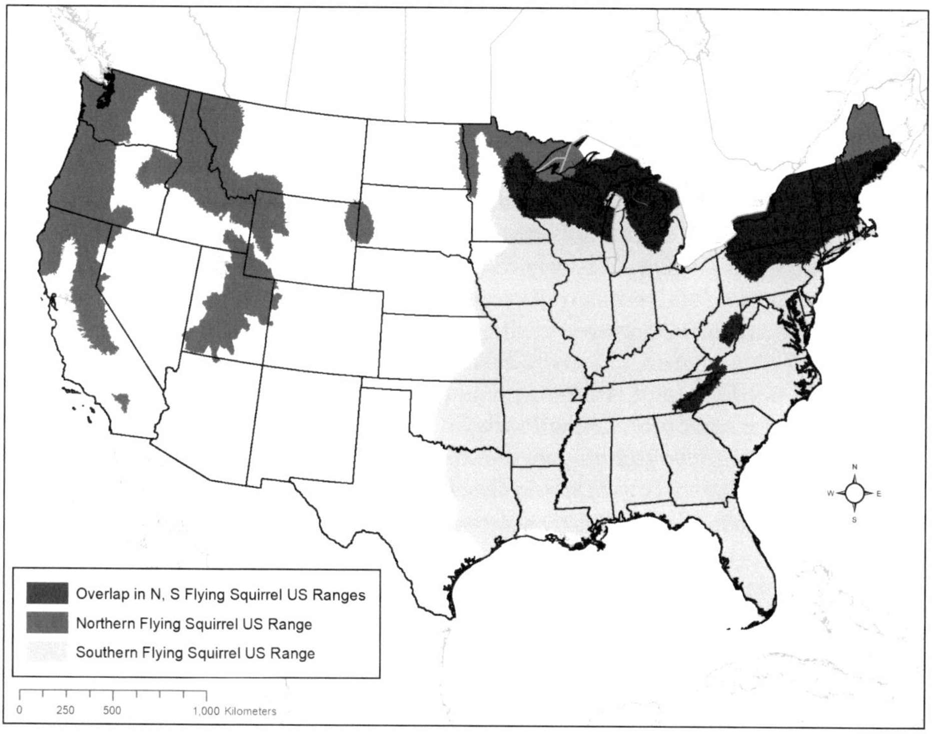

Data Source: USGS Gap Analysis Program (https://www.usgs.gov/programs/gap-analysis-project [Accessed 04 Jan 2022])

Figure 1.
*Distribution of Northern flying squirrel (*Glaucomys sabrinus*) and Southern flying squirrel (*Glaucomys volans*) in the United States, 2021.*

closely related host. In the first, the geographic range hypothesis, they predicted that species of larger geographic ranges carry more parasites and are therefore more likely to displace a similar species with a smaller range. In the second, the body-size hypothesis, Price et al. [12] hypothesize that smaller species with higher densities and higher rates of population growth are likely to displace the larger bodied species. The second hypothesis was supported in 12 of 15 cases, one of which included *G. volans* and *G. sabrinus.*

Krichbaum et al. [15] conducted a survey of gut parasite communities in sympatric populations of the two species of flying squirrel in Pennsylvania and populations of *G. sabrinus* in New York where *G. volans* is not found. Where sympatric, both flying squirrel species hosted *S. robustus* with the southern flying squirrels showing substantial numbers of the parasite and exhibiting an overdispersed distribution in the host (*G. volans*). Populations of northern flying squirrels in northern New York were not infected with *S. robustus*.

In tests of the immuno-competence hypothesis that higher levels of testosterone increase susceptibility to parasites, Waksmonski et al. [16] used high performance liquid-chromatography-ultra-violet spectroscopy (HPLC-UV) to compare testosterone levels in both species of flying squirrels infected with *S. robustus*. They observed strong qualitative evidence that testosterone levels were substantially higher in northern flying squirrels hosting *S. robustus* compared with southern flying squirrels hosting the parasite.

Even stronger evidence for repeated contact between these two species in Pennsylvania and Ontario is reported by Garroway et al. [11]. In Pennsylvania, for example, both species of Glaucomys were first captured in the same nest [14]. Soon thereafter, following an unseasonably warm period, *G. volans* was observed to move northward in Ontario and Pennsylvania, mate and produce hybrid offspring [11]. This evidence of hybridization clearly documents significant contact between the two species in the same nests where exchange of S. *robustus* is likely to occur.

Recent studies in a similar system suggest that the invasive Eastern gray squirrel in Europe [17], which is a common host for *S. robustus* may share this parasite with the endangered Eurasian red squirrel (*S. vulgaris*), potentially causing negative health effects [18]. In fact, this study represents the first experimental investigation documenting the negative effects of *S. robustus* on a potentially vulnerable host. Romeo et al. [18] conducted boldness/activity tests of individual Eurasian red squirrels infected with S. *robustus*, captured at sites where the invasive gray squirrel was found and at control sites where *S. vulgaris* was the only squirrel present. Based on these studies observers documented a negative association between the red squirrels' activity level (boldness) and infection with the invasive parasite at sites of sympatry.

Collectively the above studies provide strong evidence that *S. robustus* may mediate competition between *G. volans* and *G. sabrinus* in parts of North America and between populations of the invasive *S. carolinensis* and the native *S. vulgaris* in Europe. In both systems the affected species are considered species of conservation concern and listed as endangered in those parts of their range where *S. robustus* is potentially exerting its greatest effect.

3. *Baylisascaris procyonis* in raccoons and Allegheny woodrats: nematode-acerbated mammal decline

Ascarids are host-specific nematodes (order Ascaridida, class Secernentea) that are parasitic in the intestines of various terrestrial vertebrates. Adult ascarids live in the small intestine of their definitive host and produce eggs which are shed in the feces. Eggs are very resistant to environmental extremes and can remain infective in the environment for many years [19, 20]. Like other ascarids, *B. procyonis* has a direct and indirect life cycle and can cause zoonotic infection in a variety of paratenic hosts [20]. Although raccoon (*Procyon lotor*) is the specific host for the adult worm, there is no obligatory intermediate host. Adult female worms in the small intestines of raccoons collectively shed millions of eggs per day which are passed in the hosts' feces. After being passed, *Baylisascaris* eggs continue to develop and an infectious larva develops in 2–4 weeks. Raccoons become infected by ingesting *B. procyonis* eggs or larva during social feeding or grooming activities. In addition, raccoons may become infected by consuming flesh or droppings of other vertebrates (specifically mammals or birds) that have become infected by this roundworm. *B. procyonis* is common (prevalence rates ~65%) throughout North American wherever raccoons are found. Except for heavy infections, *B. procyonis* causes no disease in their primary host [20].

Although raccoons are the natural host for *B. procyonis*, other mammals and birds can become aberrant intermediate hosts after inadvertently ingesting eggs containing infectious larva. In these aberrant hosts, *B. procyonis* causes severe central nervous system disease that is often fatal. The life history of raccoons may contribute to the inadvertent transmission of *Baylisascaris* to non-raccoon species. Raccoon defecate in common latrines resulting in a high abundance and concentration of *B. procyonis* eggs that remain infectious for months due to their resistance to environmental extremes [19, 20].

Allegheny woodrat is a species of new world rodent that is endemic to the Appalachian mountains of eastern North America [21–23]. A decline in the numbers and range of the Allegheny woodrat was first noticed in the 1960s and the decline was considered severe by the mid-1970s. The species has since been extirpated from New York and Connecticut. Extensive surveys in Pennsylvania have revealed that woodrats have disappeared from approximately one third of their former range there [21]. Similar declines have been noted in Maryland and Ohio. Allegheny woodrat populations remained stable in West Virginia but recent data indicates that populations are declining in that state as well. This rapid decline has led to the species being listed as endangered and/or threatened by states throughout its range and is currently considered a species of conservation interest and protection by the U.S. Forest Service – although it is not listed under the Endangered Species Act [24].

Allegheny woodrats typically occur in rocky areas associated with forested mountain ridges such as cliffs, caves, talus slopes and rocky fissures. The rocky barrens where they den are generally devoid of vegetation with the exception of the occasional tree that manages to survive among the rocks. Active primarily at night, woodrats leave the security of their rocky dens to visit adjacent areas to feed on the available vegetation. They are typically found in talus fields having large sized boulders (greater than 1.2 m in diameter). Vegetative associations include birch (*Betula* spp.)/chestnut oak (*Quercus prinus*) forests, scattered birch, oaks and shrubs with herbaceous plants at the base of slopes.

Allegheny woodrats exhibit behaviors that are typical of a 'pack rat' and, besides food items, woodrats also collect and store various non-food items (e.g., feathers, snail shell, dried leaves, human items) in their rocky dens. The foraging behavior of Allegheny woodrats may increase their susceptibility to encountering *Baylisascaris* in the feces of raccoons. For example, woodrats may forage for and collect seeds present in the dried feces found in raccoon latrines. Woodrats may make repeated visits to these latrine sites, collect seeds, and subsequently store them in their food caches—resulting in repeated exposure to the parasite [21, 23].

Exposure to raccoon roundworm is considered one of many factors that act synergistically to cause the decline of this native rodent [23]. At raccoon latrine sites associated with woodrats, published prevalence rates of *B. procyonis* vary from 11% (Indiana), 22% (Maryland), and 33% (Pennsylvania) [22, 25, 26]. Accordingly, at sites where woodrats persist, raccoon roundworm was absent [22]. Furthermore, forest fragmentation and raccoon densities are also lower than at sites where woodrats have been extirpated [26–28]. In New York state, an unsuccessful woodrat reintroduction effort in 1990 was attributed to high prevalence of raccoons and *Baylisascaris* at the reintroduction site [29]. Additionally, in Indiana woodrat translocations failed at one site where the presence of raccoons and *Baylisascaris* was high [27]. However, the distribution of anhelminitic baits reduced levels of roundworm contamination permitting persistence of woodrats at additional translocation sites in Indiana [27].

Woodrat translocations should be considered at formerly-occupied sites if raccoon latrines and *B. procyonis* are removed. Anhelminitic baits can be used to reduce roundworm prevalence rates at these sites and the maintenance of continuous, mature deciduous forested habitat will reduce raccoon densities. Furthermore, protecting sites where woodrats persist from habitat alterations that will attract raccoons is important. A comprehensive regional approach to assessing the prevalence of *B. procyonis* in raccoons and the exposure level to infection in woodrat habitat is necessary. Once prevalence rates are more widely-understood, the feasibility of using anhelminitic approaches in core woodrat areas can be considered. Finally, the effects of human encroachment (highways, urban areas, agriculture) forest fragmentation on raccoon densities and woodrat habitat needs to be better understood [21]. A compilation of resources related to Allegheny woodrats, including the effects of *B. procyonis*, is available at: https://library.delval.edu/allegheny-woodrats/conservation.

4. Conclusions

Here we described two nematode parasites, *Strongyloides robustus* and *B. procyonis*, relatively common in one mammalian host that contribute to decline in another neighboring mammal species of special conservation concern. Where southern and northern flying squirrels are sympatric, *S. robustus* (commonly found in southern species) appears to contribute to poor health in threatened/endangered northern flying squirrels. Recently, *S. robustus*, also found in the invasive Eastern gray squirrel in Europe, appears to be transmitted to the now threatened Eurasian red squirrel and may contribute to its decline by modifying its behavior and limiting its ability to compete with its congener. Similarly, *B. procyonis* a common roundworm of the raccoon is often contracted by the Allegheny woodrat an inhabitant of rocky habitats on forested mountain ridges of the eastern and central U.S.A. where it feeds on and stores seeds deposited in the feces of raccoons deposited in latrines often associated with woodrat habitat. Now lost from more than a third of their original range, decline of the Allegheny woodrat is attributed largely to the presence of raccoons and this roundworm parasite.

Species distribution changes and range shifts due to climate change and/or human activity will result in the emergence of new species assemblages. Within these new assemblages, species may affect each other directly through predation or competition, or indirectly by habitat alteration or restructuring host-parasite interactions [3]. The role of climate change in restructuring host–parasite interactions through shifts in host ranges is poorly understood [4] but case studies in rodents presented here provide some predictions about the potential conservation challenges that may emerge.

Acknowledgements

We thank the Pennsylvania Game Commission, Pennsylvania Department of Conservation and Natural Resources, Wild Resources Conservation Program, State Wildlife Grants Program, Northeast Association of Fish and Wildlife Agencies, Penn State Altoona, and Wilkes University for financial support of our research. We thank John Young, U.S. Geological Survey, for creating **Figure 1**. In addition, we thank Gregory Turner, Pennsylvania Game Commission, and Dr. Peter Hudson, Huck Institutes, Penn State University, for creative leadership and insight into the interactions of wildlife and parasites.

Conflict of interest

The authors declare no conflict of interest.

Author details

Carolyn Mahan[1] and Michael Steele[2*]

1 Department of Biology, The Pennsylvania State University-Altoona College, Altoona, USA

2 Department of Biology, Wilkes University, Wilkes Barre, USA

*Address all correspondence to: msteele@wilkes.edu

References

[1] Brooks DR, Hoberg EP. How will global climate change affect parasite-host assemblages? Trends in Parasitology. 2007;**23**:571-574

[2] Polley L, Hoberg E, Kutz S. Climate change, parasites and shifting boundaries. Acta Veterinaria Scandinavica. 2010;**52**(Suppl. 1):51

[3] Lymbery AJ, Morine M, Kanani HG, Beatty SJ, Morgan DL, et al. The effects of alien parasites on native hosts. International Journal for Parasitology: Parasites and Wildlife. 2014;**3**:171-177

[4] Morales Castille I, Pappalardo P, Farrell MJ, Aguirre AA, Huang S, Gehman A-LM, et al. Forecasting parasite sharing under climate change. Philosophical Transactions of the Royal Society B. 2021;**376**:20200360

[5] Williams CF, Britton JR, Trumbull JF. A risk assessment for managing non-native parasites. Biological Invasions. 2013;**15**:1273-1286

[6] Weigl PD. The distribution of the flying squirrels, *Glaucomys volans* and *G. sabrinus*: An evaluation of the competitive exclusion idea [thesis]. Durham: Duke University; 1968. p. 247

[7] Weigl PD. Resource overlap, interspecific interactions and distribution of flying squirrels, *Glaucomos-volans* and *Glaucomos-sabrinus*. The American Midland Naturalist. 1978;**100**(1):83-96

[8] Wetzel EJ, Weigl PD. Ecological implications for flying squirrels (*Glaucomys* spp.) of effects of temperature on the in-vitro development and behavior *Strongyloides-robustus*. The American Midland Naturalist. 1994;**131**(1):43-54

[9] Santicca F, Wauters LA, Piscitelli AP, Van Dongen S, Martonili A, Preatoni D, et al. Spillover of an alien parasite reduces expression of costly behavior in native host behaviour. The Journal of Animal Ecology. 2020;**89**:1559-1569

[10] Mahan CG, Bishop JA, Steele MA, Turner G, Myers WL. Habitat characteristics and revised gap landscape analysis for the Northern flying squirrel (*Glaucomys sabrinus*), a state endangered species in Pennsylvania. The American Midland Naturalist. 2010;**164**:283-295

[11] Garroway C, Bowman JJ, Cascaden TJ, Holloway GL, Mahan CG, Malcolm JR, et al. Climate change induced hybridization in flying squirrels. Global Change Biology. 2009;**16**:113-121

[12] Price PW, Westoby M, Rice B. Parasite-mediated competition: Some predictions and tests. The American Naturalist. 1988;**131**(4):544-555

[13] Weigl PD, Knowles TW, Boynton AC. The Distribution and Ecology of the Northern Flying Squirrel (*Glaucomys sabrinus*) in the Southern Appalachians. Raleigh, NC, USA: North Carolina Wildlife Commission Nongame and Endangered Wildlife Program, Division of Wildlife Management; 1999

[14] Steele MA, Mahan C, Turner G. The Northern flying squirrel, *Glaucomys sabrinus*. In: Steele MA, Brittingham MC, Maret TJ, Merrit JF, editors. Terrestrial Vertebrates of Pennsylvania: A Complete Guide to Species of Conservation Concern. Baltimore: Johns Hopkins University Press; 2010. p. 507

[15] Krichbaum K, Mahan CG, Steele MA, Turner G, Hudson PJ. The potential role of *Strongloides robustus* on parasite mediated competition between two species of flying squirrels (*Glaucomys*). Journal of Wildlife Diseases. 2010;**46**(1):229-235

[16] Waksmonski SN, Huffman JM, Mahan CG, Steele MA. An examination of endoparasites and fecal testosterone levels in flying squirrels (*Glaucomys* spp.) using high performance liquid chromatography-ultra-violet (UV). International Journal for Parasitology: Parasites and Wildlife. 2017;**6**(2): 135-137

[17] Wauters LA, Verbeylen G, Preatoni D, Martinoli A, Matthysen E. Dispersal and habitat cuing of Eurasian red squirrels in fragmented habitats. Population Ecology. 2010;**52**(4):527-537

[18] Romeo C, Ferrari N, Lanfranchi P, Saino N, Stanticchia F, Martinoli A, et al. Biodiversity threats from outside to inside: Effects of alien grey squirrel (*Sciurus carolinensis*) on helminth community of native red squirrel (*Sciurus vulgaris*). Parasitology Research. 2013;**114**:2621-2628

[19] Kazacos KR. *Baylisascaris procyonis* and related species. In: Samuel WM, Pybus WM, Pybus MJ, Kocan KK, editors. Parasitic Diseases of Wild Mammals. Ames: Iowa State University Press; 2001. p. 559

[20] Graeff-Teixeira C, Morassutti AL, Kazacos KR. Update on *Baylisascaris*, a highly pathogenic zoonotic infection. Clinical Microbiology Reviews. 2016;**29**:375-399

[21] Wright J. History and current status of the Allegheny woodrat. In: Peles JD, Wright J, editors. The Allegheny Woodrat: Ecology, Conservation, and Management of a Declining Species. New York: Springer; 2008. pp. 3-22

[22] Page LK, Johnson SA, Swihart RK, Kazacos KR. Prevalence of *Baylisascaris procyonis* in habitat associated with Allegheny woodrat (*Neotoma magister*) populations in Indiana. Journal of Wildlife Diseases. 2012;**48**:503-507

[23] Smyser TJ, Johnson SA, Page LK, Rhodes OE Jr. Synergistic stressors and the dilemma of conservation in a multivariate world: A case study in Allegheny woodrats. Animal Conservation. 2012;**15**:205-213

[24] Monty AM, Feldhammer GA. Conservation assessment for the Eastern woodrat (*Neotoma florida*) and the Allegheny woodrat (*Neotoma magister*). Carbondale: United States Department of Agriculture, Forest Service, Southern Illinois University; 2002. p. 36

[25] Cottrell WO, Heagy RL, Johnson JB, Marcantuno R, Nolan TJ. Geographic and temporal prevalence of *Baylisascaris procyonis* in raccoons (*Procyon lotor*) in Pennsylvania, USA. Journal of Wildlife Diseases. 2014;**50**:923-927

[26] Wolfkill J, Bejarano ME, Serfass TL, Turner G, Brosi S, Steele M, et al. The prevalence of the raccoon roundworm, *Baylisascaris procyonis*, in Allegheny woodrat habitat in the mid-Atlantic region, U.S.A. The American Midland Naturalist. 2020;**185**:145-147

[27] Smyser TJ, Johnson SA, Page LK, Hudson CM, Rhodes OE Jr. Use of experimental translocations of Allegheny woodrat to decipher causal agents of decline. Conservation Biology. 2013;**27**:752-762

[28] Wright AN, Gompper ME. Altered parasite assemblages in raccoons in response to manipulated resource availability. Oecologia. 2015;**144**:148-156

[29] New York State Department of Environmental Conservation (NY DEC), Division of Fish, Wildlife, and Marine Resources. New York State Comprehensive Wildlife Conservation Strategy. Albany: New York State Department of Environmental Conservation; 2006

Chapter 15

Soil-Transmissible Helminths Infections; Diagnosis, Transmission Dynamics, and Disease Management Strategies in Low-and Middle-Income Countries

James-Paul Kretchy

Abstract

Soil-transmissible helminths (STHs) infections are the most common sanitation-related public health problems among people living in poor settlements of tropical and sub-tropical regions in low- and middle-income countries (LMICs). Though available data suggest the occurrence of disease in adults, children of school-going age bear the greatest burden, affecting their cognitive development and physical growth. The characteristic high levels of poverty, poor environmental hygiene, open defecation practices, and inadequate sanitation and waste management systems, expose residents to the risks of STH infections. Walking bare-footed, inappropriate hand hygiene behaviour, and the unavailability/improper use of personal protective equipment (PPE) can impact transmission risks in endemic communities and among occupational risk groups. These have to be properly investigated, managed, and appropriate interventions communicated to decision-makers.

Keywords: control, diagnostics, exposure, soil-transmitted helminths, low-and middle-income countries, personal protective equipment

1. Introduction

1.1 Background information and disease burden

Soil-transmissible helminths (STHs) refer to the intestinal worms infecting humans that are transmissible through faecal contaminated soil. Infections caused by STHs are widely endemic and constitute one of the major public health problems, particularly in African, South American, and Asian LMICs [1]. The geographical distribution of parasites causing these infections is known to be influenced by prevailing environmental and climatic conditions. For example, poor environmental sanitation and hygiene conditions in tropical and sub-tropical regions are major determinants of STHs. The WHO estimates that about 2.5 billion people globally, currently have no access to improved sanitation whilst close to 1.1 billion others practice open defecation [2]. Furthermore, the inequalities in socio-economic status of human populations at risk, particularly regarding access to clean water and sanitation, housing, and the access to anti-helminthic treatment, impact the observed epidemiological distribution of STH infections [3]. The transmission is by human exposures to the infective stages, either by direct skin penetration or through ingestion, which can lead to serious illness, though infections remain asymptomatic in the majority of cases with light-intensity infections. Laboratory diagnosis is the gold standard in confirming STH infections, since clinical symptoms present as non-specific gastrointestinal diseases and among persons with high intensity of infection.

The current global disease burden suggests that nearly two (2) billion people are infected, with over 80% of the disease burden found in tropical and sub-tropical regions of LMICs [4]. An estimated 870 million children live in areas of high prevalence in Africa, South Asia, and South America. The diseases are attributed to the four most prevalent STHs namely, *Ascaris lumbricoides*, *Trichuris trichiura*, or the hookworms (*Ancylostoma doudenale*/*Necator americanus*), infecting approximately 807–1121 million, 604–795 million, and 576–740 million people, respectively. *Strongyloides stercoralis*, which is the least prevalent and most neglected STH species, is responsible for an estimated 30–100 million infections globally. With the specific emphasis of the disease burden in LMICs, previous studies have found that unlike in Ghana (2.1%), *Ascaris lumbricoides* have the widest distribution reported in Nigeria (25.4%), Cameroon (30.8%), Equatorial Guinea (38.8%), and Congo (32.2%). In South America, infections with *Ascaris lumbricoides* is less widely dispersed in Ecuador (35.8%), Colombia (26.0%), and Venezuela (28.4%) compared with Asian LMICs like in the Philippines (33.6%), Afghanistan (36.0%), Malaysia (41.7%), and Bangladesh (38.4%). The hookworm infections with *Ancylostoma doudenales*/*Necator americanus*, remain common throughout African LMICs like Ghana (52.9%), in addition to the Asian LMICs, Malaysia (21.0%), Bangladesh (22.3%), Nepal (30.7%), and Papua New Guinea (60.6%). The prevalence of *Trichuris trichiura* infections in Asian LMICs like Malaysia (49.9%), and the Philippines (45.5%), as well as in the South American LMIC, Venezuela (28.4%) is more than that reported in the African LMIC Ghana, (0.8%).

It is worth considering that in addition to the single infections caused, multiple-species infections in a single individual are also common, and taken together, can cause considerable global health impacts and decrease economic productivity in vulnerable populations of many LMICs [2, 5]. The epidemiological patterns of the disease burden require consolidated efforts by governments, communities, and healthcare institutions to adopt context-specific public health interventions that would see a reduction in the rates of STH infections, if not to eliminate or completely eradicate them. Even though these infections have been reported among specific risk groups like adult food vendors [6] and sanitation workers [7] in African LMICs, the greatest burden is confirmed in children of school-going age, affecting their cognitive development and physical growth [8]. For example, an estimated 270 million pre-school children and over 568 million school-going children currently have infections that require anti-helminthic treatment and prevention interventions.

The available literature on transmission conditions of STHs, diagnostic techniques used to identify the species variety, risk factors to infections, and suggested public health interventions to reduce the risk of infection in exposed populations are inadequately published and are mostly presented in journal articles. This chapter, therefore, sought to conduct a narrative description of these aspects, plus present a case study of STH infections in an occupational risk-group in an African LMIC, to provide context-based recommendations on how STHs can be prevented and controlled in vulnerable populations living in such settings.

2. Methodology

The narrative review approach was used to draft this chapter. Information was retrieved from the internet-based search for original articles and reviews published between the years 2000 and 2021, using PubMed and Google scholar portals, and from textbooks. The keywords used for the literature search and inclusion criteria were 'control, diagnostics, exposure, soil-transmitted helminths, low-and middle-income countries, and personal protective equipment'. In-text references have been cited appropriately and full references are provided in the bibliography section.

3. Literature review

3.1 Transmission conditions and risk factors to STH infections in LMICs

Studies in Ghana and other LMICs have shown that residents in rural and peri-urban communities have higher risks for STH infections than in urban communities because of the higher proportions of poverty, poor environmental hygiene, inadequate sanitation, open defecation, and inadequate waste management systems [9, 10]. These factors perpetuate the continued existence of STHs in such settings. The infective stages of STHs persist for longer periods in human or animal faecal polluted environments and can survive a wide range of physical and chemical conditions, thereby, posing the highest disease risks to community members, particularly in pre-school children or those of school-going age, compared with other biological agents like bacteria and viruses [11, 12]. The adequate warmth and moisture in many tropical and sub-tropical LMICs also favour the survival of STH eggs and increase the risk of transmission to people living in endemic areas [13]. Researchers have also reported the persistence of STH eggs in salty beaches in Brazil [14], and Portugal [15], due to faecal contamination of the beach soil.

According to the WHO [16] although the human threadworm (*Strongyloides stercoralis*) is an important member of the STHs, it is the least prevalent. The most important STH species that infect people are the human roundworm (*Ascaris lumbricoides*), the human whipworm (*Trichuris trichiura*) and the two hookworm species (*Necator americanus* and *Ancylostoma duodenale*). These groups of STHs do not require intermediate hosts in their life cycle. Rather, the adult helminths lay eggs that hatch into larvae, grow, and then develop into adult worms inside the gastrointestinal tract of humans. The major mode of transmission is through direct faecal-oral ingestion of the eggs/ova (for *Ascaris lumbricoides*, *Trichuris trichiura*, and the hookworm, *Ancylostoma doudenale*) [17]. The *Necator americanus* is rather transmitted through direct penetration of the larvae through exposed parts of the body [18]. Government agencies and other stakeholders in the health sector of affected LMICs need to ensure the implementation of Public health intervention measures that target the blocking of the transmission chains, such as improved water, sanitation and hygiene (WASH) uptake, prevent the establishment of disease, and to improve the quality of lives, particularly of children and other occupational risk groups.

3.2 Clinical and laboratory diagnosis of STH infections

Though clinical diagnoses of STH infections are based on the signs and symptoms accompanying the disease after the establishment of an infection, infected persons usually remain clinically asymptomatic, and the diseases rarely cause mortality. When present, clinical symptoms may include non-specific gastrointestinal symptoms, such as acute abdominal pain, diarrhoea or intestinal obstruction. Chronic symptoms may present as iron-deficiency anaemia, malnutrition, retarded growth, cognitive impairment, particularly in children, and pre-term delivery, low-birth weight babies, and impaired lactation in pregnant/post-natal women. These clinical manifestations as well as self-reported cases, need to be confirmed by identifying infective stages like eggs, ova, or larvae in bowel contents collected from suspected patients with clinical illness or from asymptomatic persons.

Laboratory diagnosis for confirmation of STH infections can be done by using diverse methods with varying sensitivity and specificity [19–21]. The two most effective methods are direct parasitological, using microscopy (i.e., sedimentation concentration, McMaster, Kato Katz, FLOTAC) and molecular methods (i.e., polymerase chain reaction). The different diagnostic methods, STH detected, usefulness, and disadvantages are summarised in **Table 1**. Culture techniques and serological assays are less preferred methods in STH infection diagnosis, compared with microscopy and molecular techniques. The choice of a particular diagnostic method requires paying considerable attention to factors such as rapidity of obtaining test results, availability of infrastructure, cost of assay, ease of performance, and level of application in the field (**Table 1**). Other conditions such as proper training of laboratory personnel and strict compliance to quality control or quality assurance procedures could enhance the performance of diagnostic methods to confirm STHs. Confirmed diagnosis helps to ascertain individual infection status, and to estimate the incidence, prevalence, and intensity of infections among populations at risk. The outcomes of diagnosis can again be used to evaluate the effectiveness of parasite control measures like parasite clearance, the reduction in incidence or prevalence, and the intensity of infections. The benefit of laboratory findings is also to provide context-based policy guidance on the frequency of anti-helminthic treatment or prophylactic therapy in affected geographical areas.

3.3 The specific case of STH infections in an African LMIC

A longitudinal study conducted by Kretchy et al. [7], showed 4.3% incidence rate and low intensity of infections with the STH, *Trichuris trichiura* (*T. trichiura*) among waste handlers in a large coastal peri-urban settlement in Southern Ghana, six months post-treatment with albendazole (400 mg single oral dosage). This incidence rate for *T. trichiura* was, however, higher compared with the national average in an adult population (1.2%) and among non-school going children (0.8%) in endemic communities in Kintampo, Ghana [22, 23]. This could mean that waste handlers were at higher risk of infection with *T. trichiura* compared with the adult population of an endemic area in Ghana due to their occupational exposures. However, a similar study conducted in endemic communities in India by Narain et al. [24] among a group of teenagers found a higher incidence of infection with *T. trichiura* (43.6%), six months post-treatment with albendazole (400 mg). The most common health complaints following infections with *T. trichiura* include mainly intestinal, such as diarrhoea and abdominal pain [25]. Whilst heavy infections in adults have been found to

Diagnostic method for STH	STH detected					Usefulness	Disadvantages
	S. stercoralis	*A. lumbricoides*	*T. trichiura)*	*N. americanus*	*A. duodenale*		
Direct wet preparation/ direct microscopy	√	√	–	–	–	Rapid, inexpensive, and time saving	Low sensitivity, semi-quantitative, not often used in control programs
Kato–Katz	–	√	√	√	√	WHO "gold standard", quantification of STH eggs, high sensitivity, minimal infrastructure requirement, ability to stratify infection intensities	Requires fresh faecal specimen
Formol-ether concentration	–	√	√	√	√	Rapid, high sensitivity, Both fresh and preserved faecal specimens can be used, laboratory-acquired infection from faecal pathogens reduced	Rapid centrifugation inactivates infective stages, only qualitative, cannot be performed in laboratories with minimal infrastructure
Zinc sulphate flotation	–	–	√	–	–	Detects eggs of light intensity *T. trichiura* in faeces, less time consuming compared with other floatation methods	NI
Saturated sodium chloride flotation	–	√	–	√	√	Cost effective, useful in field surveys	NI
FLOTAC	–	√	√	√	√	Counting STH eggs in both human and veterinary faecal sample, less time consuming, highly sensitive, precise, accurate	Not useful in resource-limited settings, requires well-trained staff, uses larger amount of faecal specimen compared with Kato-Katz
McMaster	–	√	√	√	√	High sensitivity, fast and accurate results	Requires the use of a counting chamber which might not be readily available in resource-limited settings

Diagnostic method for STH	STH detected					Usefulness	Disadvantages
	S. stercoralis	*A. lumbricoides*	*T. trichiura)*	*N. americanus*	*A. duodenale*		
Antigen detection (ELISA)	√	–	–	–	–	Detects STH elements (eggs / cysts / larvae) in faecal specimen,	Not widely used in STH diagnosis
Antibody detection (ELISA)	–	√	√	√	√	Demonstrates exposure, confirms clinical findings	Can produce false positives due to previous exposure in endemic areas
Agar plate culture / Baermann	√	–	–	√	√	Detects STH in light-intensity infections	NI
Water Emergence	√	–	–	–	–	Cost-effective, suitable in resource-limited settings	Requires the use of fresh faecal specimen
Harada-Mori	√	–	–	–	–	Simple and cost-effective	Not suitable for refrigerated faecal specimen, not suitable in resource-limited settings, not suitable in field surveys where rapid results are important
Molecular (PCR)	–	√	√	√	√	High sensitivity, high specificity, species and strain level identification, detects STHs particularly in low intensity infection settings	DNA damage in faecal specimen, contaminants amplification can produce false positive results, requires well-trained staff / well-equipped laboratory, more expensive compared to Kato-Katz

√: STH detected, –: limited or not good detection of STH, ELISA: Enzyme-linked immunosorbent assay, PCR: Polymerase chain reaction, NI: None identified [19–21].

Table 1.
A summary of STH diagnostic methods, STH detected, usefulness, and disadvantages.

cause iron-deficiency anaemia [26], the light intensity infections recorded among the waste handlers may not result in this health outcome. Nevertheless, waste handlers who were infected with *T. trichiura* may serve as important reservoirs for the continued transmission of the STH among waste handlers, immediate family members and the entire peri-urban community as a whole. The findings from the study also indicated that STH infections were correlated with the type of waste handling activity performed, and that waste handlers who did not use the PPE gloves were about six times more likely to have STH infections compared to those who used gloves. This result has consolidated the knowledge on the importance of hands in the transmission of STH infections and the need to wear PPE to prevent the direct exposure of the bare hand to faecal contaminated soils/environments.

3.4 Public health interventions to reduce the risk of STH in exposed populations

In endemic populations, the risk of acquiring STH infections could be all year round however, several factors can predispose specific groups of persons to become susceptible. Specific risk factors in pre-school and children of school-going age to STH infections include having long or untrimmed fingernails, failure to wash hands before meals, walking bare-footed, nail-biting, and thumb-sucking habits. School-going children in particular, are more prone to STH infections when playing in unpaved, soil-infested school lawns. In communities, where tube-well rather than treated tap-water is used as the drinking water source, pre-school or non-school-going children become significantly vulnerable, because of the likelihood of faecal contamination from nearby latrines, seepage, or run-off water carrying faecal excrements from open defecation practices [27].

Practicing the appropriate public health intervention measures can reduce the exposure to the risk factors to STH infections in the environment and prevent disease occurrence. These can be achieved by preventive treatment with anti-helminthic drugs, adequate sanitation, and good environmental and personal hygiene practices, and by using appropriate PPE. Health education, change in health behaviour and periodic training among occupational risk groups may also be necessary preventive steps in reducing disease risks among persons living in endemic communities in resource-limited settings of African, Asian, and South American tropical, and sub-tropical LMICs.

The use of preventive anti-helminthic drugs is the current global strategy in controlling STH infections in at-risk populations [28]. In endemic countries like Ghana, albendazole (400 mg) and mebendazole (500 mg) are the anti-helminthic drugs of choice for the treatment against STH infections [29]. Albendazole and mebendazole have undergone extensive safety and efficacy testing and have been used in millions of people globally with only few and minor side effects [30]. Both drugs are effective broad-spectrum anti-helminthics, inexpensive and are easily administered by trained non-medical personnel. However, unlike mebendazole, albendazole (400 mg) is administered as a single oral dosage, which makes it easier to monitor treatment by direct observation by the researcher [16, 31]. The problem with preventive treatment with anti-helminthic drugs to at-risk populations is the inability to prevent re-infection after a short period of between three and six months [32, 33].

Other measures like proper sanitation and good personal hygiene practices are equally essential to reduce risk factors to STH infections. Good hygiene practices could also reduce the growth of other biological agents, in addition to STHs, on the hands of persons exposed to faecal contaminated soil. Wearing appropriate PPE during food vending or waste handling, and using footwear in school-going children may serve as barriers to prevent direct physical contact with the infective stages and reduce transmission risks.

Public health education and health promotion activities about keeping healthy behaviours like handwashing with soap after playing in the soil, after engaging in waste handling activities or after defecation and before eating may help to reduce transmission and re-infection rates due to STHs. Receiving periodic training about the use of appropriate PPE may also be necessary preventive steps in reducing disease risks among occupational risk groups like food vendors and waste handlers. These interventions, in addition to the use of anti-helminthic drugs, are necessary steps needed to reduce risk factors to STH infections.

It is necessary for the appropriate authorities and policymakers in endemic areas of LMICs including governments, employers, district, and local health authorities to provide appropriate and suitable PPE, replace old and worn out PPE in occupational risk groups, and also provide sufficient sanitation and hygiene facilities, such as toilets, soap, and water, and supervise their use in basic schools and poor settlements. Community members in endemic areas must be encouraged to undergo periodic medical screening and participate in deworming exercises at least once in every six months.

4. Conclusion and recommendations

Vulnerable populations particularly children and occupation risk groups in African, Asian, and South American LMICs, are predominantly faced with the hazards of STH infections. Although the burden of disease is quite high in African LMICs like Ghana and Nigeria, the highest burden of infection from hookworms, *Trichuris trichiura*, and *Ascaris lumbricoides* was reported in Asia. The high endemicity of infection in such settings and populations has huge socio-economic and developmental consequences for those infected. The ability of healthcare systems to promote strategies to block the transmission pathways, prevent infection and reduce complications arising from associated diseases is critical. Stakeholders in government and private agencies, as well as employers of occupation risk groups, need to invest adequate funds, infrastructure, and resources to support efforts in diagnosis, treatment and evaluation of WASH interventions that can mitigate the infection burden in LMICs.

It is important for future surveillance programs in the control of STHs, to consider and adopt more effective interventions that would integrate highly sensitive and specific diagnostic techniques like the polymerase chain reaction rather than microscopy-based methods so that laboratories can detect light-intensity STH infections even in areas of low endemicity. This would enable public health systems to implement appropriate curative or preventive measures against the transmission of STHs, particularly in vulnerable populations.

Acknowledgements

The Public Health (PH) Unit of the School of Medicine and Health Sciences (SMHS), Central University (CU) is greatly appreciated for its support in providing logistics and office space to conduct the narrative review in this chapter.

Conflict of interests

The author declares no conflict of interests in this chapter.

List of abbreviations

DNA	Deoxyribonucleic Acid
ELISA	Enzyme-linked Immunosorbent Assay
LMIC	Low-and Middle-Income Country
PCR	Polymerase Chain Reaction
PPE	Personal Protective Equipment
STH	Soil-transmissible Helminth
WHO	World Health Organisation

Author details

James-Paul Kretchy
Public Health Unit, School of Medicine and Health Sciences, Central University, Accra, Ghana

*Address all correspondence to: jkretchy@central.edu.gh

References

[1] Salam N, Azam S. Prevalence and distribution of soil-transmitted helminths infections in India. BMC Public Health. 2017;**17**(1):201

[2] World Health Organization. Guideline: Preventive Chemotherapy to Control Soil-Transmitted Helminthes Infections in at-Risk Population Groups. Geneva: World Health Organization; 2017

[3] Bethony J, Brooker S, Albonico M, Geiger SM, Loukas A, Diemert D, et al. Soil-transmitted helminthes infections: Ascariasis, Trichuriasis, and hookworm. The Lancet. 2006;**367**:1521-1532

[4] Strunz EC, Suchdev PS, Addiss DG. Soil-transmitted helminthiasis and vitamin a deficiency: Two problems, one policy. Trends in Parasitology. 2016;**32**(1):10-18

[5] Saki J, Khademvatan S, Foroutan-Rad M, Gharibzadeh M. Prevalence of intestinal parasitic infections in Haftkel County, southwest of Iran. International Journal of Infection Control. 2017;**4**(4):e15593

[6] Ayeh-Kumi PF, Quarcoo S, Kwakye-Nuako G, Kretchy JP, Osafo-Kantanka A, Mortu S. Prevalence of intestinal parasitic infections among food vendors in Accra, Ghana. Journal of Tropical Medicine and Parasitology. 2009;**32**:1-8

[7] Kretchy JP, Dzodzomenyo M, Ayi I, Dwomoh D, Agyabeng K, Konradsen F, et al. The incidence, intensity, and risk factors for soil-transmissible helminthes infections among waste handlers in a large coastal peri-urban settlement in southern Ghana. Journal of Environmental and Public Health. 2021;**2021**

[8] Muller O, Krawinkel M. Malnutrition and health in developing countries. Canadian Medical Association Journal. 2005;**173**(3):279-286

[9] Flores A, Estaban JG, Angles R, Mas-Coma S. Soil-transmitted helminthes infections at very high altitude in Bolivia. Transactional Royal Society of Tropical Medicine and Hygiene. 2011;**95**:272-277

[10] Mara D, Evans B. Sanitation and Water Supply in Low-Income Countries. Duncan Mara: Barbara Evans and Ventus Publishing; 2011. pp. 9-28

[11] Kone D, Cofie O, Zurbru C, Gallizzi K, Moser D, Drescher S, et al. Helminthes eggs inactivation efficiency by faecal sludge dewatering and co-composting in tropical climates. Water Research. 2007;**41**(19):4397-4402

[12] Kretchy JP, Dzodzomenyo M, Ayi I, Dwomoh D, Agyabeng K, Konradsen F, et al. Risk of faecal pollution among waste handlers in a resource-deprived coastal peri-urban settlement in southern Ghana. PLoS One. 2020;**15**(10):e0239587

[13] Brooker S, Michael E. The potential of geographical information systems and remote sensing in the epidemiology and control of human helminthes infections. Advances in Parasitology. 2000;**47**:245-287

[14] Rocha S, Pinto RMF, Floriano AP, Teixeira LH, Bassili B, Martinez A, et al. Environmental analyses of the parasitic profile found in the sandy soil from the Santos municipality beaches, sp, Brazil. Revista do Instituto de Medicina Tropical de São Paulo. 2011;**53**(5):277-281

[15] Scaini CJ, de Toledo RN, Lovatel R, Dionello MA, dos Anjos GF, Susin L,

et al. Environmental contamination by helminthes eggs and larvae in dog faeces from central area of Cassino beach, Rio Grande do Sul. Revised Social Brasil Medicine Tropical. 2003;**36**(5):617-619

[16] World Health Organisation. Soil-Transmitted Helminthes Infections. WHO Fact Sheet No. 366. Geneva; 2013

[17] Vandemark LM, Jia TW, Zhou XN. Social science implications for control of helminthes infections in Southeast Asia. Advances in Parasitology. 2010;**73**:137-170

[18] Carr R, Strauss M. Excreta-related infections and the role of sanitation in the control of transmission. In: Fewtrell L, Bartram J, editors. Water Quality: Guidelines, Standards and Health; Assessment of Risk and Risk Management for Water-Related Infectious Disease. London: International Water Association (IWA) on behalf on the World Health Organization; 2001. pp. 89-113

[19] Khurana S, Singh S, Mewara A. Diagnostic techniques for soil-transmitted helminthes- recent advances. Research and Reports in Tropical Medicine. 2021;**12**:181-196

[20] Riaz M, Aslam N, Zainab R, Aziz-Ur-Rehman RG, Ullah MI, Daniyal M, et al. Prevalence, risk factors, challenges, and the currently available diagnostic tools for the determination of helminths infections in human. European Journal of Inflammation. 2020;**18**(2020):2058739220959915

[21] Mbong Ngwese M, Prince Manouana G, Nguema Moure PA, Ramharter M, Esen M, Adegnika AA. Diagnostic techniques of soil-transmitted helminths: Impact on control measures. Tropical Medicine and Infectious Disease. 2020;**5**(2):93

[22] Tay SCK, Twum WA, Abruquah HH. Epidemiological survey of soil-transmitted helminthes in occupational risk-groups and non-school going children in the Kintampo north district of Ghana. Journal of the Ghana Science Association. 2010;**12**(2):86

[23] Humphries D, Mosites E, Otchere J, Twum WA, Woo L, Jones-Sanpei H, et al. Epidemiology of hookworm infection in Kintampo north municipality, Ghana: Patterns of malaria co-infection, anaemia, and albendazole treatment failure. American Journal of Tropical Medicine and Hygiene. 2011;**84**:792-800

[24] Narain K, Medhi GK, Rajguru SK, Mahanta J. Cure and re-infection patterns of Geohelminthic infections after treatment in communities inhabiting the tropical rainforest of Assam, India. Southeast Asian Journal of Tropical Medicine and Public Health. 2004;**35**(3):512-517

[25] Stepek G, Buttle DJ, Duce IR, Behnke JM. Human gastrointestinal nematode infections: Are new control methods required? International Journal of Experimental Pathology. 2006;**87**:325-341

[26] Gilgen D, Mascie-Taylor CGN, Rosetta L. Intestinal helminth infections, anaemia and labour productivity of female tea pluckers in Bangladesh. Tropical Medicine and International Health. 2001;**6**:449-457

[27] Kurscheid J, Laksono B, Park MJ, Clements AC, Sadler R, McCarthy JS, et al. Epidemiology of soil-transmitted helminth infections in Semarang, Central Java, Indonesia. PLoS Neglected Tropical Diseases. 2020;**14**(12):e0008907

[28] World Health Organisation / Unite Nations International Children Educational Fund. Progress on Sanitation

and Drinking-Water: 2010 Update. Geneva and New York: Joint Monitoring Programme for Water Supply and Sanitation; 2010

[29] Ghana Health Service Report. Two-Year Strategic Plan for Integrated Neglected Tropical Diseases Control in Ghana. Ghana: Ministry of Health, Republic of Ghana; 2008. pp. 2007-2008

[30] Lubis IN, Pasaribu S, Lubis CP. Current status of the efficacy and effectiveness of albendazole and mebendazole for the treatment of Ascaris lumbricoides in North-Western Indonesia. Asian Pacific Journal of Tropical Medicine. 2012;**5**(8):605-609

[31] Farmer P, Léandre F, Mukherjee J, Gupta R, Tarter L, Kim JY. Community-based treatment of advanced HIV disease: Introducing DOT-HAART directly observed therapy with highly active antiretroviral therapy. Bulletin of the World Health Organanisation. 2001;**79**:12

[32] Singer BH, de Castro MC. Bridges to sustainable tropical health. Processes of National Academy of Science USA. 2007;**104**:16038-16043

[33] Jia TW, Melville S, Utzinger J, King CH, Zhou XN. Soil-transmitted helminthes re-infection after drug treatment: A systematic review and meta-analysis. PLoS Neglected Tropical Diseases. 2012;**6**(5):e1621

Chapter 16

Zoonotic Trematode Infections; Their Biology, Intermediate Hosts and Control

Henry Madsen and Jay R. Stauffer, Jr.

Abstract

Many diseases linked with trematodes are zoonotic, including liver flukes (*Fasciola* spp., *Clonorchis*, and *Opistorchis* are the most common), intestinal flukes (some species of the Heterophyidae), lung flukes (*Paragonimus* spp.) and the blood flukes (schistosome species). A characteristic for all these species is that they have a vertebrate as final host and have freshwater snail species as the first intermediate host, and for the food-borne trematodes, also a second intermediate host where their infective stage (metacercariae) lodge or in case of the Fasciolidae, cercariae encyst on aquatic or semi-aquatic plants. We describe the biology of transmission with emphasis on the intermediate snail hosts, and the control of these.

Keywords: schistosomiasis, liver flukes, intestinal flukes, snail intermediate host

1. Introduction

Diseases resulting from zoonotic transmission of parasites are common [1]. Most parasitic zoonoses are neglected diseases despite causing a considerable global burden of ill health in humans and have a substantial financial burden on livestock industries [1]. Zoonotic trematodiasis are found worldwide and are responsible for some serious and debilitating helminthic diseases in people, particularly in rural and poor urban areas of low and middle-income countries [2, 3]. Many of the trematodes that infect humans are zoonotic or have zoonotic potential. Here we briefly discuss the most important zoonotic trematodes and focus on their first intermediate hosts, snails, and their control. Trematodes (Trematoda) belong to the phylum Platyhelminthes which also contains Turbellaria (mostly non-parasitic animals such as planarians), and three entirely parasitic groups: Cestoda, Trematoda, and Monogenea. Trematoda includes two subclasses of parasitic flatworms, also known as flukes, i.e., Aspidogastrea and Digenea. Here we focus on Digenea, which as adults are internal parasites of vertebrates. Trematodes have both sexual and asexual reproduction in different host species. Sexual reproduction occurs in the final vertebrate host, while asexual reproduction occurs in the first intermediate host, usually certain species freshwater or marine snails. Most trematodes have a second intermediate host where their infective stage (metacercariae) lodge. For the food-borne trematodes, various fish species, crustaceans, or

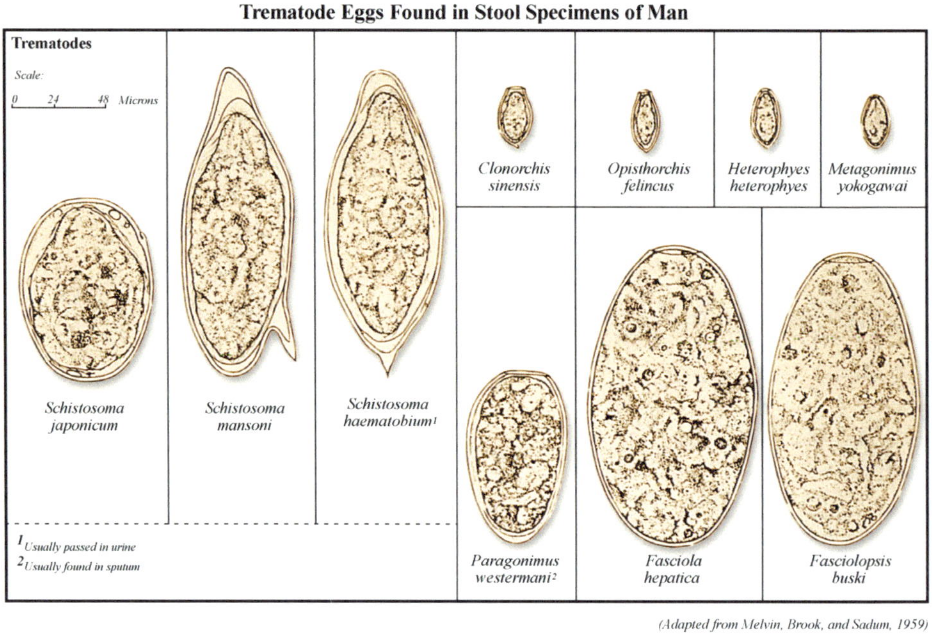

Figure 1.
Eggs of various trematodes found in human feces or urine (source: Mae Melvin, public health image library (PHIL); Centers for Disease Control and Prevention).

snails may serve as second intermediate host or in case of the Fasciolidae, cercariae encyst on aquatic or semi-aquatic plants (see more details below).

The Digenea contains about 20,000 species, within two orders, Diplostomida and Plagiorchiida. Only a few of these species infect humans, and some of the diseases they cause are briefly discussed below, i.e., schistosomiasis and several species of food-borne zoonotic trematodes (paragonimiasis, fascioliasis, clonorchiasis, opisthorchiasis, and others). Examples of eggs from these trematodes are shown in **Figure 1**. Some species of trematodes have a relatively narrow range of snail species that serve as intermediate hosts, while others have an apparently wide range (**Table 1**).

2. The diseases

2.1 Schistosomiasis

Schistosomiasis is native in many countries in Africa, South America, and Asia with an estimated number of 200 million infected people and with 800 million being at risk according to Doumenge et al. [4], but considering the population increase since then, the number of humans currently at risk must be well over a billion [5]. According to latest available information somewhere between 230 and 250 million people are actually infected [6, 7]. People become infected by contact with water harboring schistosome-infected intermediate host snails (**Figure 2**). The snails release cercariae into the water that contact and penetrate human skin.

The schistosomes belong to the trematode order Diplostomida, superfamily Schistosomatoidea and Schistosomatidae. The genus *Schistosoma* contains 23 recognized species and at least 7 of these are of medical and veterinary importance [8].

Digenean order	**Diplostomida**		**Plagiorchiida**						
				Opisthorchioidea			**Echinostomatoidea**		**Paramphistomoidea**
	Schistosomatidae		**Paragonimidae**	**Opisthorchiidae**		**Heterophyidae**	**Echino-stomatidae**	**Fasciolidae**	**Paramphistomidae**
	Schistosoma	**Other schistosomes**	***Paragonimus***	***Clonorchis***	***Opistorchis***	**Intestinal flukes**	***Echinostoma***	***Fasciola***	***Paramphistomum***
Neritomorpha									
Neritidae									
Caenogastropoda									
Viviparidae									
Ampullaridae									
Cerithiidae		x				x			
Melanopsidae									
Pachychilidae		x	x	x			x		
Paludomidae									
Potamididae									
Semisulcospiridae									
Thiaridae		x	x	x			x		
Littorinidae		x				x			
Planaxidae		x							
Amnicolidae			x			x			
Cochliopidae			x						
Bithyniidae				x	x	x			
Pomatiopsidae	x		x			x			
Stenothyridae						x			

Digenean order	**Diplostomida**		**Plagiorchiida**						
				Opisthorchioidea			**Echinostomatoidea**		**Paramphistomoidea**
	Schistosomatidae		**Paragonimidae**	**Opisthorchiidae**		**Heterophyidae**	**Echino-stomatidae**	**Fasciolidae**	**Paramphistomidae**
	Schistosoma	**Other schistosomes**	***Paragonimus***	***Clonorchis***	***Opistorchis***	**Intestinal flukes**	***Echinostoma***	***Fasciola***	***Paramphistomum***
Assimineidae			x	x					
Hydrobiidae			x			x			
Panpulmonata									
Valvatidae									
Ellobiidae									
Planorbidae	x	x					x	x	x
Bulinidae	x	x							
Physidae		x					x		x
Ancylidae									
Lymnaeidae		x					x		x
Acroloxidae									

Table 1.
Snail families involved as intermediate hosts for trematodes (flukes) causing disease in humans or domestic animals. Only certain species within a family are intermediate hosts for a given parasite.

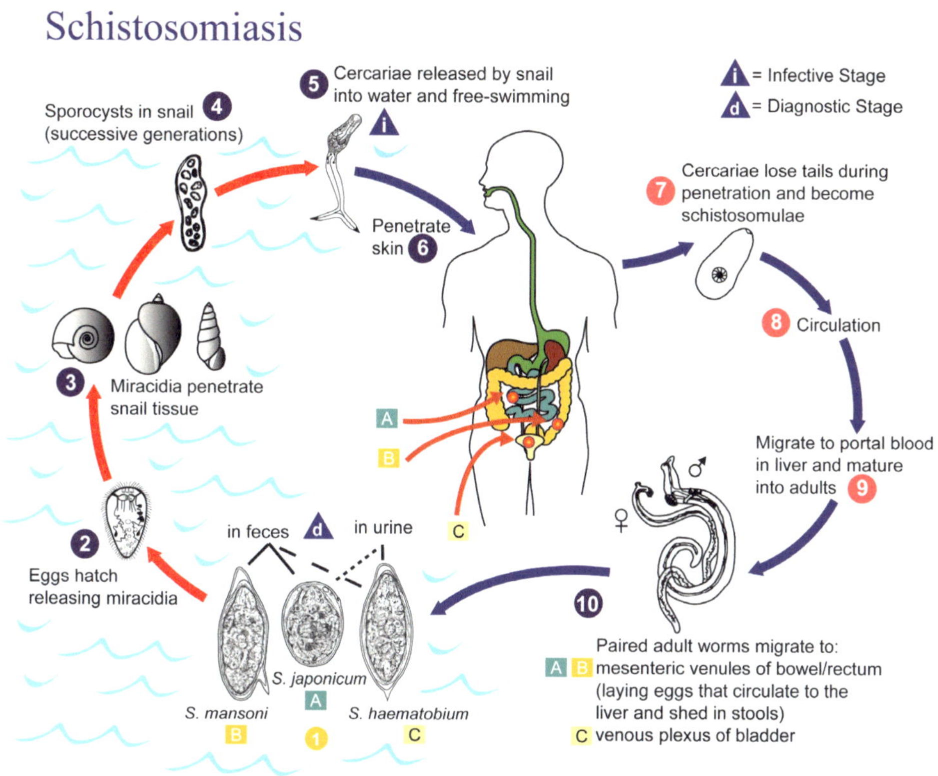

Figure 2.
Life cycle of schistosomes infecting humans (source: Alexander J. da Silva & Melanie Moser, public health image library (PHIL), Centers for Disease Control and Prevention).

The species are divided into four groups, i.e., the *S. japonicum* group, the *Schistosoma mansoni* group, the *S. indicum* group and the *S. haematobium* group [8]. Some species primarily infect humans while others primarily infect non-human animals, but infections with the former group may be found in non-human vertebrates and infections with the latter group may be found in humans [9, 10].

Species within the group of *S. japonicum* use as intermediate hosts, species of the Pomatiopsidae. *Schistosoma japonicum* is the major species of medical importance in South-East Asia and the species has many definitive hosts [6]. *Schistosoma mekongi* is found in parts of the Mekong River basin region in Cambodia, Laos, and Thailand [11]. The other species of the *S. japonicum* group are mainly parasites of rats [12] although human infection by *Schistosoma malayanum* are found [11].

The group of *Schistosoma mansoni* has 2 species, *S. mansoni* and *Schistosoma rodhaini* both using *Biomphalaria* spp. (**Figure 3**) as an intermediate host. *S. mansoni* is found throughout sub-Saharan Africa, parts of the Arabian Peninsula and it is the only *Schistosoma* spp. found in South America [8]. The two species hybridize in the wild [12]. Species of the group *S. indicum* occur in the western and southern Asian regions and are commonly found in animals, i.e., ungulates, horses, pigs, and possibly dogs [8]. The species use *Indoplanorbis exustus* as intermediate host [8]. The group associated with *S. haematobium* includes nine species that are the most widespread, i.e., Africa, Indian Ocean Islands, Arabian Peninsula, and Mediterranean regions [8]. *Schistosoma haematobium* causes urogenital schistosomiasis, while other species, *S. intercalatum* and *S. guineensis* infecting humans in this group cause intestinal

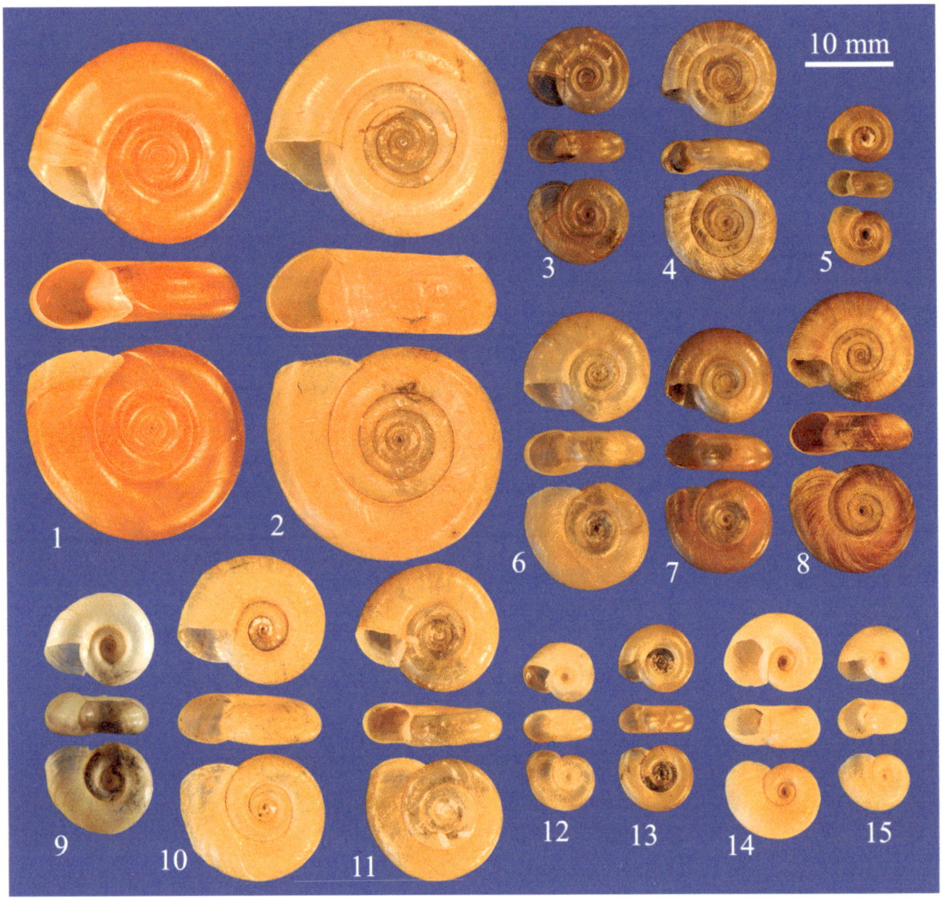

Figure 3.
Neotropical (1–5) and African (6–15) Biomphalaria species, B. glabrata (1), B. tenagophila (2), B. straminea (3), B. havanensis (4), B. helophila (5), B. alexandrina (6), B. angulosa (7), B. camerunensis (8), B. pfeifferi (9), B. salinarum (10), B. sudanica (11), B. choanomphala (12), B. rhodesiensis (13), B. smithi (14), B. stanleyi (15).

schistosomiasis [8]. Natural interactions and introgressive hybridisation between these species are common [8, 13, 14].

Each of the species of schistosomes infecting humans has a characteristic and limited intermediate snail-host spectrum. The intermediate hosts of *S. mansoni*, *S. haematobium*, *S. intercalatum*, and *S. guineensis* belong to the family Planorbidae or Bulinidae (previously a subfamily of the Planorbidae) while those of *S. japonicum*, *S. mekongi*, and *S. malayensis* are caenogastropods that belong to the Pomatiopsidae [15]. Various species of *Biomphalaria* serve as intermediate hosts for *S. mansoni* (**Figure 3**) and certain *Bulinus* spp. (**Figure 4**) are intermediate hosts for *S. haematobium*, *S. guineensis*, and *S. intercalatum*. For *S. japonicum*, species of the genus *Oncomelania* are the intermediate hosts (**Figure 4**). Species-level relationships within *Oncomelania* are not fully resolved but there seems to be four species that currently transmit *S. japonicum*, i.e., subspecies of *O. hupensis* in eastern China, *O. robertsoni* in western China, *O. quadrasi* in the Philippines and *O. lindoensis* on Sulawesi [16]. For *S. mekongi* and *S. malayensis*, the intermediate host is from the subfamily Triculinae, tribe Pachydrobiini, i.e., *Neotricula aperta* and *Robertsiella kaporensis*, respectively [17, 18] (**Figure 4**). More species can

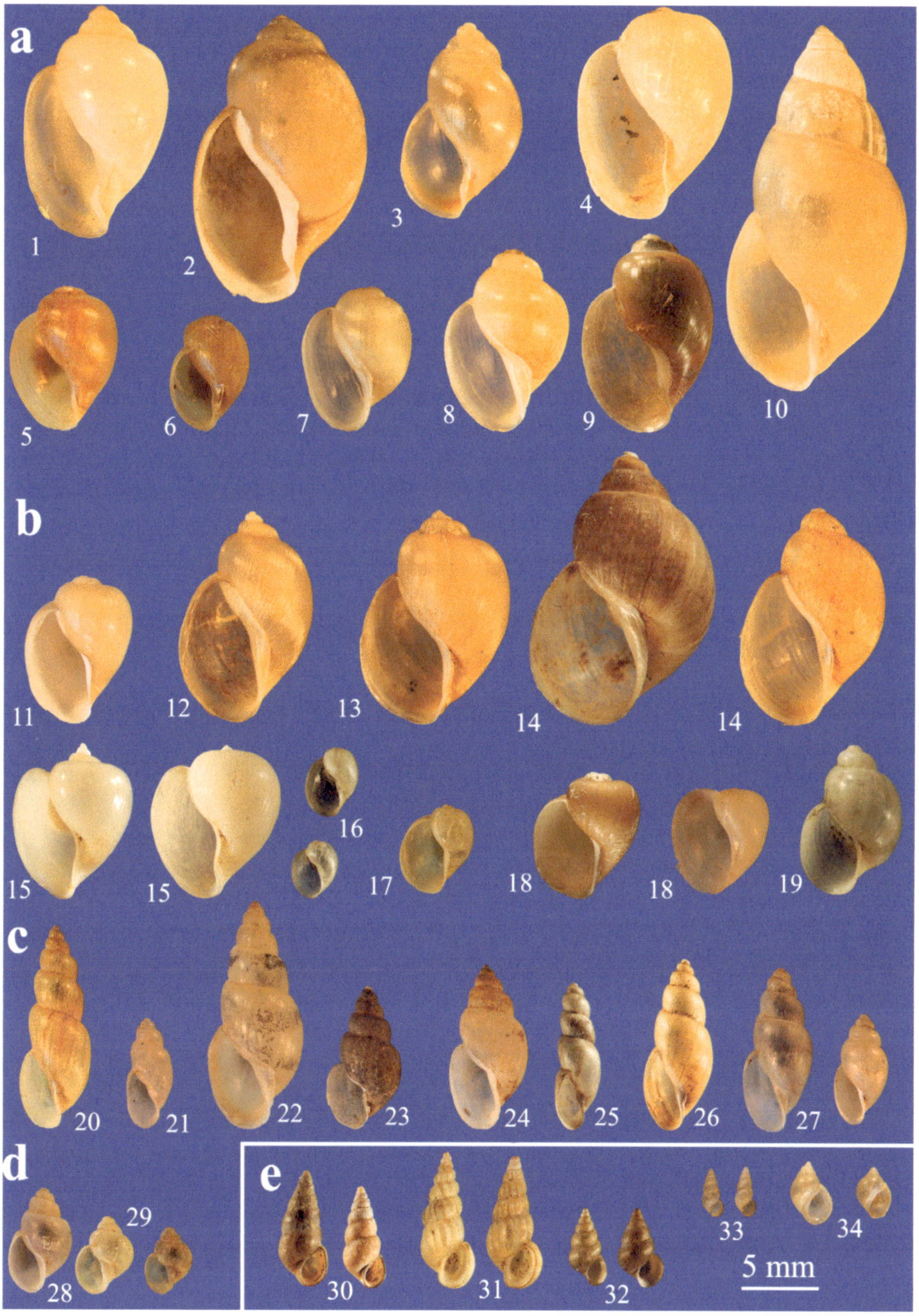

Figure 4.
Representative species of Bulinus, Oncomelania, Robertsiella and Neotricula. The B. africanus group (a): Bulinus abyssinicus (1), B. africanus (2), B. nasutus (3), B. ugandae (4), B. jousseaumei (5), B. obtusus (6), B. obtusispira (7), B. umbilicatus (8), B. globosus (9), B. productus (10). B. truncatus/tropicus complex (b): Bulinus angolensis (11), B. liratus (12), B. natalensis (13), B. tropicus (14), B. nyassanus (15), B. succinoides (16), B. transversalis (17), B. trigonus (18), B. truncatus (19). The B. forskalii group (c): Bulinus bavayi (20), B. beccarii (21), B. canescens (22), B. cernicus (23), B. crystallinus (24), B. forskalii (25), B. scalaris (26), B. senegalensis (28). The B. reticulatus group (d): B. reticulatus (28), B. wrighti (29). Asian species (e): Oncomelania hupensis smooth (30) form and ribbed form (31), O. quadrasi (32), Robertsiella kaporensis (33), Neotricula aperta (34).

be infected experimentally but they may not transmit the parasite in nature [19]. For example, there have been reports that *S. haematobium* was transmitted by *Ferrissia* in India; at least three endemic foci of human schistosomiasis have been described in India previously and sporadic autochthonous cases and cercarial dermatitis are also common (see references in [20]). Experimental exposure of *Ferrissia tenuis* to miracidia of *S. haematobium* showed that this snail could be infected and shed cercariae [21]. In the north-western extremity of Africa, *Planorbarius metidjensis* is common and although it is an experimental host for *S. mansoni* and *S. haematobium* [22, 23] there is no evidence that it is a natural host [23].

Snails may be widely distributed in an area, but there is a tendency for infected snails with *Schistosoma* spp. to be focally distributed in particular areas where infected people contaminate the water with their wastes. In some cases, human infections may be facilitated by prior contamination of habitats by reservoir hosts especially for *S. japonicum*, but also possibly for *Schistosoma mansoni* and *S. haematobium*. Snail populations undergo great seasonal variations in density and infection rates. Rainfall and/or temperature are the main causative factors. This results in the pattern of transmission commonly being of a focal and seasonal nature. Although prevalence of infection in the intermediate hosts may be low, this can result in a high percentage of human infections, e.g., in Lake Malawi [24].

2.2 Avian schistosome

Swimmer's itch or cercarial dermatitis is a short-term immune reaction occurring in the skin of humans that have been penetrated by cercariae of schistosomes (Schistosomatidae) that normally develop in birds or in mammalian hosts other than humans. Genera often associated with swimmer's itch in humans are *Trichobilharzia* and *Gigantobilharzia*, but species such as *Schistosomatium douthitti*, a parasite of rodents, may also cause swimmer's itch. In marine habitats, especially along the coasts, swimmer's itch can occur as well. Symptoms, which include itchy, raised papules, commonly occur within hours of infection and do not generally last more than a week. It is common in freshwater, brackish, and marine habitats worldwide and application of molecular diagnostic techniques has begun to unravel the many schistosome species that can be responsible [25]. Various species of Lymnaeidae, Physidae, Planorbidae, Bulinidae (see some species in **Figures 5** and **6**) and other taxa are intermediate hosts [25–28].

In Thailand, *Indoplanorbis exustus* together with *Lymnaea rubiginosa* are referred to as the "itchy snail" by rural people [29]. These snail species are hosts for a number of schistosomes including *Schistosoma spindale*, *S. indicum*, and *S. nasale*. Though these species do not develop to maturity in humans, they may cause cercarial dermatitis.

2.3 Paragonimus

Paragonimiasis, also known as pulmonary distomiasis, is a parasitic disease of humans and animals in various parts of the world, but principally in the Orient (Far East). Its etiological agents are species of the trematode genus *Paragonimus* which utilize caenogastropods (specifically superfamilies Cerithiodea and Truncatelloidea) as first intermediate hosts (see examples in **Figures 7** and **8**) and decapod crustaceans, primarily freshwater crabs and crayfish, as second intermediate hosts.

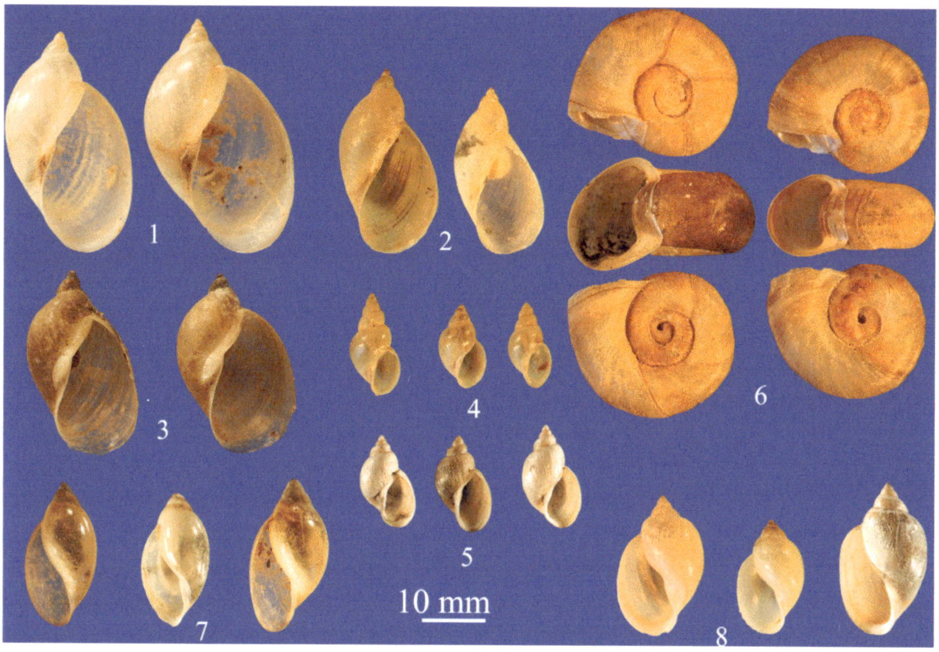

Figure 5.
Some species of the Lymnaeidae, Physidae and Bulinidae. Lymnaeidae: Radix natalensis (1), Pseudosuccinea columella (2), Radix auricularia (3), Galba truncatula (4), Austropeplea viridis (6). Bulinidae: Indoplanorbis exustus (6). Physidae: Aplexa waterloti (7), Physa acuta (8).

The genus *Paragonimus* contains several species that infect a variety of mammals and birds and some of these species affect other vertebrates. Lung fluke infections are distributed in certain parts of the World where food habits include eating raw crabs, and crayfish, which contain the infective metacercarial cysts. Several million people are thought to be infected with paragonomiasis and almost 300 million are at risk of infection [30, 31]. In Africa, *Paragonimus africanus* is important [32], while in Mexico and Central America *Paragonimus mexicanus* causes occasional human infections [30]. Similarly, in the Midwest states of the USA, a number of human infections with *Paragonimus kellicotti* have been reported. The main endemic areas are in the Orient and Southeast Asia. In these areas, the etiological agent in humans is mainly *Paragonimus westermani* [31].

The cercariae penetrate the soft body parts of the crustacean host and then invade the viscera and muscles of this host, where they usually become encysted in specific organs depending on the species of lung fluke and the species of the crustacean host (**Figure 9**). When the mammalian host, human or reservoir host ingests infected crab or crayfish meat or viscera (raw, soaked in rice wine, or salted), the metacercaria excyst in the duodenum and migrates through the intestinal wall in about an hour, reaching the abdominal cavity in 3–6 h. The larvae of various lung flukes enter and remain in the abdominal wall for several days (up to 3 weeks), then migrate through the diaphragm to the pleural cavity, where they penetrate the serosal layers of the lungs. Finally, they arrive near the bronchioles, where they develop to adult worms in pairs, and exist in tissue capsules laid down by the host, about 6–8 weeks after ingestion of the parasitized crustacean host. The lung capsules containing the worms connect with the respiratory passages of the lung, and the eggs of the parasite are moved along with lung exudates [33].

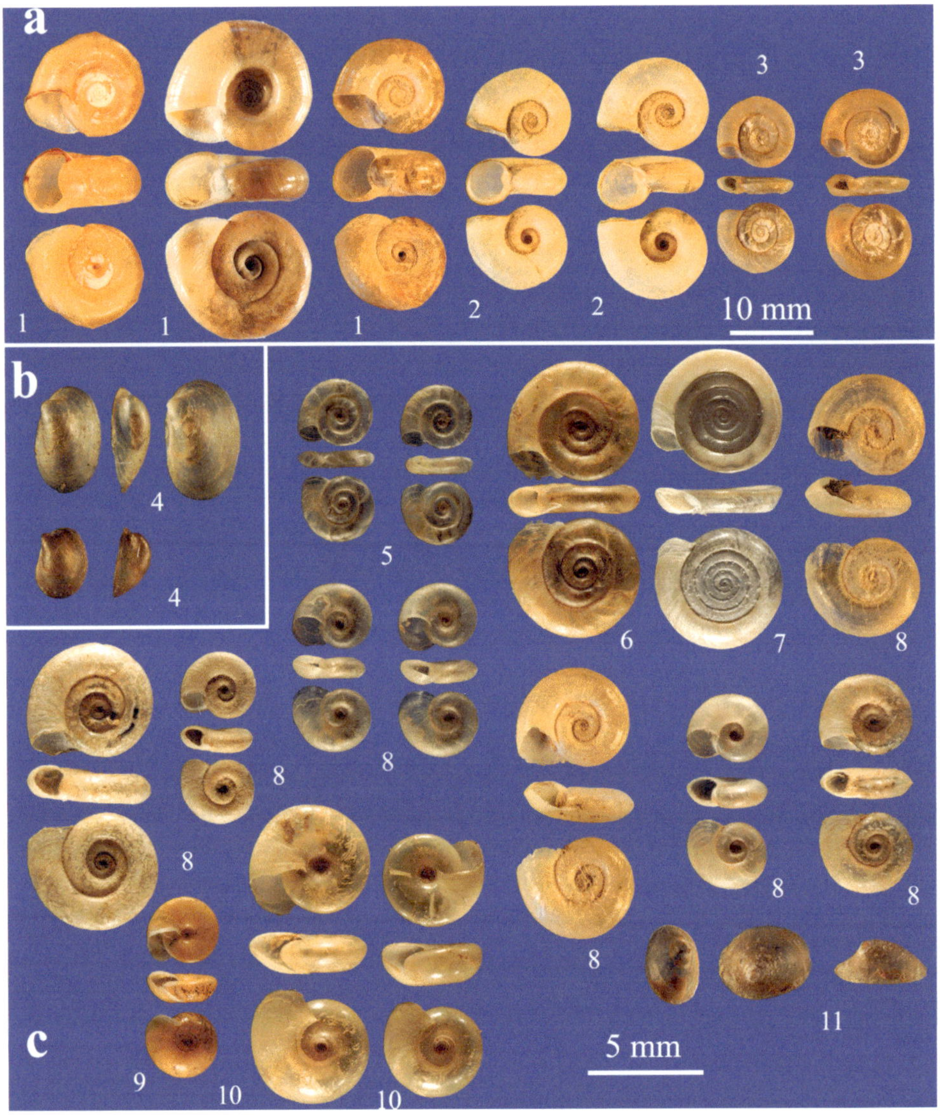

Figure 6.
Species of the Planorbidae (a and c) and Burnupiidae (b). Planorbidae: Planorbella (Helisoma) duryi (1), Planorbarius metidjensis (2), Planorbis planorbis (3), Africanogyrus coretus (5), Ceratophallus natalensis (6), Drepanotrema sp. (7), Gyraulus spp. (8), Polypylis hemisphaerula (9), Segmentorbis spp. (10), Ferrissia sp. (11). Burnupidae: Burnupia sp. (4). The scale shown in part c is also used for part b.

2.4 Fish-borne zoonotic trematodes (Clonorchiasis, Opistorchiasis, and Heterophyidiasis)

Fish-borne zoonotic trematodes utilize fish as their second intermediate host and comprise about 12 families, and five of these, Clinostomatidae, Echinostomatidae, Heterophyidae, Opisthorchiidae, and Troglotrematidae have been reported to infect humans. Among those, the opisthorchid flukes have the most public health importance [34]. It has been recognized as a Type I carcinogen, and chronic infection by this liver fluke leads to cholangiocarcinoma development. The heterophyid intestinal

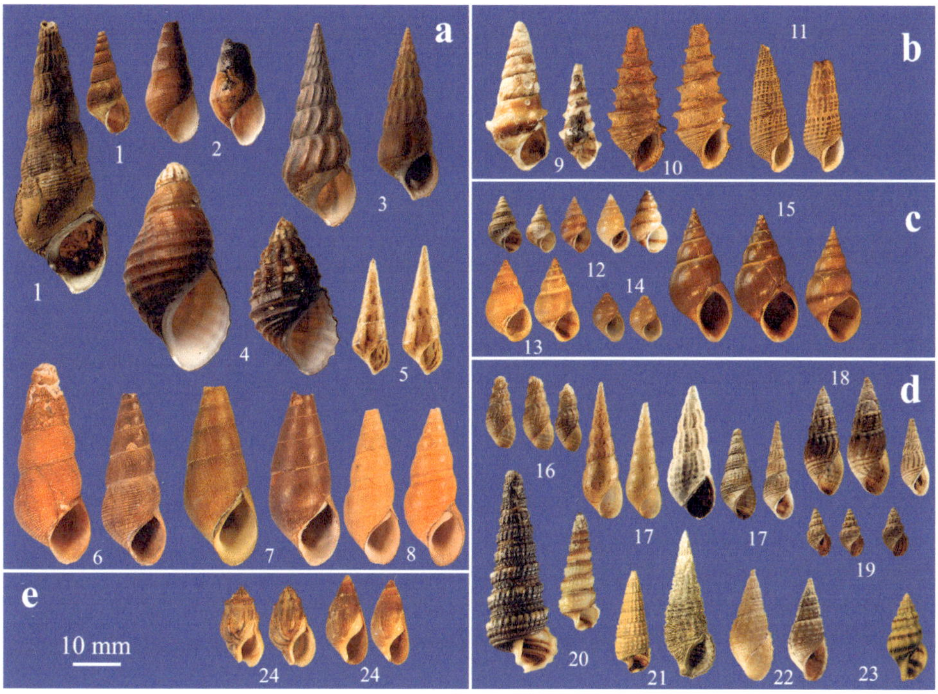

Figure 7.
Selected species of Pachychilidae (a), Heminiscidae (b), Paludomidae (c), Thiaridae (d) Potamididae (d), Melanopsidae (e) and other (d). Pachychilidae: Brotia sp. (1); Brotia costula (2); Brotia swinhoei (3); Sulcospira aubryana (4); S. housei (5); Potadoma moerchi (6); P. freethi (7); P. liricincta (8). Heminiscidae: Pachymelania aurita (9); Pachymelania fusca (10, 11). Paludomidae: Cleopatra bulimoides (12); C. nsedwensis (13), C. ferruginea (15) Pseudocleopatra togoensis (14). Thiaridae: Melanoides jugicosta (16), M. tuberculata (17), Sermyla riqueti (18), Thiara scabra (19), Tarebia granifera (22), Potamididae: Tympanotonus fuscatus (20), Cerithidea sp. (21). Melanopsidae: Melanopsis spp. (24). Other: Anentome helena (23).

fluke sometimes coexists in the endemic region of the liver fluke and can cause confusion in diagnosis and prevalence since eggs of both the opisthorchid and heterophyid flukes are similar. An overview of the various species is given in Waikagul and Thaenkham [34] and Hung et al. [35].

Fully embryonated small eggs of *C. sinensis* are found in the stools of infected humans and other mammalian hosts (e.g., dogs and cats). These eggs do not hatch until they are eaten by the snail, the first intermediate host [36]. For *C. sinensis*, the snail hosts are species of caenogastropods of the family Bithyniidae (*Parafossarulus*, *Bithynia*) or Semisulcospiridae (*Semisulcospira*). In addition, species of the Thiaridae, especially *Melanoides tuberculata* have been reported as hosts for *C. sinensis* [37] but experimental infection of this species failed [38]. The miracidia hatch in the esophagus, intestine, or rectum of the snail, and then penetrate the wall of these organs to become sporocysts developing in the hemolymph spaces of the snail (**Figure 10**). Rediae develop and migrate to the digestive gland area and form cercariae, which soon leave the snail and swim in the adjacent water [36]. They then penetrate the skin of the fish second intermediate host and become encysted metacercariae in the muscles. The metacercariae become infective within a month, and when the infected fish is ingested raw, or slightly cooked or pickled, by man or eaten by other mammalian hosts, the metacercariae excyst and make their way to the liver, which they reach in about a day or less. After reaching the bile passages, the young worms mature. The

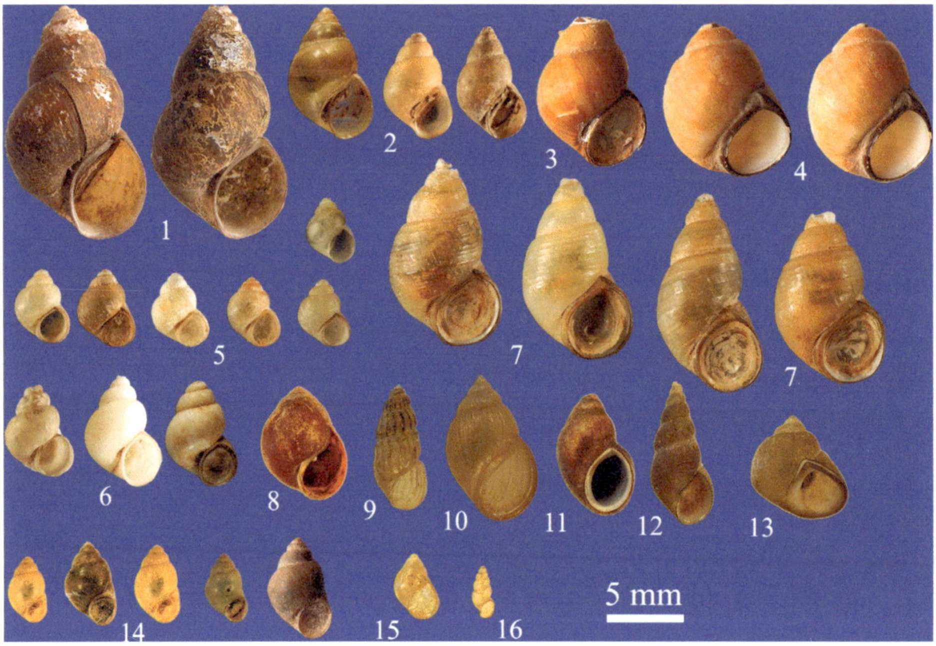

Figure 8.
Selected species of the Truncatelloidea. Bithynia fuchsiana (1), Bithynia sp. (2), Digoniostoma siamensis (3), Alocinma longicornis (4), Parafossarulus manchouricus (7), Gabbiella stanleyi (5), Gabbiella senaariensis (6), Assiminea sp. (8), Hubendickia sp. (9), Pachydrobia spp. (10, 11), Fairbankia sp. (12), Julienia sp. (13), Stenothyra spp. (14), Neotricula aperta (15), Robertsiella kaporensis (16).

first eggs are laid about 4 weeks after infection, but the worms continue to grow for some additional months. In addition to humans, dogs, cats, pigs, and rats have been found naturally infected and constitute effective reservoir hosts. In some regions where prevalence of infection among humans is very low or lacking, as in some parts of China and Vietnam, prevalence of infection is usually high among other mammals. Cats, rabbits, and guinea pigs are good experimental hosts.

Clonorchiasis is caused by the fluke *Clonorchis sinensis* (China, Japan, Korea, Russia, Thailand, and North Vietnam), and human opisthorciasis is caused by primarily *Opisthorchis viverrini* (Cambodia, Lao PDR, Thailand, Central and South Vietnam) or *O. felineus* (The Baltic States, eastern Germany, Italy, Kazakhstan, Poland, Russia, Eastern Siberia, and Ukraine) and is contracted through eating raw infected fish [34]. These trematodes have very similar life cycles.

Heterophyidae comprises several genera and species of trematodes of almost worldwide distribution. More than 25 species have been found parasitizing humans around the World [34, 35]. The heterophyid is a small-sized fluke, about 1 mm in length, and is parasitic mostly in the small intestine of birds and mammals and rarely in fish and reptiles.

The worms are usually found lodging in intestinal mucosa between villi, however, they have invaded the submucosal level in experimental immunosuppressive mice. Within a week after the metacercaria is ingested by the definitive host, metacercaria develop to mature adults in the intestine. Heterophyid adults have a short life; the reported life spans varied among different host species [34, 39].

Fish-borne zoonotic trematodes (FZT) are an important problem and fish produced in aquaculture may present a food safety risk in some areas of

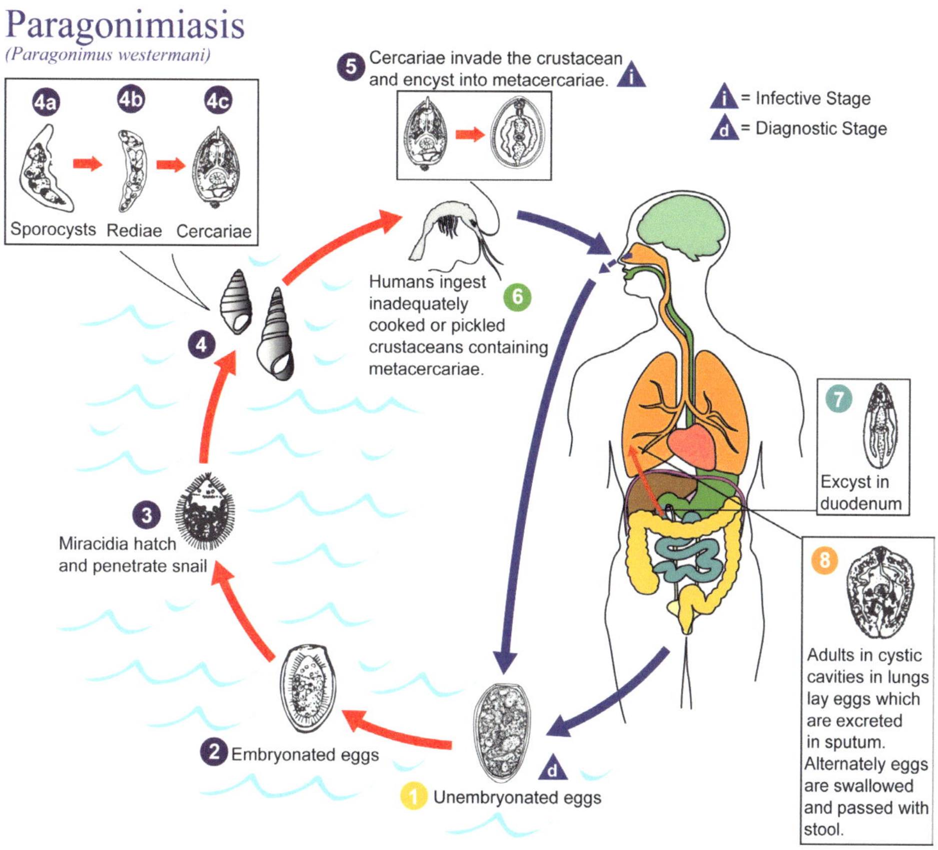

Figure 9.
Life cycle of Paragonimus westermani (source: Alexander J. da Silva & Melanie Moser, public health image library (PHIL), Centers for Disease Control and Prevention).

Southeast Asia where aquaculture is very important [36]. In at least parts of Vietnam, however, transmission of *C. sinensis* is not common in aquaculture ponds and usually occurs in natural habitats [40]. On the other hand, heterophyid trematodes are very common in aquaculture ponds. The fish culture industry may have aggravated the situation in some areas, although *C. sinensis* and *O. viverrini* mainly are transmitted in natural waterbodies. Large and small lakes and ponds are used for culturing fish, and these bodies of water are usually polluted with human and animal excreta containing eggs of FZT. Because raw fish are mainly eaten by adults, infections with clonorchiasis are, in general, more prevalent in the higher age groups (30–50 years); this is usually consistent in all endemic areas.

2.5 Echinostomatidiasis

The superfamily Echinostomatoidea is a large, cosmopolitan group of digeneans currently including nine families and 105 genera, with the vast majority parasitic, as adults, in birds with relatively few taxa parasitizing mammals, reptiles, and exceptionally, fishes [41]. Recent studies on the phylogeny of the group combining morphology and molecular data have resulted in several changes [41].

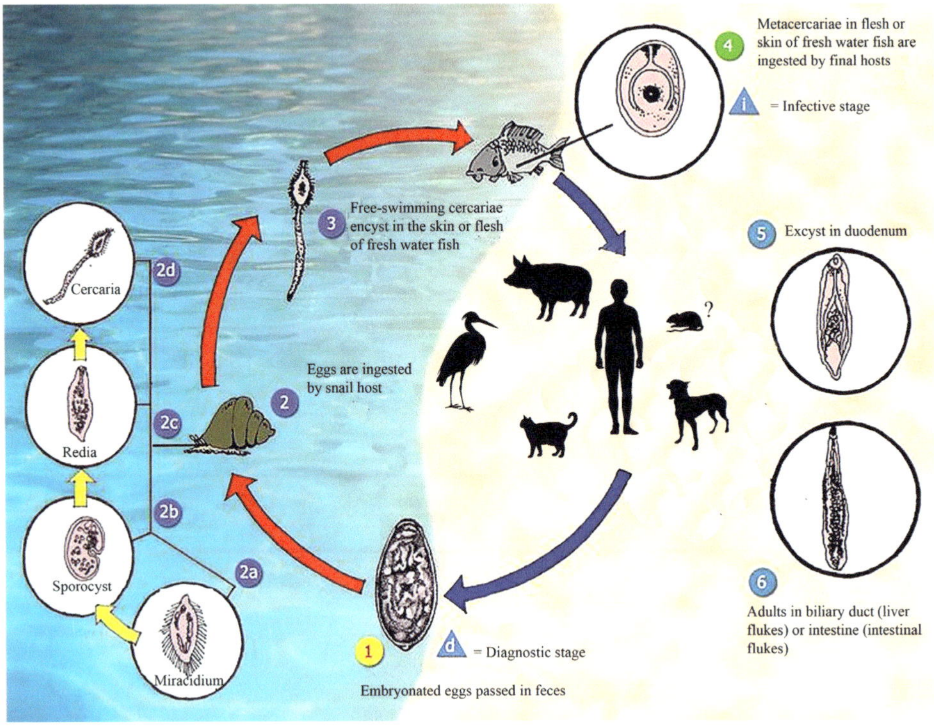

Figure 10.
Life cycle of fish-borne zoonotic trematodes (Opistchorchidae and Heterophyidae) (source Clausen et al. [36]).

Echinostomatidiasis is caused by a number of fluke species, belonging to the Echinostomatidae, which share certain morphological features, among which are the presence of a head collar surrounding the oral sucker, provided with a single or double crown of large spines which are larger than those covering the body surface. They are usually stout, fleshy, medium-sized flukes parasitizing birds and mammals in various parts of the world [42]. Several birds, during their migration, carry the infection with several echinostome species along their migratory routes. Various life cycle patterns are exhibited by echinostomes. Usually they are less specific than schistosomes as to their first or second intermediate hosts or their definitive hosts. The first intermediate hosts are several species of aquatic Hygrophila or Caenogastropods and the second intermediate hosts are the same or other species of snails, bivalves, tadpoles, or fish. The cercariae of certain species do not require a second intermediate host but, instead, encyst in the open.

Echinostomes are usually harmless flukes in the intestine of their hosts. Certain species, however, and heavy infections of the harmless species, produce some pathology and pronounced symptoms in poultry and small mammals. They are, therefore, of significance in veterinary medicine.

Transmission of the echinostome to humans is either through eating raw or undercooked fish, snails, or amphibians. Human cases have been reported mostly in Asia. Duodenum mucosal bleeding and ulceration are the main clinical findings due to mechanical damages caused by the worms. The common symptoms are abdominal pain and diarrhea followed by weakness and weight loss [42].

2.6 Fascioliasis

Fascioliasis, a disease caused by the liver flukes *Fasciola hepatica* and *Fasciola gigantica*, is cosmopolitan in distribution and occurs in sheep- and cattle-raising countries of the world, parasitizing these animals and other herbivores on almost every continent and on several islands. In Europe, diseases of sheep and cattle are found in every country, and they manifest in the form of epidemics among humans, especially in England, France, and Italy. Human fascioliasis has also been reported from Mexico, South and Central America, Asia, Africa, and Australia and is believed to be more common than has been thought. This could be ascertained if there were more accurate diagnostic methods and better reporting [43].

Fascioliasis due to *F. hepatica* generally occurs in temperate climates, and thus the disease is prevalent in Europe, North America, northern Asia, Australia, and northern Africa [44]. It is also present in the highlands of Kenya, in South Africa, and in Central and South America. *F. gigantica*, on the other hand, is the common liver fluke in widespread areas of Africa and Asia. In some parts of the world, the geographical distribution of *F. gigantica* overlaps that of *F. hepatica*.

The life cycle of *F. hepatica* is illustrated in **Figure 11**. Adults reside in the intrahepatic biliary ducts of the mammalian host. The eggs are laid in the bile

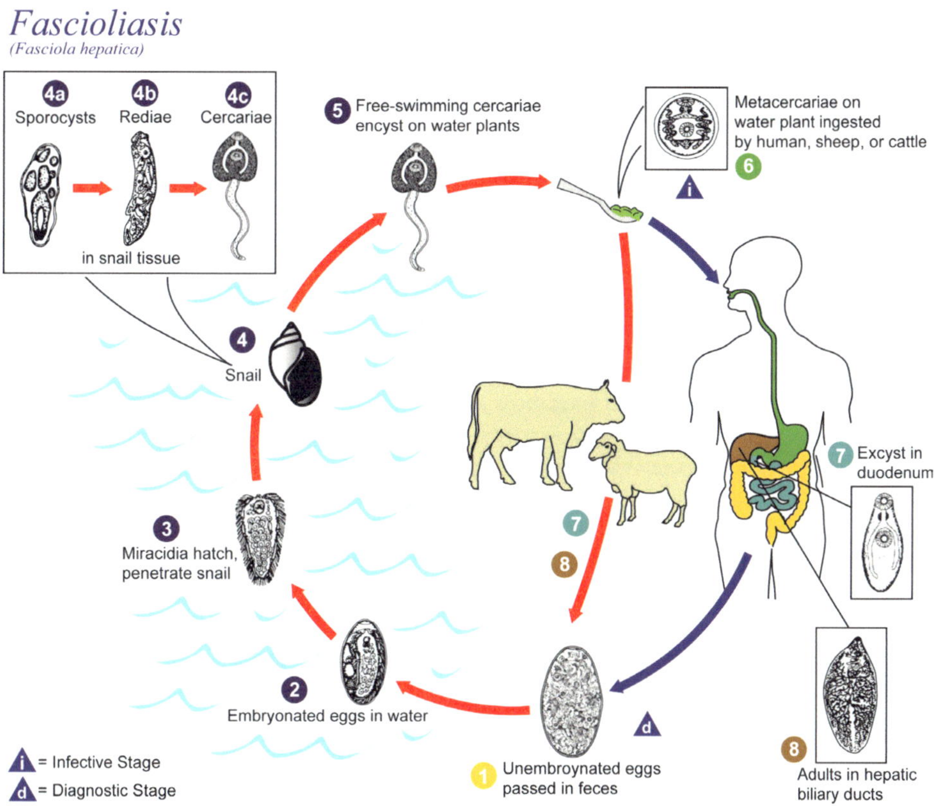

Figure 11.
Life cycle of Fasciola hepatica (source: Alexander J. da Silva & Melanie Moser, public health image library (PHIL), Centers for Disease Control and Prevention).

ducts, proceed to the intestine with the bile, and are evacuated with the feces. The development of the eggs in the water takes from 10 to 15 days at an optimal temperature of 23–25°C. The fully developed miracidium escapes from the egg. The miracidium swims actively in the water and tries to invade various snail species of the Lymnaeidae (**Figure 5**) in different geographic areas of the world. The sporocyst developing from each miracidium near the site of penetration, usually in the mantle edge, the kidney and the esophageal area, produces rediae in about 2–3 weeks. The latter move actively and migrate to the distal area of the snail, containing mainly the digestive gland. Within the body of rediae, cercariae are produced which exit the snail and actively swim in the water. Development of *Fasciola* in the snail host is affected by the environment, in particular temperature. Cercariae encyst rapidly on aquatic vegetation, grass, bark, or any floating debris, or encyst free in the water, and may either float or settle to the bottom of the water. The metacercarial cysts are resistant and remain viable for a long period but are killed by excessive heat and dryness.

Mammalian hosts, including humans, consuming aquatic vegetation with metacercariae or drinking water from contaminated snail habitats containing the metacercariae, contract the infection. The metacercariae, soon after ingestion, excyst in the small intestine. After excystment, they penetrate the wall of the small intestine to the abdominal cavity. They have been found in the latter cavity 1–3 days from the time that they have been ingested, depending on the species of the host. They wander around in the viscera and may settle and become established in ectopic sites other than the liver.

2.7 Paramphistomatidiasis

The paramphistome flukes are represented by many species throughout the world, and they are parasites of the alimentary tract (stomach and intestine) of humans, nonhuman primates, ruminants, equines, and other herbivores; only about two species occur in birds [45]. These flukes are large fleshy parasites, measuring up to 20 mm in length and 15 mm in width. Some of these flukes cause gastrodisciasis or paramphistomiasis. Whereas gastrodisciasis is restricted to Africa and Asia, paramphistomiasis occurs throughout the world [46].

Three important intestinal parasites cause gastrodisciasis: *Gastrodiscoides hominis*; *Gastrodiscus aegyptiacus*, and *Gastrodiscus secundus*. High prevalence rates have been reported from humans in various parts of India, but the parasite was also found in the Philippines, Kazakhstan, Vietnam, and from Indian immigrants in Guyana. In some countries, *G. hominis* infecting humans is a different strain from that infecting pig. *Gastrodiscus aegyptiacus* and *G. secundus* are common parasites of equines in Africa and Asia, and several pathological cases are on record in horses in Africa.

Infections with all the paramphistomatids (including the gastrodiscids) are acquired from the same habitats where the animals also contract fascioliasis, bovine schistosomiasis, and others, where various species of snails live together. The life cycle, though differing in minute details, is similar to that of *Fasciola* spp.

Like the fasciolid flukes, the paramphistomatids utilize freshwater pulmonate snails as intermediate hosts. Whereas *Fasciola* spp. utilize only lymnaeid snails throughout their wide geographical area, some rumen paramphistomes, such as those in the U.S., use lymnaeid snails, while other paramphistomes, and also gastrodiscids, utilize planorbid snails in other parts of the world.

DOI: http://dx.doi.org/10.5772/intechopen.102434

3. The first intermediate hosts (overview of major clades of the Gastropoda)

Trematodes require one or two intermediate hosts to complete their life cycle. The first intermediate host is specific species of freshwater water (and for some trematode species brackish or marine) gastropods. Due to the necessity of passing through the gastropods, control of these snails could, at least for some of zoonotic trematodes, be an important way to reduce their transmission (see later).

The class includes the snails, which are superficially asymmetrical and possess a spirally coiled shell; the limpets, which possess a low, conical un-spiraled shell; and the slugs, which possess a concealed shell or no shell at all. A recent paper [47] estimates the number of named and valid recent species as about 63,000 in 476 families. There is a great diversity among the freshwater gastropods. Gastropod taxonomy has undergone considerable revision and still undergoes revision as new DNA data become available. Here we use the classification as described in Bouchet et al. [47].

The class, Gastropoda, contains the following subclasses: Patellogastropoda, Neomphaliones, Vetigastropoda, Neritimorpha, Caenogastropoda, and Heterobranchia of which the last three are represented in freshwater. Many of the existing identification keys to freshwater gastropods follow the classification of Thiele [48] where Gastropoda was divided into three sub-classes Prosobranchia (Streptoneura, i.e. crossed nerve system), Pulmonata and Opisthobranchia (Euthyneura). Using the existing keys for species identification of freshwater snails, however, does not pose a real problem. Thus, Prosobranchia (often called prosobranchs) equates Caenogastropoda plus Neritidae and Pulmonata (often referred to as pulmonates) equates Hygrophila within the Panpulmonata. We shall restrict our discussion to primarily the freshwater gastropods.

3.1 Subclass: Neritomorpha

3.1.1 Neritidae and Neritilidae

The Neritidae are one of the most abundant groups of freshwater snails in the coastal streams of tropical and subtropical regions worldwide, as well as in the inland waters of the European continent [49]. The Neritiliidae, previously a subfamily in the Neritidae, include 23 described species in seven genera from low latitude areas of the World. Species of *Neritilia* occur in freshwater streams to brackish estuaries [50]. These are species of medium-sized snails with a characteristic shell, radula and operculum. Neritids require hard substrata for their grazing and locomotion, and some species of *Dostia* and *Septaria* can exclusively be found on branches and drift logs in estuaries and mangrove swamps [49]. These markedly euryhaline neritids have the potential to survive in fully marine conditions for some extended period of time and to disperse as benthic adults and eggs on drift logs [49]. The families are not known as intermediate hosts for medical or veterinary important trematodes, but some species may harbor other trematode or nematode infections. Examples of species are shown in **Figure 12**.

3.2 Subclass: Caenogastropoda

3.2.1 Viviparidae

The family (**Figure 12**) has a global distribution and moderate diversity [51] in the extant fauna (125–150 valid, described species). Viviparids are distributed primarily in

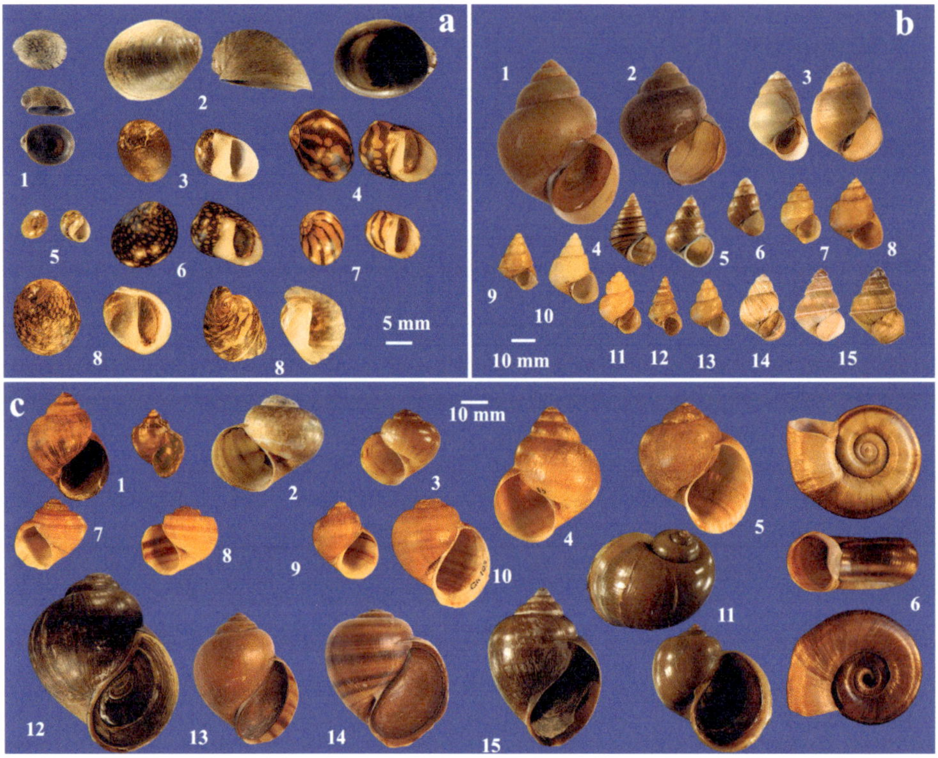

Figure 12.
Selected species of Neritidae (a), Viviparidae (b) and Ampullariidae (c). Neritidae: Dostia violacea (1, 2), Neritina afra (3, 5), N. natalensis (4, 6, 7), N. oweniana (8). Viviparidae: Cipangopaludina chinensis (1), C. lecythoides (2), Mekongia lithophaga (3), Angulyagra polyzonata (4), Filopaludina sumatrensis (5), Sinotaia aeruginosa (6), various African Bellamya spp. (7–15). Ampullariidae: Saulea vitrea (1), Lanistes spp. (2–4, 7, 8), Marisa cornuarietis (6), Pila ovata (5), Afropomus balanoidea (9), Pila africana (10), Pomacea canaliculata (11), Pila sp. (12), P. conica (13), P. ampullacea (14), P. polita (15).

lakes, rivers, and streams in temperate to tropical regions. Although they can be found in freshwater of all kinds, many species prefer, or are restricted, to one habitat type only. Their greatest diversity occurs in tropical and subtropical regions of Asia, where some 60–85 species occur. These species are medium to large snails usually with a conical shell. Tentacles are short and pointed and the right tentacle of males is transformed into a copulatory organ. The females are ovoviviparous with a uterine brood-pouch. Size and number of mature embryos may be of help to taxonomists [29]. The family is quite diverse in Asia where representatives are commonly consumed by humans. Metacercariae of the Echinostomatidae and possibly other trematodes are commonly found in viviparid snails and since many species are eaten by local people they could serve as intermediate hosts for human trematode infections if consumed insufficiently cooked. Species within the family are also reported as first intermediate hosts of some species of echinostome [51]. Some if not all species within the family are suspension feeders giving them a competitive advantage over species that only graze.

3.2.2 Ampullariidae

Ampullariidae (**Figure 12**) are predominately distributed in humid tropical and subtropical habitats in Africa, South and Central America, and Asia. The family includes 186 recent species with the majority in the three genera *Pomacea* (96 species), *Lanistes* (43 species), and *Pila* (29 species) [52]. These are large or very large species (some species can reach shell height or diameter of about 10 cm). The animal has a short rostrum that carries a tentacle-like process (pseudopodia) on either side. Tentacles are very long and thin, the eyes are placed on separate stalks beside the tentacles. The mantle cavity is separated into two parts by a septum; the right side contains the gill, the left side serves as a lung. The male has a copulatory organ formed by part of the mantle edge. Some species may harbor metacercariae of trematode species, i.e., *Echinostoma* spp. and it may also serve as first intermediate host for some avian schistosomes or echinostome species. *Pila* spp. deposit egg masses in damp soil, *Pomacea* deposit their egg masses on various objects above the water while *Lanistes* spp. deposit gelatinous egg masses in water. Only one genus, *Pila*, is represented in Asia but *Pomacea* spp., which were introduced into Asia for commercial purposes have become a very prominent element of the gastropod fauna in Asia. *Pomacea* spp. were originally introduced to Taiwan and later to other Asian countries and has become pests of wetland rice and other crops causing massive economic losses. Especially, *P. canaliculata*, the Golden Apple Snail, is effective in spreading and has become a major pest in the area. Apple snails have highly diverse feeding mechanisms (shredding, scraping and collecting) to exploit diverse food sources. *M. cornuarietis*, which has a discoid shell (**Figure 12**), has potential in biological control of schistosome intermediate hosts and it has been introduced in Africa [53–55]. Due to the unforeseeable potential impact of such introductions, further introduction or propagation of the species outside its original area of distribution should be discouraged.

3.2.3 Superfamily: Cerithioidea

The Cerithioidea (**Figure 7**) is a superfamily within the Sorbeoconcha and comprised of marine, brackish water, and freshwater gastropods containing more than 200 genera. The freshwater species are found on all continents, except Antarctica. They are dominant members of mangrove forests, estuarine mudflats, fast-flowing rivers, and placid lakes. The shell is generally turreted, sometimes ovoidal-conic, rarely subglobose. It can be smooth or with spiral and/or axial sculpture, sometimes with spiral microsculpture. The operculum is corneous, generally spiral, rarely concentric; it is retractable into the shell. The male reproductive organs are without a verge. Female reproductive organs often have a brood pouch, generally with an egg transfer groove. Many species seem to be parthenogenetic.

The superfamily contains the Hemisinidae [56], Melanopsidae [57], Pachychilidae [58], Paludomidae [59], Pleuroceridae [60], Semisulcospiridae [61], and Thiaridae [62]. Only some of these families are described further below. Some of these species are important as intermediate hosts for medically important trematodes, e.g., Semisulcospiridae is an important host for *Paragonimus westermani* and some species for *C. sinensis*.

3.2.4 Potamididae

The family has a circumtropical, distribution but is also found in moderate climates. The Potamididae (mudwhelks or mud creepers) are small to large brackish water snails that live on mud flats, mangroves, and similar habitats. The trees provide the snails with shelter, protection from predators, a solid substrate, and sometimes food [63]. Some species are intermediate hosts for some fish-borne zoonotic trematodes.

3.2.5 Pachychilidae

Pachychilidae are a group of freshwater gastropods only recently recognized as an independent freshwater radiation within the diverse and predominantly marine gastropod superfamily Cerithioidea [58]. Pachychilids were previously assigned to other cerithioidean freshwater families, such as Thiaridae or Pleuroceridae. Pachychilidae has a circumtropical distribution with the freshwater inhabiting *Pachychilus* and *Doryssa* from South and Central America, *Potadoma*, from tropical western Africa and the Congo River drainage system, and *Madagasikara* from Madagascar [58]. Asian taxa include *Paracrostoma*, *Sulcospira* and *Brotia* from Southeast Asia [58].

Pachychilid gastropods are a conspicuous element of the freshwater macroinvertebrate fauna of Southeast Asia. In this region, three spatially separated groups of pachychilids can be differentiated mostly by means of their brooding strategy [64]. Pachychilids have rather heavy, thick shells and are not eaten by molluscivores in experimental studies [65]. They often occur at very high density [66]. Some species have rather specialized habitat requirements, and this may make them more vulnerable to habitat degradation, modification, and pollution [67].

3.2.6 Thiaridae

The Thiaridae form a monophyletic group with its constituent species being probably autochthonous in Southeast and South Asia, Australia, and some Pacific Islands, as well as sub-Saharan Africa, both in lotic and lentic freshwater environments, with some species also tolerating brackish conditions in the lower courses and estuaries of rivers [62]. Some species, such as *Melanoides tuberculata*, have an extraordinarily high invasive potential and today have an almost circumglobal distribution in tropical and subtropical biomes [62]. This spread apparently has assisted in the elimination of schistosomiasis from the Caribbean [68]. The females are ovoviviparous and the young are brooded within a non-uterine subhaemocoelic brood pouch situated in the right headfoot and extending deep into the neck region above the columellar muscle. Functional males have been found in a few species.

Some populations of *M. tuberculata* are comprised of only females reproducing parthenogenetically, while males may appear only during periods of environmental stress, for example high level of infection. Relatively few studies have been done on population dynamics of thiarid snails. Dudgeon [69] found that there was a single peak in juvenile recruitment coinciding with the warmer months; hatchlings grew quickly and were sexually mature before the next breeding season. Thiarid snail species, but in particular *M. tuberculata*, are very abundant in fishponds in Vietnam and Thailand [70, 71].

The family is very important as intermediate hosts for heterophyid intestinal trematodes and possibly *Paragonimus westermani*. Some papers mention that selected species also are intermediate hosts for liver flukes [37], but this has been questioned by others [70].

3.2.7 Paludomidae

The genera and species suggested to be included in the Paludomidae have hitherto been classified as Thiaridae, especially the endemic thalassoid species from Lake Tanganyika [59]. Generic diversity of African paludomids is concentrated in the Lake Tanganyika basin and adjacent water bodies, with only two genera, *Cleopatra* and *Pseudocleopatra* recorded from outside of this region. The genus *Cleopatra* is widespread in rivers, lakes, and even temporary water bodies of sub-Saharan Africa reaching North Africa through the Nile River system and in Madagascar, while *Pseudocleopatra* is reported from Ghana and the Congo River basin [59].

3.2.8 Superfamily: Truncatelloidea

Families within this superfamily were earlier included in the Rissooidea which was one of the largest and most diverse molluscan superfamilies, with about 23 recognized recent families, including marine, freshwater, and terrestrial members. The freshwater, brackish water, and semiterrestrial families and genera were moved to Truncatelloidea [47]. Most families contain small-sized species (**Figure 8**) and several species have medical and/or veterinary importance. The following families belong to this superfamily: Amnicolidae, Assimineidae, Bithyniidae, Cochliopidae, Helicostoidae, Hydrobiidae, Lithoglyphidae, Moitessieriidae, Stenothyridae, and Tateidae. Detailed reviews of these families are found in Refs. [16, 72–79]. Here, we present a brief overview of selected families.

3.2.9 Assimineidae

The species are mostly amphibious, spending most of the time outside the water on wet mudflats under stones, on decaying wood or in the stumps of palms [29]. Some species, however, are fully aquatic [29]. They are found in drainage creeks, in the estuaries of rivers, and in trenches and ponds in freshwater within the tidal zone [29]. The animals are oviparous with free-swimming larvae. *Assiminea lutea* was reported to harbor microcercous cercariae of *Paragonimus*, probably a species infecting non-human final hosts [29]. Brandt [29] checked several thousand specimens of *A. brevicula* and *A. obtuse* from Thailand for cercariae but no infected snails were found.

3.2.10 Bithyniidae

The family (**Figure 8**) is very important in Asia because some species are intermediate hosts of liver and intestinal trematodes. Species identification based on only morphological characters may be difficult. Species are commonly found in shallow reservoirs and wetlands including rice fields and may often be exposed to desiccation. Although some snails die during desiccation, some survive through aestivation to recolonize the habitat when water returns. Species within this family may feed both by grazing and by filter feeding. Bithynid snails are often found in aquaculture ponds in the Red River and Mekong deltas and occasionally at high density but they are more commonly found in small canals and rice fields. During the spring planting of rice fields, density of *Bithynia* spp. can be extremely high in newly planted fields.

3.2.11 Pomatiopsidae

With approximately 170 species, the Pomatiopsidae is among the most species-rich freshwater gastropod families. The highest diversity can be found in Southeast Asia and the Japanese archipelago (>140 species), followed by sub-Saharan Africa with approximately 10–11 species, southern Australia with ca. 9 species, the north-western Palearctic with 1–8 species, North America with 5–6 species, and South America with ca. 2 species [80]. The Pomatiopsidae comprise two subfamilies, the

Pomatiopsinae Stimpson, 1865 and the Jullieniinae. The Asian intermediate hosts for *Schistosoma* species belong to this family.

The Triculinae in Asia is very diverse with an endemic fauna that includes over 90 species occurring along a 300 km stretch of the lower Mekong River in Thailand and Laos [29, 80–82]. Relatively few species are reported from Vietnam [83], but this is likely because relatively little work has been done on the Vietnamese part of the Mekong River. Within the Triculinae, several species have been described from Vietnam [83], i.e., *Tricula ovata*, *T. similunaris* and 11 species of a new genus *Vietricula*. Liu et al. [82], however, believed these snails to be *Pachydrobia*. Some of the pomatopsid species are intermediate host for *Paragonimus westermani* [18, 84]. Doanh et al. [85] found two *Vietricula* spp. (originally identified as *Oncomelania*) infected with *Paragonimus heterotremus* and Doanh [86] experimentally infected the two species with *P. heterotremus*.

3.2.12 Hydrobiidae

Hydrobiidae, commonly known as mud snails, is a large cosmopolitan taxonomic family of very small freshwater snails and brackish water snails. These are small snails, with a shell height of less than 8 mm. The dextrally coiled shells are smooth and renders few robust characteristics to the systematist. Furthermore, there is considerable intraspecific variation in shell characteistics. Description is mostly based on the characteristics of the operculum, radula, and penis.

3.2.13 Stenothyridae

The Stenothyridae is comprised of small-sized gastropods found in intertidal and shallow-water aquatic habitats in Asia and Australia. Also, this family is very diverse in the Mekong River. The species live in fresh or brackish water on sandy ground, on stones and decaying wood or buried in the mud where they feed on decaying organic matter. Dung et al. [70] reported, however, pleurolophocercous cercariae were shed by *Stenothyra messageri* in the Red River Delta; these cercariae were not identified to species but they could potentially be zoonotic.

3.2.14 Other caenogastropod species

Some predominantly marine species may enter rivers. For example, the neogastopod *Anentome helena* (**Figure** 7) is found in the Mekong River in Vietnam and Thailand. The species is common in the Mekong River and is exported to Europe and Americas where it is used to control snails in hobbyist's aquaria. In the wild, it probably primarily feeds on carrion rather than seeking live prey.

3.3 Heterobranchia

3.3.1 Valvatidae

Small wide-spired operculate snails, commonly referred to as valve snails. They are egg-laying and hermaphroditic [87]. Burch [88] lists 11 North American species. According to Strong et al. [89] there are 60 species in the Palaearctic region, 10 in the Nearctic, and 1 for the Afrotropical region. They have a featherlike gill, visible on the left side outside the shell when the snail is active, and a ciliated pallial tentacle extending out to the right.

3.3.2 Lymnaeidae

Lymnaeidae (**Figure 5**) is a large and diverse family of freshwater pulmonates widely distributed on all continents except Antarctica. Lymnaeidae exhibit a great diversity in shell morphology which is linked to substantial eco-phenotypic plasticity [90]. Conchological and anatomical traits cannot be taken as reliable diagnostic characters to discriminate species of Lymnaeidae as they vary largely within species [91]. At the supraspecific (genus, subgenus) level there is confusion [92], with some researchers considering numerous genera and subgenera and others only accepting the large genus *Lymnaea*, following the old classification of Hubendick [93]. Phylogenetic analyses, however, show the presence of four well defined subgenera among the genus *Lymnaea* sensu lato, *Radix*, *Galba*, *Leptolimnaea*, and *Lymnaea* [94]. For further details refer to Vinarski et al. [94].

The family is of great parasitological importance as it includes several intermediate hosts of trematodes which infect man and mammals e.g., *Fasciola* spp., and schistosomes infecting both domestic livestock, wild mammals, and birds, the cercariae of all of which can cause swimmer's itch or cercarial dermatitis.

3.3.3 Physidae

The Physidae has a Holarctic distribution, extending into Central and South America [95]. Physids have been introduced around the world and are common, particularly in lentic habitats. Physid diversity is centered in North America, where they are the most abundant and widespread freshwater gastropods [88]. Physidae are hermaphrodites and can be distinguished from other pulmonates by a high-spired sinistral shell, radula with teeth in V-shaped rows, simple jaw with no lateral processes, and lack of both hemoglobin and a pseudobranch [29]. Other unique characteristics of many species of Physidae are an extended mantle edge that can partly cover the shell, as well as the presence of a preputial gland [29]. Six major clades were uncovered in an analysis of the penial morphology [96], while four major clades, *Physa acuta*, *Physa gyrina*, *Physa fontinalis*, and *Physa pomilia* were recognized by Pip & Franck [97]. They are common hosts of avian schistosomes responsible for causing swimmer's itch. *P. acuta* which is thought to be native to North America has spread throughout the world, and this may pose some difficulties for snail identification (e.g., with confusion with *Bulinus* species) and it may cause displacement of native, disease-transmitting species.

3.3.4 Burnupiidae

The monogeneric Burnupiidae are a limpetlike group of freshwater pulmonate snails predominantly occurring in Africa. The genus *Burnupia* has traditionally been seen as member of either a freshwater limpet family Ancylidae or as a member of the Planorbidae [98]. The majority of species of *Burnupia* occur in sub-Saharan Africa, particularly in eastern and southern parts, from the isolated Ethiopian highlands down to the Cape region [98].

3.3.5 Bulinidae

Bulinidae (**Figures 4** and **5**) comprise small to medium-sized planorboid gastropods, reaching up to 25 mm in height or diameter. They are sinistral and either high-spired (e.g. *Bulinus*) or discoid (e.g. *Indoplanorbis*) and possess a large pseudobranch that is deeply folded and vascularized [99]. Buliniforme pulmonate gastropods have traditionally been a subfamily of the Planorbidae. Recent molecular phylogenetic analyses, however, have suggested a very different scenario for planorboid gastropods, in which the bulinine forms would be reduced to be represented by *Bulinus* and *Indoplanorbis* only [100, 101]. These phylogenetic suggestions were followed in the most recent classification of the worldwide gastropods [47], in which the family Bulinidae is proposed, comprising the subfamilies Bulininae and Plesiophysinae.

The classification still largely relies on the early accounts of Mandahl-Barth [102, 103], and the system is based on both shell and anatomical characters; however, the definition of the majority of the more than 30 species currently recognized is still unsatisfactory [104]. A variety of taxonomic characters have been employed in *Bulinus*, ranging from (shell) morphology to genital anatomy and radulae, chromosome numbers, and data from electrophoresis and immunodiffusion [104]. Conchological characters are of restricted value in a planorboid snail genus such as *Bulinus* that is characterized by a rather uniform shell shape largely lacking specific characters such as keels [99]. The four species groups have been basically confirmed by phylogenetic studies based on mitochondrial and nuclear markers, but all, unfortunately, suffer from unresolved or poorly supported relationships within and between the proposed species groups [99]. Clearly, many more genetic studies are needed to identify cryptic species (complexes) and to study the role of hybridization of *Bulinus* spp. [99].

Indoplanorbis exustus is an intermediate host for the *Schistosoma indicum* species group, and the role of this snail in the transmission of several other medically and veterinary important parasites has been emphasized repeatedly [99]. The species is rather ecologically flexible and thrives in unspecific freshwater habitats that are not flowing, but it requires warm climates. The species is found in Africa, and it is widespread in southern Asia.

3.3.6 Planorbidae

Planorbidae (**Figures 3** and **6**) represent the most diverse taxon of freshwater pulmonate gastropods on earth that has an almost cosmopolitan distribution [105]. After excluding the Bulinidae and Burnupiidae there are approximately 150 species globally [105]. Following the most recent classification of freshwater gastropods [47], based on various phylogenetic analyses conducted during the past two decades, the Planorbidae consist of three subfamilies, namely Planorbinae Rafinesque, 1815, Ancylinae Rafinesque, 1815, and Miratestinae P. Sarasin & F. Sarasin, 1897 [105].

Planorbidae occur in all kinds of freshwater habitats, ranging from temporary and permanent ponds, streams, rivers, and large lakes [89]. The cosmopolitan distribution of Planorbidae has been the result of a high dispersal capacity and ecological flexibility, including desiccation resistance that is particularly important for the successful passive transport via (aerial) vectors.

The snails are small to medium-sized with long slender tentacles and blood containing hemoglobin [106]. The shell is discoid, lens-shaped, or higher ovate to turreted and the animals are sinistral, that is, the genital openings and the anus are situated on the left side, but in most of the discoid forms the shell appears to be dextral, because it is carried inverted, so that the side representing the spire (apical side) in other families is the lower side of the planorbid shell and the upper side is umbilical [106].

In the Planorbinae, there are several tribes, i.e., Planorbini (almost global distribution); Segmentinini (comprise Palearctic, Oriental, and Afrotropical species); Drepanotrematini (Central and South America); Neoplanorbini (represent a likely extinct taxon endemic to river systems in the southeasten United States); Helisomatini (includes Afrotropical and American taxa); Coretini (primarily European); and Camptoceratini (southern and eastern Asia) (see references in [105]). Several species are intermediate hosts for medically or veterinary important trematodes including schistosomes.

Freshwater limpets of the subfamily Ancylinae occur on all continents. They are small species with cap- or shield-shaped shell [29]. These animals have a pallial lung, as do all pulmonate snails, but they also have a pseudobranch which serve as a gill in situations where the limpet is unable to reach the surface for air.

The subfamily Miratestinae comprises Australian high-spired planorbid species the buliniform species *Amerianna carinata* that spread widely from its Australian origin [107]. Other species of planorbid snails are global invaders as well [105].

4. Control

4.1 Changing transmission patterns

Distribution and transmission patterns for some of the zoonotic trematodes may be changing for various reason. Climate plays an important role in the transmission of many infectious diseases; it not only determines spatial and seasonal distributions, but influences inter-annual variability, including epidemics, and long-term trends [108]. Evidence of climate change includes the instrumental temperature record, rising sea levels, and decreased snow cover in the Northern Hemisphere [109]. One of the most conspicuous effects of climate is an increased frequency of extreme weather conditions, which can have devastating effects on the snail fauna in some vulnerable habitats and at least temporarily affect schistosome transmission [110]. Obviously, one of the key factors for changing transmission patterns would be temperature changes [111].

Another possibility for changing transmission patterns is introduction of intermediate hosts into new areas. There are numerous examples of snails spreading over long distances and becoming invasive. Although snails may be spread over short distances attached to other animals, in mud on feet of birds or over somewhat longer distances passing alive through the digestive channel of migratory birds, the major mean of transport is the global trade in aquatic animals and plants [108]. Asian species such as *Tarebia granifera* have spread to South Africa, *Biomphalaria straminea* from South America to Asia, *Indoplanorbis exustus* to sub-Saharan Africa, and many other examples. Apple snails were introduced to Asia for food production. Invasive species could have major impact on local biodiversity. Another reason could be parasite introduction with imported final hosts or parasites change genetically and thereby perhaps be able to use new species as intermediate hosts. Gibbs [112] listed six interconnected parameters that have increased the rate of emerging diseases including: (1) global trade and tourism; (2) speed of mass transportation; (3) exposure to new pathogens through ecosystem disruption; (4) intensification and monoculture in farming; (5) sophistication of food processing, and (6) evolutionary pressures through overpopulation.

4.2 Control

Control of the zoonotic trematode-caused diseases in people and animals must depend on the severity of pathology caused, transmission patterns, and available options for medical treatment of infection. For most of these infections, effective control needs to take a holistic approach following One-Health principles [113].

While recognizing that existing approaches to the control of zoonotic diseases will continue to benefit from their current vertical or horizontal structure, there is growing evidence for the benefits of a joint human and animal health approach [114]. The One Health concept integrates human and animal health resources and should be promoted, because many zoonoses can be better surveyed, diagnosed and controlled by considering human and animal health together [114]. In our view, the One-Health approach must take a holistic approach where all aspects of the parasite life cycle are considered and this is especially the case for zoonotic trematodes. Some of the zoonotic trematodes are closely linked to food production, and this is especially important in least developed countries.

Disease control programmes are typically integrated as there is a need to link surveillance, monitoring, and reporting all activities with actions taken by the health system and this is particularly the case for control of zoonotic diseases [114]. Such approaches may be biomedical (drug or vaccine), vector or intermediate host control (insects or snail), environmental, legislative (inspection and condemnation of infected products at slaughterhouses) or educational [114].

Some of these zoonotic trematode-caused diseases are serious problems of both public health and veterinary importance. Although infections by some of these trematodes in the final hosts can be effectively reduced through medical treatment, reinfection appears very quickly [36, 110, 115, 116]. Thus, it is necessary to take a holistic approach to control. Treatment of infections by trematodes involves the understanding of the multiple host species, environmental control, and behavior modifications and includes several scenarios. Interventions should include (1) attempts to reduce the contamination of water bodies with trematode eggs; (2) attempts to reduce the chance of eggs or miracidia infecting the first intermediate host and (3) attempts to reduce the likelihood that cercariae or metacercariae infect a final host [113].

1. The most effective means of reducing egg contamination would be medical treatment of the final hosts (humans and possibly reservoir hosts). This could be supplemented with sanitary improvements to reduce contamination of waterbodies with human feces or urine or prevention of reservoir hosts to have access to the water bodies e.g., dogs, cats, and wild birds for some of the fish-borne zoonotic trematodes [113]. Avoiding the use of untreated manure from domestic animals for fertilization of aquaculture ponds is an important way to reduce egg contamination of ponds and also prevention of rain run-off into the ponds is important [36].

2. Snail control using either habitat modification, chemical control, or biological control is important for reducing the chance of eggs or miracidia infecting the first intermediate host. Biological control should be attempted only using native species and might be a viable option in aquaculture ponds [117, 118]. Obviously, what is feasible depends on the type of habitat.

3. Snail control will also reduce cercariae production in transmission sites thus reducing infection in the final host. For schistosomiasis, transmission to people could be reduced through reducing water contact in transmission sites, e.g. through supply of safe water. For fish-borne zoonotic trematodes (FZT), behavioral changes reducing transmission include, e.g., not eating raw fish, cooking fish remains before feeding it to animals (pigs, dogs, and cats) and preventing especially cats and dogs access to the ponds [36].

Combining mass drug administration, provision of clean water and maintenance of good sanitation and hygiene, community health education towards modification of risky behaviors, surveillance, and veterinary public health interventions have been shown to be effective in combatting foodborne trematodiasis [119]. Finally, there is a need to reduce dependency on chemical compounds for control of the first intermediate hosts due to their costs and low sustainability, while management procedures could be more sustainable and long lasting.

5. Conclusions

Zoonotic trematodes cause a number of diseases some of which have major public health or animal health consequences or have huge financial implications. A key element in the parasites' life cycle are the first intermediate host which depending on the parasitic species particular species of gastropod mollusks. Control of these snails could be an important element in an integrated approach to control these diseases following the "One-Health" approach.

Author details

Henry Madsen[1]* and Jay R. Stauffer, Jr.[2,3]

1 Parasitology and Aquatic Diseases, Faculty of Health and Medical Sciences, Department of Veterinary Disease Biology, University of Copenhagen, Copenhagen, Denmark

2 Department of Ecosystem Science and Management, The Pennsylvania State University, University Park, PA, USA

3 South African Institute for Aquatic Biodiversity, Makhanda, RSA

*Address all correspondence to: hmad@sund.ku.dk

References

[1] Torgerson PR, Macpherson CNL. The socioeconomic burden of parasitic zoonoses: Global trends. Veterinary Parasitology. 2011;**182**:79-95. DOI: 10.1016/j.vetpar.2011.07.017

[2] Miranda EM. Zoonotic Trematodiasis. In: Quiroz-Castañeda RE, editor. Farm Animals Diseases, Recent Omic Trends and New Strategies of Treatment. London: IntechOpen. DOI: 10.5772/intechopen.72632

[3] Betson M, Alonteb AJI, Ancog RC, Aquino AMO, Belizario VY Jr, Bordado AMD, et al. Zoonotic transmission of intestinal helminths in Southeast Asia: Implications for control and elimination. Advances in Parasitology. 2020;**108**:49-131. DOI: 10.1016/bs.apar.2020.01.036

[4] Doumenge J, Mott KE, Cheung C, Villenave D, Chapuis O, Perrin MF, et al. WHO Atlas of the Global Distribution of Schistosomiasis. Presses Universitaires de Bordeaux Bordeaux; 1987. p. 400

[5] Bergquist R, Gray DJ. Schistosomiasis elimination: Beginning of the end or a continued march on a trodden path. Tropical Medicine and Infectious Disease. 2019;**4**:76. DOI: 10.3390/tropicalmed4020076

[6] Vos T, Flaxman AD, Naghavi M, Lozano R, Michaud C, Ezzati M, et al. Years lived with disability (YLDs) for 1160 sequelae of 289 diseases and injuries 1990-2010: A systematic analysis for the global burden of disease study 2010. Lancet. 2012;**380**(9859):2163-2196. DOI: 10.1016/S0140-6736(12)61729-2

[7] Hotez P, Alvarado M, Basáñez M, Bolliger I, Bourne R, Boussinesq M, et al. (DALYs and HALE Collaborators). The global burden of disease study 2010: Interpretation and implications for the neglected tropical diseases. PLoS Neglected Tropical Diseases. 2014;**8**:e2865. DOI: 10.1371/journal.pntd.0002865

[8] Littlewood DTJ, Webster BL. Origins and evolutionary radiation of *Schistosoma*. In: Jamieson BGM, editor. *Schistosoma*: Biology, Pathology, and Control. Boca Raton: Taylor & Francis Group, CRC Press; 2016. pp. 1-8. ISBN 9781498744263 (e-book)

[9] Standley CJ, Mugisha L, Dobson AP, Stothard JR. Zoonotic schistosomiasis in non-human primates: Past, present and future activities at the human–wildlife interface in Africa. Journal of Helminthology. 2012;**86**:131-140. DOI: 10.1017/S0022149X12000028

[10] Gower CM, Vince L, Webster JP. Should we be treating animal schistosomiasis in Africa? The need for a one health economic evaluation of schistosomiasis control in people and their livestock. Transactions of the Royal Society of Tropical Medicine and Hygiene. 2017;**111**:244-247. DOI: 10.1093/trstmh/trx047

[11] Attwood SW, Fatih FA, Upatham ES. DNA-sequence variation among *Schistosoma mekongi* populations and related taxa; phylogeography and the current distribution of Asian schistosomiasis. PLoS Neglected Tropical Diseases. 2008;**2**(3):e200. DOI: 10.1371/journal.pntd.0000200

[12] Morgan JA, DeJong RJ, Lwambo NJ, Mungai BN, Mkoji GM, Loker ES. First report of a natural hybrid between *Schistosoma mansoni*

and *S. rodhaini*. The Journal of Parasitology. 2003;**89**:416-418. DOI: 10.1645/0022-3395(2003)089[0416:FROANH]2.0.CO;2

[13] Stauffer JR, Madsen H, Rollinson D. Introgression in Lake Malaŵi: Increasing the threat of human urogenital schistosomiasis? EcoHealth. 2014;**11**:251-254. DOI: 10.1007/s10393-013-0882-y

[14] Moné H, Holtfreter MC, Allienne J-F, Mintsa-Nguéma R, Ibikounlé M, Boissier J, et al. Introgressive hybridizations of *Schistosoma haematobium* by *Schistosoma bovis* at the origin of the first case report of schistosomiasis in Corsica (France, Europe). Parasitology Research. 2015;**114**:4127-4133. DOI: 10.1007/s00436-015-4643-4

[15] Madsen H. *Schistosoma* intermediate host snails. In: Jamieson BGM, editor. *Schistosoma*: Biology, Pathology and Control. Boca Raton: Taylor & Francis Group, CRC Press; 2016. pp. 38-55

[16] Wilke T. 21. Pomatiopsidae Stimpson, 1865. In: Lydeard C, Cummings KS, editors. Freshwater Mollusks of the World. A Distribution Atlas. Baltimore: Johns Hopkins University Press; 2019. pp. 126-130

[17] Attwood SW. Mekong schistosomiasis: Where did it come from and where is it going? In: Campbell IC, editor. The Mekong: Biophysical Environment of an International River Basin. New York: Elsevier; 2009. pp. 273-295

[18] Attwood SW. Studies on the parasitology, phylogeography and the evolution of host-parasite interactions for the snail intermediate hosts of medically important trematode genera in south East Asia. Advances in Parasitology. 2010;**73**:405-440. DOI: 10.1016/S0065-308X(10)73013-X

[19] Davis GM. Snail hosts of Asian *Schistosoma* infecting man: Evolution and coevolution. The Mekong Schistosome. Malacological Review 1980;(Suppl. 2): 195-238

[20] Kali A. Schistosome infections: An Indian perspective. Journal of Clinical and Diagnostic Research. 2015;**9**(2):DE01-DE04. DOI: 10.7860/JCDR/2015/10512.5521

[21] Agrawal MC. Schistosomes and schistosomiasis in South Asia. Chapter 3. In: The Snail. New Delhi, India: Springer; 2012. pp. 51-84. DOI: 10.1007/978-81-322-0539-5_3

[22] Barbosa FS, Barbosa I, Morais RA. Laboratory infection of the snail *Planorbarius metidjensis* (Forbes) from French Morocco with a Brazilian strain of *Schistosoma mansoni*. Annals of Tropical Medicine and Parasitology. 1959;**53**:314-315

[23] Yacoubi B, Zekhnini A, Moukrim A, Rondelaud D. *Bulinus truncatus*, *Planorbarius metidjensis* and endemic bilharziosis in the southwestern Morocco. Bulletin de la Société de Pathologie Exotique. 2007;**100**:174-175

[24] Madsen H, Stauffer JR Jr. Density of *Trematocranus placodon* (Pisces: Cichlidae): A predictor of density of the schistosome Iintermediate host, *Bulinus nyassanus* (Gastropoda: Planorbidae), in Lake Malaŵi. EcoHealth. 2011;**8**:177-189. DOI: 10.1007/s10393-011-0737-3

[25] Brant SV, Loker ES. Discovery-based studies of schistosome diversity stimulate new hypotheses about parasite biology. Trends in Parasitology. 2013;**29**:449-460. DOI: 10.1016/j.pt.2013.06.004

[26] Brant SV, Bochte CA, Loker ES. New intermediate host records for the avian schistosomes *Dendritobilharzia*

pulverulenta, *Gigantobilharzia huronensis*, and Trichobilharzia querquedulae from North America. The Journal of Parasitology. 2011;**97**:946-949. DOI: 10.1645/GE-2743.1

[27] Flores V, Brant SV, Loker ES. Avian Schistosomes from the south American endemic gastropod genus *Chilina* (Pulmonata: Chilinidae), with a brief review of south American schistosome species. The Journal of Parasitology. 2015;**101**:565-576. DOI: 10.1645/14-639

[28] Horák P, Mikeš L, Lichtenbergová L, Skála V, Soldánová M, Brant SV. Avian schistosomes and outbreaks of cercarial dermatitis. Clinical Microbiology Reviews. 2015;**28**:165-190. DOI: 10.1128/CMR.00043-14

[29] Brandt AMR. The non-marine aquatic mollusca of Thailand. Archiv fuer Molluskenkunde. 1974;**105**:1-247

[30] Procop GW. North American paragonimiasis (caused by *Paragonimus kellicotti*) in the context of global paragonimiasis. Clinical Microbiology Reviews. 2009;**22**:415-446. DOI: 10.1128/CMR.00005-08

[31] Blair D. Paragonimiasis. In: Toledo R, Fried B, editors. Digenetic Trematodes. Advances in Experimental Medicine and Biology. Vol. 1154. Cham: Springer Nature Switzerland AG; 2019. pp. 105-138. DOI: 10.1007/978-3-030-18616-6_5

[32] Rabone M, Wiethase J, Clark PF, Rollinson D, Cumberlidge N, Emery AM. Endemicity of *Paragonimus* and paragonimiasis in sub-Saharan Africa: A systematic review and mapping reveals stability of transmission in endemic foci for a multi-host parasite system. PLoS Neglected Tropical Diseases. 2021;**15**(2):e0009120. DOI: 10.1371/journal.pntd.0009120

[33] Gunn A, Pitt SJ. Parasitology: An Integrated Approach. Blackwell, Chicester: John Wiley & Sons, Ltd; 2012. 442 pp

[34] Waikagul J, Thaenkham U. Approaches to Research on the Systematics of Fish-borne Trematodes. London: Elsevier, Academic Press; 2014. p. 108

[35] Hung NM, Madsen H, Fried B. Global status of fish-borne zoonotic trematodiasis in humans (invited review). Acta Parasitologica. 2013;**58**:231-258. DOI: 10.2478/s11686-013-0155-5

[36] Clausen JH, Madsen H, Van PT, Dalsgaard A, Murrell KD. Integrated parasite management: Path to sustainable control of fishborne trematodes in aquaculture. Trends in Parasitology. 2015;**31**:8-15. DOI: 10.1016/j.pt.2014.10.005

[37] De NV, Murrell KD, Cong LD, Cam PD, Chau LV, Toan ND, et al. The food-borne trematode zoonoses of Vietnam. Southeast Asian Journal of Tropical Medicine. 2003;**34**:12-34

[38] Nguyen HM, Van HH, Ho LT, Tatonova YV, Madsen H. Are *Melanoides tuberculata* and *Tarebia granifera* (Gastropoda, Thiaridae), suitable first intermediate hosts of *Clonorchis sinensis* in Vietnam? PLoS Neglected Tropical Diseases. 2021;**15**(1):e0009093. DOI: 10.1371/journal.pntd.0009093

[39] Chai J-Y, Shin E-H, Lee S-H, Rim H-J. Foodborne intestinal flukes in Southeast Asia. The Korean Journal of Parasitology. 2009;**47**(Supplement):S69-S102. DOI: 10.3347/kjp.2009.47.S.S69

[40] Phan VT, Ersbøll AK, Bui TQ, Nguyen HT, Murrell D, Dalsgaard A. Fish-borne zoonotic trematodes in cultured and wild-caught freshwater fish from the red River Delta, Vietnam. Vector-borne

and Zoonotic Diseases. 2010;**10**(9):861-866. DOI: 10.1089=vbz.2009.0134

[41] Tkach VV, Kudlai O, Kostadinova A. Molecular phylogeny and systematics of the Echinostomatoidea Looss, 1899 (Platyhelminthes: Digenea). International Journal for Parasitology. 2016;**46**:171-185. DOI: 10.1016/j.ijpara.2015.11.001

[42] Chai JY. Echinostomes in humans. In: Fried B, Toledo R, editors. The Biology of Echinostomes. Springer; 2009. pp. 147-183. DOI: 10.1007/978-0-387-09577-6_7

[43] Mas-Coma S, Bargues MD, Valero MA. Fascioliasis and other plant-borne trematode zoonoses. International Journal for Parasitology. 2005;**35**:1255-1278. DOI: 10.1016/j.ijpara.2005.07.010

[44] Mas-Coma S, Valero MA, Bargues MD. Fascioliasis in humans and animals. Reference Module in Biomedical Sciences. 2021. pp. 1-19. DOI: 10.1016/B978-0-12-818731-9.00058-6

[45] Squire SA, Yang R, Robertson I, Ayi I, Squire DS, Ryan U. Gastrointestinal helminths in farmers and their ruminant livestock from the coastal Savannah zone of Ghana. Parasitology Research. 2018;**117**:3183-3194. DOI: 10.1007/s00436-018-6017-1

[46] Lotfy WM, Brant SV, Ashmawy KI, Devkota R, Mkoji GM, Loker ES. A molecular approach for identification of paramphistomes from Africa and Asia. Veterinary Parasitology. 2010;**174**:234-240. DOI: 10.1016/j.vetpar.2010.08.027

[47] Bouchet P, Rocroi J-P, Hausdorf B, Kaim A, Kano Y, Nützel A, et al. Revised classification, Nomenclator and Typification of gastropod and Monoplacophoran families. Malacologia. 2017;**61**:1-526. DOI: 10.4002/040.061.0201

[48] Thiele J. Handbuch der systematischen Weichtierkunde. Jena, Germany: II. Verlag von GustavFischer; 1931

[49] Kano Y, Fukumori H. 3. Neritidae Rafinesque, 1815. In: Lydeard C, Cummings KS, editors. Freshwater Mollusks of the world. A distribution atlas. Baltimore: Johns Hopkins University Press; 2019. pp. 31-36

[50] Kano Y. 2. Neritiliidae Schepman, 1908. In: Lydeard C, Cummings KS, editors. Freshwater Mollusks of the World. A Distribution Atlas. Baltimore: Johns Hopkins University Press; 2019. pp. 27-30

[51] Van Bocxlaer B, Strong EE. 5. Viviparidae Gray, 1847. In: Lydeard C, Cummings KS, editors. Freshwater Mollusks of the World. A Distribution Atlas. Baltimore: Johns Hopkins University Press; 2019. pp. 43-50

[52] Cowie RH, Hayes KA. 4. Ampullariidae Gray, 1824. In: Lydeard C, Cummings KS, editors. Freshwater Mollusks of the World. A Distribution Atlas. Baltimore: Johns Hopkins University Press; 2019. pp. 37-42

[53] Nguma JFM, McCullough FS, Masha E. Elimination of *Biomphalaria pfeifferi*, *Bulinus tropicus* and *Lymnaea natalensis* by the ampullarid snail, *Marisa cornuarietis,* in a man-made dam in northern Tanzania. Acta Tropica. 1982;**39**:85-90

[54] Haridi AAM, El Safi SH, Jobin WR. Survival, growth and reproduction of the imported ampullarid snail *Marisa cornuarietis* in Central Sudan. The Journal of Tropical Medicine and Hygiene. 1985;**88**:135-144

[55] Haridi AAM, Jobin WR. Estimated risks and benefits from introducing *Marisa cornuarietis* into the Sudan. The Journal of Tropical Medicine and Hygiene. 1985;**88**:145-151

[56] Glaubrecht M, Neiber MT. 6. Hemisinidae Fischer & Crosse, 1891. In: Lydeard C, Cummings KS, editors. Freshwater Mollusks of the World. A Distribution Atlas. Baltimore: Johns Hopkins University Press; 2019. pp. 51-55

[57] Neiber MT, Glaubrecht M. 7. Melanopsidae H. Adams & A. Adams, 1854. In: Lydeard C, Cummings KS, editors. Freshwater Mollusks of the World. A Distribution Atlas. Baltimore: Johns Hopkins University Press; 2019. pp. 56-61

[58] Neiber MT, Glaubrecht M. 8. Pachychilidae Fischer & Crosse, 1892. In: Lydeard C, Cummings KS, editors. Freshwater Mollusks of the World. A Distribution Atlas. Baltimore: Johns Hopkins University Press; 2019. pp. 62-67

[59] Neiber MT, Glaubrecht M. 9. Paludomidae Stoliczka, 1868. In: Lydeard C, Cummings KS, editors. Freshwater Mollusks of the World. A Distribution Atlas. Baltimore: Johns Hopkins University Press; 2019. pp. 68-73

[60] Strong EE, Lydeard C. 10. Pleuroceridae P. Fischer, 1885. In: Lydeard C, Cummings KS, editors. Freshwater Mollusks of the World. A Distribution Atlas. Baltimore: Johns Hopkins University Press; 2019. pp. 74-80

[61] Campbell DC. 11. Semisulcospiridae Morrison, 1952. In: Lydeard C, Cummings KS, editors. Freshwater Mollusks of the World. A Distribution Atlas. Baltimore: Johns Hopkins University Press; 2019. pp. 81-85

[62] Glaubrecht M, Neiber MT. 12. Thiaridae Gill, 1871 (1823). In: Lydeard C, Cummings KS, editors. Freshwater Mollusks of the World. A Distribution Atlas. Baltimore: Johns Hopkins University Press; 2019. pp. 86-89

[63] Reid DG, Dyal P, Lozouet P, Glaubrecht M, Williams ST. Mudwhelks and mangroves: The evolutionary history of an ecological association (Gastropoda: Potamididae). Molecular Phylogenetics and Evolution. 2008;**47**:680-699. DOI: 10.1016/j.ympev.2008.01.003

[64] Köhler F, Dames C. Phylogeny and systematics of the Pachychilidae of mainland south-east asia-novel insights from morphology and mitochondrial DNA (Mollusca, Caenogastropoda, Cerithioidea). Zoological Journal of the Linnean Society. 2009;**157**:679-699. DOI: 10.1111/j.1096-3642.2009.00541.x

[65] Dudgeon D, Cheung PSC. Selection of gastropod prey by a tropical fresh-water crab. Journal of Zoology. 1990;**220**:147-155. DOI: 10.1111/j.1469-7998.1990.tb04299.x

[66] Yeung ACY, Dudgeon D. Production and population dynamics of the prosobranch snail *Sulcospira hainanensis* (Pachychilidae), a major secondary consumer in Hong Kong streams. Hydrobiologia. 2014;**724**:21-39. DOI: 10.1007/s10750-013-1703-6

[67] Köhler F, Seddon M, Bogan AE, Tu DV, Sri-Aroon P, Allen D. The status and distribution of freshwater molluscs of the indo-Burma region. In: Allen DJ, Smith KG, Darwall WRT, editors. The Status and Distribution of Freshwater Biodiversity in Indo-Burma. Cambridge, UK, Gland, Switzerland: IUCN; 2012. pp. 66-88

[68] Pointier J-P, David P, Jarne P. The biological control of the snail hosts of schistosomes: The role of competitor snails and biological invasions. In: Toledo R, Fried B, editors. Biomphalaria: Snails and Larval Trematodes. New York: Springer Science + Business Media; 2011. pp. 215-238. DOI: 10.1007/978-1-4419-7028-2_9

[69] Dudgeon D. The lifecycle, population dynamics and productivity of *Melanoides tuberculata* (Müller, 1774) (Gastropoda: Prosobranchia: Thiaridae) in Hong Kong. Journal of Zoology. 1986;**208**:37-53. DOI: 10.1111/j.1469-7998.1986.tb04707.x

[70] Dung BT, Madsen H, The DT. Distribution of freshwater snails in family-based VAC ponds and associated waterbodies with special reference to intermediate hosts of fish-borne zoonotic trematodes in Nam Dinh Province, Vietnam. Acta Tropica. 2010;**116**: 15-23. DOI: 10.1016/j.actatropica. 2010.04.016

[71] Clausen JH, Madsen H, Murrell KD, Van PT, Nguyen TTH, Dung TD, et al. Prevention and control of fish-borne zoonotic trematodes in fish nurseries, Vietnam. Emerging Infectious Diseases. 2012;**18**:1438-1445. DOI: 10.3201/ eid1809.111076

[72] Clark SA. 13. Amnicolidae Tryon, 1862. In: Lydeard C, Cummings KS, editors. Freshwater Mollusks of the World. A Distribution Atlas. Baltimore: Johns Hopkins University Press; 2019. pp. 90-93

[73] Fukuda H. 14. Assimineidae H. & A. Adams, 1856. In: Lydeard C, Cummings KS, editors. Freshwater Mollusks of the World. A Distribution Atlas. Baltimore: Johns Hopkins University Press; 2019. pp. 94-100

[74] Ponder W. Bithyniidae Gray, 1857. In: Lydeard C, Cummings KS, editors. Freshwater Mollusks of the World. A Distribution Atlas. Baltimore: Johns Hopkins University Press; 2019. pp. 101-103

[75] Stephanie A, Clark SA. Cochliopidae Tryon, 1866. In: Lydeard C, Cummings KS, editors. Freshwater Mollusks of the World. A Distribution Atlas. Baltimore: Johns Hopkins University Press; 2019. pp. 104-108

[76] Wilke T. 17. Helicostoidae Pruvot-Fol, 1937. In: Lydeard C, Cummings KS, editors. Freshwater Mollusks of the World. A Distribution Atlas. Baltimore: Johns Hopkins University Press; 2019. pp. 109-110

[77] Wilke T, Delicado D. 18. Hydrobiidae Stimpson, 1865. In: Lydeard C, Cummings KS, editors. Freshwater Mollusks of the World. A Distribution Atlas. Baltimore: Johns Hopkins University Press; 2019. pp. 111-117

[78] Clark SA. 19. Lithoglyphidae Tryon, 1866. In: Lydeard C, Cummings KS, editors. Freshwater Mollusks of the World. A Distribution Atlas. Baltimore: Johns Hopkins University Press; 2019. pp. 118-121

[79] Clark SA. 22. Stenothyridae Tryon, 1866. In: Lydeard C, Cummings KS, editors. Freshwater Mollusks of the World. A Distribution Atlas. Baltimore: Johns Hopkins University Press; 2019. pp. 131-133

[80] Davis GM. The origin and evolution of the gastropod family Pomatiopsidae, with emphasis on the Mekong River Triculinae. Monograph/Academy of Natural Sciences of Philadelphia. 1979;**20**:1-120

[81] Attwood SW, Ambu S, Meng XH, Upatham ES, Xu FS, Southgate VR. The phylogenetics of triculine snails (Rissooidea: Pomatiopsidae) from south-East Asia and southern China: Historical biogeography and the transmission of human schistosomiasis. Journal of Molluscan Studies. 2003;**69**:263-271. DOI: 10.1093/mollus/69.3.263

[82] Liu L, Huo GN, He HB, Zhou B, Attwood SW. A phylogeny

for the Pomatiopsidae (Gastropoda: Rissooidea): A resource for taxonomic, parasitological and biodiversity studies. BMC Evolutionary Biology. 2014;**14**:29. DOI: 10.1186/1471-2148-14-29

[83] Thanh DN, Hai HN. Freshwater Mollusca: Gastropoda and Bivalvia. In: Fauna of Vietnam. Hanoi: Vietnam Science and Technology Publisher (in Vietnamese); 2010

[84] Blair D, Davis GM, Wu B. Evolutionary relationships between trematodes and snails emphasizing schistosomes and paragonimids. Parasitology. 2001;**123**:S229-S243. DOI: 10.1017/S003118200100837X

[85] Doanh PN, Le NT, The DT. Distribution of *Paragonimus heterotremus* and its intermediate hosts in the northwest region of Vietnam. Journal of Biology. 2002;**3**:14-22 (in Vietnamese with English abstract)

[86] Doanh PN. Development of the *Paragonimus heterotremus* eggs and its larvae stages in the first intermediate host. Journal of Biology. 2004;**6**:6-10 (in Vietnamese with English abstract)

[87] Clewing C, Albrecht C. 24. Valvatidae Gray, 1840. In: Lydeard C, Cummings KS, editors. Freshwater Mollusks of the World. A Distribution Atlas. Baltimore: Johns Hopkins University Press; 2019. pp. 139-142

[88] Burch JB. North American freshwater snails: Identification keys, generic synonymy, supplemental notes, glossary, references, index. Walkerana. 1982;**1**:1-365

[89] Strong EE, Gargominy O, Ponder WF, Bouchet P. Global diversity of gastropods (Gastropoda; Mollusca) in freshwater. Hydrobiologia. 2008;**595**: 149-166. DOI: 10.1007/s10750-007-9012-6

[90] Correa AC, Escobar JS, Durand P, Renaud F, David P, Jarne P, et al. Bridging gaps in the molecular phylogeny of the Lymnaeidae (Gastropoda: Pulmonata), vectors of fascioliasis. BMC Evolutionary Biology. 2010;**10**:381. DOI: 10.1186/1471-2148-10-381

[91] Correa AC, Escobar JS, Noya O, Velásquez LE, González-Ramírez C, Hurtrez-Boussès S, et al. Morphological and molecular characterization of Neotropic Lymnaeidae (Gastropoda: Lymnaeoidea), vectors of fasciolosis. Infection, Genetics and Evolution. 2011;**11**:1978-1988. DOI: 10.1016/j.meegid.2011.09.003

[92] Mas-Coma S, Bargues MD. Human liver flukes: A review. Research and Reviews in Parasitology. 1997;**57**:145-218

[93] Hubendick B. Recent Lymnaeidae, their variation, morphology, taxonomy, nomenclature and distribution. Kungliga Svenska Vetenskapsakademiens Handlingar. 1951;**3**:1-223

[94] Vinarski MV, Clewing C, Albrecht C. 29. Lymnaeidae Rafinesque, 1815. In: Lydeard C, Cummings KS, editors. Freshwater Mollusks of the World. A Distribution Atlas. Baltimore: Johns Hopkins University Press; 2019. pp. 158-162

[95] Wethington AR, Lydeard C. 33. Physidae Fitzinger, 1833. In: Lydeard C, Cummings KS, editors. Freshwater Mollusks of the World. A Distribution Atlas. Baltimore: Johns Hopkins University Press; 2019. pp. 175-180

[96] Wethington AR, Lydeard C. A molecular phylogeny of Physidae (Gastropoda: Basommatophora) based on mitoghondrial DNA sequences. Journal of Molluscan Studies. 2007;**73**:241-257. DOI: 10.1093/mollus/eym021

[97] Pip E, Franck JPC. Molecular phylogenetics of Central Canadian Physidae (Pulmonata: Basommatophora). Canadian Journal of Zoology. 2008;**86**:10-16. DOI: 10.1139/Z07-112

[98] Albrecht C, Clewing C. 32. Burnupiidae Albrecht, 2017. In: Lydeard C, Cummings KS, editors. Freshwater Mollusks of the World. A Distribution Atlas. Baltimore: Johns Hopkins University Press; 2019. pp. 172-174

[99] Albrecht C, Stelbrink B, Clewing C. 31. Bulinidae P. Fischer & Crosse, 1880. In: Lydeard C, Cummings KS, editors. Freshwater Mollusks of the World. A Distribution Atlas. Baltimore: Johns Hopkins University Press; 2019. pp. 167-171

[100] Albrecht C, Kuhn K, Streit B. A molecular phylogeny of Planorboidea (Gastropoda, Pulmonata): Insights from enhanced taxon sampling. Zoologica Scripta. 2006;**36**:27-39. DOI: /10.1111/j.1463-6409.2006.00258.x

[101] Jørgensen A, Kristensen TK, Stothard JR. An investigation of the "Ancylo- planorbidae" (Gastropoda, Pulmonata, Hygrophila): Preliminary evidence from DNA sequence data. Molecular Phylogenetics and Evolution. 2004;**32**:778-787. DOI: 10.1016/j.ympev.2004.02.011

[102] Mandahl-Barth G. Intermediate hosts of *Schistosoma*. African *Biomphalaria* and *Bulinus*. 2. *Bulinus*. Bulletin of the World Health Organization. 1957;**17**:1-65

[103] Mandahl-Barth G. The species of the genus *Bulinus,* intermediate hosts of *Schistosoma*. Bulletin of the World Health Organization. 1965;**33**:33-44

[104] Brown D. Freshwater Snails of Africa and their Medical Importance. 2nd ed. London: Taylor & Francis; 1994

[105] Albrecht C, Stelbrink B. Clewing C. 34. Planorbidae Rafinesque, 1815. In: Lydeard C, Cummings KS, editors. Freshwater Mollusks of the World. A Distribution Atlas. Baltimore: Johns Hopkins University Press; 2019. pp. 181-186

[106] Mandahl-Barth G. Intermediate Hosts of *Schistosoma*. African *Biomphalaria* and *Bulinus*. World Health Organization Monograph Series No. 37. Geneva: World Health Organization; 1958. 132 pp

[107] Madsen H, Frandsen F. The spread of freshwater snails including those of medical and veterinary importance. Acta Tropica. 1989;**46**:139-146. DOI: 10.1016/0001-706X(89)90030-2

[108] Kelly-Hope L, Thomson MC. Climate and infectious diseases. In: Thomson MC et al., editors. Seasonal Forecasts, Climatic Change and Human Health. Dordrecht: Springer Science + Business Media BV; 2008

[109] Lotfy WM. Climate change and epidemiology of human parasitosis in Egypt: A review. Journal of Advanced Research. 2014;**5**:607-613. DOI: 10.1016/j.jare.2013.06.009

[110] Kariuki HC, Madsen H, Sturrock RF, Ouma JH, Butterworth AEB, Dunne D, et al. Focal molluscicididing using niclosamide (Bayluscide) in stream habitats and its effect on transmission of schistosomiasis mansoni following community-based chemotherapy at Kibwezi in Makueni District, Kenya. Parasites & Vectors. 2013;**6**:107. DOI: 10.1186/1756-3305-6-107

[111] Kalinda C, Chimbari M, Mukaratirwa S. Implications of changing temperatures on the growth, fecundity and survival of intermediate host snails of schistosomiasis: A systematic review. International Journal of Environmental

Research and Public Health. 2017;**14**:80. DOI: 10.3390/ijerph14010080

[112] Gibbs EP. Emerging zoonotic epidemics in the interconnected global community. The Veterinary Record. 2005;**157**:673-679

[113] Stauffer JR, Madsen H. A one health approach to reducing schistosomiasis transmission in Lake Malawi. Preventive Medicine and Community Health. 2018;**1**:1-4. DOI: 10.15761/PMCH.1000115

[114] Research Priorities for Zoonoses and Marginalized Infections. Technical Report of the TDR Disease Reference Group on Zoonoses and Marginalized Infectious Diseases of Poverty. WHO Technical Report Series 971

[115] Wilkins HA. Reinfection after treatment of schistosome infections. Parasitology Today. 1989;**5**:83-88. DOI: 10.1016/0169-4758(89)90008-2

[116] Lier T, Do DT, Johansen MV, Nguyen TH, Dalsgaard A, Asfeldt AM. High reinfection rate after preventive chemotherapy for fish borne zoonotic trematodes in Vietnam. PLoS Neglected Tropical Diseases. 2014;**8**:e2958. DOI: 10.1371/journal.pntd.0002958

[117] Hung NM, Nguyen VD, Stauffer JR Jr, Madsen H. Use of black carp (*Mylopharyngodon piceus*) in biological control of intermediate host snails of fish-borne zoonotic trematodes in nursery ponds in Vietnam. Parasites & Vectors. 2013;**6**:142. DOI: 10.1186/1756-3305-6-142

[118] Makoni P, Chimbari MJ, Madsen H. Interactions between fish and snails in a Zimbabwe pond, with particular reference to *Sargochromis codringtonii* (Pisces: Cichlidae). African Journal of Aquatic Science. 2005;**30**(1):45-48. DOI: 10.2989/16085910509503833

[119] Tenorio JCB, Molina EC. Monsters in our food: Foodborne trematodiasis in the Philippines and beyond. Veterinary Integrative Sciences. 2021;**19**(3):467-485. DOI: 10.12982/VIS.2021.038

Chapter 17

Biology of the Human Filariases

Jesuthas Ajendra, Achim Hoerauf and Marc P. Hübner

Abstract

Filarial nematodes are parasitic worms transmitted by blood-feeding insects. Mainly found in tropical and subtropical areas of the developing world, diseases such as lymphatic filariasis and onchocerciasis represent major public health issues. With millions of people infected and billions at risk of infection, these diseases can stun economic growth and impair the life quality, hence the WHO classified both lymphatic filariasis and onchocerciasis as Neglected Tropical Diseases. The lesser known filarial disease loiasis is not only affecting millions of people, but represents a huge obstacle during mass drug administration programmes targeting other filarial diseases. Even less is known about mansonellosis, potentially the most widespread of the human filariases, but underestimated due to the lack of clinical symptoms. Large scale intervention as well as mass drug administration programmes are undertaken with the long term goal of eliminating the filarial diseases lymphatic filariasis and onchocerciasis. However, there is still neither a vaccination nor short term macrofilaricidal treatments available. The following chapter will encompass the different filarial diseases, the biology of the parasite and their vector, the epidemiology as well as pathology of the filariases, highlighting the impact of these diseases is still immense and further research in understanding and combating these diseases is needed.

Keywords: *Brugia*, filariasis, ivermectin, *Loa loa*, loiasis, lymphatic filariasis, *Mansonella*, mansonellosis, neglected tropical diseases, *Onchocerca volvulus*, onchocerciasis, parasitic diseases, *Wolbachia*, *Wuchereria bancrofti*

1. Introduction

Listed as a Neglected Tropical Disease (NTD) by the WHO, lymphatic filariasis (LF) is a debilitating infectious disease of the developing world. This disease is caused by three species of lymph-dwelling filarial nematodes, *Wuchereria bancrofti*, *Brugia malayi* and *Brugia timori* (see **Table 1**). These worms are transmitted by mosquitoes and infections can lead to severe clinical manifestations such as elephantiasis, hydrocele, and lymphedema. It is these serious outcomes, which makes LF one of the leading causes of disability in the endemic regions, ultimately impairing life quality and stunning economic growth. Due to the massive negative effect LF has on public health, the WHO coordinates programmes with the aim to eliminate LF as a public health problem in 80% of the endemic countries by 2030 [1].

Disease	Causative agent	Vector	Infection rate (estimations)	Geographical distribution
Lymphatic filariasis	*Wuchereria bancrofti, Brugia malayi, B. timori*	*Aedes spp., Anopheles spp., Culex spp., Mansonia spp.,*	65 million	Africa, South and Southeast Asia, South America, Pacific Islands
Onchocerciasis	*Onchocerca volvulus*	*Simulium spp.,*	20.9 million	Sub-Saharan Africa, South America, Yemen
Loiasis	*Loa loa*	*Chrysops spp.*	10 million	Western and Central Africa
Mansonellosis	*Mansonella perstans, M. streptocerca, M. ozzardi*	*Culicoides spp., Simulium spp., Ceratopogonidae*	114 million	Sub-Saharan African, Central and South America

Overview of the human filarial diseases, their causative agents with the nematode-transmitting arthropod vectors as well as estimations of currently infected people and the endemic regions for the disease.

Table 1.
Overview of the human filarial diseases.

1.1 Biology of the parasites

The three species of filarial nematodes causing LF are transmitted to its human host by different mosquito species. *W. bancrofti* is transmitted by mosquitos of the genera *Aedes*, *Anopheles*, *Culex* and *Mansonia*. *B. malayi* by *Mansonia* and *Anopheles spp*., and *B. timori* is transmitted by *Anopheles barbirostris* [2–4]. To date, no reservoir host is known, but subperiodic forms have been found in domestic and wild animals such as cats and monkeys. Development and replication of the filarial nematodes requires both the mammalian host and the arthropod vector. During the blood meal of the mosquito infective L3 larvae are transmitted into the mammalian host. These L3 larvae reach lengths up to 1.5 mm and 18–23 μm in diameter. Within their host, the L3 larvae migrate to the lymphatics, where they molt and become adult worms within 5–18 months. In these filarial nematodes display sexual dimorphism with females being longer than their male counterparts. Females of *W. bancrofti* are 8–10 cm long and between 0.24–0.30 mm in diameter, while males reach 4 cm in length and up to 1 mm in diameter. Compared to *W. bancrofti*, *Brugia ssp*. adult worms are smaller in length with females measuring 4.3–5.5 cm in length and 130–170 μm in diameter and males reaching 1.3–2.3 cm in length and 70–80 μm in width. When gravid, female worms release sheathed microfilaria (MF) in the lymphatic vessels that drain into the blood stream. The MF of *W. bancrofti* are larger in size compared to those of *Brugia ssp*.. *W. bancrofti* MF are 244–296 μm long and 7.5–10 μm wide, while *Brugia* MF are 177–230 μm and 5–7 μm wide (see **Table 2**). MF release by female worms follows a nocturnal or diurnal periodicity that is in tune with the biting behavior of the mosquito vector in the endemic area [5]. While *W. bancrofti* and *B. malayi* mostly follow a nocturnal periodicity with peak MF blood counts around midnight, diurnal patters have been observed in the Pacific regions, where *Aedes* mosquitoes (e.g. *Aedes polynesiensis*) are the common vector [6]. This coordinated behavior between parasite and vector is a

Species	Residency of adult worms	Size of adult worms	Microfilariae	Presence of *Wolbachia*	Major severe forms of pathology
Wuchereria bancrofti	Lymphatic vessels and lymph nodes; scrotal tissue	♂4 cm ♀ 8–10 cm	Blood, nocturnal, sheathed, 244–296 μm	Yes	Lymphangitis, elephantiasis, hydrocele
Brugia malayi	Lymphatic vessels and lymph nodes	♂ 1.3–2.3 cm ♀4.3–5.5 cm	Blood, nocturnal, sheathed, 177–230 μm	Yes	Lymphangitis, elephantiasis
Brugia timori	Lymphatic vessels and lymph nodes	♂ 1.3–2.3 cm ♀4.3–5.5 cm	Blood, nocturnal, sheathed, 177–230 μm	Yes	Lymphangitis, elephantiasis
Onchocerca volvulus	Subcutaneous nodules	♂ 2–5 cm, ♀ 33–70 cm	Skin (upper dermis), unsheathed, 220–360 μm	Yes	Blindness, dermatitis, Sowda
Loa loa	Subcutaneous tissue	♂ 3–3.4 cm, ♀ 4–7 cm	Blood, diurnal, sheathed, 230–300 μm	No	Calabar swelling, Eye worm, Angioedema,
Mansonella streptocerca	Dermal skin layer	♂ 1.7 cm, ♀ 2.7 cm	Skin (upper dermis), unsheathed, 180–240 μm	?	Mild dermatitis
Mansonella perstans	Peritoneal, pleural, and pericardial cavity	♂ 4.5 cm, ♀ 7–8 cm	Blood, unsheathed, 200 μm	Yes	Mainly asymptomatic
Mansonella ozzardi	Peritoneal and pleural cavity	♂ 2.6 cm, ♀ 3.2–6 cm	Blood and skin, unsheathed, 207–232 μm	Yes	Mainly asymptomatic

This table gives an overview over the discussed filarial nematodes species with facts about their biology, size and associated disease pathology.

Table 2.
Overview of the human-pathogenic filarial nematodes.

great example of co-evolution. Estimations for the life span for adult female worms of the aforementioned filarial nematode species range between 5 and 10 years, MF have a lifespan of 6–24 months [7, 8]. Female worms produce up to several thousand MF per day which remain in the lymphatics or in blood vessels, preferably under the skin. During a blood meal, MF are ingested by the female mosquitos. The MF penetrate the midgut and thereby shed their sheaths and migrate on to the thoracic muscles, where they molt twice and develop to the infective L3 stage. The L3 migrate through the haemocoel to the mosquito's proboscis and from there is transmitted to the mammalian host during a blood meal of the mosquito. The development rate of the larvae within the mosquitoes is temperature-dependent and takes between 10 and 12 days [3, 9–11]. Of note, no sexual reproduction or replication occurs within the arthropod vector.

1.2 Epidemiology

Currently, an estimated 858 million people live in 50 endemic countries [12, 13]. Of these, 65 million people are infected with LF. The majority of these infections, around 90%, are thereby caused by *W. bancrofti*. An estimated 19 million cases with hydrocele and 17 million lymphedema cases exist, leading to 1.3 million disability-adjusted life years (DALYs) [12, 14, 15]. Most infections with *W. bancrofti* occur in South and Southeast Asia as well as in Sub-Saharan Africa, but also Central and South America, the Middle East as well as the Pacific Islands are endemic regions. *B. malayi* has its distribution in South and Southeast Asia, found in India, Indonesia, Thailand, Vietnam, Malaysia, and the Philippines. *B. timori* is limited to Eastern Indonesia and Timor-Leste. Despite the wide distribution of LF, the prevalence rate has been decreasing in many areas, mainly due to the impact of the Global Programme to Eliminate Lymphatic Filariasis (GPELF). This programme has even led to the elimination of LF in several countries including Togo, Egypt, Maldives, Sri Lanka, Thailand, Cambodia, Cook Island, Marshall Islands, Niue, Palau, Tonga, Vanuatu, Vietnam, Japan, Korea and China [16, 17]. In the last two decades, GPELF has distributed more than 8.2 billion treatments, ultimately leading to this success. GPELF has ended in 2020, but MDAs targeting LF are still ongoing in 45 endemic countries. While the initial goal to globally eliminate LF by 2020 was missed, GPELF has created a good foundation for endemic countries to achieve the goal which the WHO has stated in their NTD roadmap 2021–2030: to eliminate LF as a public health problem in 80% of the endemic countries by 2030 [14, 18, 19]. Further major challenges for the future are increasing population numbers in endemic countries and the associated unplanned urbanization combined with poor sanitary [20].

1.3 Pathology

LF is a chronic and persistent disease, but the majority of infected individuals remain asymptomatic and do not develop clinical symptoms. However, LF can cause a broad spectrum of clinical manifestations including the most severe forms seen in patients with elephantiasis or hydrocele. The most common symptoms are lymphedema of the legs, lymphangitis, elephantiasis, and only in *W. bancrofti*-infected individuals, hydrocele [21, 22]. Interestingly, even asymptomatic patients display some degree of subclinical disease with microscopic haematuria/proteinuria, dilated lymphatics and presence of scrotal lymphangiectasia. The most prevalent symptoms are caused by the presence of worms and their products in the lymphatic system, which leads to the induction of endothelial cell proliferation and lymphangiectasia, the dilatation of lymphatic vessels. Furthermore, host proteins such as vascular endothelial growth factors, matrix metalloproteinases and angiopoietins are involved. Studies have demonstrated that lymphedema development is associated with genetic risk factors and nucleotide polymorphisms for genes encoding for the proteins mentioned above [23–25]. The dilated lymph vessels and the associated impaired lymph function leads to lymph fluids no longer being pumped against gravity, resulting in elevated tissue pressure. Progression of lymphedema can take many years during which leg skin thickens and loses elasticity, develop deep folds accompanied with development of dermatosclerosis and skin lesions. The lesions additionally can lead to secondary bacterial and fungal infections, further accelerating the development of chronic and severe lymphedema and elephantiasis [26–28]. Hydrocele is a common clinical symptom in men infected with *W. bancrofti*. Hydrocele is characterized by fluid accumulation inside the tunica vaginalis and swelling of the groin and scrotal area. Acute hydrocoel is a result of worm death, both naturally and medically, leading to temporary clogging of the lymphatics due to disintegrating worms [29], whereas chronic hydrocoel develops after years of infection due to impaired lymph transport. A rare, but serious manifestation of LF is the so-called tropical pulmonary eosinophilia (TPE). TPE is caused by immunological hyperresponsiveness to MF in the lungs, associated with coughing and wheezing, extremely high eosinophil counts and high levels of serum IgE. TPE can lead to further manifestations such as lymphadenopathy as well as spleno- and hepatomegaly [30].

2. Onchocerciasis

Another neglected tropical disease caused by a filarial nematode is onchocerciasis, also known as river blindness. This disease is caused through infections with *Onchocerca volvulus*, a filarial nematode transmitted by bites of *Simulium* blackflies (see **Table 1**). These blackflies breed usually along fast-flowing and oxygen-rich rivers, hence the term river blindness. Similar to LF, onchocerciasis is a major public health problem in endemic areas due to the risk to develop severe dermatitis, vision impairment and blindness. With new diagnostic tools and the aid of MDAs, onchocerciasis was successfully eliminated in many foci of its endemic region [31]. The WHO targets elimination of transmission for onchocerciasis, set for 2022 in the Americas and for 12 African countries by 2030 [31].

2.1 Biology of the parasite

The life cycle of *O. volvulus* is similar to the LF-causing nematodes. Humans harbor the adult worms while blood-feeding arthropod vectors transmit the larval stages. Onchocerciasis is closely associated with fast-flowing rivers that serve as breeding grounds for *Simulium* blackflies. The predominant *Simulium* vector in Africa is *S. damnosum*, with *S. naevei* driving transmission in parts of East and Central Africa [32–34]. In South and Central America, the disease is transmitted mainly by *S. ochraceum* [35] with other species have been active in transmission before elimination of the disease in most countries [36]. Female blackflies transmit the infectious L3 stage of *O. volvulus* during the blood meal into the human body. Within 10 days, the L3 larvae molt once to become L4, which then persists in the host for 6–12 months before molting into an adult worm. The adult worms reside in so called onchocercomata, subcutaneous nodules commonly located around the hip regions of an infected person, but also on head and torso [36]. Onchocercomata are granulomatous reactions around the adult worms, they are painless for the infected person and have a diameter of 0.5–3 cm. They often consist of separate chambers with thick fibrous walls and cellular infiltration around the adult worms residing in the chambers. The ratio of females and males residing in a nodule is approximately 3:1. The worms mate here and gravid females produce and subsequently release thousands of unsheated MF into the subcutaneous tissue [37]. Female worms are long-lived, with their reproductive life span being an estimated 9–11 years, in extreme cases up to 15 years [38, 39]. The MF of *O. volvulus* are 220–360 μm long and 5–9 μm wide, female adult worms are 33–70 cm long and 270–440 μm wide, adult males are significantly smaller with 19–42 mm length and a width of 130–210 μm (**Table 2**). MF migrate and reside within the host's skin for 6–30 months and can be taken up by the aforementioned insect vector during a blood meal. MF do not exhibit any form of periodicity. Therefore skin snips for diagnostics can be collected at any time. The MF can also be found in the lymphatics, sputum, urine and blood and it is their migration into the ocular regions which causes ocular pathology. Within the blackflies, the MF penetrate the membranes of the mid gut and migrate through the haemolymph where they then settle in the syncytial cells of the thoracic longitudinal flight muscles. The MF molt twice to become the infectious L3 larvae [40]. Similar to other human-pathogenic filariae, *O. volvulus* contain the endosymbiontic bacteria *Wolbachia*. These bacteria are found in the hypodermis and are essential for filarial development, embryogenesis and survival [41, 42]. Depleting these endosymbionts using doxycycline leads to inhibition of filarial embryogenesis and death of adult worms, currently representing the macrofilaricidal drug for onchocerciasis [43].

2.2 Epidemiology

As of 2017, 20.9 million individuals were infected with *O. volvulus* [15]. Of these, 14.6 million are cases of severe forms of skin disease and 1.2 million were suffering from visual impairment and blindness, accounting for an estimated 205 million DALYs [15, 35]. 99% of all onchocerciasis cases are found in 31 countries of tropical sub-Saharan Africa. Rigorous Ivermectin distribution programs have eliminated onchocerciasis in most areas in South and Central America. Isolated transmission sites of this disease exist in the border region of Brazil and Venezuela as well in the western parts of Yemen [1, 35]. Taken together, 218 million people live in areas that are endemic for onchocerciasis [1]. The endemicity of onchocerciasis can be classified in hypoendemic, mesoendemic and hyperendemic areas according to the MF prevalence rates. In hypoendemic areas, less than 30% of the patients have microfilaridermia [44], in mesoendemic areas microfilaridermia is 30–60% and nodules are detectable in around 20% of the patients [44]. In hyperendemic areas with more than 60% microfilaridermia, 30–40% of patients have skin pathology. This classification is a very helpful tool to predict effects of treatment and vector control programmes as well as transmission dynamics [45]. As such, the activity of the Onchocerciasis Control Programme and the African Programme for Onchocerciasis Control (APOC) focused mainly on mesoendemic to hyperendemic areas, so areas where the disease risk is the highest [44]. Since its launch in 1995, the APOC has prevented an estimated 8.2 million onchocerciasis associated DALYs from 1995 to 2010 and another 9.2 million DALYs by 2015 [46]. However, in future hypoendemic areas must be included meet the formulated goal of onchocerciasis elimination. Based on the success of APOC and the following ESPEN (the Expanded Special Programme to Eliminate Neglected Tropical Diseases) program, the WHO targets the elimination of the transmission of onchocerciasis by 2030 as part of their roadmap 2021–2030 [1, 13].

2.3 Pathology

The vast majority of individuals infected with *O. volvulus* are associated with mild clinical symptoms. The adult worm-containing nodules contribute little to morbidity but can be uncomfortable and cosmetically bothersome. Individuals with onchocercomata formation, high parasite burden and mild dermatitis are referred to as generalized onchocerciasis (GEO). Clinically significant onchocerciasis results from inflammatory responses to MF and its *Wolbachia* in the skin and the eyes. Early symptoms of *O. volvulus*-induced dermatitis are itching or rash due to immune responses against dead or dying MF. While the rash can disappear shortly after, in some cases the rash persists and results in intense pruritus with secondary infections with bacteria or fungi due to extensive scratching. As a consequence, repeated inflammation can lead to chronic onchodermatitis including large papules. Chronic skin inflammation can lead to severe dermatological changes including loss of elasticity, lichenification and thickening of skin ("lizard skin") as well as depigmentation and hyperpigmentation ("leopard skin") [47]. The most severe form of skin pathology is "Sowda", which presents hyperpigmented papules and plaques and local lymphadenopathy, accompanied by enlarged lymph nodes with prominent follicular hyperplasia [48–51]. This disease manifestation is called hyperreactive onchocerciasis (HO). interestingly, HO patients usually harbor low worm burden, but exhibit increased immune effector mechanisms [48]. These increased effector responses eliminate the MF, however simultaneously elicit dermatitis and the "Sowda" pathology [52]. Besides the skin pathology, onchocerciasis is commonly associated with blindness. In fact, onchocerciasis is the second most prominent infectious cause of blindness in the tropics. Loss of vision is due to immune responses against dead or dying MF and its exposed *Wolbachia* endosymbionts in the cornea and anterior chamber with keratitis and iridocyclitis, respectively. Opacity develops from the corners of the cornea to the center and permanent exposure to inflammation can lead to irreversible sclerosing keratitis which can develop into blindness [53, 54]. Laboratory studies have demonstrated a role for the *Wolbachia* endosymbionts in the ocular pathology of onchocerciasis [55]. Dying MF release *Wolbachia* which leads to infiltration and activation of fibroblasts, dendritic cells and macrophages which in turn induce neutrophil recruitment in a chemokine-dependent manner [54]. The neutrophilic responses, mostly degranulation but potentially also the release of DNA-mediated trap formation results in degradation of the corneal matrix. This leads to corneal haze, which can cause visual impairment and in worst cases blindness. The exact route of how the MF get into the eye is still unclear, but authors suggested that blood sheaths of the posterior ciliary arteries as well as cerebrospinal fluids as entry points [56, 57].

3. Loiasis

Commonly known as the "African eye-worm", the filarial nematode *Loa loa* is the causative agent of Loiasis (**Table 1**). While this disease is not yet listed as a NTD by the WHO, it still represents a public health issue in endemic regions. It especially became prominent because Ivermectin and diethylcarbamazine (DEC) treatment during MDA programmes against LF and ivermectin MDA for onchocerciasis can lead to in co-infected individuals with high *L. loa* MF loads. Loiasis is also known under names like Calabar swelling, fugitive swelling and filaria lacrimalis and in contrast to other filarial nematodes, *L. loa* does not possess *Wolbachia* [58, 59].

3.1 Biology of the parasite

Like mentioned before, loiasis is caused by the tissue-dwelling nematode *L. loa*. This worm gets transmitted through a bite of deer fly species *Chrysops silacea*, *C. dimidiate* and *C. langi*, which are restricted to Africa [60, 61]. Similar to other vector species, deer flies transmit infective L3 during a blood meal into their host. Humans are the only known host for *L. loa* although *in vivo* experiments are possible with Drills (*Mandrillus leucophaeus)* and immunocompromised mice [62, 63]. Upon entering the host, the L3 migrate through the subcutaneous tissues and molt to adult worms. Adult female of *L. loa* can reach lengths of 40–70 mm and are 0.5 mm wide while males are smaller with 30–34 mm lengths and 0.35–0.43 widths. Fecund females release sheathed MF (230–300 μm) that are found in peripheral blood but also in spinal fluid, urine, lung and sputum (**Table 2**). Lifespan estimations of adult worms are rare, but range from at least 9 years to as long as 15–21 years [64]. Adapted to their insect vectors, *L. loa* MF are diurnal, so appear in the peripheral blood during the day. They reside overnight in the lung tissues. During another blood meal, the deer flies ingest the MF. The MF lose their sheaths and migrate from the midgut into the thoracic muscles of the arthropods. Upon developing into the L3, the larvae migrates to the proboscis of the fly to get transmitted during the next blood meal [60, 61].

3.2 Epidemiology

Loiasis is restricted to the rain forest areas of 12 countries of Western and Central Africa. These are namely Angola, Cameroon, the Central African Republic, Chad, the Republic of Congo and the Democratic Republic of Congo, Equatorial Guinea, Ethiopia, Gabon, Nigeria, Sudan and South Sudan [65]. Although large sections of these countries have low or no prevalence of loiasis, an estimated 14 million people reside in high-risk areas, where the prevalence of *L. loa* is greater than 40%. An estimated 10 million people are currently infected with *Loa loa* [64, 65]. The vector species are more common during the rainy season and usually bite during the day [66]. But these insects can also be found in rubber and palm oil plantations as well as mangrove swamps [67]. Travelers are more likely to become infected if they are exposed to bites for many months.

3.3 Pathology

The majority of infected individuals remain asymptomatic. However, clinical symptoms of loiasis may take years to develop and due to the lack of severe pathology, this disease is even more neglected [68–71]. One common clinical symptom is the Calabar swelling, a localized angioedema caused by transient subcutaneous swellings which mark the migratory course of the nematode [70]. Interestingly, only around 16% of endemic patients develop this symptom, which are usually located on the face, limbs or joints [27]. It is hypothesized that these swellings are a result of an allergic reaction to the migrating adult filariae or MF [71]. Associated symptoms also include local or disseminated pruritus, urticaria and restricted movement patterns. Symptoms usually resolve after 2–4 days, but they can persist or even reoccur [71]. *L. loa* is known as the "African eye-worm" because of its migration across the eye. This eye migration is found in 10–20% of infected individuals and can result in inflammation, itching, light sensitivity, congestion and severe pain [69]. Similar to the aforementioned symptoms, these signs of infection usually last for several days and the ensuing damage is not permanent. Due to the removal of high MF loads, patients may also present proteinuria and hematuria. Other described, but rare pathologies include inflammation of the lymph glands [72], arthritis [73], scrotal swellings [74], eosinophilic lung infiltrates [75] and endomyocardial fibrosis [71]. Attention to loiasis was raised due to reports about severe adverse effects including fatal cases of encephalopathy after ivermection or DEC treatment during MDA for LF or onchocerciasis [76–79]. These serious events were connected with patients with high peripheral blood MF loads of *L. loa* (>30,000 MF/ml) and the associated inflammatory responses to dying MF [80–82].

Therefore, in regions where onchocerciasis and LF elimination programmes are ongoing, the co-endemicity with *L. loa* represents a major obstacle [20, 83], leading to a test-and-not-treat scenario. Currently, the focus in these areas is on alternative strategies including a better understanding of the micro-epidemiology, integrated vector management and new *L. loa* tests [84].

4. Mansonellosis

Mansonellosis is caused by four different species of the nematode genus *Mansonella*. Knowledge about epidemiology, pathology and even just the general biology of the parasite is very limited. Mansonellosis is not listed as a NTD and further research is urgently needed not only in understanding the immune response of infected patients, but also in developing better diagnostic tools. In contrast to the aforementioned filarial diseases, *Mansonella* infections lack a distinct clinical picture and infections appear mild or asymptomatic—a feature that probably comes with an optimal adaptation to the human host. Currently, mansonellosis can be considered the most neglected of the human filarial diseases.

4.1 Biology of the parasite

Mansonellosis is caused by four species of *Mansonella*, named *Mansonella perstans*, *M. ozzardi* and *M. streptocerca* (**Table 1**) as well as the newly discovered molecular clade of *M. perstans* named *Mansonella sp.* "DEUX" [85, 86]. Latter could represent a new species with a pathogenic role. It has been detected only in febrile children in Gabon [86]. Most of our knowledge about mansonellosis is based on *M. perstans* infections. Transmission of *M. perstans* is associated with midges of the genus *Culicoides*. *M. streptocerca* and *M. ozzardi* can also be transmitted by *Simulium* blackflies and *M. ozzardi* is additionally transmitted by *Ceratopogonidae* midges in South America and the Caribbeans [87–89]. The life cycle of the *Mansonella* species is similar to the other tissue-dwelling nematodes. L3 get transmitted onto the skin during the blood meal of the insect vector and they penetrate into the bite wound. The L3 eventually develop into adult worms which reside in body cavities like the peritoneum, the pleura and the pericardium. Female worms of *M. perstans* are 70–80 mm long and 120 μm wide, males are smaller, reaching 45 mm in length and being 60 μm wide. *M. ozzardi* is smaller and more slender than *M. perstans*, reaching 32–61 mm for females and 24–28 mm for males. *M. ozzardi* also resides in subcutaneous tissues. Gravid females release unsheated MF, which are sub-periodic for *M. perstans*, meaning they are present in the blood at all times, and non-periodic for *M. ozzardi* and *M. streptocerca* (MF size: *M. perstans;* 200 μm long and 4.5 μm wide, *M. ozzardi:* 207–232 μm long and 3–4 μm wide and *M. streptocerca:* 180–240 μm long and 3–5 μm wide, **Table 2**). The MF can be taken up again by their vectors during a blood meal and there they migrate from the midgut to the thoracic muscles to develop from L1 to L3 [85, 90–92]. MF of *Mansonella* species do not exhibit periodicity.

4.2 Epidemiology

More than 600 million people live at high risk of infection with *M. perstans* in 33 countries of sub-Saharan Africa as well as in tropical regions of Central and South America. Studies have also brought up evidence for *M. perstans* infections by migrants from Africa living in Spain [93]. It is estimated that 114 million individuals in total are infected with *M. perstans*. While only a few epidemiological studies have been carried out for *M. perstans* infections so far, it has been shown that MF prevalence rates are higher in adults than in children and that males are more frequently infected than females [94]. Endemic areas for *M. streptocerca* are the tropical rainforests of West, Central and Eastern Africa. *M. ozzardi* is found in South America and in the Caribbean. Also in these areas, a high prevalence is suggested. A recent study from Ecuador showed a high prevalence of >20% for *M. ozzardi* [95]. Although once again the actual number of infected patients is unknown, up to 70% of patients in endemic areas are MF+ [96]. Transmission of mansonellosis is strongly associated with the abundance and seasonal occurrence of the vector. The vector species themselves rely on aquatic or semi-aquatic habitats, animal dung as well as banana stems, rotting fruits or cacti that are required as breeding sites and essential for insect development [97, 98].

4.3 Pathology

Generally, mansonellosis is not associated with severe clinical symptoms and is therefore not considered a public health problem. Infections with both *M. perstans* and *M. ozzardi* are usually asymptomatic and only transient itching, skin swellings and rashes occur. *M. streptocerca* was reported to induce dermatological pathology similar to *O. volvulus* with spotty depigmentations around thorax and shoulders, coinciding with areas where MF are often detected [99]. Further clinical studies also report symptoms like fever, headache, tiredness, joint pain and lymph node enlargement [100–102]. Serological tests to diagnose *Mansonella* infections are not yet available. The current method for diagnosis is identifying the unsheated MF in blood (*M. perstans* and *M. ozzardi*) and skin biopsy (*M. streptocerca* and *M. ozzardi*).

5. Current treatments and future perspectives

The United Nations Sustainable Development Goals and the WHO NTD road map 2021–2030 stated the goal of confirmed elimination of transmission for onchocerciasis and as a public health problem for LF by 2030. MDAs with ivermectin in combination with albendazole within Africa, or diethylcarbamazine (DEC) plus albendazole outside of Africa for LF and ivermectin alone for onchocerciasis were used. As mentioned above, the goal of eliminating LF by 2020 was missed by WHO's GPELF. However, over 8 billion doses of the annual MDA treatments were distributed to more than 923 million people. The result is that 17 countries are currently under surveillance to confirm the elimination of LF transmission [18, 19, 103, 104]. The main intervention strategy for LF consists of annual, single dose MDAs with ivermectin plus albendazole or DEC plus albendazole targeting the MF stage. These treatments do not efficiently kill the adult worms, but removes MF from peripheral blood and inhibit MF release for a few months [105, 106]. A new approach for LF in areas that are that are not co-endemic for onchocerciasis and loiasis, is the now WHO-recommended MDA using a triple therapy. This therapy consists of a single dose of ivermectin (200 μg/kg), DEC (6 mg/kg) and albendazole (400 mg) [107]. The triple therapy was shown to reduce microfilaremia for more than 2 years and may have some macrofilaricidal efficacy. While the triple therapy can be seen as a game changer for LF, it is not recommended in co-endemic areas for onchocerciasis and loiasis. DEC can lead to severe adverse effects in onchocerciasis patients and *L. loa* patients with high MF loads can experience severe adverse effects due to ivermectin [107]. In loiasis co-endemic areas, people with high MF loads have to be identified and excluded from treatment, or pretreated with albendazole. In onchocerciasis co-endemic areas the MDAs consist of a combination of ivermectin and albendazole. A treatment that can be used safely in patients with LF and *L. loa* co-infection is doxycycline. A treatment for four weeks with 200 mg/kg of doxycycline is sufficient to clear the *Wolbachia* endosymbionts, leading to a permanently inhibited filarial embryogenesis. *L. loa* worms are not affected by this treatment since they do not harbor *Wolbachia*. Doxycycline also slowly kills the adult worms [108]. Furthermore, doxycycline treatment has been shown to improve lymphedema pathology, probably due to its immunomodulatory and anti-inflammatory properties. For the treatment of lymphedema, doxycycline should be given daily at 200 mg/kg for 6 weeks, with intervals every 12–24 months [109].

Targeting the *Wolbachia* endosymbionts using doxycycline is also a proven treatment for *O. volvulus* patients. Similar to LF, depleting *Wolbachia* in *O. volvulus* leads to permanent inhibition of filarial embryogenesis and death of adult worms after 1.5–2 years [110–112]. No MF-induced adverse effects are observed and MF clearance happens over time due to natural removal of MF combined with the lack of filarial embryogenesis. Macrofilaricidal efficacy is achieved with 200 mg/day for 6 weeks. In order to accelerate the clearance of MF, doxycycline treatment can be combined with a single dose of ivermectin. The disadvantage of doxycycline is that its use is not recommended in pregnant as well as breast-feeding women and in children below the age of 8. Current research is focused on identifying anti-wolbachials with shorter treatment regimens. As such, the tylosin analogue ABBV-4083 is currently tested in phase 2 clinical studies with onchocerciasis patients [113, 114]. Current WHO supported MDA for onchocerciasis rely on ivermectin [1]. Treatment with this macrocyclic lactone (150 μg/kg) leads to clearance of MF and a temporary inhibition of female embryogenesis [115]. This results in interruption of transmission for several months [116]. However, ivermectin has no macrofilaricidal effect and has to be repeated every 6–12 months for the fecund life span of *O. volvulus*, which means for 10 years or more. Additionally, ivermectin treatment is—similar to doxycycline—not indicated in pregnant and breast-feeding women as well as in little children, although circumstantial evidence suggests that it has been inadvertently administered millionfold in early yet undetected pregnancies without overt pathologies [117]. Furthermore, side effects caused by ivermectin-induced dying MF can lead to inflammatory immune responses resulting in rashes, fever, and itching skin. Yet, in comparison to DEC, adverse effects caused by ivermectin treatment are less severe as compared to permanent visual impairment which has been reported following DEC treatment [118]. More recently, another macrocyclic lactone has been registered for onchocerciasis treatment—moxidectin. It works similar to ivermectin with clearing MF and inhibiting filarial embryogenesis. However, moxidectin leads to an extended absence of lasting up to one year [119], so that it may replace ivermectin in some settings in the future. Another drug which has successfully passed the clinical phase I trials and is currently evaluated for its macrofilaricidal and long-term sterilizing activity in onchocerciasis patients is emodepside [120].

In contrast to LF and onchocerciasis, loiasis cannot be treated with anti-wolbachials such as doxycycline due to the lack of *Wolbachia* in *L. loa* [59]. The standard treatment is DEC, given at 5–10 mg/kg for 2–4 weeks, clearing microfilaremia with some macrofilaricidal efficacy. A single oral treatment of ivermectin also clears microfilaremia. However, both these treatments can lead to severe adverse effects associated with high MF counts in patients [121]. Adverse effects range from fever, nausea and itching (especially with DEC) to life-threatening events such as neurological symptoms, encephalopathy, coma and even death after ivermectin treatment. Therefore it is recommend that patients with more than 20,000 MF/ml are not treated with ivermectin. Patients with high MF loads can instead be treated with 200 mg albendazole twice a day for 21 days [122]. The risk of these aforementioned serious adverse effects is also one of the major obstacles during onchocerciasis elimination programs. Before treatment with ivermectin, patients require a so-called "test-and-not-treat" measure [123]. MDA activities are still continuing in *L. loa* co-endemic areas, but the co-infection represents a major challenge going forward. For mansonellosis, treatment and success of treatment differs between the three *Mansonella* species. *M. ozzardi* MF are not susceptible for DEC treatment, but a single ivermectin dose leads to reduction of MF counts [124]. For *M. streptocerca*, DEC was demonstrated to eliminate both MF and adult worms, but side effects such as severe pruritus and urticaria has been reported [125]. A single treatment of ivermectin has led to long-lasting reduction of *M. streptocerca* MF load [99]. On the other hand, single treatment of ivermectin or albendazole had very small or no effect on *M. perstans* microfilaremia [94, 126]. MF were however cleared in clinical trials using 200 mg doxycycline for 6 weeks [127].

Author details

Jesuthas Ajendra[1]*, Achim Hoerauf[1,2] and Marc P. Hübner[1,2]

1 Institute for Medical Microbiology, Immunology and Parasitology, University Hospital Bonn, Bonn, Germany

2 German Center for Infection Research (DZIF), Partner Site Bonn-Cologne, Bonn, Germany

*Address all correspondence to: jesuthas.ajendra@ukbonn.de

References

[1] World Health Orgaization. 2020. Elimination of Human Onchocerciasis: Progress Report, 2019-2020

[2] Manguin S, Bangs MJ, Pothikasikorn J, Chareonviriyaphap T. Review on global co-transmission of human *Plasmodium* species and *Wuchereria bancrofti* by *Anopheles* mosquitoes. Infection, Genetics and Evolution. 2010. DOI: 10.1016/j.meegid.2009.11.014

[3] Bizhani N, Hashemi Hafshejani S, Mohammadi N, Rezaei M, Rokni MB. Lymphatic filariasis in Asia: A systematic review and meta-analysis. Parasitology Research. 2021. DOI: 10.1007/s00436-020-06991-y

[4] Atmosoedjono S, Partono F, Dennis DT, Purnomo. *Anopheles barbirostris* (Diptera: Culicidae) as a vector of the Timor filaria on Flores island: Preliminary observations. Journal of Medical Entomology. 1977. DOI: 10.1093/jmedent/13.4-5.611

[5] Simonsen PE, Niemann L, Meyrowitsch DW. *Wuchereria bancrofti* in Tanzania: Microfilarial periodicity and effect of blood sampling time on microfilarial intensities. Tropical Medicine and International Health. 1997. DOI: 10.1046/j.1365-3156.1997.d01-237.x

[6] Moulia-Pelat JP et al. Periodicity of *Wuchereria bancrofti* var. Pacifica filariasis in French Polynesia. Tropical Medicine and Parasitology. 1993

[7] Dreyer G, Addiss D, Norões J. Does longevity of adult *Wuchereria bancrofti* increase with decreasing intensity of parasite transmission? Insights from clinical observations. Transactions of the Royal Society of Tropical Medicine and Hygiene. 2005. DOI: 10.1016/j.trstmh.2005.05.006

[8] Stolk WA, de Vlas SJ, Habbema JDF. Advances and challenges in predicting the impact of lymphatic filariasis elimination programmes by mathematical modelling. Filaria Journal. 2006. DOI: 10.1186/1475-2883-5-5

[9] Edeson JFB. Filariasis. British Medical Bulletin. 1972. DOI: 10.1093/oxfordjournals.bmb.a070895

[10] Srividya A, Subramanian S, Jambulingam P, Vijayakumar B, Dinesh Raja J. Mapping and monitoring for a lymphatic filariasis elimination program: A systematic review. Research and Reports in Tropical Medicine. 2019. DOI: 10.2147/rrtm.s134186

[11] Nutman TB, Kazura JW. Lymphatic filariasis. Tropical Infectious Diseases. 2011

[12] Global Programme to Eliminate Lymphatic Filariasis: Progress Report, 2019

[13] World Health Organization. Ending the neglect to attain the Sustainable Development Goals: A road map for neglected tropical diseases 2021-2030. Geography Review. 2020

[14] Ramaiah KD, Ottesen EA. Progress and Impact of 13 years of the global programme to eliminate lymphatic filariasis on reducing the burden of filarial disease. PLoS Neglected Tropical Diseases. 2014. DOI: 10.1371/journal.pntd.0003319

[15] James SL et al. Global, regional, and national incidence, prevalence, and years lived with disability for 354 diseases and injuries for 195 countries and territories;2017: A systematic analysis for the Global Burden of Disease Study 2017. Lancet. 2018;**392**(10159):1789-1858. DOI: 10.1016/S0140-6736(18)32279-7

[16] Il Cheun H, Lee JS, Cho SH, Kong Y, Kim TS. Elimination of lymphatic filariasis in the Republic of Korea: An epidemiological survey of formerly endemic areas, 2002-2006. Tropical Medicine and International Health. 2009. DOI: 10.1111/j.1365-3156.2009.02240.x

[17] De-jian S, Xu-li D, Ji-hui D. The history of the elimination of lymphatic filariasis in China. Infectious Diseases of Poverty. 2013. DOI: 10.1186/2049-9957-2-30

[18] Hooper PJ, Chu BK, Mikhailov A, Ottesen EA, Bradley M. Assessing progress in reducing the at-risk population after 13 years of the global programme to eliminate lymphatic filariasis. PLoS Neglected Tropical Diseases. 2014;**8**(11):e3333. DOI: 10.1371/journal.pntd.0003333

[19] Ichimori K et al. Global programme to eliminate lymphatic filariasis: The processes underlying programme success. PLoS Neglected Tropical Diseases. 2014. DOI: 10.1371/journal.pntd.0003328

[20] Addiss D. The 6th meeting of the global alliance to eliminate lymphatic filariasis: A half-time review of lymphatic filariasis elimination and its integration with the control of other neglected tropical diseases. Parasites & Vectors. 2010. DOI: 10.1186/1756-3305-3-100

[21] Rebollo MP, Bockarie MJ. Can lymphatic filariasis be eliminated by 2020? Trends in Parasitology. 2017. DOI: 10.1016/j.pt.2016.09.009

[22] G. Dreyer, D. Addiss, J. Bettinger, P. Dreyer, J. Norões, and F. Rio, Lymphoedema Staff Manual: Treatment and Prevention of Problems Associated with Lymphatic Filariasis. WHO; 2001

[23] Debrah LB et al. Single nucleotide polymorphisms in the angiogenic and lymphangiogenic pathways are associated with lymphedema caused by *Wuchereria bancrofti*. Human Genomics. 2017. DOI: 10.1186/s40246-017-0121-7

[24] Bennuru S, Nutman TB. Lymphangiogenesis and lymphatic remodeling induced by filarial parasites: Implications for pathogenesis. PLoS Pathogens. 2009. DOI: 10.1371/journal.ppat.1000688

[25] Taylor MJ. Wolbachia in the inflammatory pathogenesis of human filariasis. Annals of the New York Academy of Sciences. 2003. DOI: 10.1111/j.1749-6632.2003.tb07409.x

[26] Dreyer G, Medeiros Z, Netto MJ, Leal NC, De Castro LG, Piessens WF. Acute attacks in the extremities of persons living in an area endemic for bancroftian filariasis: Differentiation of two syndromes. Transactions of the Royal Society of Tropical Medicine and Hygiene. 1999. DOI: 10.1016/S0035-9203(99)90140-2

[27] Dreyer G, Addiss D, Gadelha P, Lapa E, Williamson J, Dreyer A. Interdigital skin lesions of the lower limbs among patients with lymphoedema in an area endemic for bancroftian filariasis. Tropical Medicine and International Health. 2006. DOI: 10.1111/j.1365-3156.2006.01687.x

[28] Olszewski WL et al. Bacteriological studies of blood, tissue fluid, lymph and lymph nodes in patients with acute dermatolymphangioadenitis (DLA) in course of 'filarial' lymphedema. Acta Tropica. 1999. DOI: 10.1016/S0001-706X(99)00029-7

[29] Noroes J, Addiss D, Cedenho A, Figueredo-Silva J, Lima G, Dreyer G. Pathogenesis of filarial hydrocele: Risk associated with intrascrotal nodules caused by death of adult Wuchereria

bancrofti. Transactions of the Royal Society of Tropical Medicine and Hygiene. 2003. DOI: 10.1016/S0035-9203(03)80029-9

[30] Ottesen EA, Nutman TB. Tropical pulmonary eosinophilia. Annual Review of Medicine. 1992. DOI: 10.1146/annurev.me.43.020192.002221

[31] Albert H et al. Developing strategies for onchocerciasis elimination mapping and surveillance through the diagnostic network optimization approach. Frontiers in Tropical Diseases. 2021. DOI: 10.3389/fitd.2021.707752

[32] Fischer P, Kipp W, Bamuhiga J, Binta-Kahwa J, Kiefer A, Buttner DW. Parasitological and clinical characterization of Simulium neavei-transmitted onchocerciasis in Western Uganda. Tropical Medicine and Parasitology. 1993

[33] Fischer P, Garms R, Buttner DW, Kipp W, Bamuhiiga J, Yocha J. Reduced prevalence of onchocerciasis in Uganda following either deforestation or vector control with DDT. East African Medical Journal. 1997

[34] Makunde WH, Salum FM, Massaga JJ, Alilio MS. Clinical and parasitological aspects of itching caused by onchocerciasis in Morogoro, Tanzania. Annals of Tropical Medicine and Parasitology. 2000. DOI: 10.1080/00034980020017051

[35] Basáñez MG, Pion SDS, Churcher TS, Breitling LP, Little MP, Boussinesq M. River blindness: A success story under threat? PLoS Medicine. 2006. DOI: 10.1371/journal.pmed.0030371

[36] Brattig NW, Cheke RA, Garms R. Onchocerciasis (river blindness)—More than a century of research and control. Acta Tropica. 2021. DOI: 10.1016/j.actatropica.2020.105677

[37] Schulz-Key H. Observations on the reproductive biology of *Onchocerca volvulus*. Acta Leidensia. 1990

[38] Udall DN. Recent updates on onchocerciasis: Diagnosis and treatment. Clinical Infectious Diseases. 2007. DOI: 10.1086/509325

[39] Specht S, Brattig N, Büttner M, Büttner DW. Criteria for the differentiation between young and old *Onchocerca volvulus* filariae. Parasitology Research. 2009. DOI: 10.1007/s00436-009-1588-5

[40] Murdoch ME. Mapping the burden of onchocercal skin disease*. British Journal of Dermatology. 2021. DOI: 10.1111/bjd.19143

[41] Taylor MJ, Hoerauf A, Townson S, Slatko BE, Ward SA. Anti-Wolbachia drug discovery and development: Safe macrofilaricides for onchocerciasis and lymphatic filariasis. Parasitology. 2014;**141**:119-127. DOI: 10.1017/S0031182013001108

[42] Hoerauf A et al. Endosymbiotic bacteria in worms as targets for a novel chemotherapy in filariasis. Lancet. 2000. DOI: 10.1016/S0140-6736(00)02095-X

[43] Hoerauf A, Mand S, Adjei O, Fleischer B, Büttner DW. Depletion of *Wolbachia* endobacteria in *Onchocerca volvulus* by doxycycline and microfilaridermia after ivermectin treatment. Lancet. 2001. DOI: 10.1016/S0140-6736(00)04581-5

[44] Hoerauf A, Pfarr K, Mand S, Debrah AY, Specht S. Filariasis in Africa-treatment challenges and prospects. Clinical Microbiology and Infection. 2011;**17**(7):977-985. DOI: 10.1111/j.1469-0691.2011.03586.x

[45] Basáñez MG, Walker M, Turner HC, Coffeng LE, de Vlas SJ, Stolk WA. River

blindness: Mathematical models for control and elimination. Advances in Parasitology. 2016. DOI: 10.1016/bs.apar.2016.08.003

[46] Coffeng LE et al. African programme for onchocerciasis control 1995-2015: Model-estimated health impact and cost. PLoS Neglected Tropical Diseases. 2013. DOI: 10.1371/journal.pntd.0002032

[47] Kipp W, Bamhuhiiga J. Onchodermal skin disease in a hyperendemic onchocerciasis focus in Western Uganda. The American Journal of Tropical Medicine and Hygiene. 2002. DOI: 10.4269/ajtmh.2002.67.475

[48] Katawa G et al. Hyperreactive onchocerciasis is characterized by a combination of Th17-Th2 immune responses and reduced regulatory T cells. PLoS Neglected Tropical Diseases. 2015;**9**(1):e3414. DOI: 10.1371/journal.pntd.0003414

[49] Murdoch ME et al. A clinical classification and grading system of the cutaneous changes in onchocerciasis. The British Journal of Dermatology. 1993. DOI: 10.1111/j.1365-2133.1993.tb11844.x

[50] Edungbola LD, Watts SJ, Kayode OO. Endemicity and striking manifestations of onchocerciasis in Shao, Kwara State, Nigeria. African Journal of Medicine and Medical Sciences. 1987

[51] Njim T, Ngum JM, Aminde LN. Cutaneous onchocerciasis in Dumbu, a pastoral area in the north-west region of Cameroon: Diagnostic challenge and socio-economic implications. The Pan African Medical Journal. 2015. DOI: 10.11604/pamj.2015.22.298.7707

[52] Hoerauf A, Brattig N. Resistance and susceptibility in human onchocerciasis—Beyond Th1 vs Th2. Trends in Parasitology. 2002. DOI: 10.1016/S1471-4922(01)02173-0

[53] Abiose A. Onchocercal eye disease and the impact of Mectizan treatment. Annals of Tropical Medicine and Parasitology. 1998. DOI: 10.1080/00034983.1998.11813361

[54] Tamarozzi F, Halliday A, Gentil K, Hoerauf A, Pearlman E, Taylor MJ. Onchocerciasis: The role of Wolbachia bacterial endosymbionts in parasite biology, disease pathogenesis, and treatment. Clinical Microbiology Reviews. 2011;**24**(3):459-468. DOI: 10.1128/CMR.00057-10

[55] Andre AS et al. The role of endosymbiotic Wolbachia bacteria in the pathogenesis of river blindness. Science (80-.). 2002. DOI: 10.1126/science.1068732

[56] Basak SK, Hazra TK, Bhattacharya D. Persistent corneal edema secondary to presumed dead adult filarial worm in the anterior chamber. Indian Journal of Ophthalmology. 2007. DOI: 10.4103/0301-4738.29501

[57] Budden FH. Route of entry of *Onchocerca volvulus* microfilariae into the eye. Transactions of the Royal Society of Tropical Medicine and Hygiene. 1976. DOI: 10.1016/0035-9203(76)90066-3

[58] Desjardins CA et al. Genomics of *Loa loa*, a Wolbachia-free filarial parasite of humans. Nature Genetics. 2013;**45**(5):495-500. DOI: 10.1038/ng.2585

[59] Büttner DW, Wanji S, Bazzocchi C, Bain O, Fischer P. Obligatory symbiotic *Wolbachia* endobacteria are absent from *Loa loa*. Filaria Journal. 2003. DOI: 10.1186/1475-2883-2-10

[60] Padgett JJ, Jacobsen KH. Loiasis: African eye worm. Transactions of the

Royal Society of Tropical Medicine and Hygiene. 2008. DOI: 10.1016/j.trstmh.2008.03.022

[61] Wanji S, Tendongfor N, Esum ME, Enyong P. Chrysops silacea biting densities and transmission potential in an endemic area of human loiasis in south-west Cameroon. Tropical Medicine and International Health. 2002. DOI: 10.1046/j.1365-3156.2002.00845.x

[62] Pionnier NP et al. Mouse models of *Loa loa*. Nature Communications. 2019. DOI: 10.1038/s41467-019-09442-0

[63] Duke BOL. Experimental transmission of *Loa loa* from man to monkey. Nature. 1957. DOI: 10.1038/1791357c0

[64] Whittaker C, Walker M, Pion SDS, Chesnais CB, Boussinesq M, Basáñez MG. The population biology and transmission dynamics of *Loa loa*. Trends in Parasitology. 2018. DOI: 10.1016/j.pt.2017.12.003

[65] Zouré HGM et al. The geographic distribution of *Loa loa* in Africa: Results of large-scale implementation of the rapid assessment procedure for Loiasis (RAPLOA). PLoS Neglected Tropical Diseases. 2011. DOI: 10.1371/journal.pntd.0001210

[66] Noireau F, Apembet JD, Nzoulani A, Carme B. Clinical manifestations of loiasis in an endemic area in the Congo. Tropical Medicine and Parasitology. 1990

[67] Davey JT, O'Rourke FJ. Observations on chrysops silacea and c. dimidiata at benin, southern nigeria. Annals of Tropical Medicine and Parasitology. 1951. DOI: 10.1080/00034983.1951.11685477

[68] Boussinesq M. Loiasis. Annals of Tropical Medicine and Parasitology. 2006. DOI: 10.1179/136485906X112194

[69] Churchill DR, Morris C, Fakoya A, Wright SG, Davidson RN. Clinical and laboratory features of patients with loiasis (*Loa loa* filariasis) in the U.K. The Journal of Infection. 1996. DOI: 10.1016/S0163-4453(96)93005-4

[70] Klion AD, Massougbodji A, Sadeler BC, Ottesen EA, Nutman TB. Loiasis in endemic and nonendemic populations: Immunologically mediated differences in clinical presentation. The Journal of Infectious Diseases. 1991. DOI: 10.1093/infdis/163.6.1318

[71] Nutman TB, Miller KD, Mulligan M, Ottesen EA. *Loa loa* infection in temporary residents of endemic regions: Recognition of a hyperresponsive syndrome with characteristic clinical manifestations. The Journal of Infectious Diseases. 1986. DOI: 10.1093/infdis/154.1.10

[72] Paleologo FP, Neafie RC, Connor DH. Lymphadenitis caused by *Loa loa*. The American Journal of Tropical Medicine and Hygiene. 1984. DOI: 10.4269/ajtmh.1984.33.395

[73] Bouvet JP, Thérizol M, Auquier L. Microfilarial polyarthritis in a massive *Loa loa* infestation. A case report. Acta Tropica. 1977

[74] C.-C. for D. C. and Prevention. 2019. CDC - Loiasis - Disease

[75] Klion AD, Eisenstein EM, Smirniotopoulos TT, Neumann MP, Nutman TB. Pulmonary involvement in loiasis. The American Review of Respiratory Disease. 1992. DOI: 10.1164/ajrccm/145.4_pt_1.961

[76] Carme B, Boulesteix J, Boutes H, Puruehnce MF. Five cases of encephalitis during treatment of loiasis with diethylcarbamazine. The American Journal of Tropical Medicine and

Hygiene. 1991. DOI: 10.4269/ajtmh.1991.44.684

[77] Duke BO. Overview: Report of a Scientific Working Group on Serious Adverse Events following Mectizan(R) treatment of onchocerciasis in *Loa loa* endemic areas. Filaria Journal. 2003. DOI: 10.1186/1475-2883-2-S1-S1

[78] Nieves-Moreno M, Bañeros-Rojas P, Díaz-Valle D, Gegúndez-Fernández JA. Encephalitis secondary to diethylcarbamazine treatment in a patient with ocular loiasis. Journal Français d'Ophtalmologie. 2017. DOI: 10.1016/j.jfo.2015.12.012

[79] Twum-Danso NAY, Meredith SEO. Variation in incidence of serious adverse events after onchocerciasis treatment with ivermectin in areas of Cameroon co-endemic for loiasis. Tropical Medicine and International Health. 2003. DOI: 10.1046/j.1365-3156.2003.01091.x

[80] Gardon J, Gardon-Wendel N, Demanga-Ngangue J, Kamgno J, Chippaux P, Boussinesq M. Serious reactions after mass treatment of onchocerciasis with ivermectin in an area endemic for *Loa loa* infection. Lancet. 1997. DOI: 10.1016/S0140-6736(96)11094-1

[81] Boussinesq M, Gardon J, Gardon-Wendel N, Kamgno J, Ngoumou P, Chippaux JP. Three probable cases of *Loa loa* encephalopathy following ivermectin treatment for onchocerciasis. The American Journal of Tropical Medicine and Hygiene. 1998. DOI: 10.4269/ajtmh.1998.58.461

[82] Boussinesq M, Gardon J, Kamgno J, Pion SDS, Gardon-Wendel N, Chippaux JP. Relationships between the prevalence and intensity of *Loa loa* infection in the Central province of Cameroon. Annals of Tropical Medicine and Parasitology. 2001. DOI: 10.1080/00034980120073184

[83] Amazigo UV et al. The challenges of community-directed treatment with ivermectin (CDTI) within the African Programme for Onchocerciasis Control (APOC). Annals of Tropical Medicine and Parasitology. 2002. DOI: 10.1179/000349802125000646

[84] Kelly-Hope LA, Cano J, Stanton MC, Bockarie MJ, Molyneux DH. Innovative tools for assessing risks for severe adverse events in areas of overlapping *Loa loa* and other filarial distributions: The application of micro-stratification mapping. Parasites & Vectors. 2014. DOI: 10.1186/1756-3305-7-307

[85] Simonsen PE, Onapa AW, Asio SM. Mansonella perstans filariasis in Africa. Acta Tropica. 2011. DOI: 10.1016/j.actatropica.2010.01.014

[86] Mourembou G et al. Mansonella, including a Potential New Species, as Common Parasites in Children in Gabon. PLoS Neglected Tropical Diseases. 2015. DOI: 10.1371/journal.pntd.0004155

[87] Crosskey RC. The Natural History of Blackflies. Chichester: John Wiley & Sons; 1990 Rev. la Soc. Entomológica Argentina, 1996

[88] Shelley AJ, Coscarón S. Simuliid Blackflies (Diptera: Simuliidae) and Ceratopogonid Midges (Diptera: Ceratopogonidae) as Vectors of Mansonella ozzardi (Nematoda: Onchocercidae) in Northern Argentina. Memórias do Instituto Oswaldo Cruz. 2001. DOI: 10.1590/S0074-02762001000400003

[89] Linley JR, Hoch AL, Pinheiro FP. Biting midges (Diptera: Ceratopogonidae) and human health.

Journal of Medical Entomology. 1983. DOI: 10.1093/jmedent/20.4.347

[90] Lima NF, Veggiani Aybar CA, Dantur Juri MJ, Ferreira MU. Mansonella ozzardi: A neglected New World filarial nematode. Pathogens and Global Health. 2016. DOI: 10.1080/20477724.2016.1190544

[91] Mediannikov O, Ranque S. Mansonellosis, the most neglected human filariasis. New Microbes and New Infections. 2018. DOI: 10.1016/j.nmni.2018.08.016

[92] Ta-Tang T-H, Crainey J, Post RJ, Luz SL, Rubio J. Mansonellosis: Current perspectives. Research in Reports Tropical Medicine. 2018. DOI: 10.2147/rrtm.s125750

[93] Puente S et al. Imported Mansonella perstans infection in Spain. Infectious Diseases of Poverty. 2020. DOI: 10.1186/s40249-020-00729-9

[94] Asio SM, Simonsen PE, Onapa AW. Mansonella perstans: Safety and efficacy of ivermectin alone, albendazole alone and the two drugs in combination. Annals of Tropical Medicine and Parasitology. 2009. DOI: 10.1179/136485909X384929

[95] Calvopina M, Chiluisa-Guacho C, Toapanta A, Fonseca D, Villacres I. High prevalence of *Mansonella ozzardi* infection in the Amazon Region, Ecuador. Emerging Infectious Diseases. 2019. DOI: 10.3201/eid2511.181964

[96] Marinkelle CJ, German E. Mansonelliasis in the Comisaría del Vaupes of Colombia. Tropical and Geographical Medicine. 1970

[97] Wanji S et al. Update on the biology and ecology of Culicoides species in the South-West region of Cameroon with implications on the transmission of Mansonella perstans. Parasites & Vectors. 2019. DOI: 10.1186/s13071-019-3432-9

[98] Meiswinkel R, Venter GJ, Nevill EM. Vectors: Culicoides spp. Infectious Diseases of Livestocks. 2004

[99] Fischer P, Bamuhiiga J, Büttner DW. Treatment of human Mansonella streptocerca infection with ivermectin. Tropical Medicine and International Health. 1997. DOI: 10.1046/j.1365-3156.1997.d01-233.x

[100] Sondergaard J. Filariasis caused by Acanthocheilonema perstans. Archives of Dermatology. 1972. DOI: 10.1001/archderm.106.4.547

[101] Holmes GKT, Gelfand M, Boyt W. A study to investigate the pathogenicity of a parasite resembling acanthocheilonema perstans. Transactions of the Royal Society of Tropical Medicine and Hygiene. 1969. DOI: 10.1016/0035-9203(69)90035-2

[102] Adolph PE, Kagan IG, McQUAY RM. Diagnosis and treatment of Acanthocheilonema perstans filariasis. The American Journal of Tropical Medicine and Hygiene. 1962. DOI: 10.4269/ajtmh.1962.11.76

[103] Ottesen EA, Horton J. Setting the stage for a Global Programme to Eliminate Lymphatic Filariasis: The first 125 years (1875-2000). International Health. 2021. DOI: 10.1093/inthealth/ihaa061

[104] Ramaiah KD, Ottesen EA. Progress and impact of 13 years of the Global Programme to eliminate lymphatic filariasis on reducing the burden of filarial disease. PLoS Neglected Tropical Diseases. 2014;**8**(11):e3319. DOI: 10.1371/journal.pntd.0003319

[105] Cao WC, Van Der Ploeg CPB, Plaisier AP, Sivera Van Der Sluijs IJ, Habbema JDF. Ivermectin for the chemotherapy of bancroftian filariasis: A meta- analysis of the effect of single treatment. Tropical Medicine and International Health. 1997. DOI: 10.1111/j.1365-3156.1997.tb00157.x

[106] Eberhard ML, Hightower AW, Addiss DG, Lammie PJ. Clearance of *Wuchereria bancrofti* antigen after treatment with diethylcarbamazine or ivermectin. The American Journal of Tropical Medicine and Hygiene. 1997. DOI: 10.4269/ajtmh.1997.57.483

[107] World Health Organization (WHO), Guideline: Alternative Mass Drug Administration Regimens to Eliminate Lymphatic Filariasis. WHO; 2017

[108] Hoerauf A et al. Macrofilaricidal activity in *Wuchereria bancrofti* after 2 weeks treatment with a combination of rifampicin plus doxycycline. Journal of Parasitology Research. 2011. DOI: 10.1155/2011/201617

[109] Mand S et al. Doxycycline improves filarial lymphedema independent of active filarial infection: A randomized controlled trial. Clinical Infectious Diseases. 2012. DOI: 10.1093/cid/cis486

[110] Hoerauf A et al. Doxycycline in the treatment of human onchocerciasis: Kinetics of Wolbachia endobacteria reduction and of inhibition of embryogenesis in female Onchocerca worms. Microbes and Infection. 2003. DOI: 10.1016/S1286-4579(03)00026-1

[111] Hoerauf A et al. Wolbachia endobacteria depletion by doxycycline as antifilarial therapy has macrofilaricidal activity in onchocerciasis: A randomized placebo-controlled study. Medical Microbiology and Immunology. 2008. DOI: 10.1007/s00430-007-0062-1

[112] Hoerauf A et al. Efficacy of 5-week doxycycline treatment on adult *Onchocerca volvulus*. Parasitology Research. 2009. DOI: 10.1007/s00436-008-1217-8

[113] Taylor MJ et al. Preclinical development of an oral anti-Wolbachia macrolide drug for the treatment of lymphatic filariasis and onchocerciasis. Science Translational Medicine. 2019. DOI: 10.1126/scitranslmed.aau2086

[114] David Hong W et al. AWZ1066S, a highly specific anti-Wolbachia drug candidate for a short-course treatment of filariasis. Proceedings of the National Academy of Sciences of the United States of America. 2019. DOI: 10.1073/pnas.1816585116

[115] Gardon J, Boussinesq M, Kamgno J, Gardon-Wendel N, Ngangue D, Duke BOL. Effects of standard and high doses of ivermectin on adult worms of *Onchocerca volvulus*: A randomised controlled trial. Lancet. 2002. DOI: 10.1016/S0140-6736(02)09456-4

[116] Duke BOL, Zea-Flores G, Munoz B. The embryogenesis of *Onchocerca volvulus* over the first year after a single dose of ivermectin. Tropical Medicine and Parasitology. 1991

[117] Gyapong JO, Chinbuah MA, Gyapong M. Inadvertent exposure of pregnant women to ivermectin and albendazole during mass drug administration for lymphatic filariasis. Tropical Medicine and International Health. 2003. DOI: 10.1046/j.1360-2276.2003.01142.x

[118] Greene BM et al. Comparison of ivermectin and diethylcarbamazine in the treatment of onchocerciasis. The New England Journal of Medicine. 1985. DOI: 10.1056/nejm198507183130301

[119] Opoku NO et al. Single dose moxidectin versus ivermectin for *Onchocerca volvulus* infection in Ghana, Liberia, and the Democratic Republic of the Congo: A randomised, controlled, double-blind phase 3 trial. Lancet. 2018. DOI: 10.1016/S0140-6736(17)32844-1

[120] Krücken J et al. Development of emodepside as a possible adulticidal treatment for human onchocerciasis-The fruit of a successful industrial-academic collaboration. PLoS Pathogens. 2021. DOI: 10.1371/journal.ppat.1009682

[121] Gobbi F et al. Comparison of different drug regimens for the treatment of loiasis—A TropNet retrospective study. PLoS Neglected Tropical Diseases. 2018. DOI: 10.1371/journal.pntd.0006917

[122] Klion AD et al. Albendazole in Human Loiasis: Results of a Double-Blind, Placebo-Controlled Trial. The Journal of Infectious Diseases. 1993. DOI: 10.1093/infdis/168.1.202

[123] Pion SD et al. Implications for annual retesting after a test-and-not-treat strategy for onchocerciasis elimination in areas co-endemic with *Loa loa* infection: An observational cohort study. The Lancet Infectious Diseases. 2020. DOI: 10.1016/S1473-3099(19)30554-7

[124] Ferreira MU, Crainey JL, Luz SLB. *Mansonella ozzardi*. Trends in Parasitology. 2021. DOI: 10.1016/j.pt.2020.03.005

[125] Meyers WM, Connor DH, Harman LE, Fleshman K, Moris R, Neafie RC. Human streptocerciasis. A clinico-pathologic study of 40 Africans (Zairians) including identification of the adult filaria. The American Journal of Tropical Medicine and Hygiene. 1972. DOI: 10.4269/ajtmh.1972.21.528

[126] Wanji S et al. Update on the distribution of Mansonella perstans in the southern part of Cameroon: Influence of ecological factors and mass drug administration with ivermectin. Parasites & Vectors. 2016. DOI: 10.1186/s13071-016-1595-1

[127] Debrah LB et al. The efficacy of doxycycline treatment on mansonella perstans infection: An open-label, randomized trial in Ghana. The American Journal of Tropical Medicine and Hygiene. 2019. DOI: 10.4269/ajtmh.18-0491

Section 5

Advances in Vaccines against Helminth Parasites

Chapter 18

Perspective Chapter: Advances in the Development of Anti-*Trichinella spiralis* Vaccine, Challenges, and Future Prospective

Muhammad Tahir Aleem, Ruofeng Yan, Asad Khan, Rida Asrar, Amna Shakoor, Areej Asif, Zhaohai Wen, Zhengqing Yu, Muhammad Abdullah Malik, Tauseef-ur-Rehman, Rao Zahid Abbas, Muhammad Mohsin, Xiaokai Song, Lixin Xu and Xiangrui Li

Abstract

Trichinellosis is a food-borne, zoonotic disease that causes infection by a nematode parasite belonging to the genus *Trichinella*. This is an important disease, and its causative agent is prevalent throughout the world (cosmopolitan). More clinical awareness of *trichinellosis* is required due to its many outbreaks, increase in the consumption of pork meat and its by-products. *Trichinellosis* is an epizootic in nature and its economic burden is associated with the prevention of this disease from the human food chain. This disease is transmitted from animals to humans through the consumption of raw or undercooked meat containing encapsulated muscle larvae of *Trichinella spiralis*. This paper demonstrates the direct effect of progesterone (P4) and mifepristone (RU486) on the progesterone receptors of *T. spiralis*. Also, studied the challenges in the preparation of DNA and recombinant protein vaccination to control trichinellosis. It is simply done this study at different life cycle developmental stages of *T. spiralis*. Vaccines development against *T. spiralis* infection is the new paradime shift from prevention of trichinellosis to fulfilling the food safety requirements.

Keywords: *Trichinella spiralis*, immune response, progesterone receptor, hormones, vaccine

1. Introduction

The phylum Nematoda consists of non-segmented invertebrates commonly known as roundworms that occur in a wide range of habitats around the globe and lack jointed appendages. The causative agent of *trichinellosis* is *Trichinella* species including

Trichinella spiralis (*T. spiralis*) which belongs to the superfamily Trichinelloidea of the phylum Nematoda. At present, the recognized number of species and genotypes in the genus *Trichinella* are nine and three respectively based on the larvae appearance in muscle cells [1, 2]. The most pathogenic and prevalent pathogen in this genus is *T. spiralis* [3]. This is a most serious zoonotic food-borne parasite which can infect a wide range of hosts, is liable for *trichinellosis* disease in humans, and can infect more than 150 species of animals such as carnivores and omnivores including human beings worldwide [4, 5]. *Trichinellosis* occurs around many parts of the world and infects a huge number of human beings. Its ranges from Europe, North America, China, Japan, and Tropical Africa. However, China is the most affected country [1, 6].

The definitive hosts of nematode *Trichinella* include many domestic animals such as pigs, horses, and wild animals like bears, rats, and wild pigs. Each intermediate host of *Trichinella spiralis* is also its definitive host and serves as a source of infection for any other definitive host species by carnivorism [2]. Humans can acquire infection by the ingestion of undercooked, or raw meat of these animals contaminated with the larvae of *T. spiralis* [7]. The important preventive measure (to limit people from getting *trichinellosis*) is to disrupt the transmission of infective *Trichinella* larvae encapsulated in meat to human beings [8, 9]. However, in some countries, this disease is also transmitted by wild animals [10]. Since an enormous amount of pork and its by-products are consumed in China, that results in increased issues in the country [5, 11]. Unlike many other helminth parasites, the survival of *T. spiralis* nematodes is only direct host-to-host transmission adapting normal cellular functions and host immunity at all the stages of infection [12, 13].

The life cycle of *T. spiralis* starts when an adult female and male worms reproduce sexually in the small intestine of the host. The unique characteristic of *T. spiralis* among other parasites is that it passes all the stages of its life cycle within a single host including all phases of adult worm, newborn larvae, and muscle larvae [10, 14, 15]. Humans acquire the infection when they ingest *Trichinella* larvae that are encapsulated in the striated muscles of domestic or wild animals [5]. After the consumption of infected meat, parasitic larvae which are encysted in the meat are then released into the host stomach by acid-pepsin digestion [16]. Columnar epithelial cells of the intestine at the base of the villus are invaded by muscular larvae. Previously released into the stomach from meat and each molts four times to reach sexual maturity [7, 9, 17]. Approximately 1500 newborn larvae are produced by each fertilized female *T. spiralis* within 2–3 weeks and up to 10,000 over 4 months period. These larvae penetrate the intestinal lining with the help of unique sword-like stylet they possess and migrate to the striated (skeletal) muscles via the circulatory and lymphatic system [15]. These larvae can enter any type of cells but only survive in skeletal muscles. In the striated muscles, these previously migrated newborn larvae develop into infective muscle larvae and transform the skeletal muscle cells into a new type of cells known as nurse cells which maintain the larval life and for many species of *Trichinella* changes into capsules or cysts made up of hyaline and collagen fiber [8]. These capsules containing the muscle larvae can persist for many years and calcification occurs in most of the cysts and dies within a few months (see **Figure 1**). The life span of live adult worms in the mucosa of the intestine is 4–6 weeks in human beings while the muscle larvae encapsulated in the striated muscle fibers persist for months to years [1].

Immunity is the defensive mechanism against any pathogenic organisms that invade the victimized host. When the host consumes contaminated meat containing nurse cells, an immune-mediated inflammatory response starts due to the development of the adult worms in the epithelium of the intestine to expel the parasites. The

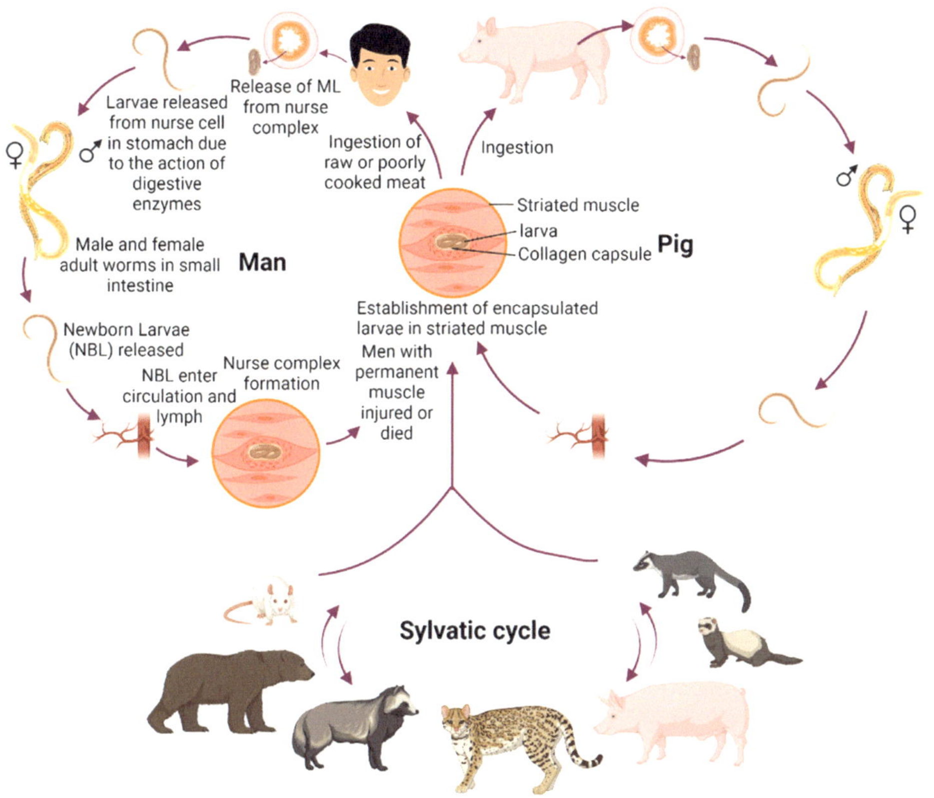

Figure 1.
Life cycle of T. spiralis *[10].*

level of antibody IgE which defends the body against parasitic organisms starts to increase. The inflammatory infiltrates containing mast cells and eosinophils present there pathologically. Both these immune cells are involved in the clearance of parasites. Toxic oxygen molecules and major basic proteins are elaborated by eosinophil to kill invaded organisms but also cause to damage the host body tissues. While mast cell protease-1 (MCP-1) is produced by mast cells that are also lethal to worms. There is widespread inflammation, edema if worm load is high and cells death occurs frequently during the parenteral stage of infection [18, 19].

Trichinellosis infection is classified into three stages depending upon the life cycle of the pathogenic worm; **(1)** as an **invasive stage**, in which larvae grow into adult worms and after fertilization females begin to release newborn larvae which then migrate to blood circulation via the Lymphatic system [9]. This stage is characterized by nausea, diarrhea, abdominal cramps, and seldom vomiting. Constipation is also seen in some of the individuals instead of diarrhea. All these symptoms appear within 2–30 h of post-eating infected food. **(2)** As **migratory phase**; characterized by the encapsulation of larvae in the muscles of the host. The main symptoms observed in this stage include fever, face edema, swelling, muscle pain, and weakness of the infected muscles [14, 16]. (3) As **encystment stage**; characterized by the calcification of cysts in the striated muscles only and results in everlasting injury [1]. As this parasite shows nonspecific signs and symptoms of the disease, its clinical diagnosis is difficult [15]. For the diagnosis of *Trichinellosis*, the digestion method is the best method reported by World Organization for Animal Health (OIE) but to better detect the *Trichinella* parasites molecular biology and serologic methods have been developed [5]. Currently, *Trichinellosis* diagnosis is based on larvae detection in muscle biopsy or immunodiagnostic tests which are highly specific. Many antigens are expressed during the developmental stages of the *T. spiralis* and are useful for the serodiagnosis of *trichinellosis*. However, due to limited *T. spiralis* antigens availability testing is not extensively available [15, 16].

Trichinellosis is not only responsible for public health casualties but also cause the economic problem in food safety and swine animal production. Due to a large number of people infected with *T. spiralis*, this disease is regarded as re-emerging in many regions of the world [2, 15]. If transmission of this disease is not under control, it can lead to serious public health problems [10].

2. Status of anti-*T. spiralis* vaccine

It is a promising method for the control of parasites in pigs to develop a vaccine against *T. spiralis* infection. However, most of the studies for the development of vaccines against *Trichinella* have been performed in lab animals (Mouse models) so far. Only a few studies are performed on pigs for the development of vaccines against *Trichinella* infection. To prevent and control the transmission of *T. spiralis* infection from pigs to humans vaccine exploitation is an important step [20]. *Trichinella* is a tissue-lodging, enteral, and multicellular parasite. Its life cycle is complex and has a diverse developmental phase. *Trichinella* worms have stage-specific antigens [21]. It is necessary to develop an effective vaccine against *Trichinella* to interrupt the transmission of parasites among animals and the cycle of pathogen transmission from swine to humans [5].

Till now, various practices and strategies have been used in the prevention and eradication of parasites including the application of chemicals. The chemical methods are not well signed and have certain limitations such as continuous use of antiparasitic drugs resulting in rising resistance, have risks related to the environment, health, and their potential effects on the host or non-target organisms. Chemotherapy and antiparasitic drugs are used to prevent *T. spiralis* infection, but when we compare the vaccination of animals with chemotherapy treatment, we found that it has several advantages. A single dose of vaccine can provide lifelong prevention of *T. spiralis* infection, reduce the risk of drug residues in meat and other by-products, and decline the emergence of *T. spiralis* drug-resistant parasites [2].

Anti-*Trichinella* vaccines will provide a substantial contribution to the control, prevention, and elimination of *Trichinellosis*. The eradication of *Trichinella* spp. infections in animals is a difficult task as vaccines against *Trichinella* that act as a preventive weapon are not currently available except for rats and pig models [6]. For the past three decades, significant improvements have been made for the recognition of several antigens from *T. spiralis*. It will lead toward a better understanding of the formulation of novel vaccine developments. A variety of vaccines such as subunit vaccines, recombinant proteins vaccines, inactivated vaccines, synthesized epitope vaccines, DNA vaccines, viral or bacterial vector vaccines can elicit an immune response against *Trichinella* and provide effective protection. Scientists have used different antigens to formulate recombinant protein vaccines and many of them have provided some effective protection against *Trichinella* infection [4, 10].

Preventive vaccine development against *Trichinella* infection in domestic pigs is valuable to control and prevent this parasite [21]. The diseases can also be controlled in animals through a veterinary vaccine. To induce long-term intestinal immunity the appropriate route for immunization against *Trichinellosis* is oral as the infection occurs due to the ingestion of poorly cooked meat containing encapsulated infective larvae [20]. Proteases (enzymes) are widely distributed in viruses, prokaryotes, and eukaryotes participate in different events of the parasite's life cycle. In the process of causing infection, parasites serine proteases are thought to be a key factor and exist in the *T. spiralis* excretory-secretory (ES) products [20, 22]. The hydrolyzing enzyme Elastase (trypsin-like serine protease) helps the parasites in the penetration of host tissue through the hydrolysis of laminin, fibronectin, elastin, and type IV collagen. Elastases also participate in the immune evasion process. This enzyme is also involved in the digestion and molting of parasites and has an important role in parasitic worm intrusion of victimized hosts. It might be a target for a novel vaccine [21]. Recently, many anti-*T. spiralis* vaccines have been developed to interrupt the transmission of parasites from animals to humans. Many vaccine candidates which are effective against *T. spiralis* were selected from ES products and recombinant proteins. Serine protease enzymes (from *T. spiralis*) provide partial protection against *T. spiralis* larvae challenges [20].

T. spiralis exerts an immunomodulatory effect through ES products on the immune response of the host [22]. *T. spiralis* Nudix hydrolase (TsND) is a protein that binds to intestinal epithelial cells of normal mice (up-regulated gene). The size of this gene is about 1248 bp. A partial protective immunity against *Trichinella* infection was observed when mice were vaccinated with recombinant TsND protein [22, 23]. Vehicle (delivery system) and antigen are important elements that are responsible for the protection level induced by the candidate vaccine [24].

3. *T. spiralis* -associated immune mechanism

T. spiralis (Helminth) establishes infection which is long-lasting in the striated muscles of the host. Depending on the longevity of the host. It can persist successfully until the end of life in rodents and in higher species including humans can persist over several months to years following infection. They do not kill the host striated muscles cells during their stay, unlike some other intracellular parasites. This characteristic makes them one of the most successful symbiotic parasites [25]. Parasitic nematode *T. spiralis* completes its entire life cycle in one host and each stage of its life cycle provokes the immune system of the host differently [14, 15]. For the establishment of the life cycle successfully, this parasite with the help of its defensive mechanism manages to escape the host immune system responses. The excretory-secretory products of *T. spiralis* play a crucial role in the establishment of parasitism and modulation of host immune response to protect both host and the parasite [22]. When the host acquired the infection of *T. spiralis*, at early-stage cellular immunity of the host is inhibited but later recovery of host cellular immune function occurs, and humoral immunity starts its role in resisting the infection of *T. spiralis.* During the infection, both the cells Th1 (T helper cell) and Th2 play a major role in maintaining the immune system function. They are involved in the eradication of pathogens. When the maintenance of the host immune system disrupts it gets infected [18]. Nitric oxide (NO) is a molecule in the immune system which acts as an immunomodulator and immunotoxin. It is a gaseous molecule and has appropriate lipid membranes solubility. Without binding to any specific receptor of viruses and bacteria, it exerts lethal effects on them. NO is involved in the selective killing of parasites including infected cells and has a major role in the adult worm expulsion during *Trichinella spiralis* infection in mice (see **Figure 2**) [12].

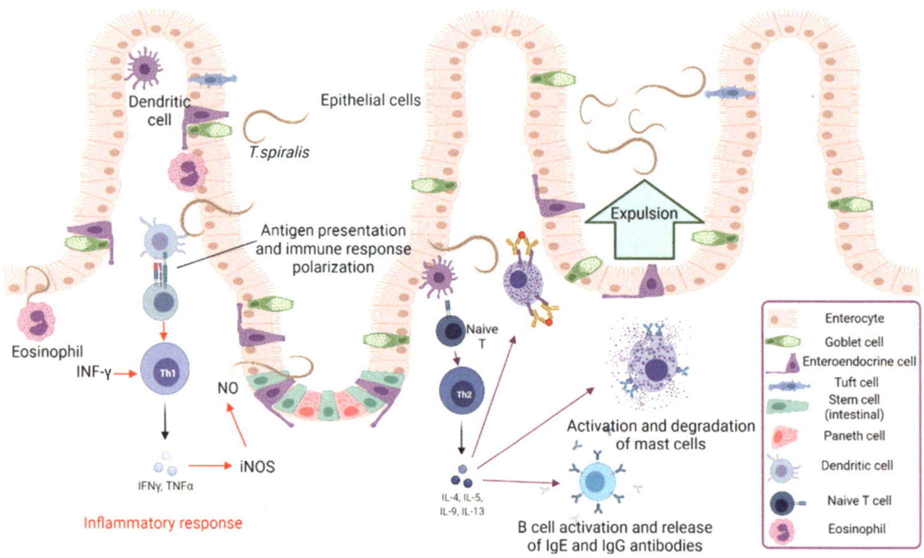

Figure 2.
Immune response against T. spiralis.

Infection of *T. spirilis* has an immunosuppressive effect on the innate immune system of the host. Larvae release secretory antigens that elicit a protective strong immune response which is specific to invading parasites [20]. ES products reduce inflammation when parasites invade the muscle cells, modulate the host immune system response in a way to protective for both the host and the parasites. For survival inside the organism, *T. spiralis* build a unique place for their living and their niche contains a cyst or capsule composed of nurse cell (cellular components) and collagenous wall [22, 25, 26]. Both the wall and nurse cell are originated from the host, provide protection and maintenance of the parasite's metabolism respectively [14].

Macrophages play a major role in the immune response of the host against various pathogens [22]. In vitro, ES products from different phases of the life cycle of *T. spiralis* can modulate macrophage's function by inhibiting cytokine production. In chronic helminth infections, macrophages are activated by Th2 cytokines such as interleukin-4 (IL-4) and interleukin-13 (IL-13). Many immune mediator molecules are released such as IL-6, IL-12, nitric oxide (NO), and tumor necrosis factor (TNF-α) when in macrophages the signaling pathways are triggered by Th2 cytokines [22, 25, 27].

4. Genomic and proteomic profile of *T. spiralis*

There are 12 species and genotypes of *Trichinella* which are distributed worldwide and cause serious disease *Trichinellosis* in humans which leads to morbidity and mortality [1, 2, 12]. Based on larvae appearance in the muscle cells of the host only encapsulated and non-encapsulated clades (morphological distinct) *Trichinella* is recognized. Based on molecular studies, nine species and three genotypes of *Trichinella* show a wide biological diversity. Based on genetic data, only *Trichinella* encapsulated clade infects mammals includes *Trichinella spiralis* (T1), *Trichinella nativa* (T2), *Trichinella britovi* (T3), *Trichinella murrelli* (T5), *Trichinella nelson* (T7), and *Trichinella patagoniensis*(T12). The three *Trichinella* genotypes includes T6, T8, and

T9. The *Trichinella* non-encapsulated clade includes *Trichinella pseudospiralis* (T4), which infects birds and mammals only, *Trichinella papuae* (T10), and *Trichinella zimbabwensis* (T11), they infect reptiles and mammals [1].

Proteomics (because of bioinformatics and mass spectrometry) is an effective technique to examine the modifications after the translation of genes such as proteolysis or glycosylation. These are powerful techniques to examine the samples obtained from pathogens to find the possible proteins involved in the pathogenesis of the disease [12]. *Trichinella* is substantially different in molecular and biological characteristics from other crown groups. The assembly of *Trichinella* is 64 million bp in length and about 15,808 proteins are encoded by this genome assembly. In *T. spiralis* genome, the estimation of repeat content is about 18% having low GC content (about 27%) relative to the overall genome (34%) and protein-coding region (43%) of *Trichinella spiralis* [14]. Microsatellites are present in the entire genome and many are distributed in the non-coding sequence of the genome. It leads to genetic diversity due to mutation [28]. During the early stage of *Trichinella* infection, *Trichinella spiralis* 14-3-3 protein is a strong immunogenic antigen [29]. Ts14-3-3 is an immunodominant antigen and this protein is also used to detect the whole period of infection with *Trichinella.* During the early phase of *Trichinella* infection, HSP70, cysteine protease, and Ts14-3-3 play a crucial role in balancing the host–parasite relationship. Therefore, these proteins are a good target for the development of vaccines and early immunodiagnostic measures [15].

4.1 DNA based vaccine

DNA vaccines got a glare in the early 1990s and evoked both humoral and cellular responses, when tested and identified, particularly induced cytotoxic T cell response, and abolished the safety concerns associated with the live vaccine [17]. Such vaccines tend to sustain host immune system stimulation in comparison to the Recombinant protein-based vaccines [6]. DNA vaccines emerged as a strong way of eliciting a humoral and cellular immune response against many parasitological antigens in small animal models. Moreover, DNA vaccines produce a concurrent Th1 and Th2 immune response against *T. spiralis* [30, 31].

The TspE1gene encoding a 31 kDa antigen of *T. spiralis* has been cloned to an expression vector pcDNA3 and administered in a mouse as a DNA vaccine [31]. Naturally, *T. spiralis* challenge suppresses the type 2 immune system response which inhibits them [17]. The mice immunized with the TspE1-pcDNA3 presented a significant larval reduction rate and an increased serum anti-*Trichinella* antibody level, hence this DNA vaccine proved to be partially protective against *T. spiralis* challenges [31]. Spleen cells after stimulation with the TspE1 recombinant protein exhibited a lympho-proliferative response, which is an indication of cellular response elicited by the DNA vaccine. Sequence of a serine protease (Ts-NBLsp) cDNA from newborn larvae of *T. spiralis*, cDNA sequence of recombinant TsNd (*Trichinella spiralis* nudix hydrolases) has been cloned to the plasmid pcDNA3.1 [17, 31, 32]. The antibody response against the serine protease of *T. spiralis* inhibits the protease activity thus hindering invasion of the parasite. The DNA vaccines Ts-NBLsp-pcDNA3.1 and pcDNA3.1-TsNd presented a balanced systemic Th1\Th2 immune response. The immunization with recombinant TsNd DNA vaccine resulted in an increased intestinal IgA and total IgG response with an exalted IgG1 than that of IgG2a [31]. To compare the recombinant nudix hydrolase DNA vaccine, the Ts-NBLsp-pcDNA3.1 vaccine showed a dominant IgG2a anti *trichinella* antibody and a predominantly Th1 immune response [17]. DNA vaccines elevated IFN gamma, IL-2, IL-4, and IL-10 levels [31]. Secretory IgA causes a significant reduction in the female worm fecundity and this response is enhanced by cytokine IL-10 specifically. The intestinal mucosa of the infected animals produces a specific antibody response against *T. spiralis*. Ts-NBLsp-pcDNA3.1 and reduces the muscle larvae burden (77.93%) greater than that of the TsNd vaccine (53.9%).

In another study of the TsDNase II, the complementary DNA sequence of *T. spiralis* serine protease 2.1 has been cloned to the eukaryotic expression vector pcDNA3.1 and administered as a DNA vaccine through an attenuated *Salmonella typhimurium* to avoid degradation [30]. To elicit a persistent systemic and mucosal immune response against *T. spiralis*, attenuated salmonella is an effective live carrier that gives an efficient mode of vaccination. *T. spiralis* DNase II is an excretory-secretory product associated with adult worms and IIL which is expressed in the cuticle of IIL. *T. spiralis* serine protease appeared to be present in the spliceosome and cuticle of adult worms and intestinal infective larvae. Both of these vaccine candidates against *T. spiralis* resulted in the significant rise of specific IgG responses. IgG1 titer after the first dose of vaccination and then an increased level of IgG2a after the second dose of vaccination, furthermore they produced mixed Th1\Th2 response which can be described through elicited cytokines response as Th1(IFN gamma) and Th2 cytokines (IL-4, IL10) [30]. TsSP 1.2-pcDNA3.1 vaccine resulted in a 71.84% reduction in the muscle larvae in comparison to the TsDNase II DNA vaccine which caused a 59.26% reduction in the muscle larvae [30].

T. spiralis adult-specific DNase II-1 (TsDNase II-1) and DNase II-7 recognized in the excretory-secretory proteins of the AW [30] has been analyzed for their immune response against the worm. Antibody-dependent cell-mediated cytotoxicity assay (ADCC) revealed that both recombinant anti-TsDNase II-1 and anti-TsDNase II-7 sera mediated the attachment of mouse peritoneal exudate cells (PECs) to NBL and finally killing of the NBL. Paramyosin is a thick myofibrillar protein [6, 30, 33], which is an immunomodulatory protein that evades host immune response by inhibiting complement C1q and C8\C9. TsPmy and Ts87 both are efficient vaccine candidates against *T. spiralis*. The DNA encoding TsPmy and Ts87 have been cloned in a eukaryotic vector pVAX1 and the recombinant DNA was transformed in the *S. typhimurium* strain SL7207. The resulting DNA vaccines produced protective immunity against *T. spiralis* when administered in mice, both resulted in mucosal sIgA response in the intestine and systemic anti TsPmyIgG response. The antibody-secreting cells from the spleen and mesenteric lymph nodes of the mice immunized with TsPmy vaccine expressed the intestinal homing receptors CCR9 and CCR10. [30] determined that SL7207\ pVAX1-TsPmy vaccine came out with a 44.8% reduction in muscle larvae and a 46.6% reduction in adult worms. While SL7207\ pVAX1-Ts87 caused a 34.2% reduction in muscle larvae and a 29.8% reduction in adult worm burden. By using B and T cell epitopes from TsPmy a novel multi-epitope vaccine has been designed which elicits an immune response more efficiently as compared to traditional vaccines, TsPmy MEP vaccine reduced the muscle larvae up to 55.4% [33].

DNA vaccines have many advantages as they are inexpensive, focused immune response against the antigen of interest, heat stable and a broad-spectrum vaccine can be developed by mixing plasmids.

4.2 Protein-based vaccine

In recent studies, it is reported that specific protein molecules from numerous *T. spiralis* life cycle stages have been considered and expressed properly, so that their immune protection was also estimated, such as paramyosin (Ts-Pmy) obtained from an adult cDNA library [21], TspGST and fructose-1,6-bisphosphate aldolase (Ts-FBPA) taken from the *T. spiralis* draft genome utilizing high expression at the ML stage, Ts31 from the ML ES proteins, serine protease (TsSP) from IIL (intestinal offensive stage) and ML surface proteins and cathepsin B (TsCB) from the *T. spiralis* draft genome [8]. On the other hand, when these recombinant proteins were used for vaccinating mice, they showed only 36.2–53.50% ML reduction following the *T. spiralis* challenge. In the current study, we determine the protective immunity persuaded by vaccination through a novel TsE protein. TsE is highly expressed and acts as a secretory protein at the *T. spiralis* intestinal offensive stage (IIL), TsE shows potency to be exposed first to the host's intestinal mucosa and then produce the local immune response through its working. It is observed that vaccination with rTsE persuaded significantly high levels of TsE-specific sIgA, which can simplify adult worm removal from the intestine. TE immune protection having 64.06% ML reduction, with this novel TsE vaccination was considered superior to those of the above-mentioned other *T. spiralis* proteins act as candidate vaccine target molecules. This study also recognized a foundation to develop polyvalent anti-*T. spiralis* vaccines in the upcoming period.

The immune response stimulated by a vaccine based on an exclusive antigen and multi-epitope (that work more efficiently than the large protein molecules) vaccines against *T. spiralis* has now been proposed. Therefore, the amalgamation of three selected epitopes from Ts-Pmy and Ts87 from *T. spiralis* adult produced in immunized mice IgG and IgG1 production and higher protection of about 35% in contrast to the parasite challenge in comparison to that encouraged by individual epitope peptides [8]. To achieve higher shielding immune responses counter to *T. spiralis*, it will be essential to propose a vaccine with multi-epitopes from different parasite stages focusing on NBL and adult stages (**Table 1**).

Antigen	Database ID	Strain	Developmental stage	Function	Reference
Cathepsin B [*T. spiralis*]	XP_003373289	ISS 195	Muscle larvae(ML) and adult worm (AW)	Has important function in worm invading, migrating, molting and immune escape	[5]
Cysteine protease ATG4C [*T. spiralis*]	XP_003367319	ISS 195	Intestinal infective L1 larvae (IIL1)	Participates in IIL1 intrusion of the enteral epithelium	[5]
Putative serine protease [*T. spiralis*]	XP_003369429	ISS 195	AW	Involved in the processes of immune evasion	[17]
Paramyosin [*T. spiralis*]	XP_003371652	ISS 195	AW	Plays an important role in the evasion of the host complement attack	[10]
Conserved hypothetical protein, partial [*T. spiralis*]	XP_003369591	ISS 195	AW		[10]

Antigen	Database ID	Strain	Developmental stage	Function	Reference
Serpin B4 [*T. spiralis*]	XP_003375999	ISS 195	AW, NBL, ML	Initiates acute inflammatory response	[7]
Putative nudix hydrolase 6 [*T. spiralis*]	XP_003378071	ISS 195	IIL	Catalyzes the hydrolysis of nucleoside diphosphate	[23]
Cystatin-B [*T. spiralis*]	XP_003379766	ISS 195	AW	Has immunomodulatory functions and helps the parasites to evade the host immune responses	[34]
Antigen targeted by protective antibodies [*T. spiralis*]	AAA20539	Library lambda ZAP	ML	Regulates host immune response	[31]
Membrane-associated progesterone receptor component 2 [*T. spiralis*]	XP_003375934	ISS 195	AW, ML	Play a role in adipocyte function and systemic glucose homeostasis	[11]

Table 1.
Immunoregulatory kinetics of different T. spiralis *based protein after binding with host immune cells.*

5. Role of progesterone receptor in *trichinella spiralis*

Progesterone (P4) is a sex steroid hormone that plays roles in the physiology of the reproductive system such as corpus luteum of the ovary and placenta in females, while testes and adrenal cortex in males also participate in many other functions such as brain activity, immune modulation, metabolism of bones heart and lungs physiology. P4 is also responsible for the maintenance of pregnancy and shows an immunosuppressive effect [35]. when a high level of progesterone is present during the luteal phase of the estrus/menstrual cycle in females. Recent studies showed that these hormones also influence the course of parasites infections and also restrict the invasion of parasites when a high level of P4 in female animals is produced. Restricts the invasion of parasites [11]. P4 has an immunomodulatory effect on fetal antigens during pregnancy by suppressing the maternal immune response. However, progesterone can be either an inhibitory or stimulatory effect on the immune response mechanism depending upon cell type, concentration, and exposure time to steroids. It has nematotoxicity against newborn larvae of *T. spiralis*. Progesterone is responsible for decreased parasite load during pregnancy [11].

Sex steroids are known as immune response modulators and play a major role in *T. spiralis* susceptibility at two levels viz. (1) protective immune response and (2) direct effect on the development of worms. Besides, P4 up-regulates many molecules expressions from major histocompatibility complex class I and it also participates in the down-regulation of genes that are responsible for the fecundity and oviposition of the worms and inhibits the nuclear factor kappa B (NFƙB) activation in innate immunity [11].

6. Role of progesterone and mifepristone against *T. spiralis*

Progesterone is a gonadal hormone primarily involved in the preparation of the endometrium for implantation of an embryo and necessary for the maintenance of pregnancy, while mifepristone is a drug that works as an antagonist of progesterone and glucocorticoid. It has an abortifacient effect and terminates early pregnancy by binding to intracellular progesterone receptors. Mifepristone has an antagonistic effect on the *T. spiralis* (Ts) membrane-associated progesterone receptor component-2 (Ts-MAPRC2). It also down-regulates the expression of the Ts-MAPRC2 gene and results in the abortion of the pregnant adult female worms [11].

Mifepristone (RU486) can be taken as an example that works as an antagonist in contrast to the progesterone receptor (PR) and glucocorticoid receptor (GR) with some lethal properties such as aborting agent and anticancer activities in the body. In the case of helminths, several research studies are concentrated on PGRMC receptors. Similarly, RU486 was one of the first medications accepted for surgical abortion and is frequently used to terminate an early or midterm pregnancy. Hereafter, PR and binding of P4 molecules (agonist) and RU486 (antagonist) can be helpful to elaborate *T. spiralis* species regarding differentiation and reproductive development as well as creating potential pharmacological targets that might be used as a drug therapy against *Trichinellosis*.

Progesterone is known for its immune-modulatory effects, which happen during pregnancy that is done by suppressing the response from the mother toward paternal antigens expressed in the fetus [11]. Taking into the description, we can conclude that progesterone is an adequate inducing activation of the effector cell populations responsible for cell death in an antibody-independent cytotoxic mechanism. This cytotoxicity should also be activated by soluble antigens released by the parasite because at constant self-aggression of tissues by these activated cells 0% NBL mortality 10 10 100 Progesterone (ng/ml) cells [35] .

7. Challenges to developing an efficient vaccine against *T. spiralis*

The control of helminths in animals is usually through anthelmintics. Vaccine development against *T. spiralis* infection in pigs is an alternate method for the prevention of parasite *T. spiralis* from zoonosis. Effective vaccine development against *Trichinellosis* is conducted in mice instead of pigs. Effective development of a vaccine, is not only due to high price of experimental pigs but also due to poorly satisfied antigens detected from the mice. Moreover, the immune response induced by the same antigen in swine and mice is extremely different. So, [2]. concluded that in mice, poor immunogenic vaccine candidates are not capable to induce a strong protective immune response against *T. spiralis* infection in pigs.

TsT was a *T. spiralis* somatic antigen and at adult-stage with specific surface antigen it had a good antigenicity. If vaccination of mice is done with TsT, it will induce a systemic mixed Th1/Th2 response and an intestinal local sIgA response, which can produce partial protection against *T. spiralis* larval challenge. Then these results suggested that TsT plays a role in *T. spiralis* growth and survival in the host, and it might be deliberated as a potential target antigen for anti-*T. spiralis* vaccines. However [9], revealed that oral anti-Trichinella vaccines comprised of multiple antigenic epitopes of various *T. spiralis* life cycle phases should be recognized.

7.1 Diversity within *T. spiralis* parasites

T. spiralis is a nematode parasite that is prevalent throughout the world and translocated by humans and their animals. They occupy well-defined geographic ranges [36]. There is a big diversity among the *T. spiralis* parasites present in different geographic locations [24]. *T. spiralis* nematode belongs to the clade that diverged early in the phylum Nematoda evolution [14]. *T. britovi* parasitizes many sylvatic mammals such as Felidae, Canidae, Ursidae, Mustelidae, Suidae, Viverridae and is endemic to Northern-western Africa and Eurasia while *T. murrelli* is the only present in wild animals in North America. Millions of years ago, *Trichinella* could infect human beings evidenced by the ingestion of other parasites in meat [36].

The nematode *T. spiralis* is involved in the most common cause of human *trichinellosis*, which is considered a zoonotic disease worldwide. The heredity of *T. spiralis* giving rise to the genus *Trichinella* and reported that the last shared common ancestor was approximately 275 million years ago (Lower Permian Period) identified, however the modification of extant *Trichinella* species happened about 16–20 million years ago [14].

We compare the molecular physiognomies of nematodes and former metazoans by using the *T. spiralis* genome as standard. This comparative approach by using the *T. spiralis* permitted us to categorize conserved protein and gene sequences through the superficial model, particularly for the phylum Nematoda. We bring an approach that intrachromosomal modifications were common all over the phylum. However, this was in divergence to other features such as births and deaths of a protein family, which exhibited clear discrimination among the parasitic and non-parasitic nematodes. The identification of well-maintained physiognomies predicated based on this work will advance the more accurate research on pathogens from a phylum embracing thousands of pathogens that are mainly to infect humans, animals, and plants and behaves like infectious agent. The advances possibly will one day be responsible for complete strategies to prevent and control diseases that are caused by pathogens from across the Nematoda family around the globe [14, 36, 37].

Commencing from the time of the discovery of *Trichinella* which is in 1835 in anticipation of the middle of the next century. During the last decade, the use of molecular and biochemical methods in combination with experimental studies on biology, have resulted in the identification of seven *Trichinella* species that have different epidemiological and topographical distributions. Even though these species are very difficult to differentiate morphologically, this can be done with the molecular and positive biological characters for further identification [16].

7.2 Genetic diversity related to multiple hosts

A total of 30 species of *T. spiralis* having mtDNA genomes has 20 unique haplotypes that were observed containing 86 isolating sites. So, with four out of five shared haplotypes taking place in European and North American samples. Samples from North America had one haplotype, which is present in each geographic sampling site [38]. Out of the total, mostly the variations were limited to the Asian *T. spiralis* samples. There are about 7 Asian samples, and from these 8 haplotypes were identified; these differed on an ordinary by 24.9 nucleotides. In comparison to this, western samples are averaged with only 3.2 nucleotide differences per haplotype with only 13 haplotypes in 23 samples; the most different pair of western haplotypes differed by only 6 nucleotide differences between any two isolates. Similarly, nucleotide diversity (pi) was 0.00016 in western samples while Asian nucleotide diversity was 10-fold greater (0.00179). As a result, we can say that all Asian samples are different from the western samples by at least 45 bp and averaged 49 bp differences [24].

The most noticeable properties of this parasite's epidemiology are its requisite transmission by mode of meat ingestion in consumers. There is another important feature, which is present in two normally isolated ecological systems, which are sylvatic and domestic. In certain situations, the two biotopes are connected from end to end man's activities, which results in the revelation of humans to *Trichinella* species [38]. Usually, it is restricted to sylvatic animals. The species furthermost often associated with human infection is *T spiralis*, which is the reported species that is usually found in the meat of domestic pigs. The life cycle of *T spiralis* includes a multipart set of possible routes. Farm transmission can be the result of predation on or hunting other animals for food purposes (rodents), hog anthropophagy, and the feeding of uncooked meat leftovers [16].

Most outbreaks resulting from ingesting of *T spiralis* infected pigs can lead to its outbreak through local single-source but, progressively, the mass marketing of meat can distribute the disease-causing parasite in the entire population. There has been a great increase in the reported cases due to Trichinella species, just because of having so many species that are involved in the food chain. The reason for having genetic diversity is also stated that we are lacking in vaccines to eradicate it. The main source is considered as the meat from the game and domestic animals. From recent reports, we can conclude that it also specifies that infected herbivores including horses, sheep, goats, and cattle have been the source of the outbreak [14, 16].

7.3 Multiple stage complexity of *T. spiralis*

*T. spiralis*also has several stages of the complex life cycle that completes in two niches viz. intra-multicellular niche occurs in the intestine epithelium of host where adult male and female worms are involved with the help of (proteolytic digestive enzymes and become mature adult worms). Whereas intracellular niche occurs in the striated muscles of the organism where muscle larvae participate in the development of nurse cells [16], *T. spiralis* life cycle represents different antigens specific for a particular stage, where these antigens elicit immune responses and facilitate the developmental cycle of the parasites by modifying the host immune responses. To complete their life cycle, they skip the defensive mechanism of the host against invading the foreign body.

Once newborn larvae invade the lymphatic or circulatory system, they can drive anywhere in the organism and survive only in the skeletal muscles of the host. Humans can acquire *T. spiralis* infection only if they consume undercooked or raw meat containing muscle larvae [36]. Several genes are differentially expressed among the life cycle stages and up-regulated genes in the newborn larvae. The genome of *T. spiralis* is regulated in the developmental stages [34].

8. Future perspective

Trichinella infection is an emerging zoonosis in many countries and where it become the reason for *trichinellosis* disease. Due to its widespread prevalence and high amount of pork meat consumption more clinical awareness is required. The acute infection is characterized by two phases viz. enteral which disrupt intestinal functions and parenteral phases are associated with the inflammatory and allergic reaction. The diagnosis of this disease contains new specific serological tests such as immunoblot or ELISA. Anthelmintics and anti-inflammatory drugs are the drug of choice for *Trichinella* infection [16]. Vaccines formulated for veterinary purposes have made a great impact not only on animal welfare, production, and health but also on human health. Vaccines are considered reliable, efficient, and sustainable for the control and prevention of parasitic infection.

In *Thrichinellosis*, induction of protective and therapeutic responses should evoke both innate and adaptive immune systems to prevent the establishment of parasites in the organism. The life cycle of *T. spiralis* is complex, and the immune response is not strong that induced by a vaccine containing specific antigen to overcome the challenging infection. Therefore, a vaccine containing multiple epitopes against *T. spiralis induces higher immunity* [24]. Probiotics such as *Lactobacillus* keep the environment of the intestine healthy and prevent enteric infections. Probiotic *Lactobacillus casei* is most commonly used for protection against *Trichinellosis*. *L. casei* is involved in the production of IL-4, IgA, and IgG (anti-*T. spiralis* antibodies) and has a preventive role against high infection of *T. spiralis*. Some strains of *L. casei* include *L. casei* ATCC 469, *L. casei* ATCC 7469, and *L. casei* Shirota have proven efficacy against *T. spiralis* infection. For the control of *Trichinellosis*, Probiotics and plants-based veterinary vaccines are a new approach and can be used as treatment and edible vaccines for various parasitic diseases in animals. Due to the low cost of plants production, sterile delivery, and transportation at a suitable temperature, plants are considered as a suitable vehicle for veterinary vaccines [1].

Antigens in the vaccines administered orally are subject to proteolysis by the proteolytic enzymes present in the digestive tract of the organism. It will decrease the bioavailability of the vaccines and will induce a low immune response [1]. On the other hand, in plant-based vaccines antigens are protected from proteolytic enzymes by the cell wall of the plant cells and enable antigens to reach their desired destination (gut-associated lymphoid tissue). Various plants and vegetable species such as potato, tomato, tobacco, alfalfa, rice, spinach, beans, maize, strawberries, and carrots can be used in the biotechnology of plants for the expression and production of recombinant proteins.

For the prevention and control of diseases in animals and their transmission from animals to humans, plant-based vaccines seem to be an excellent tool. More research is required to thoroughly understand the applications of medical plant extracts, probiotics, and other biological agents [24].

9. Conclusion

At least twelve species and genotypes of *Trichinella* genus can cause veterinary or medical health hazards in a wide geographical range throughout the world. The main etiological agent of *Trichinellosis* in humans is only *T. spiralis* parasite and can result in mild to severe clinical signs and symptoms. Numerous antigens are used as candidate vaccines from different stages of *T. spiralis and* can be used as DNA vaccines or recombinant protein vaccines. The role of progesterone and mifepristone against *T. spiralis* is also very helpful as they penetrate the vaccine into the target of *T. spiralis*. Altogether, we can get different strains for specific vaccines with molecular physiognomies of different Trichinella species.

Acknowledgements

The author wishes to thank all other co-authors for providing guidance and support.

Conflict of interest

The authors declare that they have no conflict of interest.

Author details

Muhammad Tahir Aleem[1], Ruofeng Yan[1*], Asad Khan[1], Rida Asrar[2], Amna Shakoor[2], Areej Asif[2], Zhaohai Wen[1], Zhengqing Yu[1], Muhammad Abdullah Malik[3], Tauseef-ur-Rehman[4], Rao Zahid Abbas[3], Muhammad Mohsin[5], Xiaokai Song[1], Lixin Xu[1] and Xiangrui Li[1]

1 MOE Joint International Research Laboratory of Animal Health and Food Safety, College of Veterinary Medicine, Nanjing Agricultural University, Nanjing, China

2 Faculty of Veterinary Science, University of Agriculture, Faisalabad, Pakistan

3 Faculty of Veterinary Science, Department of Parasitology, University of Agriculture, Faisalabad, Pakistan

4 Faculty of Veterinary and Animal Sciences, Department of Parasitology, The Islamia University of Bahawalpur, Pakistan

5 College of Animal Science, College of Life Sciences, Fujian Agriculture and Forestry University, Fuzhou, China

*Address all correspondence to: yanruofeng@njau.edu.cn

References

[1] Korhonen P, Pozio E, La Rosa G, et al. Phylogenomic and biogeographic reconstruction of the *Trichinella* complex. Nature Communications. 2016;7:10513. DOI: 10.1038/ncomms10513

[2] Zhang N, Li W, Fu B. Vaccines against Trichinella spiralis: Progress, challenges and future prospects. Transboundary and Emerging Diseases. 2018;**65**(6):1447-1458. DOI: 10.1111/tbed.12917

[3] Yr Y, Yf Q. Progress in Treatment and Prevention of Trichinellosis. Journal of Infectious Diseases & Therapy. 2015;**03**(06). DOI: 10.4172/2332-0877.1000251

[4] Bai X, Hu X, Liu X, Tang B, Liu M. Current research of trichinellosis in China. Frontiers in Microbiology. 2017;**8**(AUG):1-7. DOI: 10.3389/fmicb.2017.01472

[5] Cui J, Han Y, Yue X, Liu F, Song YY, Yan SW, et al. Vaccination of mice with a recombinant novel cathepsin B inhibits Trichinella spiralis development, reduces the fecundity and worm burden. Parasites and Vectors. 2019;**12**(1):1-12. DOI: 10.1186/s13071-019-3833-9

[6] Qi X, Han Y, Jiang P, Yue X, Ren HN, Sun GG, et al. Oral vaccination with Trichinella spiralis DNase II DNA vaccine delivered by attenuated Salmonella induces a protective immunity in BALB/c mice 11 Medical and Health Sciences 1107 Immunology. Veterinary Research. 2018;**49**(1):1-12. DOI: 10.1186/s13567-018-0614-y

[7] Jin X, Liu X, Ding J, Zhang L, Yang Y, Wang X, et al. Lentinan improved the efficacy of vaccine against trichinella spiralis in an nlrp3 dependent manner. PLoS Neglected Tropical Diseases. 2020;**14**(9):1-13. DOI: 10.1371/journal.pntd.0008632

[8] Ehsan M, Hu RS, Liang QL, Hou JL, Song X, Yan R, et al. Advances in the development of anti-haemonchus contortus vaccines: Challenges, opportunities, and perspectives. Vaccines. 2020;**8**(3):1-18. DOI: 10.3390/vaccines8030555

[9] Zhang Y, Zeng J, Song YY, Long SR, Liu RD, Jiang P, et al. Vaccination of mice with a novel trypsin from trichinella spiralis elicits the immune protection against larval challenge. Vaccines. 2020;**8**(3):1-20. DOI: 10.3390/vaccines8030437

[10] Gu Y, Wei J, Yang J, Huang J, Yang X, Zhu X. Protective Immunity against *Trichinella spiralis* Infection Induced by a Multi-Epitope Vaccine in a Murine Model. PLoS ONE. 2013;**8**(10):e77238. DOI: 10.1371/journal.pone.0077238

[11] Aleem MT, Shi J, Yu Z, Wen Z, Zhang Y, Liang M, et al. Characterization of membrane-associated progesterone receptor component-2 (MAPRC2) from trichinella spiralis and its interaction with progesterone and mifepristone. Vaccines. 2021;**9**(8):934. DOI: 10.3390/vaccines9080934

[12] Wang X, Li L, Wei X, et al. Proteomic analysis of the response of Trichinella spiralis muscle larvae to exogenous nitric oxide. Plos One. 2018;**13**(6):e0198205. DOI: 10.1371/journal.pone.0198205

[13] White RR, Miyata S, Papa E, Spooner E, Gounaris K, Selkirk ME, et al. Characterisation of the Trichinella spiralis deubiquitinating enzyme, TsUCH37, an evolutionarily conserved

proteasome interaction partner. PLoS Neglected Tropical Diseases. 2011;**5**(10):e1340. DOI: 10.1371/journal.pntd.0001340. Epub 2011 Oct 4

[14] Mitreva M, Jasmer DP, Zarlenga DS, Wang Z, Abubucker S, Martin J, et al. The draft genome of the parasitic nematode Trichinella spiralis. Nature Publishing Group. 2011;**43**(3). DOI: 10.1038/ng.769

[15] Yang J, Pan W, Sun X, et al. Immunoproteomic profile of *Trichinella spiralis* adult worm proteins recognized by early infection sera. Parasites Vectors. 2015;**8**:20. DOI: 10.1186/s13071-015-0641-8

[16] Bruschi F, Murrell KD. New aspects of human trichinellosis: the impact of new Trichinella species. Postgraduate Medical Journal. 2002;**78**(915):15-22. DOI: 10.1136/pmj.78.915.15

[17] Xu D, Bai X, Xu J, Wang X, Dong Z, Shi W, et al. The immune protection induced by a serine protease from the trichinella spiralis adult against trichinella spiralis infection in pigs. PLoS Neglected Tropical Diseases. 2021;**15**(5):1-15. DOI: 10.1371/journal.pntd.0009408

[18] Song Y, Xu J, Wang X, et al. Regulation of host immune cells and cytokine production induced by Trichinella spiralis infection. Parasite (Paris, France). 2019;**26**:74. DOI: 10.1051/parasite/2019074

[19] Wakelin D, Lloyd M. Immunity to primary and challenge infections of Trichinella spiralis in mice: A re-examination of conventional parameters. Parasitology. 1976; **72**(Pt 2):173-182

[20] Hafez EN, Kholy W. A. E. S. El, Amin MM, Hafez EN, Kholy W. A. E. S. El, & The, M. M. A. The potential protective role of gamma-irradiated vaccine versus Punica granatum treatment against murine trichinellosis. Journal of Radiation Research and Applied Sciences. 2020;**13**(1):560-567. Doi: 10.1080/16878507.2020.1777659

[21] Zhang XZ, Sun XY, Bai Y, Song YY, Hu CX, Li X, et al. Protective immunity in mice vaccinated with a novel elastase - 1 significantly decreases Trichinella spiralis fecundity and infection. Veterinary Research. 2020:1-12. DOI: 10.1186/s13567-020-00767-z

[22] Han C, Yu J, Zhang Z, Zhai P, Zhang Y, Meng S, et al. Immuno-modulatory effects of *Trichinella spiralis* excretory-secretory antigens on macrophages. Experimental Parasitology. 2018. DOI: 10.1016/j.exppara.2018.10.001

[23] Liu P, Cui J, Liu RD, et al. Protective immunity against Trichinella spiralis infection induced by TsNd vaccine in mice. Parasites & Vectors. 2015;**8**:185. DOI: 10.1186/s13071-015-0791-8

[24] Thompson PC, Bilska-zajac E, Zarlenga DS, Liu M, Cencek T. Divergence at mitochondrial and ribosomal loci indicates the split between Asian and European populations of Trichinella spiralis occurred prior to swine domestication. Infection , Genetics and Evolution. 2021;**88**(December 2020):4-10. DOI: 10.1016/j.meegid.2021.104705

[25] Ilic N, Gruden-Movsesijan A, Sofronic-Milosavljevic L. *Trichinella spiralis*: shaping the immune response. Immunologic Research. 2012;**52**:111-119. DOI: 10.1007/s12026-012-8287-5

[26] Han C, Yu J, Zhang Z, Zhai P, Zhang Y, Meng S, et al. Experimental Parasitology Immunomodulatory e ff ects of Trichinella spiralis excretory-secretory antigens on macrophages. Experimental Parasitology.

2019;**196**(March 2018):68-72. DOI: 10.1016/j.exppara.2018.10.001

[27] Sun X, Li Y, Naqvi MA, Naqvi SZ, Chu W. Succinate coenzyme A ligase beta-like protein from trichinella spiralis suppresses the immune functions of rat PBMCs in vitro and inhibits the secretions of interleukin-17 in vivo. Vaccines. 2019;7:167. DOI: 10.3390/vaccines7040167

[28] Zhang X, Han LL, Hong X, Jiang P, Niu YF, Wang ZQ, et al. Genotyping and Phylogenetic Position of Trichinella spiralis Isolates from Different Geographical Locations in China. Frontiers in Genetics. 2019;**10**(October):1-10. DOI: 10.3389/fgene.2019.01093

[29] Love RJ, Ogilvie BM, Mclaren DJ. The immune mechanism which expels the intestinal stage of Trichinella spiralis from rats. Immunology 1976. 1976;**30**(1):7-15

[30] Wang L, Wang X, Bi K, Sun X, Yang J, Gu Y, et al. Oral Vaccination with Attenuated *Salmonella typhimurium*-Delivered *Ts*Pmy DNA Vaccine Elicits Protective Immunity against *Trichinella spiralis* in BALB/c Mice. PLoS Neglected Tropical Diseases. 2016;**10**(9):e0004952. DOI: 10.1371/journal.pntd.0004952

[31] Wang ZQ, Cui J, Wei HY, Han HM, Zhang HW, Li YL. Vaccination of mice with DNA vaccine induces the immune response and partial protection against T. spiralis infection. Vaccine. 2006;**24**:1205-1212. DOI: 10.1016/j.vaccine.2005.08.104

[32] Xu J, Bai X, Wang LB, Shi HN, Van Der Giessen JWB, Boireau P, et al. Immune responses in mice vaccinated with a DNA vaccine expressing serine protease-like protein from the new-born larval stage of Trichinella spiralis. Parasitology. 2017;**144**(6):712-719. DOI: 10.1017/S0031182016002493. Epub 2017 Jan 10

[33] Gu Y, Sun X, Li B, Huang J, Zhan B, Zhu X. Vaccination with a paramyosin-based multi-epitope vaccine elicits significant protective immunity against trichinella spiralis infection in mice. Frontiers in Microbiology. 2017;**8**(August):1-9. DOI: 10.3389/fmicb.2017.01475

[34] Liu X, Song Y, Jiang N, Wang J, Tang B, Lu H, et al. Global Gene Expression Analysis of the Zoonotic Parasite *Trichinella spiralis* Revealed Novel Genes in Host Parasite Interaction. PLoS Neglected Tropical Diseases. 2012;**6**(8):e1794. DOI: 10.1371/journal.pntd.0001794

[35] Nuñez G, Gentile T, Costantino S, Sarchi M, Venturiello S. In vitro and in vivo effects of progesterone on Trichinella spiralis newborn larvae. Parasitology. 2005;**131**(2):255-259. DOI: 10.1017/S0031182005007468

[36] Rosenthal BM, Larosa G, Zarlenga D, Dunams D, Chunyu Y, Mingyuan L, et al. Human dispersal of Trichinella spiralis in domesticated pigs. Infection, Genetics and Evolution. 2008;**8**:799-805. DOI: 10.1016/j.meegid.2008.07.008

[37] Liu X, Feng Y, Bai X, Wang X, Qin R, Tang B, et al. Comparative multi-omics analyses reveal differential expression of key genes relevant for parasitism between non-encapsulated and encapsulated Trichinella. Communications Biology. 2021:1-12. DOI: 10.1038/s42003-021-01650-z

[38] Ren HN, Guo KX, Zhang Y, et al. Molecular characterization of a 31 kDa protein from Trichinella spiralis and its induced immune protection in BALB/c mice. Parasites & Vectors. 2018 Dec;**11**(1):625. DOI: 10.1186/s13071-018-3198-5

Chapter 19

Perspective Chapter: Multi-Omic Approaches to Vaccine Development against Helminth Diseases

Vrushabh Daga, Evangeline Green, Priyanka Ravichandran, Meagan Short and Meghan May

Abstract

Though the past three decades have led to a renaissance in vaccine design, the development of vaccines that protect against helminth diseases remains elusive. The need for protective vaccines for humans and livestock remains urgent because of the side-effect profiles of anti-helminthic drugs and the growing incidence of antimicrobial resistance and declining efficacy. The "-omics" era has led to renewed interest in vaccine development against helminth diseases, as candidate vaccines can now be designed, evaluated, and refined in a fraction of the time previously required. In this chapter, we describe and review genomic, transcriptomic, and proteomic approaches to the design of vaccines against helminth diseases.

Keywords: omics, vaccine, proteomics, parasitic helminth, onchocerciasis, lymphatic Filariasis, soil-transmitted helminths, schistosomiasis

1. Introduction

Parasitic helminths that cause human and veterinary diseases can be found in two phyla: *Nematoda* and *Platyhelminthes*. Helminth diseases carry a significant global burden and collectively infect over 1 billion people [1], and cause a disproportionate number of neglected tropical diseases (NTDs). They are a significant cause of morbidity, and often result in permanent disabilities, impaired responses to other infections leading to worse outcomes, and significant social and economical burden upon patients [2–5]. Helminth diseases of livestock further threaten human health and economic development by adversely affecting food security. Antimicrobial treatments are available for helminth infections; however, they come with significant challenges. The number of available drug classes is small, and the ones that are available cause significant side effects and do not protect against reinfection [6]. As drug resistance has been observed in animal nematode models, the catastrophic potential for treatment-refractory infections exists [7, 8]. These challenges indicate that the ideal strategy for

 IntechOpen

helminth disease control is prevention rather than treatment. Despite this, there are no known effective vaccines to protect humans against diseases, such as filariasis which carry a high morbidity rate [9, 10]. While practical measures, such as skin coverings (*i.e.*, shoes, waders) and vector control, aid in prevention; these strategies would optimally be coupled with vaccination to ultimately meet the goals of reducing or eliminating disease burden. Continuity of care, treatment side effects, and the potential for drug resistance underscore the urgent need for anti-helminth vaccine development.

Vaccine development against helminth diseases has historically been challenging for a variety of reasons. Helminths are diploid organisms with multiple life stages that are notoriously immunomodulatory. They are able to migrate to multiple tissues and possess numerous immune evasion strategies. The combination of the transient antigen profiles and complex Type 2 immune responses have rendered efforts to immunize patients with killed organisms, attenuated organisms, or single immunogens unsuccessful [11–13]. Many experimental vaccines for ruminant helminth diseases, such as echinococcosis and fascioliasis, have been described, and a vaccine that protects sheep and goats from Barber's pole worm (Barbervax®, developed by the Moredun Foundation) has been licensed in the United Kingdom, Australia, and South Africa. The development of Barbervax® was a lengthy process because of the technology available at the time. Additionally, Barbervax® and other experimental vaccines suffer from modest efficacy and at times complicated dosing regimens. Vaccines for human helminth diseases have yet to be licensed due to failures of traditional vaccine design approaches.

The advent of the "-omics" era has led to renewed enthusiasm for vaccine development against helminth diseases and other NTDs. Vaccines similar to Barbervax® can now be designed and modified in a fraction of the time required. Research efforts utilizing genomics, transcriptomics, and proteomics have been undertaken to identify potential antigens and evaluate their expression kinetics during infection and chronic disease as well as their potential to evolve in response to vaccinated populations. Ultimately, multi-omics approaches to vaccine design for helminth infections have the potential to address a multitude of complex factors that are involved in the host–parasite interaction, the intricacies of vaccine design, and the evolutionary implications that follow the introduction of any and all selective pressures. In this chapter, we explore genomic, transcriptomic, and proteomic approaches to the design of vaccines against helminth diseases.

2. "Omic" technologies and reverse vaccinology

Vaccine design was historically approached by manipulating whole infectious agents or their toxins, either by inactivating them or attenuating them. Next-generation vaccines (*i.e.*, those deriving from molecular and synthetic biology) are rooted in reverse vaccinology, wherein design begins by examining the complete genomes, transcriptomes, or proteomes of pathogens. Advances made toward anti-helminth vaccines will undoubtedly rely on reverse vaccinology via multi-omic analysis.

The field of genetic and genomic studies has significantly progressed in the last few decades. Scientists have progressed from analyzing single genes and their functions to studying the entire genetic complements—genomes—of organisms. The field of pathogen genomics has facilitated the development of numerous precise diagnostics and vaccines. These vaccines almost exclusively target viral or bacterial pathogens, however [14]. While it is possible to identify potential antigens based on gene sequences, actual transcribed and translated epitopes may look vastly different, and may not elicit the expected immune response. As such, genomics alone may not be the most reliable informant of a potential vaccine target, due to variations in transcription and protein processing that take place. Section 3 of this chapter aims to review genomic approaches to vaccine development against helminth diseases and elucidate critical concepts and issues related to this approach.

As opposed to a genome, a transcriptome is a collection of all non-ribosomal RNA within a cell type, tissue, or organism under a specific set of circumstances or at a specific stage of the life cycle. The study of transcriptomics allows for the focus to be placed on gene expression throughout various steps of the life cycle and under different conditions [15]. Recently, the availability of sequencing technologies has made both genomics and transcriptomics relatively low-cost analyses that can be routinely performed in many laboratories. Transcriptomic analysis of helminths suffered from a bottleneck due to a lack of publicly available genomic databases for parasitic helminths until recently. Some of these challenges still persist, however, because helminths contain many unique sequences that have not previously been annotated with correlation to an associated protein in other organisms [16]. Additionally, transcriptomics can be used to provide insight into immunomodulation and thus vaccine interference mechanisms by being used as profiling tools to screen infected hosts. While transcriptomic analysis provides greater sensitivity in predicting potential antigens that will be expressed during infection, it cannot account for post-transcriptional regulation of protein expression or any non-canonical post-translational modifications. Section 4 of this chapter aims to review transcriptomic approaches to vaccine development against helminth diseases and elucidate critical concepts and issues related to this approach.

Thematically similar to a transcriptome, a proteome is the full complement of mature, modified proteins present under specific conditions within specific cells or tissues [17]. The proteomic analysis allows target-based approaches to parasite interventions, including the development of anti-helminth vaccines. Previously, transcriptomes of pathogens have been used to identify vaccine targets; however, proteomics allows for a greater likelihood of true representation of potential antigens present during infection. This is especially important for helminths and other parasites because protein expression varies greatly based on the life-cycle stage [18, 19]. By describing a parasitic helminth's proteome, we can gain a better insight into antigenic targets that are present at each life stage of the parasite. Similar to transcriptomic analysis, proteomic studies of infected hosts can also aid in understanding and circumventing helminth immunomodulatory mechanisms that could adversely affect vaccine efficacy. These studies can be critical in aiding complex vaccine designs such that poor or adverse responses can be avoided. Section 5 of this chapter aims to review proteomic approaches to vaccine development against helminth diseases and elucidate critical concepts and issues related to this approach.

3. Genomic approaches to vaccine development for helminth diseases

The advent of high-throughput genome sequencing has fundamentally changed the approach to vaccine design, enabling the evaluation and fine-scale targeting of potential vaccine antigens throughout the parasite life cycle. Structural genomic, functional genomic, and epigenomic approaches allow for the identification of an estimated 10- to 100-fold more new antigens for vaccine design and drug target candidates as compared to conventional methods in the same time frame [20].

Furthermore, the completion of the Human Genome Project allows for the evaluation of potential antigens for molecular mimicry by parasites that could cause pathological responses to vaccines, and for a thorough understanding of host-pathogen interactions during active infection that could impact vaccine-derived protection [21].

The use of genome-wide applications for human vaccine development has already been observed for bacterial and viral pathogens. The complete genome sequence of *Neisseria meningitidis* Group B, the agent of meningococcal meningitis, was used to identify several candidate vaccine antigens [22]. Potential antigens were later successfully narrowed down using reverse vaccinology approaches [23]. More recently, the development of both mRNA and Adenovirus-vectored vaccines for the viral pathogen SARS-CoV-2 relied exclusively on viral genomics [24].

The first parasitic nematode, whose genome was sequenced, was *Brugia malayi* [25], and technological advances have allowed for the sequencing of several more human and animal parasites over the past two decades [26–31]. The continually expanding amount of genomic data is available in numerous public databases, including generalized repositories, such as GenBank and EBI, and specialized resources, such as WormBase and HelmDB [16, 32–34]. Additionally, veterinary parasites, such as *Haemonchus contortus*, serve as a model for genomically-based vaccine development due to its status as the only helminth with a commercially available vaccine and its phylogenetic position that makes it an excellent candidate to be compared to *Caenorhabditis elegans*, a model organism closely related to numerous human parasites [35, 36].

Despite their numerous advantages, genomic analyses have several drawbacks. Genomic analyses allow for the identification of numerous potential vaccine antigens; however, antigen target selection for vaccine development can be clouded by the immense number of options, many of which may be nonfunctional or promote regulatory responses in helminths and should be eliminated from vaccine formulations [37]. This was previously observed in the development of candidate vaccines against *Schistosoma mansoni*, where genomic analyses and reverse vaccinology yielded multiple antigen sites and peptides for vaccine development, none of which were protective [38, 39]. Genome sequences also include noncoding intron sections that have to be eliminated during the development process leading to more time-consuming than necessary. Similarly, genomic technology may recommend the creation of monovalent vaccines for helminths that may prove ineffective, as the vaccines may only confer partial immunity [12], or may prove ineffective in human candidates [40].

4. Transcriptomic approaches to vaccine development for helminth diseases

Transcriptomic analysis with a view toward vaccine design circumvents some of the challenges posed by relying on genomic analysis alone. Traditionally, to annotate a transcriptome, the transcriptome of interest is run using a pairwise homology-based analysis with other known curated and annotated genome sequence data sets from other organisms. Initially, the transcripts and genes of parasitic helminths were not able to be annotated in this manner as they did not correlate with data that were publicly available [16]. Analysis of transcriptomic data for various parasites identified several categories of genes that encode proteins without similarity to other organisms. It is likely that these genes are exclusive to the parasite they are found in and likely play a role in parasite survival and adaptation. The uniqueness of these genes found in the transcriptome at various life stages may also provide targets for vaccine development [41]. Mangiola *et. al* sought to centralize these unique genes in annotated parasite transcriptomes through the creation of HelmDB [16]. This database was initially created by annotating the transcriptomes of 11 parasitic helminths with socioeconomic importance. Though HelmDB is no longer functional, transcriptomes for numerous species can be freely accessed via WormBase [35].

The creation of annotated transcriptome databases and the relative availability of transcriptome sequencing has created an opportunity for researchers to explore the difference in gene expression across the life cycle of various helminths. Vaccine development targeting multiple life stages of many parasitic helminths can be pursued by understanding the changes in gene expression throughout the life cycle [41–45]. These analyses have been carried out with different species of parasitic helminths and have been able to identify differentially expressed genes throughout the life cycle related to parasite infection, survival, and immune evasion. Genes that are differentially expressed in transcriptome analysis between life-cycle stages in relation to their role in the host infection process may be relevant to the survival of the parasite and can serve as targets for vaccine development that will prevent against infectious stages, or therapeutics that will protect against pathologic life stages [42]. The importance of this is apparent with the success of Barbervax®. The complex life cycle of *H. contortus* lasts 3 weeks. The first larval stage (L1) develops within an egg and hatches to molt to the second larval stage (L2) followed by a third larval stage (L3). It is the L3 stage that is ingested by the host and develops into the fourth larval stage (L4) to become adults [44]. Barbervax® consists of two adult-stage proteins present in the worm gut and is effective because worms ingest antibodies with each blood meal. The antibodies bind the proteins and disrupt gut function, leading to starvation and detachment (**Figure 1**) [46, 47]. While effective at reducing worm burden,

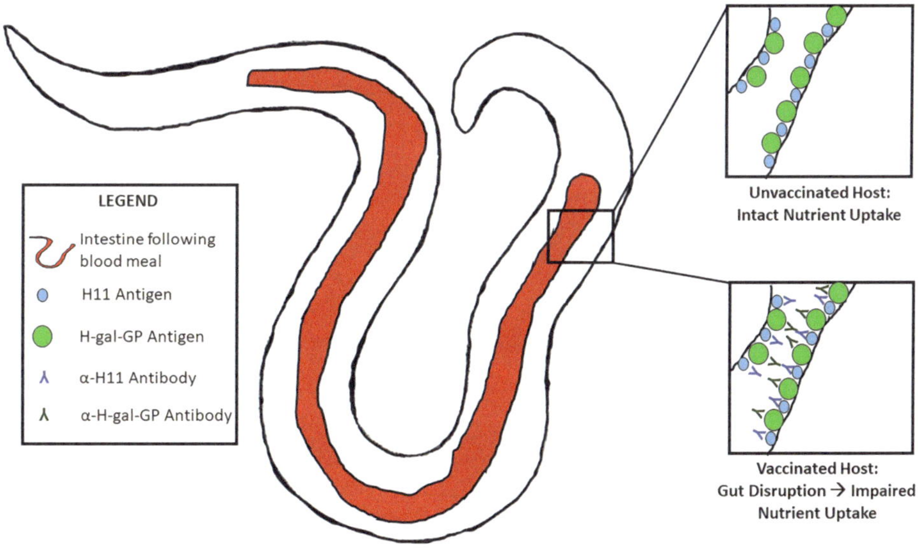

Figure 1.
Mechanistic view of worm burden reduction in BarberVax®-immunized hosts. Vaccinated individuals raise IgG antibodies against the H. contortus *intestinal proteins H11 and H-gal-GP. Upon infection and taking a blood meal, antibodies in the blood of vaccinated hosts disrupt the intestinal surface of the worm (lower inset) and interfere with normal nutrient uptake (upper inset). Adult worms in vaccinated animals produce fewer ova, eventually, succumb to starvation, and detach.*

vaccine-derived immunity does not protect immunized animals from infection with L3 parasites. The worms must mature through the L4 stage and into adulthood for protection to manifest. Schwartz *et al.* found that once ingested, the transition from L3 to L4 and adult is accompanied by a massive alteration of differentially transcribed genes [44]. These changes in gene expression notably did not inform the design of Barbervax®. It is plausible that subunit vaccines targeting L3 stage antigens could prevent the establishment of infection. A polyvalent vaccine consisting of L3 antigens, L4 antigens, and adult phase gut proteins would be maximally effective at both preventing infection and reducing worm burden should it occur (**Figure 2A**).

Transcriptomic analysis can also be used to examine the host–parasite interactions. On the helminth side, transcriptomic analysis can identify specific gene expression patterns in locations of interest in the parasite body. For example, Foth et al described transcripts found in the anterior region of *Trichuris muris*, which likely facilitate host–parasite interactions, nutrient uptake, and digestion [48]. An understanding of the relationship between the host and the parasite can identify vaccine candidates that

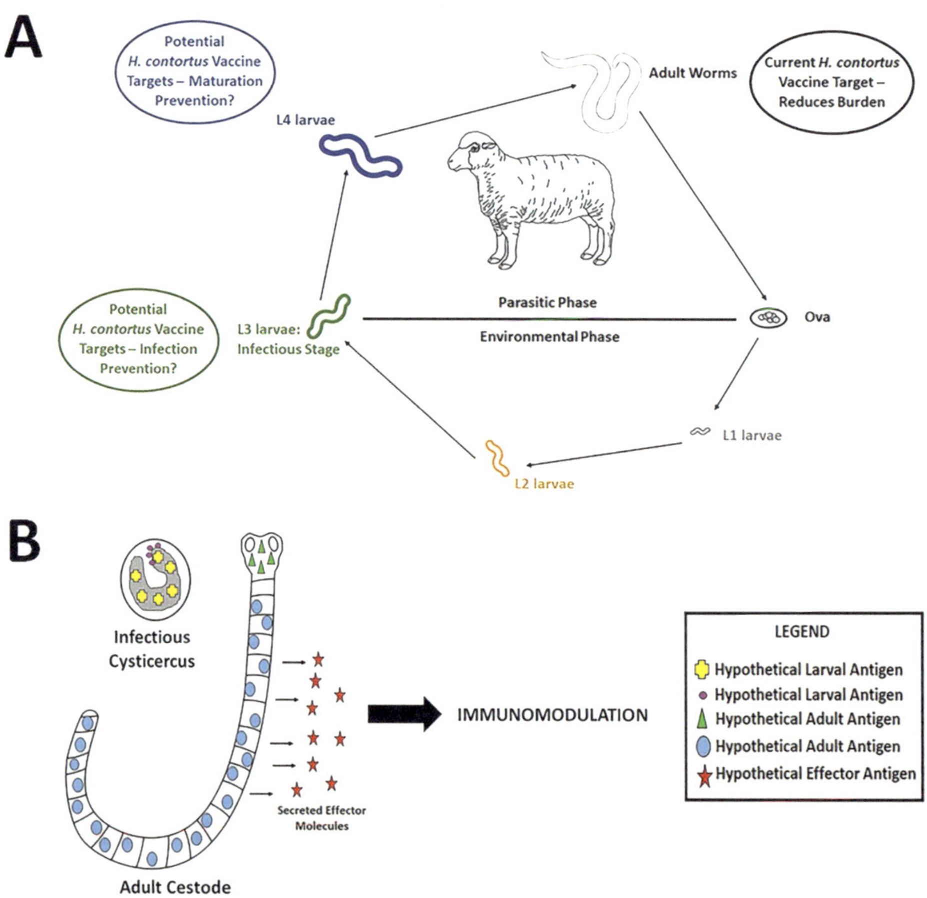

Figure 2.
Potential omics-guided vaccine design. The current vaccination strategy against H. contortus *(A) can be expanded to include antigens expressed in the L3 and/or L4 life stages, potentially preventing infection in addition to reducing worm burden should it occur. A proteomics-guided approach to vaccination against a hypothetical cestode (B) could target antigens present in the infectious stage (the cysticercus) and the adult worms, immunizing hosts against the infection or persistence of parasitic helminths. This approach could also include immunomodulatory effector proteins as antigens, maximizing the potential of a robust response to vaccination.*

target transcription products that play a role in immunomodulation or metabolism [49]. Transcriptomic analysis can also illuminate host responses by examining gene expression changes in host tissue during infection. Most notably, these analyses can aid in the understanding of the immunomodulation that allows for chronic parasite infections to occur. Parasitic effects on the host immune system have made vaccine development difficult, and it is, therefore, critical to understand mechanisms of immunomodulation exhibited by each parasitic helminth. For example, *Fasicola hepatica* infection was shown to inhibit natural killer cells and IgE production at the transcriptomic level, likely aiding *Fasciola hepatica* in evading cytotoxicity [50]. Vaccines targeting *F. hepatica* must, therefore, be designed and suitably adjuvanted in anticipation of the parasite's ability to strongly downregulate these protective activities post-challenge. Taken together, an ideal vaccine formulation would include not only protective *F. hepatica* antigens but antigens from the immunosuppressive effector proteins as well so that they are neutralized immediately upon infection of a vaccinated host.

A newer area of interest in vaccine development for parasitic helminths is the analysis of excretory/secretory products. These are various molecules released at the host–parasite interface and likely play a role in the manipulation of the host response. These products can be proteins, lipids, nucleic acids, metabolites, and extracellular vessels [51]. The microRNA (miRNA) present in extracellular vessels appears to play a role in the regulation of gene expression and immunomodulation of the host response. Understanding this miRNA will aid in identifying the ways that helminth infections are able to induce differing expressions within the host [52]. The ability of concentrated, purified versions of this miRNA may be able to be used to augment responses to subunit antigen vaccines.

Transcriptomic analysis from parasite life cycles and infected hosts is a useful tool in the development of anti-helminth vaccines. These analyses can contribute to all aspects of vaccine design, from identification of antigens to identifying (and thus circumventing) mechanisms with which parasitic helminths are able to evade adaptive immunity.

5. Proteomic approaches to vaccine development for helminth diseases

Proteomic analysis is among the most powerful tools for the identification of potential protective antigens against helminth diseases. The advent of proteomic technologies provided the opportunity not only to identify potential antigens but to detect any post-translational modifications as well. In addition, proteomic analyses identify all potential antigens, not simply those targeted by patient immune responses during infection. To ensure long-term survival, helminths tend to modulate and subdue immune responses, and the ability of these organisms to undergo host immune evasion poses a challenge for vaccine development [53]. Evaluating the adaptive immune responses of infected patients to identify potential antigens may be misleading, because these responses may be directed at non-neutralizing or variable antigens. Proteomic analyses can identify secreted proteins (*i.e.*, the secretome) expressed by helminths that modulate host immune responses and promote parasite survival [18, 54]. Anti-helminthic vaccine design guided by proteomics holds the promise to target both protective helminth body antigens and to neutralize immune evasion proteins generated by the parasite (**Figure 2B**).

A small number of vaccines designed following proteomics, immunomics, and reverse vaccinology analyses have been described; however, few have moved into animal trials to evaluate their efficacy. Potential antigens have been identified for *Schistosoma* spp. [19, 55], *Ascaris lumbricoides* [56, 57], *Trichuris trichiura*, *Necator americanus*, *Ancylostoma duodenale* [57], *Strongyloides stercoralis* [58], *Taenia solium* [59], *Toxocara canis* [60], *Onchocerca volvulus*, *Brugia malayi* [61], and *Echinococcus granulosus* [62, 63]. The number of experimental vaccines developed and tested for both immunogenicity and protection against challenge following *in vivo* proteomic analyses is vanishingly small. A recombinant protein vaccine targeting two surface glycoproteins of adult *Fasciola hepatica* lead to robust production of IgG antibodies, but failure to protect vaccinated cattle against infectious challenge [64]. A similarly designed recombinant protein vaccine targeting *T. canis* also resulted in seroconversion of immunized mice, and in this instance, worm burdens were significantly reduced compared to sham-vaccinated controls [60]. An experimental vaccine targeting secreted effector molecules of *Cooperia oncophora* initially seemed to provide some protection to vaccinated cattle, though subsequent studies found protection to be minimal [65]. However, another vaccine targeting secreted proteins of *Ostertagia ostertagi* resulted in a significant reduction of egg shedding by experimentally infected cattle [66]. These variable approaches across vaccine design strategies indicate that ideal formulations may require combining approaches and/or tailoring strategies as well as antigens to each parasitic helminth species. Consistent with this notion is the experimental vaccine against *Teladorsagia circumcincta*, which is a cocktail of larval stage antigens identified by reverse vaccinology, secreted immunomodulatory effector proteins, and adult-stage antigen identified by multi-omic analysis [65]. Vaccinated sheep showed significant reductions in both egg shedding and worm burden [67]. Though proteomic-guided development of immunizations against helminth diseases is a field in its infancy, it holds outstanding promise to craft vaccines that feature precise alignment with parasite life stages and the potential to raise immune responses that can neutralize immunomodulatory effector molecules.

6. Conclusions

Vaccines that protect against helminth diseases remain largely elusive in human and veterinary medicine. The successful licensure and deployment of the subunit vaccine Barbervax® provide evidence that the development of next-generation vaccines against parasitic helminths is an attainable goal. Multi-omic approaches allow for the design and evaluation of rationally designed subunit vaccines. The development of successful candidate vaccines has enormous potential to provide protection for the billions of people impacted by helminth diseases.

Author details

Vrushabh Daga†, Evangeline Green†, Priyanka Ravichandran†, Meagan Short† and Meghan May*

University of New England College of Osteopathic Medicine Biddeford, Maine, United States

*Address all correspondence to: mmay3@une.edu

† These authors contributed equally.

References

[1] James SL, Abate D, Abate KH, Abay SM, Abbafati C, Abbasi N, et al. Global, regional, and national incidence, prevalence, and years lived with disability for 354 diseases and injuries for 195 countries and territories, 1990-2017: A systematic analysis for the global burden of disease study 2017. The Lancet. 2018;**392**(10159):1789-1858

[2] Hotez PJ. Forgotten People, Forgotten Diseases: Neglected Tropical Diseases and their Impact on Global Health and Development. 3rd ed. Washington, DC, USA: ASM Press; 2021

[3] Salgame P, Yap GS, Gause WC. Effect of helminth-induced immunity on infections with microbial pathogens. Nature Immunology. 2013;**14**(11):1118-1126

[4] Babu S, Nutman TB. Helminth-tuberculosis co-infection: An immunologic perspective. Trends in Immunology. 2016;**37**(9):597-607

[5] Law AE, Shears RK, Lopez Rodas AA, Grencis RK, Cooper PJ, Neill DR, et al. Intestinal helminth co-infection is an unrecognised risk factor for increased pneumococcal carriage density and invasive disease. Scientific Reports. 2021;**11**(1):6984

[6] Albonico M, Smith PG, Ercole E, Hall A, Chwaya HM, Alawi KS, et al. Rate of reinfection with intestinal nematodes after treatment of children with mebendazole or albendazole in a highly endemic area. Transactions of the Royal Society of Tropical Medicine and Hygiene. 1995;**89**(5):538-541

[7] Albonico M, Wright V, Bickle Q. Molecular analysis of the β-tubulin gene of human hookworms as a basis for possible benzimidazole resistance on Pemba Island. Molecular and Biochemical Parasitology. 2004;**134**(2):281-284

[8] Geerts S, Coles GC, Gryseels B. Anthelmintic resistance in human helminths: Learning from the problems with worm control in livestock. Parasitology Today. 1997;**13**(4):149-151

[9] Hotez PJ, Brindley PJ, Bethony JM, King CH, Pearce EJ, Jacobson J. Helminth infections: The great neglected tropical diseases. Journal of Clinical Investigation. 2008;**118**(4):1311-1321

[10] Prabhu PR, Madhumathi J, Kaliraj P. Immunotechnological advancements in developing vaccines for lymphatic Filariasis. In: Tyagi B, editor. Lymphatic Filariasis. Singapore: Springer; 2018

[11] Loukas A, Giacomin P. Developments in the design of anti-helminth vaccines. In: Gause W, Artis D, editors. The Th2 Type Immune Response in Health and Disease. New York, NY: Springer; 2016

[12] Maizels RM, Holland MJ, Falcone FH, Zang X-X, Yazdanbakhsh M. Vaccination against helminth parasites–the ultimate challenge for vaccinologists? Immunological Reviews. 1999;**171**(1):125-147

[13] Maizels RM. Identifying novel candidates and configurations for human helminth vaccines. Expert Review of Vaccines. 2021;**20**(11):1389-1393

[14] Sautto GA, Kirchenbaum GA, Diotti RA, Criscuolo E, Ferrara F. Next generation vaccines for infectious diseases. Journal of Immunology Research. 2019;**2019**:5890962

[15] Dong Z, Chen Y. Transcriptomics: Advances and approaches. Science China. Life Sciences. 2013;**56**:960-967

[16] Mangiola S, Young ND, Korhonen P, Mondal A, Scheerlinck JP, Sternberg PW, et al. Getting the most out of parasitic helminth transcriptomes using HelmDB: Implications for biology and biotechnology. Biotechnology Advances. 2013;**31**(8):1109-1119

[17] Tyers M, Mann M. From genomics to proteomics. Nature. 2003;**422**:193-197

[18] Maizels RM, Smits HH, McSorley HJ. Modulation of host immunity by helminths: The expanding repertoire of parasite effector molecules. Immunity. 2018;**49**(5):801-818

[19] Rehman A, Ahmad S, Shahid F, Albutti A, Alwashmi ASS, Aljasir MA, et al. Integrated core proteomics, subtractive proteomics, and immunoinformatics investigation to unveil a potential multi-epitope vaccine against schistosomiasis. Vaccine. 2021;**9**(6):658

[20] Seib KL, Dougan G, Rappuoli R. The key role of genomics in modern vaccine and drug design for emerging infectious diseases. PLoS Genetics. 2009;**5**(10):e1000612

[21] Gay CG, Zuerner R, Bannantine JP, Lillehoj HS, Zhu J, Green RB, et al. Genómica y Desarollo de Vacunas. Revue Scientifique et Technique de l'OIE. 2007;**26**(1):49-67

[22] Pizza M, Scarlato V, Masignani V, Giuliani MM, Aricò B, Comanducci M, et al. Identification of vaccine candidates against Serogroup B Meningococcus by whole-genome sequencing. Science. 2000;**287**(5459):1816-1820

[23] Welsch JA, Moe GR, Rossi R, Adu-Bobie J, Rappuoli R, Granoff DM. Antibody to genome-derived Neisserial antigen 2132, a Neisseria meningitidis candidate vaccine, confers protection against bacteremia in the absence of complement-mediated bactericidal activity. The Journal of Infectious Diseases. 2003;**188**(11):1730-1740

[24] Knyazev S, Chhugani K, Sarwal V, Ayyala R, Singh H, Karthikeyan S, et al. Unlocking capacities of viral genomics for the COVID-19 pandemic response. 2021;ArXiv, arXiv:2104.14005v2

[25] Ghedin E, Wang S, Foster JM, Slatko BE. First sequenced genome of a parasitic nematode. Trends in Parasitology. 2004;**20**(4):151-153

[26] Zerlotini A, Aguiar ERGR, Fudong Y, Huayong X, Li Y, Young ND, et al. SchistoDB: An updated genome resource for the three key schistosomes of humans. Nucleic Acids Research. 2013;**41**(D1):D728-D731

[27] Huang Y, Chen W, Wang X, Liu H, Chen Y, et al. The carcinogenic liver fluke, *Clonorchis sinensis*: New assembly, reannotation and analysis of the genome and characterization of tissue transcriptomes. PLoS One. 2013;**8**(1):e54732

[28] Desjardins C, Cerqueira G, Goldberg J, et al. Genomics of *Loa loa*, a *Wolbachia*-free filarial parasite of humans. Nature Genetics. 2013;**45**:495-500

[29] Zheng H, Zhang W, Zhang L, et al. The genome of the hydatid tapeworm *Echinococcus granulosus*. Nature Genetics. 2013;**45**:1168-1175

[30] Hunt V, Tsai I, Coghlan A, et al. The genomic basis of parasitism in the *Strongyloides* clade of nematodes. Nature Genetics. 2016;**48**:299-307

[31] Small ST, Reimer LJ, Tisch DJ, King CL, Christensen BM, Siba PM, et al. Population genomics of the filarial nematode *Parasitewuchereria bancrofti* from mosquitoes. Molecular Ecology. 2016;**25**(7):1465-1477

[32] Benson DA, Cavanaugh M, Clark K, Karsch-Mizrachi I, Ostell J, Pruitt KD, et al. GenBank. Nucleic Acids Research. 2018;**46**(D1):D41-D47

[33] Madeira F, Park YM, Lee J, Buso N, Gur T, Madhusoodanan N, et al. The EMBL-EBI search and sequence analysis tools APIs in 2019. Nucleic Acids Research. 2019;**W1**(02):W636-W641

[34] Howe KL, Bolt BJ, Shafie M, Kersey P, Berriman M. WormBase parasite—a comprehensive resource for helminth genomics. Molecular and Biochemical Parasitology. 2017;**215**:2-10

[35] Laing R, Kikuchi T, Martinelli A, et al. The genome and transcriptome of *Haemonchus contortus*, a key model parasite for drug and vaccine discovery. Genome Biology. 2013;**14**:R88

[36] Markaki M, Tavernarakis N. Modeling human diseases in *Caenorhabditis elegans*. Biotechnology Journal. 2010;**5**(12):1261-1276

[37] Hewitson JP, Maizels RM. Vaccination against helminth parasite infections. Expert Review of Vaccines. 2014;**13**(4):473-487

[38] Carvalho GB, Silva-Pereira RA, Pacífico LG, Fonseca CT. Identification of *Schistosoma mansoni* candidate antigens for diagnosis of schistosomiasis. Memórias do Instituto Oswaldo Cruz. 2011;**106**(7):837-843

[39] Carvalho GB, Pacífico LG, Pimenta DL, Siqueira LM, Teixeira-Carvalho A, Coelho PM, et al. Evaluation of the use of C-terminal part of the *Schistosoma mansoni* 200kda tegumental protein in schistosomiasis diagnosis and vaccine formulation. Experimental Parasitology. 2014;**139**:24-32

[40] Riveau G, Schacht AM, Dompnier JP, Deplanque D, Seck M, et al. Safety and efficacy of the rSh28GST urinary schistosomiasis vaccine: A phase 3 randomized, controlled trial in Senegalese children. PLoS Neglected Tropical Diseases. 2018;**12**(12):e0006968

[41] Farias LP, Tararam CA, Miyasato PA, et al. Screening the *Schistosoma mansoni* transcriptome for genes differentially expressed in the schistosomulum stage in search for vaccine candidates. Parasitology Research. 2011;**108**:123-135

[42] Marcilla A, Garg G, Bernal D, et al. The transcriptome analysis of *Strongyloides stercoralis* L3i larvae reveals targets for intervention in a neglected disease. PLoS Neglected Tropical Diseases. 2012;**6**(2):e1513

[43] Laing R, Kikuchi T, Martinelli A, et al. The genome and transcriptome of *Haemonchus contortus*, a key model parasite for drug and vaccine discovery. Genome Biology. 2013;**14**(8):R88

[44] Schwarz EM, Korhonen PK, Campbell BE, et al. The genome and developmental transcriptome of the strongylid nematode *Haemonchus contortus*. Genome Biology. 2013;**14**(8):R89

[45] Zhang S. Comparative transcriptomic analysis of the larval and adult stages of *Taenia pisiformis*. Genes. 2019;**10**(7):507

[46] Kabagambe EK, Barras SR, Li Y, Peña MT, Smith WD, Miller JE. Attempts to control haemonchosis in grazing ewes by vaccination with gut membrane

proteins of the parasite. Veterinary Parasitology. 2000;**92**(1):15-23

[47] Smith WD, Smith SK, Pettit D. Evaluation of immunization with gut membrane glycoproteins of *Ostertagia ostertagi* against homologous challenge in calves and against Haemonchus contortus in sheep. Parasite Immunology. 2000;**22**(5):239-247

[48] Foth BJ, Tsai IJ, Reid AJ, et al. Whipworm genome and dual-species transcriptome analyses provide molecular insights into an intimate host-parasite interaction. Nature Genetics. 2014;**46**(7):693-700

[49] Mangiola S, Young ND, Sternberg PW, et al. Analysis of the transcriptome of adult *Dictyocaulus filaria* and comparison with *Dictyocaulus viviparus*, with a focus on molecules involved in host-parasite interactions. International Journal of Parasitology. 2014;**44**(3-4):251-261

[50] Naranjo-Lucena A, Correia CN, Molina-Hernández V, et al. Transcriptomic analysis of ovine hepatic lymph node following *Fasciola hepatica* infection–inhibition of NK cell and IgE-mediated Signaling. Frontiers in Immunology. 2021;**12**:687579

[51] Sánchez-López CM, Trelis M, Bernal D, Marcilla A. Overview of the interaction of helminth extracellular vesicles with the host and their potential functions and biological applications. Molecular Immunology. 2021;**134**:228-235

[52] Tritten L, Geary TG. Helminth extracellular vesicles in host-parasite interactions. Current Opinion in Microbiology. 2018;**46**:73-79

[53] Robinson MW, Cwiklinski K. Proteomics of host-helminth interactions. Pathogens. 2021;**10**(10):1317

[54] Garg G, Ranganathan S. Helminth secretome database (HSD): A collection of helminth excretory/secretory proteins predicted from expressed sequence tags (ESTs). BMC Genomics. 2012;**13**(7):S8

[55] Neves LX, Wilson RA, Brownridge P, Harman VM, Holman SW, Beynon RJ, et al. Quantitative proteomics of enriched Esophageal and gut tissues from the human blood fluke. Journal of Proteome Research. 2020;**19**(1):314-326

[56] Kaur R, Arora N, Rawat SS, Keshri AK, Singh N, Show SK, et al. Immunoinformatics driven construction of multi-epitope vaccine candidate against. Expert Review of Vaccines. 2021;**20**(12):1637-1649

[57] Montaño KJ, Cuéllar C, Sotillo J. Rodent models for the study of soil-transmitted helminths: A proteomics approach. Frontiers in Cellular and Infection Microbiology. 2021;**11**:639573

[58] Culma MF. *Strongyloides stercoralis* proteome: A reverse approach to the identification of potential immunogenic candidates. Microbial Pathogenesis. 2021;**152**:104545

[59] Kaur R, Arora N, Jamakhani MA, Malik S, Kumar P, Anjum F, et al. Development of multi-epitope chimeric vaccine against. Expert Review of Vaccines. 2020;**19**(1):105-114

[60] Salazar Garcés LF, Santiago LF, Santos SPO, Jaramillo Hernández DA, da Silva MB, Alves VDS, et al. Immunogenicity and protection induced by recombinant *Toxocara canis* proteins in a murine model of toxocariasis. Vaccine. 2020;**38**(30):4762-4772

[61] Devoe NC, Corbett IJ, Barker L, Chang R, Gudis P, Mullen N, et al. Differential evolutionary selection and natural evolvability observed in ALT

proteins of human filarial parasites. PLoS One. 2016;**11**(2):e0148611

[62] Miles S, Portela M, Cyrklaff M, Ancarola ME, Frischknecht F, Durán R, et al. Combining proteomics and bioinformatics to explore novel tegumental antigens as vaccine candidates against *Echinococcus granulosus* infection. Journal of Cellular Biochemistry. 2019;**120**(9): 15320-15336

[63] Pourseif MM, Moghaddam G, Saeedi N, Barzegari A, Dehghani J, Omidi Y. Current status and future prospective of vaccine development against *Echinococcus granulosus*. Biologicals. 2018;**51**:1-11

[64] McCusker P, Toet H, Rathinasamy V, Young N, Beddoe T, Anderson G, et al. Molecular characterisation and vaccine efficacy of two novel developmentally regulated surface tegument proteins of *Fasciola hepatica*. Veterinary Parasitology. 2020;**286**:109244

[65] Matthews JB, Geldhof P, Tzelos T, Claerebout E. Progress in the development of subunit vaccines for gastrointestinal nematodes of ruminants. Parasite Immunology. 2016;**38**(12):744-753

[66] Geldhof P, Vercauteren I, Vercruysse J, Knox DP, Van Den Broeck W, Claerebout E. Validation of the protective *Ostertagia ostertagi* ES-thiol antigens with different adjuvantia. Parasite Immunology. 2004;**26**(1):37-43

[67] Nisbet AJ, McNeilly TN, Wildblood LA, Morrison AA, Bartley DJ, Bartley Y, et al. Successful immunization against a parasitic nematode by vaccination with recombinant proteins. Vaccine. 2013;**31**(37):4017-4023